Palliative Care
Core Skills and
Clinical Competencies

LINDA L. EMANUEL, MD, PhD
Buehler Professor of Medicine
Director, Buehler Center on Aging, Health & Society Principal,
The Education in Palliative and End-of-Life Care (EPEC) Project
Northwestern University Feinberg School of Medicine
Chicago, Illinois

S. LAWRENCE LIBRACH, MD, CCFP, FCFP
W. Gifford-Jones Professor
Professor and Head, Division of Palliative Care
Department of Family and Community Medicine
University of Toronto
Director, Temmy Latner Centre for Palliative Care
Mount Sinai Hospital
Toronto, Ontario, Canada

Palliative Care

Core Skills and Clinical Competencies

SECOND EDITION

ELSEVIER
SAUNDERS

3251 Riverport Lane
St. Louis, Missouri 63043

Notices

Knowledge and best practice in this field are constantly changing. As new research and experience broaden our understanding, changes in research methods, professional practices, or medical treatment may become necessary.

Practitioners and researchers must always rely on their own experience and knowledge in evaluating and using any information, methods, compounds, or experiments described herein. In using such information or methods they should be mindful of their own safety and the safety of others, including parties for whom they have a professional responsibility.

With respect to any drug or pharmaceutical products identified, readers are advised to check the most current information provided (i) on procedures featured or (ii) by the manufacturer of each product to be administered, to verify the recommended dose or formula, the method and duration of administration, and contraindications. It is the responsibility of practitioners, relying on their own experience and knowledge of their patients, to make diagnoses, to determine dosages and the best treatment for each individual patient, and to take all appropriate safety precautions.

To the fullest extent of the law, neither the Publisher nor the authors, contributors, or editors assume any liability for any injury and/or damage to persons or property as a matter of products liability, negligence or otherwise, or from any use or operation of any methods, products, instructions, or ideas contained in the material herein.

Library of Congress Cataloging-in-Publication Data

Palliative care : core skills and clinical competencies / [edited by] Linda L. Emanuel, S. Lawrence Librach. — 2nd ed.
    p. ; cm.
    "Expert consult online and print."
    Includes bibliographical references and index.
    ISBN 978-1-4377-1619-1 (pbk.)
  1. Palliative treatment. I. Emanuel, Linda L. II. Librach, S. Lawrence.
    [DNLM: 1. Palliative Care. 2. Clinical Competence. WB 310]
    R726.8.P3427 2011
    616′.029—dc22

                    2011006018

Acquisitions Editor: Pamela Hetherington   *Project Manager:* Jessica Becher
Developmental Editor: Jessica Pritchard   *Design Manager:* Ellen Zanolle
Publishing Services Manager: Anne Altepeter

Printed in the United States of America

Last digit is the print number: 9 8 7 6 5 4 3

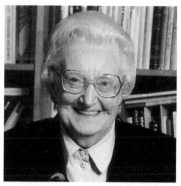

Courtesy St. Christopher's Hospice, London, UK

"The last stages of life should not be seen as defeat, but rather as life's fulfillment. It is not merely a time of negation but rather an opportunity for positive achievement. One of the ways we can help our patients most is to learn to believe and to expect this."

Cicely Saunders, 1965
—First published in *American Journal of Nursing*;
republished in *Cicely Saunders: selected writings by David Clark*
Oxford University Press, 2006

We dedicate this book to the memory of Dame Cicely Saunders. In its pages, we have sought to provide for the core skills that a clinician needs to make it possible for every man, woman, and child that, when dying is necessary, it becomes life's fulfillment.

Linda L. Emanuel, S. Lawrence Librach

CONTRIBUTORS

Carla S. Alexander, MD
Assistant Professor of Medicine, Department of Medicine, University of Maryland
  School of Medicine, Institute of Human Virology, Baltimore, Maryland
HIV/AIDS

Wendy G. Anderson, MD, MS
Assistant Professor, Division of Hospital Medicine and Palliative Care Program,
  University of California, San Francisco, San Francisco, California
Withholding and Withdrawing Life-Sustaining Therapies

Peter Angelos, MD, PhD
Professor and Chief of Endocrine Surgery, Associate Director of the MacLean
  Center for Clinical Medical Ethics, Department of Surgery, University of
  Chicago, Chicago, Illinois
Principles of Palliative Surgery

Robert M. Arnold, MD
Professor of Medicine, Division of General Internal Medicine, Chief, Section of
  Palliative Care and Medical Ethics, Director, Institute for Doctor-Patient
  Communication, University of Pittsburgh School of Medicine, Pittsburgh,
  Pennsylvania
Leo H. Criep Chair in Patient Care, School of Medicine, University of Pittsburgh,
  Pittsburgh, Pennsylvania
Withholding and Withdrawing Life-Sustaining Therapies

F. Amos Bailey, MD
Associate Professor Division of Geriatrics, Gerontology and Palliative Care,
  Internal Medicine, University of Alabama, Birmingham, Alabama
Director, Safe Harbor Palliative Care Program, Internal Medicine, Birmingham VA
  Medical Center, Birmingham, Alabama
Veterans, Veterans Administration Health Care, and Palliative Care

Al B. Benson III, MD, FACP
Professor of Medicine Division of Hematology/Oncology, Northwestern University
  Feinberg School of Medicine, Chicago, Illinois
Gastrointestinal Malignancies

Ann M. Berger, MD, MSN
Bethesda, Maryland
Nausea and Vomiting

Richard H. Bernstein, MD, FACP
Adjunct Associate Professor, Baruch/Mount Sinai MBA Program in Health Care
    Administration, Zicklin School of Business of the City University of New York,
    New York, New York
Associate Professor of Clinical Medicine, Department of Medicine, Associate
    Professor of Clinical Preventive Medicine, Department of Preventive Medicine,
    The Mount Sinai School of Medicine, New York, New York
Chief Medical Officer, VNSNY CHOICE Health Plan, Visiting Nurse Service of New
    York, New York, New York
Integrating Palliative Care Guidelines into Clinical Practice

Susan Blacker, MSW
Adjunct Lecturer, Division of Palliative Care, Department of Family and
    Community Medicine, University of Toronto
Director, Cancer Services Planning & Performance, St. Michael's Hospital, Toronto,
    Ontario, Canada
Supporting the Family in Palliative Care

Alexander A. Boni-Saenz, JD, MSc
Skadden Fellow/Staff Attorney, Chicago Medical-Legal Partnership for Seniors, Legal
    Assistance Foundation of Metropolitan Chicago, Chicago, Illinois
The Economic Burden of End-of-Life Illness

Robert O. Bonow, MD
Max and Lily Goldberg Distinguished Professor of Cardiology, Chicago, Illinois
Vice Chairman, Department of Medicine, Chicago, Illinois
Director, Center for Cardiovascular Innovation, Chicago, Illinois
Northwestern University Feinberg School of Medicine, Chicago, Illinois
Heart Failure and Palliative Care

Kerry W. Bowman, MSW, PhD
Assistant Professor, Department of Family and Community Medicine, University
    of Toronto, Toronto, Ontario, Canada
Clinical Bioethicist, Department of Bioethics, Mount Sinai Hospital, Toronto,
    Ontario, Canada
Understanding and Respecting Cultural Differences

Eduardo Bruera, MD
Professor, Department of Palliative Care and Rehabilitation Medicine, Chair,
    Department of Palliative Care and Rehabilitation Medicine, The University of
    Texas MD Anderson Cancer Center, Houston, Texas
Palliative Care in Developing Countries

Robert Buckman, MB, PhD
Professor, Department of Medicine, University of Toronto, Toronto, Ontario, Canada
Adjunct Professor, The University of Texas MD Anderson Cancer Center, Houston,
    Texas
Medical Oncologist, Department of Medical Oncology, Princess Margaret Hospital,
    Toronto, Ontario, Canada
Communication Skills

Toby C. Campbell, MD, MSCI
Assistant Professor, Department of Medicine, University of Wisconsin, Madison,
    Wisconsin
Hematology/Oncology

Elizabeth K. Chaitin, MSW, DHCE
Assistant Professor of Medicine, Department of Medicine, University of Pittsburgh,
    Pittsburgh, Pennsylvania
Director, Department of Medical Ethics and Palliative Care Services, University of
    Pittsburgh Medical Center Shadyside, Pittsburgh, Pennsylvania
Withholding and Withdrawing Life-Sustaining Therapies

Anita Chakraborty, MD, CCFP
Lecturer, Department of Family and Community Medicine, Division of Palliative
    Care, University of Toronto, Toronto, Ontario, Canada
Consultant, Department of Palliative Care, Sunnybrook Health Science Centre,
    Toronto, Ontario, Canada
Neurodegenerative Diseases

Harvey Max Chochinov, MD, PhD
Professor of Psychiatry, Community Health Sciences, and Family Medicine,
    Division of Palliative Care, University of Manitoba
Director of the Manitoba Palliative Care Research Unit, CancerCare Manitoba,
    University of Manitoba, Manitoba, Canada
The Therapeutic Implications of Dignity in Palliative Care

Alexie Cintron, MD, MPH
Director, Pain and Palliative Care Fellowship, Memorial-Sloan Kettering Cancer
    Center, New York, New York
Palliative Care Services and Programs

Kenneth E. Covinsky, MD, MPH
Professor of Medicine, Department of Medicine, University of California, San
    Francisco, San Francisco, California
The Economic Burden of End-of-Life Illness

Maria Danilychev, MD
Geriatrician, San Diego, California
Last Hours of Living

Liliana De Lima, MS, MHA
Executive Director, International Association for Hospice and Palliative Care,
    Houston, Texas
Palliative Care in Developing Countries

Christopher Della Santina, MD
Mid-Atlantic Permanente Medical Group, Rockville, Maryland
Integrating Palliative Care Guidelines into Clinical Practice

Arthur R. Derse, MD, JD
Director, Center for Bioethics and Medical Humanities, Julia and David Uihlein
    Professor of Medical Humanities, and Professor of Bioethics and Emergency
    Medicine, Institute for Health and Society, and Department of Emergency
    Medicine, Medical College of Wisconsin, Milwaukee, Wisconsin
Chair, Ethics Committee, and Emergency Physician, Department of Emergency
    Medicine, Froedtert Hospital, Milwaukee, Wisconsin
Emergency Physician, Emergency Department, Zablocki Veterans Administration
    Hospital, Milwaukee, Wisconsin
Chair, National Ethics Committee, Veterans Health Administration, Washington, DC
Legal and Ethical Issues in the United States

G. Michael Downing, MD
Clinical Associate Professor, Department of Family Medicine, Division of Palliative
    Care, University of British Columbia, Vancouver, British Columbia, Canada
Adjunct Assistant Professor, School of Health Information Science, University of
    Victoria, Victoria, British Columbia, Canada
Palliative Medicine, Director of Research and Development, Victoria Hospice
    Society, Victoria, British Columbia, Canada
"Who Knows?" 10 Steps to Better Prognostication

Deborah J. Dudgeon, MD, FRCPC
W. Ford Connell Professor of Palliative Care Medicine, Departments of Medicine
    and Oncology, Queen's University, Kingston, Ontario, Canada
Dyspnea

Geoffrey P. Dunn, MD, FACS
Medical Director, Palliative Care Consultation Service, Hamot Medical Center,
    Erie, Pennsylvania
Consultant, Department of Surgery, Hamot Medical Center, Erie, Pennsylvania
Principles of Palliative Surgery

Linda L. Emanuel, MD, PhD
Buehler Professor of Medicine
Director, Buehler Center on Aging, Health & Society Principal, The Education in
    Palliative and End-of-Life Care (EPEC) Project, Northwestern University
    Feinberg School of Medicine, Chicago, Illinois
*Palliative Care: A Quiet Revolution in Patient Care; Comprehensive Assessment; Loss,
    Bereavement, and Adaptation; Addressing the Social Suffering Associated with
    Illness: A Focus on Household Economic Resilience*

Robin L. Fainsinger, MD
Director/Professor, Division of Palliative Care Medicine, Department of Oncology,
    University of Alberta, Edmonton, Alberta, Canada
Director, Tertiary Palliative Care Unit, Grey Nuns Hospital, Edmonton, Alberta,
    Canada
Clinical Director, Edmonton Zone, Palliative Care Program, Alberta Health
    Services, Edmonton, Alberta, Canada
Pain

Frank D. Ferris, MD, FAAHPM, FAACE
Clinical Professor, Departments of Family & Preventative Medicine, University of
    California, San Diego School of Medicine, San Diego, California
Assistant Professor, Adjunct, Departments of Family and Community Medicine,
    University of Toronto, Toronto, Ontario, Canada
Director, International Programs, Institute for Palliative Medicine at San Diego
    Hospice, San Diego, California
Last Hours of Living

Russell Goldman, MD, MPH, CCFP
Assistant Professor, Department of Family and Community Medicine, Faculty of
    Medicine, University of Toronto, Toronto, Ontario, Canada
Assistant Director, Temmy Latner Centre for Palliative Care, Mount Sinai Hospital,
    Toronto, Ontario, Canada
Home Palliative Care

Hunter Groninger, MD
Staff Clinician, Pain and Palliative Care Department, National Institutes of Health,
    Bethesda, Maryland
Pulmonary Palliative Medicine

Liz Gwyther, MBChB, FCFP, MSc Pall Med
Senior Lecturer, School of Public Health & Family Medicine, University of Cape
    Town, South Africa
CEO, Hospice Palliative Care Association of South Africa
Trustee, Worldwide Palliative Care Alliance
Palliative Care in Developing Countries

Melissa J. Hart, MA
Chaplain, Department of Spiritual Care, Horizon Hospice & Palliative Care,
    Chicago, Illinois
Spiritual Care

Joshua M. Hauser, MD
Assistant Professor, Palliative Care Department of Medicine, Northwestern
    University Feinberg School of Medicine, Chicago, Illinois
Attending Physician, Palliative Care, Department of Medicine, Northwestern
    Memorial Hospital, Chicago, Illinois
*Heart Failure and Palliative Care; Veterans, Veterans Administration Health Care,
    and Palliative Care*

Laura A. Hawryluck, MSc, MD, FRCPC
Associate Professor, Department of Medicine/Critical Care, University of Toronto,
    Toronto, Ontario, Canada
Toronto General Hospital, University Health Network, Toronto, Ontario, Canada
Palliative Care in the Intensive Care Unit

Susan Hunt, MD, FACP
Professor of Medicine, Division of General Internal Medicine, Section of Palliative
    Care and Medical Ethics, University of Pittsburgh Medical Center, Pittsburgh,
    Pennsylvania
Withholding and Withdrawing Life-Sustaining Therapies

Amna F. Husain, MD, MPH
Assistant Professor, Department of Family and Community Medicine, Division of
    Palliative Care, Associate Member, School of Graduate Studies, Faculty of
    Nursing, University of Toronto, Toronto, Ontario, Canada
Associate Staff, Department of Family Medicine, Mount Sinai Hospital, Toronto,
    Ontario, Canada
Palliative Care Physician, Temmy Latner Centre for Palliative Care, Mount Sinai
    Hospital, Toronto, Ontario, Canada
Cachexia; Fatigue

Bridget Margaret Johnston
Senior Research Fellow, School of Nursing and Midwifery, University of Dundee,
    Dundee, Scotland
The Therapeutic Implications of Dignity in Palliative Care

Jennifer M. Kapo, MD
Assistant Professor of Clinical Medicine, Division of Geriatrics, Department of
    Medicine, Penn VA Palliative Medicine Fellowship Director, University of
    Pennsylvania, Philadelphia, Pennsylvania
Medical Director, Palliative Care Service, Department of Medicine, Philadelphia
    Veteran's Administration Medical Center, Philadelphia, Pennsylvania
Dementia; Palliative Care in Long-Term Care Settings

Nuala P. Kenny, OC, MD, FRCP(C)
Emeritus Professor, Department of Bioethics, Dalhousie University, Halifax, Nova
    Scotia, Canada
Responding to Requests for Euthanasia and Physician-Assisted Suicide

Sara J. Knight, PhD
Associate Professor, Departments of Psychiatry and Urology, University of
    California at San Francisco, San Francisco, California
Acting Director, Health Services Research Program, San Francisco Department of
    Veterans Affairs Medical Center, San Francisco, California
Loss, Bereavement, and Adaptation

Tapas Kundu, PhD
Post Doctoral Fellow, Economics Department & Centre of Equality, Social
    Organization, and Performance, University of Oslo, Oslo, Norway
*Addressing the Social Suffering Associated with Illness: A Focus on Household
    Economic Resilience*

Stephen Liben, MD
Associate Professor, Department of Pediatrics, McGill University, Montreal,
    Quebec, Canada
Director, Pediatric Palliative Care Program, The Montreal Children's Hospital,
    Montreal, Quebec, Canada
Pediatric Palliative Care

S. Lawrence Librach, MD, CCFP, FCFP
W. Gifford-Jones Professor, Professor and Head, Division of Palliative Care,
    Department of Family and Community Medicine, University of Toronto
Director, Temmy Latner Centre for Palliative Care, Mount Sinai Hospital, Toronto,
    Ontario, Canada
*Palliative Care: A Quiet Revolution in Patient Care; Multiple Symptoms and Multiple
    Illnesses; Constipation; Urinary Incontinence; Sexuality; Addressing the Social
    Suffering Associated with Illness: A Focus on Household Economic Resilience;
    Appendix I: Medication Tables; Appendix II: Resources for Palliative and
    End-of-Life Care*

Matthew J. Loscalzo, LCSW
Liliane Elkins Professor in Supportive Care Programs, Administrative Director,
    Sheri & Les Biller Patient and Family Resource Center, Executive Director,
    Department of Supportive Care Medicine, Professor, Department of Population
    Sciences, Department of Supportive Care Medicine, City of Hope, National
    Medical Center, Duarte, California
Social Work Practice in Palliative Care: An Evolving Science of Caring

Bill Mah, MA, MD, FRCPC
Lecturer, Department of Psychiatry, University of Toronto, Toronto, Ontario,
    Canada
Consultant Psychiatrist, Department of Psychiatry, Mount Sinai Hospital, Toronto,
    Ontario, Canada
Depression and Anxiety; Delirium

Denise Marshall, BSc, MD, CCFP, FCFP
Assistant Professor, Assistant Dean, Faculty of Health Sciences, McMaster
    University, Hamilton, Ontario, Canada
Palliative Care Physician, Hamilton Health Sciences, Hamilton, Ontario, Canada
Palliative Care Physician, West Lincoln Memorial Hospital, Grimsby, Ontario,
    Canada
The Role of the Physician in Palliative and End-of-Life Care

Jeanne Marie Martinez, FPCN, CHPN, RN, MPH
Quality Specialist, Home Hospice Program, Northwestern Memorial Hospital,
    Chicago, Illinois
Palliative Care Nursing

Rohtesh S. Mehta, MD, MPH
Instructor of Medicine, Departments of General Internal Medicine and Palliative
    Care, University of Pittsburgh Medical Center, Pittsburgh, Pennsylvania
Withholding and Withdrawing Life-Sustaining Therapies

Diane E. Meier, MD
Professor of Geriatrics and Internal Medicine, Departments of Geriatrics and
    Palliative Medicine, Mount Sinai School of Medicine, New York, New York
Director, Lilian and Benjamin Hertzberg Palliative Care Institute, New York, New
    York
Director, Center to Advance Palliative Care, New York, New York
Palliative Care Services and Programs

Seema Modi, MD
Department of Family Medicine, Baylor Medical Center at Carrollton, Carrollton,
    Texas
Palliative Care in Long-Term Care Settings

Sandra Y. Moody, BSN, MD
Associate Professor of Medicine, Department of Medicine, University of California,
    San Francisco, San Francisco, California
Medical Director, Home Based Primary Care, Department of Medicine, Division of
    Geriatrics, San Francisco Veterans Affairs Medical Center, San Francisco,
    California
The Economic Burden of End-of-Life Illness

Daniela Mosoiu, MD
Director, Hospice Casa Sperantei, Brasov, Romania
Palliative Care in Developing Countries

Alvin H. Moss, MD, FAAHPM
Professor of Medicine, Department of Medicine, West Virginia University School
    of Medicine, Morgantown, West Virginia
Executive Director, West Virginia Center for End-of-Life Care, Morgantown, West
    Virginia
Kidney Failure

Timothy J. Moynihan, MD
Associate Professor of Medical Oncology, Department of Medical Oncology, Mayo
    Clinic, Rochester, Minnesota
Hospice Medical Director, Mayo Clinic, Rochester, Minnesota
Sexuality

J. Cameron Muir, MD, FAAHPM
Assistant Professor of Oncology, Johns Hopkins Medicine, Baltimore, Maryland
Executive Vice President, Quality and Access, Capital Hospice, Fairfax, Virginia
Pulmonary Palliative Medicine

Jeff Myers, MD, MSEd
Assistant Professor and Associate Head, Division of Palliative Care, Department of Family and Community Medicine, University of Toronto, Toronto, Ontario, Canada
Head, Department of Palliative Care, Sunnybrook Health Sciences Centre, Toronto, Ontario, Canada
Neurodegenerative Diseases

Judith A. Paice, PhD, RN
Director, Cancer Pain Program, Division of Hematology/Oncology, Northwestern University Feinberg School of Medicine, Chicago, Illinois
The Interdisciplinary Team

Robert Allan Pearlman, MD, MPH
Professor, Departments of Medicine, Health Services, and Bioethics and the Humanities, University of Washington, Seattle, Washington
GRECC, VA Puget Sound Health Care System, Seattle, Washington
Chief, Ethics Evaluation, National Center for Ethics in Health Care, Department of Veterans Affairs, Seattle, Washington
Advance Care Planning

Tammie E. Quest, MD
Associate Professor, Department of Emergency Medicine, Emory University School of Medicine, Atlanta, Georgia
Emergency Medicine and Palliative Care

M.R. Rajagopal, MD
Physician, Departments of Pain and Palliative Medicine, Trivandrum Institute of Palliative Sciences, S.U.T Hospital, Trivandrum, Kerala, India
Chairman, Pallium India, Trivandrum, Kerala, India
Palliative Care in Developing Countries

Eva B. Reitschuler-Cross, MD
Instructor in Medicine, Harvard Medical School, Boston, Massachusetts
Chief Resident, Department of Internal Medicine, Mount Auburn Hospital, Cambridge, Massachusetts
Addressing the Social Suffering Associated with Illness: A Focus on Household Economic Resilience

Karen Glasser Scandrett, MD, MPH
Assistant Professor of Geriatrics, Buehler Center on Aging, Health & Society, Northwestern University Feinberg School of Medicine, Chicago, Illinois
Assistant Professor of Geriatrics, Department of Medicine, Northwestern Medical Faculty Foundation, Chicago, Illinois
Addressing the Social Suffering Associated with Illness: A Focus on Household Economic Resilience

Corinne D. Schroder, MD, MEd, CCFP, FCFP

Associate Professor, Departments of Oncology and Family Medicine, Queen's
University, Kingston, Ontario, Canada

Palliative Medicine Consultant, Palliative Care Medicine Program, Kingston
General Hospital, Kingston, Ontario, Canada

Dyspnea

R. Gary Sibbald, MD, FRCPC, ABIM, DABD

Professor, Public Health Sciences and Medicine, Director International
Interprofessional Wound Care Course, University of Toronto, Director of
Toronto Regional Wound Clinics, Toronto, Ontario, Canada

President, World Union of Wound Healing Societies

Local Wound Care for Palliative and Malignant Wounds

Arthur Siegel, MD

Medical Director, Halquist Memorial Inpatient Center, Capital Hospice, Falls
Church, Virginia

Last Hours of Living

Melissa Simon, MD, MPH

Assistant Professor, Department of Obstetrics and Gynecology, Northwestern
University Feinberg School of Medicine, Chicago, Illinois

*Addressing the Social Suffering Associated with Illness: A Focus on Household
Economic Resilience*

Eliezer Soto, MD

Bethesda, Maryland

Nausea and Vomiting

Helene Starks, PhD, MPH

Associate Professor, Departments of Bioethics and Humanities, University of
Washington, Seattle, Washington

Advance Care Planning

Regina M. Stein, MD

Oncology Palliative Medicine Fellow, Northwestern University Feinberg School of
Medicine, Chicago, Illinois

Gastrointestinal Malignancies

Vincent Thai, MBBS

Associate Clinical Professor, Department of Oncology, Division of Palliative Care
Medicine, University of Alberta, Edmonton, Alberta, Canada

Director, Palliative Care Services, University of Alberta Hospitals, Edmonton,
Alberta, Canada

Visiting Consultant, Departments of Pain and Symptom Management, Cross
Cancer Institute, Edmonton, Alberta, Canada

Pain

Maxwell T. Vergo, MD
Assistant Professor of Medicine, Division of Hematology/Oncology, Northwestern
University Feinberg School of Medicine, Chicago, Illinois
Palliative Medicine Attending, Department of Medicine, Northwestern Memorial
Hospital, Chicago, Illinois
Gastrointestinal Malignancies

Elizabeth K. Vig, MD, MPH
Assistant Professor, Departments of Medicine and Gerontology and Geriatric
Medicine, University of Washington, Seattle, Washington
Staff Physician, VA Puget Sound Health Care System, Seattle, Washington
Advance Care Planning

Annette M. Vollrath, MD
Voluntary Assistant Clinical Professor of Medicine, Department of Medicine,
University of California, San Diego, San Diego, California
Clinical Medical Director, San Diego Hospice and The Institute for Palliative
Medicine, San Diego, California
Consultant in Palliative Medicine, Scripps Mercy Hospital, San Diego, California
Negotiating Goals of Care: Changing Goals Along the Trajectory of Illness

Charles F. von Gunten, MD, PhD
Clinical Professor of Medicine, School of Medicine, University of California, San
Diego, San Diego, California
Provost, Institute for Palliative Medicine at San Diego Hospice, San Diego, California
Negotiating Goals of Care: Changing Goals Along the Trajectory of Illness

Jamie H. von Roenn, MD
Professor of Medicine, Department of Medicine, Division of Hematology/Oncology,
Northwestern University Feinberg School of Medicine, Chicago, Illinois
Attending Physician, Department of Medicine, Division of Hematology/Oncology,
Medical Director, Home Hospice Program, Department of Medicine, Division of
Hospital Medicine, Northwestern Memorial Hospital, Chicago, Illinois
Hematology/Oncology

Roberto Daniel Wenk, MD
Director, Programa Argentino de Medicina Paliativa, Fundación FEMEBA, Buenos
Aires, Argentina
Chairman, International Association for Hospice and Palliative Care, Houston,
Texas
Palliative Care in Developing Countries

Kevin Y. Woo, PhD, RN, ACNP, FAPWCA
Assistant Professor, Department of Nursing, Queen's University, Toronto, Ontario,
Canada
Nursing Director, Villa Colombo, Home for the Aged, Toronto, Ontario, Canada
Wound Care Consultant, Department of Professional Practice, West Park Health
Centre, Toronto, Ontario, Canada
Local Wound Care for Palliative and Malignant Wounds

FOREWORD TO THE FIRST EDITION

Balfour M. Mount, OC, MD, FRCSC
Emeritus Professor of Palliative Medicine, Department of Oncology,
McGill University, Montreal, Quebec, Canada

We emerge deserving of little credit, we who are capable of ignoring the conditions which make muted people suffer. The dissatisfied dead cannot noise abroad the negligence they have experienced.[1]

JOHN HINTON

The Roots of Hospice/Palliative Care

With these searing words, British psychiatrist John Hinton proclaimed the societal neglect and deficiency in end-of-life care that he documented in his research during the 1960s. As a champion for change, he was not alone. Cicely Saunders, an Oxford-trained nurse, had also noted the plight of the dying and, in particular, the need for improved pain control. Her commitment was unswerving. When a back injury ended her nursing career, she became an almoner (social worker) and finally, on the advice of a medical mentor (*"Go read Medicine. It's the doctors who desert the dying"*),[2] she "read Medicine," qualifying as a doctor in 1957 at the age of 39. With this she became a one-person interdisciplinary team, a breadth of perspective that was to serve her well.[3,4]

Cicely Saunders brought a unique spectrum of personal qualities, including unstoppable determination, to the task of redressing the care of those with far-advanced disease. Her published 1959–1999 correspondence[5] sheds light on the many reasons for her success as a health care reformer: her keen intellect, an inquiring mind given to attention to detail; an articulate tongue, capable of infectious persuasiveness; a tendency to consult wisely and widely with world authorities on each successive issue under the scrutiny of her "beady eye"; personal warmth, coupled with confident humility; and natural leadership skills of epic proportions!

The result of this providential mix was St. Christopher's Hospice in London, the first center of academic excellence in end-of-life care. Dame Cicely saw St. Christopher's as being "founded on patients."[6] The evolution of her dream was painfully slow. David Tasma, a young Polish cancer patient whom she had nursed in February 1948, had famously remarked to her, "I only want what is in your mind and in your heart,"[7] thus indicating to Cicely's discerning ear the twin pillars on which she would construct her refined approach to whole-person care. There must be all the diagnostic and therapeutic skills of the mind, but also an empathic, caring, presence of the heart, a presence that is willing to accompany into the uncertain terrain where both sufferer and caregiver may learn that "there is great strength in weakness accepted."[8]

Dame Cicely recognized that, as health care providers, we don't always "make it all better." Indeed, we don't *ever* make it all better. As she expressed it,

> However much we can ease distress, however much we can help the patients to find a new meaning in what is happening, there will always be the place where we will have to stop and know that we are really helpless . . . . It would be very wrong indeed if, at that point, we tried to forget that this was so and to pass by. It would be wrong if we tried to cover it up, to deny it and to delude ourselves that we are always successful. Even when we feel that we can do absolutely nothing, we will still have to be prepared to stay. "Watch with me" means, above all, just be there.[8]

Nineteen long years of careful planning, fundraising, and the evolving clarity of her vision passed between David Tasma's prophetic comment and the admission of the first patient to St. Christopher's in June 1967. Dame Cicely was leading global health care into a paradigm shift: from disease to illness[9]; from quantity of life to a broader perspective that included quality of life; from the reductionism of the biomedical model, to Engel's biopsychosocial model[10]; and beyond, to include consideration of the determinants of suffering and the existential/spiritual issues implicit in "Total Pain,"[11] whole-person care and healing.

The Legacy and the Challenge

Now, four decades later, we marvel at the wisdom of Cicely Saunders' planning and the richness of her legacy. At this writing, St. Christopher's addresses the needs of 1600 patients and families per year with its 48 beds, 500 patients per day on the Home Care Service, and 20 patients per day in the Day Care Centre. Their education and research programs continue in Cicely's fine tradition of excellence. They host 2000 visitors and convene 80 conferences and workshops annually. But her legacy reaches far beyond South East London; she has been the critical catalyst for the international modern hospice movement, with the creation to date of at least 8000 hospice and palliative care programs in more than 100 countries and the academic field of palliative medicine.

The progress in palliative care diagnosis and therapeutics over the decades since 1967 has been remarkable.[12] With our increasing sophistication as "symptomatologists"[13] and the trend toward specialization, however, are we in palliative care in danger of losing touch with Dame Cicely's challenge to see our mandate as "a characteristic mixture of tough clinical science and compassion"?[14] Do we see palliative medicine as going "beyond symptom control to creating conditions where healing at a deep personal level may occur for the individual patient,"[15] or are we progressively less effective as we attempt to stretch our perspective from biomedical model, to biopsychosocial model, to whole-person care with its notion of "healing"?[16] Each practitioner must answer this question for himself or herself.

Our answer to that question is important. The *whole-person* approach to understanding the patient's needs is gaining increasing credibility as research repeatedly identifies major pieces of evidence of its validity. It is becoming clear that *the whole-person care model* has greater explanatory power than either the biomedical or the biopsychosocial models alone. For instance, there is now evidence to support the following:

- The existential/spiritual domain is a significant determinant of quality of life (QOL) throughout the disease trajectory in cancer patients[17,18] and is the most important QOL determinant once patients with human immunodeficiency virus (HIV) have acquired immunodeficiency syndrome (AIDS).[19]

- Cognitive processing of loss that leads to increased perception of meaning is associated with increased CD4 counts and enhanced survival among grieving men with HIV—the first study to show a link between meaning and mortality and the first to report an association between meaning and physical health indexes that does not appear to be mediated by health behaviors.[20]
- QOL is not dependent on the physical domain alone. For example, 2 out of 3 cancer patients who were aware of their diagnosis (and most were on active therapy at the time) assessed their own health to be "very healthy"—including 12 who died during the study.[21] Similarly, in a study of emotional well-being, persons with malignant melanoma had emotional well-being levels similar to those of the general population.[22] Furthermore, in a study of life satisfaction, seriously disabled persons, including some who were paralyzed following trauma, had life satisfaction levels equal to those of the general population.[23]
- Telomere shortening compatible with cellular aging of a full decade has been found in premenopausal women with chronic stress.[24]
- Those able to find equanimity in the face of impending death are distinguished from those with anguish and suffering by several themes. They commonly experience: a sense of "healing connection" to self, others, the phenomenal world experienced through the five senses, or ultimate meaning as perceived by that person; a sense of meaning in the context of their suffering; a capacity to enter the present moment; a sympathetic connection to the cause of their suffering; and an openness to finding potential in the moment that is greater than their need for control.[25]

Clinicians must, it would seem, take seriously Kearney's insightful observation that we need to aim "beyond symptom control to creating conditions where healing at a deep personal level may occur for the individual patient,"[15] and do so with a growing understanding of the potential involved. If human life is, as the world's great Wisdom Traditions remind us, body, mind, and spirit, and the agreed goal of palliative care is to improve the quality of life, then how can we *possibly* do this without considering the whole person?

Today, the multiplicity of challenges that face those who would follow in Dame Cicely's footsteps are as varied as the cultural, geopolitical, and economic realities that frame the communities they work in. How different are the demands and constraints in the isolated communities of the Canadian Arctic from the teeming cities of India. Yet the root causes of suffering are the same. This book is offered in the hope that a well-referenced, reader-friendly guide to palliative care principles and practices in a wide range of clinical settings will be of assistance to you.

As you provide your patients with palliative care, keep the whole-person care model in mind and create care plans that truly integrate the comprehensive assessment that it demands. Offer care that reaches for perfection in symptom management and in care for the psychosocial and spiritual forms of suffering that life-limiting and serious illnesses entail, and consider ways of working with the innate healing potential that resides within each individual, and which, paradoxically, appears to be catalyzed by approaching death.[26] Whether you are a surgeon in a tertiary care center (as I have been), or a nurse or social worker (both of which Dame Cicely Saunders was before she became a doctor), or any other health care provider, may you find in the following pages what you need to accomplish the noble task of caring for the seriously ill person and his or her family "with tough clinical science and compassion."

References

1. Hinton J: *Dying*, ed 2, London, 1972, Penguin Books, p 159.
2. Du Boulay S: *Cicely Saunders: the founder of the modern hospice movement*, London, 1984, Hodder and Stoughton, p 63.
3. Saunders C: Dying of cancer, *St. Thomas Hosp Gazette* 56(2), 1957.
4. Saunders C: The treatment of intractable pain in terminal cancer, *Proc Royal Soc Med* 56:195, reprinted, 1963.
5. Clark D: *Cicely Saunders, founder of the hospice movement: selected letters 1959–1999*, London, 2002, Oxford University Press.
6. Saunders C: Watch with me, *Nursing Times* 61(48):1615–1617, 1965.
7. Du Boulay S: *Cicely Saunders: the founder of the modern hospice movement*, London, 1984, Hodder and Stoughton, p 56.
8. Saunders C: *Watch with me: inspiration for a life in hospice care*, Sheffield, UK, 2003, Mortal Press, p 15.
9. Reading A: Illness and disease, *Med Clin North Am* 61(4):703–710, 1977.
10. Engel GL: The need for a new medical model: a challenge for biomedicine, *Science* 196(4286): 129–136, 1977.
11. Saunders C: The philosophy of terminal care. In Saunders C, editor: *The management of terminal malignant disease*, ed 2, Baltimore, 1984, Edward Arnold, pp 232–241.
12. Doyle D, Hanks G, Cherny N, Calman K, editors: *Oxford textbook of palliative medicine*, ed 3, Oxford, UK, 2004, Oxford University Press.
13. Ahmedzai SH: Editorial: Five years, five threads, *Prog Palliat Care* 5(6):235–237, 1997.
14. Saunders C: Foreword. In Doyle D, Hanks G, Cherny N, et al, editors: *Oxford textbook of palliative medicine*, ed 3, Oxford, UK, 2004, Oxford University Press, pp xvii–xx.
15. Kearney M: Palliative medicine: just another specialty? *Palliat Med* 6:39–46, 1992.
16. Kearney M: *A place of healing*, Oxford, UK, 2000, Oxford University Press.
17. Cohen SR, Mount BM, Tomas J, et al: Existential well-being is an important determinant of quality of life: evidence from the McGill quality of life questionnaire, *Cancer* 77(3):576, 1996.
18. Cohen SR, Mount BM, Bruera E, et al: Validity of the McGill Quality of Life Questionnaire in the palliative care setting: a multi-center Canadian study demonstrating the importance of the existential domain, *Palliat Med* 11:3–20, 1997.
19. Cohen SR, Hassan SA, Lapointe BJ, et al: Quality of life in HIV disease as measured by the McGill Quality of Life Questionnaire, *AIDS* 10:1421–1427, 1996.
20. Bower JE, Kemeny ME, Taylor SE, et al: Cognitive processing, discovery of meaning, CD4 decline, and AIDS-related mortality among bereaved HIV-seropositive men, *J Consult Clin Psychol* 66(6):979–986, 1998.
21. Kagawa-Singer M: Redefining health: living with cancer, *Soc Sci Med* 295–304, 1993.
22. Casselith BR, Lusk EJ, Tenaglia AN: A psychological comparison of patients with malignant melanoma and other dermatologic disorders, *J Am Acad Derm* 7:742–746, 1982.
23. Kreitler S, Chaitchik S, Rapoport Y, et al: Life satisfaction and health in cancer patients, orthopedic patients and healthy individuals, *Soc Sci Med* 36:547–556, 1993.
24. Epel ES, Blackburn EH, Lin J, et al: Accelerated telomere shortening in response to life stress, *Proc Natl Acad Sci USA* 101(49):17312–17315, 2004.
25. Mount B, Boston P: *Healing connections: a phenomenological study of suffering, wellness and quality of life* (in press).
26. Edinger E: *Ego and archetype*, Boston, 1972, Shambala, p 115.

PREFACE

Linda L. Emanuel, MD, PhD
S. Lawrence Librach, MD, CCFP, FCFP

Palliative care comprises at least half of medicine. It is the art and science of providing relief from illness-related suffering. Every medical declaration binds medical professionals not only to cure when it is possible, but also to care always. Alleviation of suffering is needed for all who have a curable illness as well as for those who have an incurable illness, and it is certainly needed for those with chronic, serious illnesses. Palliative care developed in the modern era as a set of skills for care of those near the end of life. This hospice movement's achievements have provided much. It afforded dignity and comfort to those who were dying and to the families of the dying and, with the cognitive and technical skill set that has developed within hospice, it is now augmenting the quality of care provided by all disciplines and specialties within medicine.

Never in the history of medicine has our knowledge and technical capacity to manage symptoms and address other forms of suffering been so sophisticated. Palliative care combines a growing understanding of the molecular, physiological, and psychological mechanisms of suffering at the end of life with interventions that are increasingly subjected to rigorous evaluations. These care interventions are provided with interdisciplinary care delivery models that are human-centered (rather than technology- or pathophysiology-centered) and grounded in a network of community-specific, therapeutic relationships that take into account the whole picture of the origins of the patient's suffering and its consequences.

Palliative care can provide something else that society sorely needs: the ability to make life transitions and sustain tragedies without being entirely decimated. By accepting the concept of a good death, palliative care can focus on the journey at the end of life and the possibilities for continuing contributions of the patient to his or her family and society. By managing symptoms and attending to mental health, spiritual well-being, and social needs, palliative care allows the patient to continue living life to the fullest extent possible for the longest possible time. It allows the patient to stay out of the dependent, sick role and continue in the role of a productive member of society, including staying in the work force if it is helpful to do so, for as long as possible. Palliative care also supports the caregiver and, after the patient's death, the bereaved. Caregivers can perform better and sustain their prior roles better with this type of support. Bereaved families can grieve and learn to go on without their loved one in a healthier, more viable way if they have the type of preparation and support that palliative care offers. These approaches combine to provide potentially tremendous improvement in what is known in medical economics as the realm of indirect costs. As such, societies ravaged by tragedies such as the current HIV/AIDS (human immunodeficiency virus/acquired immunodeficiency syndrome) epidemic or other sources of widespread loss may need palliative care for societal survival and future well-being.

It is hoped that the present textbook will help spread the practices of palliative care to those areas of medical care and regions of the world that need it. The first section provides a practical rendition of the framework philosophy and core skills—cognitive and technical—of palliative care. The second section examines how palliative care can be integrated into some of the major illness categories that encompass chronically disabling and life-shortening conditions. The third section is about care delivery; palliative care can be delivered in settings that range from specialty consultation services to home care and each has its own common and unique challenges. Finally, the fourth section sets out some features of the range of social settings in which palliative care must be delivered and considers some of the policy options that affect palliative care and, in turn, the social impact that palliative care can have.

The content of this book has been gathered from pioneers of palliative care and is offered to all those who serve their fellow human beings with care: professionals, policy makers, service delivery administrators, and family and community members.

CONTENTS

PART C   Personal Contexts

PART D   Specific Situations and Skill Sets

SECTION 2
Specific Types of Illness and Sites of Care

SECTION 3
Service Delivery

SECTION 4
The Social Context

Appendixes

Appendixes can be found online at www.expertconsult.com.

SECTION 1

Palliative Care: Core Skills

PART A

General Foundations

3

CHAPTER 1

Palliative Care: A Quiet Revolution in Patient Care

LINDA L. EMANUEL and S. LAWRENCE LIBRACH

In some respects, this century's scientific and medical advances have made living easier and dying harder.[1]

The opening quote from the Institute of Medicine stands in stark contrast to the reality that dying can be the last great time of living. Sadly, multiple studies have confirmed the poor quality of end-of-life care in North America.[2-4] If the health care system is part of what stands between people and their ability to access the potential qualities of that time of life, the system needs to ask, What happened? Part of the answer comes from the fact that the way people die has changed over the past 100 years. Most people now die with one or more chronic illnesses and often demonstrate a predictable, slow decline in function.[5] Another part of the answer must note that the emphasis in medical care has been on technology, cure, and life prolongation, and some societal expectations have also been youth-oriented and similarly disinclined to afford dying its place. The medical and social cultures offered little that was appropriate for those who were dying. Therefore, these patients stayed in the sick role rather than entering the dying role, and they received interventions designed for cure and recovery.

4

Both the health care system and society have great capacity to react, however, and a set of countermovement initiatives began. In a parallel to the home birthing movement, which was a reaction to the intense focus on technology in obstetrics, people facing the other end of life also began to seek control over their dying. Some pushed for assisted suicide, whereas others sought and found ways to protect the human meaning that could be found in dying; this approach was supplied by hospice palliative care, and more people began to seek home hospice and palliative care at the end of life.[6,7] The pioneers and leaders of hospice and palliative care constructed a coherent analysis of what needed to be fixed. It was a radical list, as the Foreword by Mount describes. Hospice and palliative care developed rapidly in a movement that made *hospice* a household word and *palliative care* a type of care that people now know they can demand from their health care delivery organization. Looking back at three decades of progress, it seems fair to say that the early decades of hospice and palliative care can be understood as a successful call to action to address the observed deficiencies in end-of-life care that had come to characterize the modern North American health care systems.[8]

This chapter delineates what constitutes palliative care and what is quality end-of-life care. It illustrates how palliative care seeks to change the norms of health care so that palliative care can be integrated into all of health care, summarizes some remaining challenges in palliative care for both the practicing clinician and the health care system, and explores challenges for palliative care in the global setting.

This book goes on to outline the following: the core competencies of end-of-life care, which can now be taught to future generations of health care professionals; essential palliative care skills for specialty settings, which can now be taught in specialty training programs; and service delivery features in palliative care that should be essential knowledge for all health care administrators and community practitioners of all professions. This book ends with a broad overview of the social setting in which palliative care is still facing major challenges, including a hard look at the role of financial devastation in the illness experience and a look at global challenges. Finally, the Appendixes (available online at www.expertconsult.com) offer a drug formulary, further resources for professionals, and further resources for patients and their informal caregivers.

Definition of Palliative Care

The terms *hospice* and *end-of-life care* can be seen as synonyms for *palliative care*. Although each term has distinguishing features, for simplicity we use *palliative care* throughout this book to denote either or both.

The World Health Organization (WHO) has defined palliative care as follows[9]:

Palliative care is an approach that improves the quality of life of patients and their families facing the problem associated with life-threatening illness, through the prevention and relief of suffering by means of early identification and impeccable assessment and treatment of pain and other problems, physical, psychosocial and spiritual.

Palliative care:

- provides relief from pain and other distressing symptoms
- affirms life and regards dying as a normal process
- intends neither to hasten or postpone death
- integrates the psychological and spiritual aspects of patient care

- offers a support system to help patients live as actively as possible until death
- offers a support system to help the family cope during the patient's illness and in their own bereavement
- uses a team approach to address the needs of patients and their families, including bereavement counselling, if indicated
- will enhance quality of life, and may also positively influence the course of illness
- is applicable early in the course of illness, in conjunction with other therapies that are intended to prolong life, such as chemotherapy or radiation therapy, and includes those investigations needed to better understand and manage distressing clinical complications

The attributes of palliative care have been articulated in a consensus document from Canada.[10] These attributes support the WHO definition and guide all aspects of care at the end of life. They are as follows:

1. *Patient-family focused.* Because patients are typically part of a family, when care is provided, the patient and family are treated as a unit. All aspects of care are provided in a manner that is sensitive to the patient's and family's personal, cultural, and religious values, beliefs, and practices; their developmental state; and their preparedness to deal with the dying process.
2. *High quality.* All hospice palliative care activities are guided by the following: the ethical principles of autonomy, beneficence, nonmaleficence, justice, truth telling, and confidentiality; standards of practice that are based on nationally accepted principles and norms of practice and standards of professional conduct for each discipline; policies and procedures that are based on the best available evidence or opinion-based preferred practice guidelines; and data collection and documentation guidelines that are based on validated measurement tools.
3. *Safe and effective.* All hospice palliative care activities are conducted in a manner that is collaborative; ensures confidentiality and privacy; is without coercion, discrimination, harassment, or prejudice; ensures safety and security for all participants; ensures continuity and accountability; aims to minimize unnecessary duplication and repetition; and complies with laws, regulations, and policies in effect within the jurisdiction, host, and palliative care organizations.
4. *Accessible.* All patients and families have equal access to timely hospice palliative care services, wherever they live at home or can access services within a reasonable distance from their home.
5. *Adequately resourced.* The financial, human, information, physical, and community resources are sufficient to sustain the organization's activities and its strategic and business plans. Sufficient resources are allocated to each of the organization's activities.
6. *Collaborative.* Each community's needs for hospice palliative care are assessed and addressed through the collaborative efforts of available organizations and services in partnership.
7. *Knowledge based.* Ongoing education of all patients, families, caregivers, staff, and stakeholders is integral to the provision and advancement of high-quality hospice palliative care.

8. *Advocacy based.* Regular interaction with legislators, regulators, policy makers, health care funders, other palliative care providers, professional societies and associations, and the public is essential to increase awareness about and to develop palliative care activities and the resources that support them. All advocacy is based on nationally accepted norms of practice.
9. *Research based.* The development, dissemination, and integration of new knowledge are critical to the advancement of high-quality hospice palliative care. When possible, all activities are based on the best available evidence. All research protocols comply with legislation and regulations in effect within the jurisdiction that govern research and the involvement of human subjects.

Concepts of Quality of Life and Quality of Dying

As palliative care made its case and consolidated its progress, it had to respond to those who saw no need and asked, Why should care be changed? It also had to respond to the skeptics who asked, Is it possible to have a quality of life at the end of life or a quality of dying? For those who wanted change but needed direction, it had to respond to the question, What are those issues that are important to patients and families at the end of life? The following studies, among others, identify guiding answers to these questions.

One study interviewed 385 U.S. residents in 32 cities using a qualitative interview and focus group–based method. Those who were interviewed were not yet facing a terminal illness and reflected mixed demographics, including age, race, culture, and religion. These persons articulated their concerns, hopes, and beliefs about the process of dying.[10] They feared being hooked up to machines at the end of life and preferred a natural death with loved ones in familiar surroundings. They did not believe that the current health care system supported their ideal concept of dying, and although they thought it was important to plan for dying and death, they were uncomfortable with the topic and resisted taking action. They said that family consideration was their primary concern in making end-of-life decisions. Finally, they reported that the current planning options did not support the way they wanted to manage dying and the death experience.

In another study,[11] 126 patients from three groups (patients undergoing dialysis, patients with human immunodeficiency virus [HIV] disease, and chronic care patients) were interviewed to explore their views about what constitutes good end-of-life care. A qualitative analysis was done, and certain themes were identified. These included receiving adequate pain and symptom management, avoiding inappropriate prolongation of dying, achieving a sense of control, relieving burden, and strengthening relationships with loved ones.

Similarly, in March 1999 through August 1999, another study[12] conducted a cross-sectional, stratified, random, national survey of seriously ill patients ($n = 340$), recently bereaved family ($n = 332$), physicians ($n = 361$), and other care providers (nurses, social workers, chaplains, and hospice volunteers; $n = 429$) and found similar themes. The investigators also identified items that were consistently rated as important (>70% responded that the item is important) across all four groups, including pain and symptom management, preparation for death, a sense of completion, decisions about treatment preferences, and being treated as a "whole person." Eight items received strong importance ratings from patients but were not rated as highly by physicians ($P < .001$). These items included being mentally aware, having funeral arrangements planned, not being a burden, helping others, and coming to peace with God. Ten items had broad variation within, as well as among, the four groups, including decisions about life-sustaining treatments, dying at home, and talking about the meaning of death. Participants ranked freedom from pain most important and dying at home least important among nine major attributes.

Palliative Care as a Revolution

The palliative care movement has been revolutionary in that it insisted on a return to the professional values of health care that seemed to have been too much overlooked at the time. The changes required were applicable to most settings of health care. So perhaps it is ironic that it began as a movement on the fringes of the system, providing hospice care as a charity. Palliative care is based on a clear and coherent philosophy of care that Dame Cicely Saunders first articulated as care of the whole person.[13] This comprehensive model of care was interprofessional from the beginning in that it recognized the need to meet physical, psychological, social, and spiritual needs of dying patients and their families. An important goal in palliative care is to educate the patient and family about dying and death. Another goal is to integrate care across the continuum of care stages, even when the doctors or sites of care change; palliative care seeks to bridge these changes by communicating and transferring the patient's goals of care and resultant care plans from one team to another. Care is also extended beyond the patient's death to reflect a concern for the grief outcomes of family members.

In this new model of care, death is not seen as the "enemy" but rather as an acceptable outcome. The dying are seen as having an important role, complete with tasks and expectations, that is different from the sick role when recovery is expectable.[14] The goal is not to prolong or shorten life; rather, the process of dying is to be freed of as much unnecessary suffering as possible. The inevitable dimensions of suffering that do accompany dying and death can be soothed by finding meaning and purpose in the life lived and by enhancing quality of life and the quality of the dying process. The model is not technology based, but it does accept technology when it reduces suffering. The model is based on a comprehensive, humanistic approach to suffering and dying. It attempts to make end-of-life care as comprehensive and important as care at the beginning of life. The philosophy of palliative care is remarkably similar throughout many countries; this reality may be understood as evidence for the fundamental need and place of palliative care in medicine and medicine's mandate to care for people who face illness-related suffering.

Palliative care has grown progressively as an international movement and has many national and international organizations that promote better care for the dying across all continents. Specialists have developed in all health care professions, and a large volunteer component has emerged to support care for patients and families. There has been a tremendous growth in knowledge about dying and death in our society, and research is now taking on a level of sophistication that parallels any other area in medicine. The public, especially in developed nations but also those that are resource constrained, has become more aware of the option of palliative care. For professionals, many new text and web resources, comprehensive education programs, research efforts, and specialty journals are devoted to enhancing end-of-life care.

Challenges for the Practicing Clinician

The palliative care movement has seen dramatic progress, and in this sense, as characterized earlier, the call to action has been successful. However, major challenges remain, some of which are listed and discussed here.

DEVELOPING COMPETENCIES

Much still has to be done to incorporate competencies in end-of-life care into curricula of undergraduate and postgraduate professional training programs. All practicing clinicians must have at least basic competence in this area, with support from specialists as necessary. Continuing professional development in palliative care needs to be more in evidence in conferences and other professional development activities.

DEALING WITH ONE'S OWN FEELINGS AND OUTLOOK

Death anxiety among professionals appears to play a strong role in the way clinicians interact with dying patients.[15,16] This probably results, in part, from training that emphasized death as the enemy. When clinicians see patients and families suffer greatly and feel helpless to intervene, they may feel powerfully compelled to walk away if they have had no training in how to deal with their own (in part, transferred) suffering. If clinicians cannot access their intuitive capacities for empathic healing through presence, it may be impossible to offer the kind "being there" that Mount describes in the Foreword of this book as one of Dame Cicely Saunders' founding insights and premises for palliative care. Better training and care are necessary.

PROVIDING PALLIATIVE CARE FOR ALL LIFE-LIMITING ILLNESSES

Cancer is only one cause of death, and although the prevalence of cancer is increasing, other illnesses such as heart disease, lung disease, and Alzheimer's disease account for a larger proportion of deaths. Palliative care has grown up in the midst of cancer care; more attention must now be paid to providing palliative care to patients dying of other diseases too.

Palliative care needs to be integrated into the care of all chronic, progressive illnesses and some acute illnesses in which the prognosis is quite poor. This integration should take place much earlier in the course of the illness than it often currently does. Patients and families need to deal with many issues from diagnosis on and not only after some magic line is crossed into acknowledged dying. Clinicians can integrate palliative care into any disease management guideline as described in Chapter 44. Clinicians also need to be aware that reducing palliative care into symptom management alone avoids the desired comprehensive, humanistic approach to dying patients and their families.

WHEN TO INVOLVE A PALLIATIVE CARE SPECIALIST

The knowledge base in palliative care has grown progressively. Specialists who focus on complex issues in end-of-life care have emerged in all health care professions. These professionals have provided necessary research, education, and advocacy, but this should not mitigate the need for every professional to have some basic competencies in end-of-life care. Palliative care specialists are not needed for every patient, and these specialists will never be able to meet the increasing need for care for the dying. Moreover, specialized palliative care should not be confined to freestanding hospices or palliative care units; rather, it must be present across the continuum of the health care system, in part to avoid the abrogation of others in providing better care.

MAINTAINING THE INTERPROFESSIONAL NATURE OF THE WORK

No one profession or discipline can provide all the care necessary to meet the physical, psychological, functional, social, and spiritual needs of a dying patient and family. Interprofessional teamwork is essential both for the patient and family and for the professionals.

Challenges for the Health Care System

The challenges that still face the palliative care movement are not limited to those that must be shouldered by individual clinicians. The health care systems, and those who design, manage, advise, and influence them also face challenges. Some are listed and discussed here.

INTEGRATING PALLIATIVE CARE INTO THE SYSTEM

The Institute of Medicine landmark report in 2001[17] laid out the components of a quality health care system. These components include the following:

- A safe system that avoids harming patients by care that is intended to help them
- An effective system that provides services based on scientific knowledge to all who could benefit and that refrains from providing services to those not likely to benefit (avoiding underuse and overuse)
- Patient-centered care that is respectful and responsive to individual patient preferences, needs, and values and that ensures that these guide all clinical decision making
- Timely assistance so that harmful delays are avoided for both those who receive care and those who give care
- Efficient care to avoid waste of equipment, supplies, ideas, and energy
- Equitable care so that care provision does not vary in quality because of personal characteristics, such as gender, ethnicity, geographic location, and socioeconomic status

Palliative care must heed these issues as it enters the mainstream of health care.

DEVELOPING STANDARDS AND QUALITY IMPROVEMENT PROCESSES

The standards for palliative care set out by National Consensus Project for Quality Palliative Care[17] in the United States and the norms of practice developed in Canada have started to set standards for palliative care organizations. Certification of practitioners in palliative care is evolving rapidly in the United States, so fellowship requirements for specialty board certification, which will occur through the American Board of Medical Specialties, will be in place over the next few years. In addition, there are guidelines in palliative care and recommendations on how to incorporate palliative care into other disease management guidelines.[18,19] A need exists, however, for accreditation standards and quality improvement strategies for all organizations and agencies involved in end-of-life care, whether they be acute care hospitals, cancer centers, long-term care facilities, home health agencies, or others. The Joint Accreditation Commission of Healthcare Organizations' standards for hospitals have been examined by the Center to Advance Palliative Care, and a detailed cross-walk has been provided so that facilities can build according to established standards.[20] In Canada, Accreditation Canada, the agency that accredits almost every health care organization and agency, has developed a palliative care section in their accreditation instrument. Implementation may spur the development of high-quality end-of-life care across the spectrum of health care. For the health care system in general, attention to at least the following areas is necessary.

PROVIDING SUPPORT FOR FORMAL INTERDISCIPLINARY TEAMS

All palliative care organizations, whether national, regional, or local, recognize the need for interdisciplinary formal teams. However, the challenge is for the system to recognize and support formal teams (organized interdisciplinary teams devoted to palliative care), rather than relying on the informal teams that form around a patient and family but that have no consistent existence or commitment to work as a team with palliative care expertise and focus.

Many palliative care services already rely on nursing care to a greater extent than other specialties. Over the long term, it may be necessary to adjust the ratio of professionals involved because much more counseling is needed than can be provided by the current workforce of social workers and pastors in most medical service delivery systems.

PROVIDING SUPPORT FOR EDUCATION AT ALL LEVELS

Across the care continuum, there is a need for basic competencies in end-of-life care for all who work with terminally ill patients and their families. This includes not only health care professionals but also volunteers, health care aides, personal support workers, and administrative personnel who come into direct contact with palliative care patients and their families. The Canadian Strategy on Palliative and End of Life Care Education Work Group has developed a list of six basic, common competencies for any professional:

1. Address and manage pain and symptoms.
2. Address psychosocial and spiritual needs.
3. Address end-of-life decision making and planning.
4. Attend to suffering.
5. Communicate effectively.
6. Collaborate as a member of an interdisciplinary team.

This framework has been used to develop a national education program for medical students and postgraduate trainees in Canada. Health care curricula in North America must incorporate such competencies and must ensure that they are taught and evaluated in the clinical milieu. Health care organizations need to incorporate palliative care into orientation sessions for new employees and new care providers. Continuing professional development in palliative care is also important. Organizations such as the Education in Palliative and End-of-Life Care

Project in the United States and its focused educational projects in oncology and emergency medicine and the Pallium Project in Canada have been leaders in developing comprehensive, basic education materials and educational and high-quality train-the-trainer programs. In some jurisdictions (e.g., California), palliative care professional development is required for renewal of medical licensure. It is important to develop opinion leaders or champions in institutions and regions to sustain education and skills development. Communities of practice lead to better and more rapid change. Effective knowledge transfer methods must be used.

PROVIDING SUPPORT FOR RESEARCH

Although much research is done on curative or life-prolonging treatments, many agencies that support research have not devoted funding to end-of-life care research until recently. The recently formed National Center for Palliative Care Research in the United States is a promising development.

There are a number of challenges that need special support in order for palliative care research to progress. One challenge arose when commentators questioned whether palliative care patients who are often quite ill can participate in research ethically. Others argued that it was a right and essential for progress that palliative care patients be included in research. The ensuing debate made it is clear that such research can be ethical as long as the basic precepts of autonomy, informed consent, privacy, confidentiality, and justice are observed. It has been observed that patients and families are frequently open to participating in research in palliative care environments because they are often grateful for the care they have received.

Another challenge arose from the practical realities involved in doing research on people who are so sick that they often cannot participate in research for long. Special methods for collecting and analyzing data are needed to mitigate this problem.[21]

Furthermore, research in symptom management aspects of palliative care is challenged by the reality that palliative care patients have a wide diversity of illnesses and usually have multisystem failure and multiple symptoms. Research on health care delivery and indicators of quality end-of-life care is essential.

Moreover, palliative care needs to go beyond medical interventions in pain and symptom management to include research on the psychosocial and spiritual needs of patients and families. Much of the necessary research in those areas requires social and behavioral research techniques that are often qualitative or ethnographic or economic, research types not well represented in health care environments and often not adequately supported by national health care research funding agencies. Interdisciplinary research networks and partnerships need to be developed that include experienced researchers from those areas as well as medical, nursing, social worker, pastoral, and pharmaceutical researchers. This will reflect the diverse needs of patients and the interdisciplinary care that characterizes high-quality end-of-life care.

Finally, to foster the development of research in end-of-life care and the training of required personnel, palliative care must become part of research at academic institutions. Centers, units, or departments must be fostered.

INTEGRATING PALLIATIVE CARE THROUGHOUT HEALTH CARE SERVICES

Palliative care should not be seen as a transfer of care out of the usual care system. Palliative care can be successfully integrated much earlier into the course of patients with progressive, life-threatening illness without any negative effects on patients and families. The commonly held view that patients will give up hope and "stop fighting" their illness is wrong and often prevents or delays high-quality end-of-life care until just a few weeks or days before death. This short period of intervention may mean that patients and families suffer unnecessarily for months. Diagrammatic care models (e.g., that provided in Figure 23-1 of Chapter 23, by Ferris and associates) and models of adjustment (e.g., those described by Knight and Emanuel in Chapter 18) have been developed to demonstrate how transitions can happen effectively, enhance patient and family satisfaction, and lead to outcomes such as better quality of life during the process of dying and, for families, after death has occurred.

Transitions between services remain a challenge. Constraints on the provision of palliative care exist in some jurisdictions in the United States and Canada; they are inherently harmful and without scientific basis. These and other challenges can be met through local and national initiatives of government, accreditation bodies, health care organizations and agencies, academic institutions, professional organizations, and research funding agencies.

Palliative Care and the Global Setting

The threat of future pandemics, the current pandemic of HIV disease, and the health consequences of poverty and violence that have plagued populations through the ages show no sign of abatement, and all pose considerable challenges, the response to which must include providing better palliative care.

In resource-limited nations, family members, community volunteers, or health care workers are often not available in sufficient numbers to provide adequate care without overburdening individual caregivers. However, palliative care is potentially the kind of low-cost, high-impact approach to maximizing function until inevitable death that resource-limited countries need. Ideally, a mix of family, volunteers, and health care workers will be used, perhaps with hospital- or clinic-based health care workers providing initial teaching to families and volunteers who can follow up with most of the care in the home. Palliative care should be included in the curricula of medical, nursing, and other health professional students to ensure that health care workers are sufficiently prepared to care in all settings and are able to train family members and community volunteers.[22]

Good palliative care also requires that standards, policies, and guidelines be in place at the system and institutional level to ensure that adequate palliative care is integrated into health care systems. In many countries, especially resource-constrained countries, restrictive regulations regarding the use of morphine and other opioids constitute obstacles to pain control. Even in the United States, where palliative care is relatively well developed, some jurisdictions have regulations (e.g., triplicate prescriptions for opioids) that inhibit physicians from prescribing these analgesics for terminally ill patients. In both resource-constrained and wealthier environments, good palliative care can be cost-effective and can result in fewer hospital days, more home care, and fewer high-technology investigative and treatment interventions, with responsibility of care given to an interdisciplinary care team that includes volunteers.

PEARLS

- The goal of palliative care is quality of life for the dying and their families.
- Palliative care is well defined, has clear content areas, and has well-specified guidelines.
- Palliative care demands sophisticated skills that have warranted its acceptance as a full specialty in medicine in the United States.
- Challenges to implementing high-quality palliative care involve internal barriers within the clinician as well as system barriers.[23]

PITFALLS

- Palliative care is not a soft discipline.
- Lack of competence in the area is a barrier to high-quality palliative care.
- Lack of training and lack of adjustment to the clinician's own mortality are barriers to high-quality palliative care.
- Lack of institutional support for palliative care makes it difficult to provide high-quality care to the dying.

Summary

The accurate observation of the Institute of Medicine that "in some respects, this century's scientific and medical advances have made living easier and dying harder" has a silver lining. The fundamental humanity in members of society and the ability of the medical system to see the need for change have fostered a rebalancing movement that has made significant progress in returning to high-quality health care for the dying. Palliative care is now a component of health services, and it is replete with skill sets and the capacity to deliver its desired outcomes. The remaining chapters of this book outline the following: the core competencies of end-of-life care, which can now be taught to future generations of clinicians; essential palliative care skills for specialty settings, which can now be taught in specialty training programs; and service delivery features in palliative care that should be essential knowledge for all health care administrators and community practitioners of all professions. This book ends with a broad overview of the social setting in which palliative care is still facing major challenges, including a hard look at the role of financial devastation in the illness experience and a look at global challenges. Finally, the Appendixes (available online at www.expertconsult.com) offer a drug formulary, information on the practicalities of reimbursement for clinicians in the United States, further resources for professionals, and further resources for patients and their informal caregivers.

References

1. Committee on Care at the End of Life, Division of Health Services, Institute of Medicine, Cassel CK, Field MJ, editors: *Approaching death: improving care at the end of life*, Washington, DC, 1997, National Academy Press, p 14.
2. Emanuel EJ, Emanuel LL: The promise of a good death, *Lancet* 351(Suppl II):21–29, 1998.
3. Emanuel EJ, Fairclough D, Slutsman J, et al: Assistance from family members, friends, paid care givers, and volunteers in the care of terminally ill patients, *N Engl J Med* 341:956–963, 1999.
4. Tyler BA, Perry MJ, Lofton TC, Millard F: *The quest to die with dignity: an analysis of Americans' values, opinions, and attitudes concerning end-of-life care*, Appleton, WI, 1997, American Health Decisions, p 5.

5. Covinsky KE, Eng C, Lui LY, et al: The last 2 years of life: functional trajectories of frail older people, *J Am Geriatr Soc* 51:492–498, 2003.
6. Naisbitt J: *Megatrends: ten new directions transforming our lives*, New York, 1982, Warner Books, pp 39–54.
7. Naisbitt J: *Megatrends: ten new directions transforming our lives,* New York, 1982, Warner Books, p 139.
8. Jennings B: Preface. Improving end of life care: why has it been so difficult? *Hastings Cent Rep* 35:S2–S4, 2005.
9. World Health Organization: Available at http://www.who.int/cancer/palliative/definition/en/. Accessed November 30, 2010.
10. Ferris FD: *A model to guide hospice palliative care*, Ottawa, Canada, 2002, Canadian Hospice Palliative Care Association.
11. Singer PA, Martin DK, Kelner M: Quality end-of-life care: patients' perspectives, *JAMA* 281:163–168, 1999.
12. Steinhauser KE, Christakis NA, Clipp EC, et al: Factors considered important at the end of life by patients, family, physicians, and other care providers, *JAMA* 284:2476–2482, 2000.
13. Saunders C: The philosophy of terminal care. In Saunders C, editor: *The management of terminal malignant disease*, ed 2, Baltimore, 1984, Edward Arnold.
14. Emanuel L, Dworzkin K, Robinson V: The dying role, *J Palliat Med* 10(1):159–168, 2007.
15. Viswanathan R: Death anxiety, locus of control, and purpose of life in physicians: Their relationship to patient death notification, *Psychosomatics* 37:339–345, 1996.
16. Schulz R, Aderman D: Physician's death anxiety and patient outcomes, *Omega (Westport)* 9:327–332, 1978–1979.
17. Committee on Quality Health Care in America, Institute of Medicine: *Crossing the quality chasm: a new health system for the 21st century*, Washington DC, 2001, National Academy Press.
18. National Consensus Project for Quality Palliative Care: Available at http://www.nationalconsensusproject.org. Accessed November 30, 2010.
19. National Comprehensive Cancer Network (NCCN): Clinical Practice Guidelines in Oncology v2. 2005: Available at http://www.nccn.org/professionals/physician/gls/PDF/palliative.pdf. Accessed November 30, 2010.
20. Emanuel L, Alexander C, Arnold R, et al: Integrating palliative care into disease management guidelines, *J Palliat Med* 7:774–783, 2004.
21. Center to Advance Palliative Care: Available at http://www.capc.org/jcaho-crosswalk. Accessed November 30, 2010.
22. Chang C-H, Boni-Saenz Aa, Durazo-Arvizu RA, et al: A system for interactive assessment and management in palliative care, *Pain Symptom Manage* 33(6):745–755, 2007.

CHAPTER 2

Comprehensive Assessment

LINDA L. EMANUEL

Medical care depends on the traditional patient history and physical examination, an approach to patient assessment that has developed gradually over the course of the modern medical era. Variants that emphasize diverse aspects of a person's situation are used in different disciplines in medicine, such as nursing, social work, and pastoral assessments. Furthermore, different specialties (e.g., family medicine, rehabilitation medicine, cardiology, and infectious disease) also use their own variants that emphasize different aspects of a person's situation. Many components of patient assessment have been evaluated for efficacy. As a whole, however, the assessment has received sparse attention in research, and its variants are often not well codified or researched. Palliative care has adopted its own distinctive approach based on the whole-patient assessment. Early in the evolution of the discipline, the palliative care assessment was founded on its specific purposes, and soon thereafter on research.

Palliative care aims at improving the quality of both life and dying by ameliorating or relieving physical symptoms and psychological, social, and existential suffering for the patient and family within the community context. This comprehensive care is demanding in that it depends on global information. Palliative care professionals also assert that it is important to have some meaningful human interaction during the assessment, yet the practicalities of real-life care depend on efficient collection of concise information. Although these demands also characterize other areas of medicine, palliative care in particular emphasizes the global picture of human meaning in the setting of serious and terminal illness. In addition, palliative care tries to minimize uncomfortable physical examinations and inconvenient, expensive, or invasive tests by avoiding those that are unlikely to change the management plan. Because palliative care also specifies an interdisciplinary approach that can respond to a comprehensive assessment of needs, its assessments should be conducted in such a way that they can link directly to the interdisciplinary team's care plan.

Palliative care has recently engaged in some of the research necessary to bring rigor to this comprehensive assessment of patients with advanced, life-limiting illnesses. This rigor has been made possible in part because palliative care is based on an articulated philosophy and framework of care that identifies domains of need. In what follows, the framework is described, followed by a description of how to approach comprehensive assessment in palliative care. The approach is based on both experience among the discipline's experts and supportive evidence from research of its efficacy.

It may require two or more visits to complete the initial comprehensive assessment for the seriously ill patient because persons in this circumstance may have limited ability to interact, at least until the most consuming sources of suffering are controlled. Once the complete assessment is accomplished, it will need to be revisited on a regular basis with a brief screening question and a review of active concerns so that the whole picture is always retained as the most important guide to the continuously updated and tailored care plan.

Framework

The existence of a clear framework and of identified domains of experience in which suffering can occur has allowed systematic identification of areas that need assessment. The first study of the dying was conducted by William Oser at the turn of the twentieth century.[1] These studies were to be of great interest to Cicely Saunders,[2] who later defined the domains of need for the first decades of the modern hospice and palliative care movement. She defined the field as attending to what could become "total pain," or pain in the physical, mental, social, and spiritual domains of experience. Beginning in the late 1990s, palliative care researchers began again to empirically identify domains of illness-related suffering, and areas within them, that constitute the components of the palliative care framework.

These empirical identifications were grounded in rigorously researched experiences of patients and family caregivers. They therefore differed from the origins of the traditional medical history, which evolved over time, mostly from the insights of physicians about the origin of illness, and in the modern era emphasized the biomedical aspects of the causes of illness. These palliative care studies were conducted on populations with serious and advanced illness, so they tend to apply more appropriately to patients facing the end of life than to those with better prognoses. Although differences existed among findings, they all confirmed that patient and family illness-related experiences were consistent with the whole-person, full-picture approach.[3-6] More recent standards of care and clinical guidelines provide another source for identifying the content areas that should be included in a comprehensive assessment. These also use the whole-person, full-picture approach.[7,8] Most recently, some research has become available on the feasibility, validity, and efficacy of systematic instruments to guide assessment. Those instruments that are validated for specific areas can be used if an overall evaluation so indicates. Some instruments also provide for an initial overall approach to guide more specific evaluations.

The Unfolding Approach: Screening Queries Guide Evaluative Questions

In all general assessments, the key is first to ask sensitive screening questions that will reveal the existence of needs in a general domain. This first step allows the clinician to judge whether an indication of need exists so additional time will not be wasted by asking further questions to which a negative answer is almost ensured. Conversely, if need is indicated, more evaluative questions are posed that become progressively more specific for a set of conditions that are among the possibilities raised by the detected need. Enough screening questions must be asked so, as often as possible, no relevant or important need is left undetected and yet no needless negative inquiry of a specific, evaluative kind is prompted. Decision sciences have underscored the reality that testing for something that is unlikely commonly leads to false-positive results. Poorly applied screening questions divert attention away from the real needs and require the expenditure of time, energy, and resources in populations that have little to spare, all in pursuit of irrelevant matters and possibly producing their own negative side effects.

The first systematic, comprehensive palliative care assessment was provided by Higginson.[9] Originally named for its use as an outcomes scale, it is also offered as an assessment instrument and has shown acceptable reliability and validity as both a clinical assessment tool and an outcomes measure. Known as the Palliative Care Outcomes Scale, or POS, this instrument is a list of survey-type questions.

The next step in systematic, comprehensive assessment approaches involved the creation of a nested guide to the use of sensitive screening items that, when responded to in a way that indicates a need, lead to further, more specific, evaluative items for needs in the screened area. This approach was first reported in the field of geriatrics, another discipline that has promoted the comprehensive assessment, in the form of the nursing home Resident Assessment Instrument (RAI). In a parallel line of thinking in palliative care, the Needs at the End of Life Screening Test (NEST) was developed.[10] A palliative care version of the RAI followed: the Resident Assessment Instrument for Palliative Care (RAI-PC).[11] Other instruments are less comprehensive.[12,13]

Linear survey-type approaches to caregiver comprehensive assessment are available,[14] in addition to numerous caregiver outcomes assessment instruments that evaluate areas such as burden and gratification. An unfolding approach is under development in the form of the Multidimensional Aspects Related to Caregiving Experience (MARCE).[15] MARCE also links to NEST, thus allowing coordinated assessments for the patient and caregiver with purpose-designed, partner instruments.

Because of their brevity, forms such as the POS or the initial screening questions from an unfolding instrument such as NEST or RAI-PC can be used not only for the patient intake comprehensive assessment but also for continuous assessment. A brief assessment for caregivers, such as that developed by Glajchen and associates or the MARCE,[14,15] can be used for intake and update assessment of family caregivers.

Conducting the Comprehensive Assessment for the Patient

In starting a therapeutic relationship, the clinician should greet the patient and caregiver respectfully and should introduce himself or herself and use formal titles for all present. Although more a matter of suitable courtesy, the introduction can also provide something of a rapid screen for norms of communication, whether personal, family, or cultural norms, that should be observed to optimize the therapeutic alliance. The clinician can then ask, "Is there a different way you like to be addressed, or is [Mr/s ___] fine with you?" This inquiry can make future communication about how to discuss subsequent, more specific issues more comfortable.

The palliative care clinician should then learn about the disease, the history, and the clinical management approaches taken to date, including who has provided care and where it was provided. To make the process efficient, this information should be gathered from previous records whenever possible. However, a point should be made of asking the patient and family members what they know about the illness, its significance to them, and what they see as the issues that need attention. This will provide an initial insight into their understanding and how to communicate with them, and it may also indicate their priorities. It also communicates to them that their perceptions are important in guiding care. Overall, the face-time component of this start to comprehensive assessment can be brief, even for longstanding illnesses; the main goal of this phase of an initial palliative care assessment is to begin the relationship on a good footing, orient to the medical background, and ascertain the perceived situation.

NEEDS IN THE SOCIAL DOMAIN

For efficiency, it can be helpful to ask screening questions in all the main areas before going to more specific evaluation questions. Both screening queries and deeper questions can be taken from the NEST or the RAI-PC. The clinician may want to start by memorizing the areas and questions. Eventually the questions will flow smoothly as part of a give-and-take interaction between the patient or family member and the clinician.

Functional and Caregiving Needs

Asking about day-to-day functioning and caregiving needs is a reasonable area in which to start an assessment. It is neither too personal nor too technical, and it affirms the nature of the therapeutic alliance, namely, to help meet their needs.

It is often fairly clear from a first visual impression of a person's condition the level of assistance that will be needed with activities of daily living. A question such as "When you need help, how often can you count on someone for house cleaning, groceries, or a ride?"[16] can screen for instrumental needs. A follow-up question such as "When you need assistance in bathing, eating, dressing, transfer, or toileting, how often can you count on someone being there for you?" can screen for needs with basic activities of daily living. This question may be asked in the past tense ("When you needed help, how often could you count on someone ...?") for patients who are in the hospital and are not expected to leave, because it will provide a gauge of how much stress existed in this area before the hospitalization. For patients who are expected to return home and who are being visited in another setting, asking them to describe their home will give further clues to functional and practical issues.

Isolation

From this point in the assessment, and especially if family members are not present, the atmosphere may be comfortable enough to screen for isolation with a question such as "How much do you have the sense of being acknowledged and appreciated?"[10] or "In the last two weeks, how often would you say someone let you know they care about you?"[17] Much of the ability to accept mortality, to rally despite the burden of illness, and to achieve the quality states of mind that can be attained by the terminally ill and their families probably depends on intergenerational and community visits. Therefore, assessment in this area is important.

Economic and Access Needs

The question "How much of an economic or financial hardship is the cost of your illness and medical care for you or your family?" screens sensitively for financial needs. Asking "How much of a problem have you had getting to see a specialist?" screens reasonably well for difficulty in accessing care. If it feels premature to ask these questions on a first visit, the clinician should follow his or her intuition; it will probably be seen as prying or too personal to the patient or family member as well. The question should be saved for another visit.

NEEDS IN THE EXISTENTIAL DOMAIN

All people have a spiritual dimension in that we all relate in some fashion to the universe beyond us and have a reaction to knowing that we are mortal. Susceptibility to life-threatening illness is obvious to most patients in need of palliative care, and existential issues may have taken on new urgency. Approaches that worked for the patient while he or she was in good health may not be adequate for coping during serious illness. "How much does a spiritual or religious community help in your personal spiritual journey?" is a good screening question, both for unmet needs in that area and for the importance of spirituality to the person. The question "How much does your relationship with God contribute to your sense of well-being?" may seem not obviously relevant for nontheists, but nonetheless a negative answer, on empirical evaluation among patients in the United States near the end of life, appears to correlate with spiritual distress.

In addition, the question "How much have you settled your personal relationships with the people close to you?" screens for a sense of equanimity and a feeling of peace that people value highly near the end of life. The absence of such feelings may indicate need. The counterpart question "Since your illness, how much do you live life with a special sense of purpose?" screens for a sense of having a meaningful role in the current situation. This can be heightened rather than diminished near the end of life. A negative answer may also indicate need.

SYMPTOM MANAGEMENT NEEDS

Physical and Mental Symptoms

A general question such as "How much do you suffer from physical symptoms such as pain, shortness of breath, fatigue, and bowel or urination problems?" can screen for any physical suffering. Asking "How often do you feel confused or anxious or depressed?" can screen for mental suffering. Because some patients tend to not report symptoms unless asked about the specific symptom, it is wise also to screen for the most common symptoms directly, at least until such point as a routine expectation allows the clinician to be confident that the patient will identify symptoms with a general prompt.

For a patient who is unlikely to be symptom free, it makes sense to skip directly to symptom-specific questions. The Edmonton Symptom Assessment Scale (ESAS) provides quick and sensitive screening questions for the 10 most common physical and mental symptoms among palliative care patients. This scale, designed for patients to fill out themselves, can be a time-saving approach if the patient is given the form ahead of time. If incorporating the ESAS into the verbal interview, the clinician should ask the patient to rate how he or she feels about each symptom on a scale of 0 to 10 (with 10 being the worst possible) and list the symptoms: painful, tired, nauseated, depressed, anxious, drowsy, (lost) appetite, (lost) feeling of well-being, and shortness of breath. At the end of the interview, the patient should be asked if there are any other physical symptoms.

THE THERAPEUTIC ALLIANCE

Goals of Care

No amount of understanding of a person's needs will result in an optimal care plan if that person's goals for care are not understood. The clinician should screen right away, and then on a continuous basis, for any mismatch between goals and actual care, so the care can be progressively adjusted to meet the patient's goals as much as possible. The clinician should ask a question such as "How much do you feel that the medical care you are getting fits with your goals?" If the answer is not the equivalent of "Completely," then he or she should probe for and settle on realistic goals that are compatible with medical care so the team can consider how to adjust the care to meet the patient's goals (see Chapter 4, Negotiating Goals of Care). Goals change over time, depending on the physical realities and the mental, spiritual, and social circumstances of the patient.

Because goals do change and patients near the end of life can readily become too sick to communicate, inquiry about advance care planning is also necessary. As part of comprehensive assessment, it is sufficient to know if advance planning discussions or documents have been completed and, if so, whether changes have occurred since then (see Chapter 20 on Advance Care Planning).

Therapeutic Relationships

As patients and caregivers become more dependent on medical care, the professional team becomes more and more a part of their day-to-day life. These relationships can have a profound impact on quality of life. Needs in this area should be screened for with questions that ask about the relationship, such as "How much do you feel your doctors and nurses respect you as an individual?" and about their information needs by using a question such as "How clear is the information from the medical team about what to expect regarding your illness?"

PROBING ISSUES RAISED ON SCREENING

A focused inquiry begins once issues have been identified on screening. Selection of questions that have steadily increasing specificity while retaining as much sensitivity as possible will allow the clinician to zero in on the evaluation without missing related issues along the way. For instance, if a patient with abdominal pain is presented with questions related to cholecystitis but not questions related to adherence to the bowel regimen prescribed to go along with opioid use for bone pain, the clinician may miss the possibility of constipation. Similarly, consider a patient who responds to the screening question that his or her relationship with God does not contribute to his or her sense of well-being. If the clinician immediately infers that the patient needs a visit from the hospital chaplain, the clinician may miss something important, merely for lack of a suitable follow-up question. For example, a question about what does help may reveal that members of a local religious community can be of much greater help in identifying and fostering a resolution to, say, a ruptured family relationship that has been blocking spiritual peace. Similarly, for mental health symptoms and social needs, such poorly chosen questions can lead to wasted time and effort and possibly to negative impact from the ill-fitting diagnoses and interventions.

The unfolding screening-evaluation approach can be illustrated for any area, but it is described here in the area of symptom management. The general approach is as follows: Starting with the first layer of screening questions from an instrument such as NEST or RAI-PC, suppose that the clinician identifies symptoms that need further evaluation. The clinician therefore follows with questions taken from ESAS. Once a symptom has been clearly identified, the clinician can follow the recommendations for symptom evaluation outlined in specific chapters of this textbook and other palliative care resources. The Memorial Symptom Assessment Scale Short Form (MSAS-SF) covers 32 symptoms.[18] After evaluation is complete and management is under way, the palliative care clinician can use the relevant MSAS questions for monitoring progress in symptom management over time.

To illustrate this point with specific questions, consider a patient who responds to the initial screening question for mental symptoms, "How often do you feel confused or anxious or depressed?" with "Most of the time." The clinician can go on to ask each mental symptom question in the ESAS. If the patient's responses indicate no problem except in relation to the question "How would you describe your feelings of depression during the last 3 days?" to which he or she answers "Very depressed," then the clinician will continue to probe the history and possible sources of depression. In this situation, the clinician will also gather baseline answers to the questions in the MSAS-SF, by asking, for instance, "In the last week, how often have you felt sad? Rarely, occasionally, frequently, or almost constantly?" and then "How severe was it usually? Slight, moderate, severe, or very severe?" and finally, "How much did it distress or bother you? Not at all, a little bit, somewhat, quite a bit, or very much?" After treatment has begun, the clinician may repeat the last set of the MSAS-SF questions periodically to monitor the symptom and the efficacy of treatment. Analogous progression can be used for any physical or mental symptom. In sum, by using this approach the clinician will have efficiently moved from (a) the shortest available screening question set (e.g., from the NEST or the RAI-PC); to (b) intermediate questions (e.g., from the ESAS); then (c) in-depth evaluation questions and tests as needed; and finally to (d) a specific validated scale (e.g., the MSAS) for monitoring the progression of the symptom and its management.

Content Areas for Family Caregiver Comprehensive Assessment

PROXY PERSPECTIVES ABOUT THE PATIENT

An interview with the family caregiver can provide a second perspective on the needs of the patient. This interview can be the sole source of information other than the medical record for patients who are unable to respond to questions. Questions posed to the caregiver are largely the same as those posed to the patient, except all are framed in the third person, to ask the caregiver's perception of the patient's circumstance and experience.

Family caregiver perspectives tend to differ from those of the patient. Some differences are relatively predictable. For instance, caregivers tend to underemphasize the burden to themselves relative to the patient's report and to overemphasize patient pain relative to the patient's report.[19] Other differences are less predictable, and all individual patient–family caregiver dyads differ, so clinicians need to take proxy perspective as relevant but less certain to represent the patient's perspective than patient-provided information.

FAMILY CAREGIVER ASSESSMENT

A second, equally important function of the family caregiver interview is to find out how the caregiver himself or herself is doing. Because caregiver well-being appears to correlate strongly with patient well-being[20] and with the future health of the caregiver, because the caregiver is an essential member of the whole care team, and because intolerable caregiving burdens tend to have an adverse impact on other members of the family and even on the community,[21] it is also crucial to interview the family caregiver about himself or herself.

Some areas of need in the patient interview should lead the clinician to probe more deeply in the family caregiver interview. For instance, needs in the social domain of the patient interview are especially likely to indicate needs for the family caregiver. In addition, the caregiver often starts out with a brave face, in keeping with the role of providing for needs rather than seeking help. The caregiver may not admit to needs unless he or she is reassured that it is important to take care of his or her needs as well as those of the patient.

The areas of evaluation that go into a caregiver assessment are not as well established as those that comprise the patient assessment. One researcher recommended seven possible areas to evaluate:

1. Preparedness for the tasks of the role
2. Competence or performance quality in the role
3. Rewards of the role
4. Social support
5. Self-efficacy or belief that he or she can manage the situation
6. Reactions to caregiving, whether by sense of burden or gratification
7. Optimism

The MARCE suggests use of slightly different areas, which are roughly followed here.

Burden/Gratification of the Caregiving Role

An early sense of how the family caregiver is doing in the role can be ascertained by asking whether the patient needs more help with nursing care than the caregiver can provide. The family caregiver's comfort level with the role seems to be fairly well indicated by being able to talk with the patient about how to handle the patient's physical care needs.

Care Skills and Understanding Illness Information

Caregiving by family members requires some special skills and an understanding of the illness. Research indicates that patients are often bewildered by the medical system and do not know how to access the information or resources they need. The health care provider should ask questions such as "Do you get help from us in knowing what [patient name] needs?" or "Do you get enough clear information from us about what to expect regarding [patient name's] illness and outcome?" or "… about the risks and side effects of [patient name's] treatment?" Responses to these questions allow the clinician to determine whether the caregiver is receiving enough comprehensible information and assistance from the clinical team to perform the role and can guide the clinician to fill any gaps in needed understanding or skill.

Psychological Issues, Including Adaptation to Losses

Family caregivers face many losses, including perhaps loss of their hopes for the future, loss of their own activities in favor of caregiving tasks, loss of aspects of the patient who may well have been different before the illness, and eventually loss of the patient to death. Family caregivers need to employ many skills of adaptation and creative reintegration to maintain a quality of life, and these challenges often overwhelm their personal resources and result in depression. The clinician can ask how well caregivers are adapting and can screen for anxiety and depression with questions such as "How often have you felt downhearted and blue in the last weeks?"

Social Issues

Family caregivers are at risk for isolation. The clinician should ask whether "other family members provide help with caring for [patient's name]" and whether he or she sometimes feels "alone or abandoned." If it has not been covered earlier in the interview as described previously, then as soon as feels reasonable, it is important to ask about economic stresses and difficulties in accessing medical services, especially if the family caregiver has had to cut back on work or stop working to care for the patient.

PROBING ISSUES RAISED ON SCREENING

A progressive approach to probing issues can be used for caregivers and patients alike. However, the clinician's obligation to diagnose and therapeutically intervene for the caregiver is more limited because no patient–clinician fiduciary therapeutic relationship is in place; the caregiver has not sought medical care. Nonetheless, some probing is reasonable and necessary to allow the care team to provide suitable information and skills to the caregiver, as well as recommendations for care. Therefore, it is reasonable that the clinician follow the progression over time once the early screening and deeper evaluation questions have identified an issue. The clinician can do this by using items from validated scales to assess an area more quantitatively. Numerous instruments for caregiver assessment have been studied and have achieved standards for validity.[22]

Connecting the Assessment to an Interdisciplinary Team's Care Plan

A comprehensive assessment is of some independent worth if the patient and family caregiver receive therapeutic effect from being heard and from the empathic exchange of the interaction. However, most of the potential impact depends on effective translation of detected needs into a care plan for those needs. Several issues are important in making this an effective translation.

PATIENT AND FAMILY AS PART OF THE TEAM

Confidentiality Issues

Palliative care seeks to include the family. At the same time, the patient is the key figure in the situation, and his or her confidentiality needs to be honored to the greatest extent possible. The patient should be asked at the outset how he or she likes to have information shared with family members.

Ensuring Accessibility for the Patient and Family

Even taking into account the variations among people, patients and families tend to do well if they feel a sense of choice and control over their care options. Drawing them into the comprehensive assessment and its connection to the care team's deliberated plan of care, to whatever level is suitable for the particular patient and family, is one mechanism that can help to provide the best balance for them.

DIFFERENT SOURCES AND HOW INFORMATION IS GATHERED AND RECORDED

The approach to comprehensive assessment that relies on the interdisciplinary team and on the inclusion of the patient and family in the total care team has both strengths and hazards. In many systems of care, multiple professionals take their own version of the comprehensive assessment. The strength of this method of care delivery is derived from the full picture that multiple sources of information provide. However, the burden involved in information gathering and the potential to lose track of much of that information or to favor one source over another when the findings are disparate also need to be considered. Approaches such as that used by the NEST instrument, which is designed for use by anyone, provide a mechanism by which all members of the interdisciplinary team and the family caregiver can derive the same full picture of the patient's needs. In some service delivery situations, this may provide improved coordination and quality of care.

TEAM MEETINGS

The interdisciplinary team is distinct from the multidisciplinary team, in which interactions among the perspectives of each are less clearly emphasized. Palliative care has strongly emphasized the interdisciplinary team, and most palliative care services honor this by holding regular interdisciplinary team meetings. A chance to share perspectives is essential in translating the comprehensive assessment into high-quality care. The family meeting may also be a setting in which valuable perspectives and exchanges can occur so that the assessment is both comprehensive and, to whatever level is appropriate, shared by all relevant parties.

CONTINUOUSLY ADJUSTED PLANS OF CARE

As noted earlier, the situation of seriously ill patients tends to change rapidly. The comprehensive assessment therefore needs to be periodically administered and reviewed by the team for an adjusted care plan.

Special Issues

DIFFICULT FAMILIES, DIFFICULT PATIENTS

Some families and some patients seem intent on avoiding the difficult realities of serious illness. Others have emotional reactions that can be hard for clinicians, patients, and families. Simple, genuine acknowledgment of the difficult nature of the situation and the feelings it causes can help the clinician to form a productive relationship with the patient and family. If this fails, it can be difficult to collect the needed information and to translate it into an effective care plan; seek help from colleagues.

PATIENTS WITH COGNITIVE IMPAIRMENT

Cognitive impairment need not preempt all aspects of a comprehensive assessment. Direct inquiry of the patient with as many of the screening and specific evaluation questions as possible should be attempted. Cognitive impairments may be quite variable, and some ability to give useful information can be retained even when other aspects of cognitive function are lost. Family caregivers can provide proxy information, although, as discussed earlier, the clinician must take into account that proxy information tends to be inaccurately correlated with patients' reports.

LANGUAGE AND CULTURAL BARRIERS

When language is a barrier, the services of a medical translator should be employed. The clinician should pay attention to the physical location of the translator, who should be seated to the side of the clinician and patient so the clinician and patient can make eye contact and the translator does not "get in between." If the translator starts to add supplemental explanations or to ask questions him or herself, the clinician should ask for a full translation, so nothing is assumed and inaccurate extrapolations or inferences are prevented.

Open acknowledgment of cultural differences can help the clinician to ask the patient or family caregiver about his or her expectations for health care and communication and about those expectations that may have already had a poor (or good) outcome. The clinician should assure the patient and the caregiver that the goal is to meet all possible expectations and to try to close the gap if some expectations have not been met. Because only the patient and family know their unique culture, they should be asked to help the care team honor it by sharing information about it.

Outcome Measures in Palliative Care

Many of the assessment questions used for screening and evaluation are in a format that elicits a scaled response and are also valid for use as outcomes measures. These questions are often sufficient for the practicing clinician. Individual assessment questions that can double as outcomes measures are useful not only in chronicling the progress of individual patients but also for research and continuous quality improvement activities.

In addition, for researchers, specific areas may have not only validated outcome measures but also large databases that contain data from those instruments. A compendium of approximately 160 assessment and outcomes instruments is found in the End-of-Life Care Toolkit, and a recent compilation of areas of relevant information in palliative care and database sources for that information has been provided by the Institute of Medicine.[23,24]

Information Technology in Comprehensive Assessment

The comprehensive assessment is well suited to a form of computer-assisted technology that has been developed in the field of educational assessment. Computer-assisted testing (CAT) in education examinations uses item response theory to select test items that progressively assess the respondent's knowledge or capacity. If the respondent evidences superior knowledge in response to a difficult item, the easier items are skipped, and more difficult items are given. Conversely, if the respondent fails to answer an item correctly, the computer selects easier items to determine what the respondent does know. A similar approach to sensitive screening items followed by specific, deeper evaluation items as described in the unfolding approach in this chapter can be programmed into a CAT system. Such a system could allow for completion of assessments by a range of clinicians and by patients and caregivers. Tablet-based self-response assessments have proven effective in some settings.[25] Comprehensive information management systems that connect patients and caregivers with clinical teams across distances could be set up using such CAT-based assessments,[26] and clinicians should expect that such progress may occur rapidly.

PEARLS

- A good comprehensive assessment is the foundation of high-quality palliative care. Devote effort to developing and honing the needed skills.
- To make comprehensive assessment efficient, start by asking screening questions for the major areas of illness-related suffering: physical, mental, social, and spiritual.
- If need be, take more than one session to complete a comprehensive assessment.
- After the initial comprehensive assessment, periodic reassessment is essential because things change rapidly with seriously ill patients. Make a point of asking screening questions on a regular basis.
- Use validated questions for screening whenever possible.

PITFALLS

• Omitting any major area of a comprehensive assessment is a mistake. Diagnoses may be misguided as a result.

• Do not try to cover everything in detail at one session. The patient may lose stamina, and eventually so will you.

• Do not avoid areas of inquiry that you find difficult. Ask yourself why it is difficult for you; talk about it with a friend, a colleague, or a counselor.

• When taking a patient transfer from a colleague, do not accept assessments that are not comprehensive. Ask questions about what he or she should have investigated.

Summary

Comprehensive assessments in palliative care are the cornerstone of high-quality care. However, they are demanding by their nature, requiring as they do rapid but accurate assessment of a very broad range of sensitive issues that vary widely among people. Nonetheless, use of a systematic method that covers established domains with questions that have been selected for the ability to screen sensitively for problems, followed by more specific items to identify and evaluate the issues, provides for an efficient and reliable approach. Information technology may soon allow for computer-assisted approaches that will make comprehensive assessments even more efficient.

References

1. Mueller PS: William Osler's "Study of the Act of Dying": an analysis of the original data, *J Med Biogr* 2007 (in press).
2. Personal communication from Paul Mueller, December 2006.
3. Lynn J: Measuring quality of care at the end of life: a statement of principles, *J Am Geriatr Soc* 45:526–527, 1997.
4. Committee on Care at the End of Life, Division of Health Services, Institute of Medicine, Cassel CK, Field MJ, editors: *Approaching death: improving care at the end of life*, Washington, DC, 1997, National Academy Press.
5. Emanuel EJ, Emanuel LL: The promise of a good death, *Lancet* 351(Suppl 2):21–29, 1998.
6. Singer PA, Martin DK, Kelner M: Quality end-of-life care: patients' perspectives, *JAMA* 281:163–168, 1999.
7. A model to guide hospice palliative care: Based on national principles and norms of practice. Ottawa, Canada, 2002, Canadian Hospice Palliative Care Association.
8. National Consensus Project: Clinical Practice Guidelines for Quality Palliative Care. Pittsburgh, National Consensus Project, 2004–2006. Available at http://www.nationalconsensusproject.org/Guidelines_Download.asp.
9. Higginson I: Palliative Care Outcomes Scale (P.O.S.). London, Department of Palliative Care, Policy and Rehabilitation, King's College, University of London: Available at https://www.kcl.ac.uk/schools/medicine/depts/palliative/qat/pos-form.html.
10. Emanuel LL, Alpert H, Emanuel EJ: Concise screening questions for clinical assessments of terminal care: the needs near the end of life care screening tool (NEST), *J Palliat Med* 4:465–474, 2001.
11. Steel K, Ljunggren G, Topinkova E, et al: The RAI-PC: an assessment instrument for palliative care in all settings, *Am J Hosp Palliat Care* 20:211–219, 2003.
12. Okon TR, Evans JM, Gomez CF, Blackhall LJ: Palliative educational outcome with implementation of PEACE tool integrated clinical pathway, *J Palliat Med* 7:279–295, 2004.

13. Lo B, Quill T, Tulsky J: Discussing palliative care with patients: ACP-ASIM End-of-Life Care Consensus Panel, American College of Physicians–American Society of Internal Medicine, *Ann Intern Med* 130:744–749, 1999.

14. Glajchen M, Kornblith A, Komel P, et al: Development of a brief assessment scale for caregivers of the medically ill, *J Pain Symptom Manage* 29:245–254, 2005.

15. Chang C-H, Emanuel LL: Multidimensional aspects related to caregiving experience (MARCE). Invited paper presented at the 2005 Joint Statistical Meetings, Minneapolis.

16. Seeman TE, Berkman LF: Structural characteristics of social networks and their relationship with social support in the elderly: who provides support, *Soc Sci Med* 26:737–749, 1988.

17. Turner RJ, Marino F: Social support and social structure: a descriptive epidemiology, *J Health Soc Behav* 35:193–212, 1994.

18. Chang VT, Hwang SS, Feuerman M, et al: The Memorial Symptom Assessment Scale Short Form (MSAS-SF), *Cancer* 89:1162–1171, 2000.

19. Hauser J, Baldwin D, Alpert H, et al: Who's caring for whom? Differing perspectives between seriously ill patients and their family caregivers, *J Hosp Palliat Med* 23:105–112, 2006.

20. Christakis NA, Allison PD: Mortality after the hospitalization of a spouse, *N Engl J Med* 354:719–730, 2006.

21. Boni-Saenz A, LoSasso A, Emanuel LL, Dranove D: Measuring the economics of palliative care, *Clin Geriatr Med* 21:147–163, 2005.

22. Hudson PL, Hayman-White K: Measuring the psychosocial characteristics of family caregivers of palliative care patients: psychometric properties of nine self-report instruments, *J Pain Symptom Manage* 31:215–228, 2006.

23. TIME: A Toolkit of Instruments to Measure End-of-life Care. Available at http://www.chcr.brown.edu/pcoc/choosing.htm.

24. Institute of Medicine Executive Summary: *Describing death in America: what we need to know*, Washington, DC, 2003, National Academy of Sciences, pp 1–15. Available at http://www.nap.edu/books/0309087252/html.

25. Fortner B, Baldwin S, Schwartzberg L, Houts AC: Validation of the cancer care monitor items for physical symptoms and treatment side effects using expert oncology nurse evaluation, *J Pain Symptom Manage* 31:207–214, 2006.

26. Chang C-H, Boni-Saenz AA, Durazo-Arvizu RA, et al: A System for Interactive Assessment and Management in Palliative Care (SIAM-PC), *J Pain Symptom Manage* Mar 13, 2007. (online publication ahead of print; PMID:17360148).

CHAPTER 3

Communication Skills

ROBERT BUCKMAN

Introduction: The Role of Communication in Palliative Care

Palliative care is all about the relief of suffering; most tangibly, palliative care aims to relieve the symptoms associated with terminal illness. Symptoms are complex entities that the patient experiences. In other words, symptoms, like all experiences, unpleasant or pleasant, require processing by the brain (or, more precisely, by its main function, the mind). Assessing symptoms is therefore crucially different from assessing an objectifiable disease process. Whereas a disease process such as a bone metastasis can be visualized objectively and measured on a radiograph or in a computed tomography scan, the pain provoked by that metastasis can be assessed only by talking to the patient and finding out how much it hurts. As has often been said, there is no blood test that measures pain. Hence, to assess the patient's symptoms (and subsequently the effect of treatment on those symptoms), the health care professional must have good communication skills. It is through communication that

30

we assess how the patient is feeling and whether our interventions for symptom control are effective. However, in addition to assessing the patient's symptoms and the effects of therapy, communication also has a therapeutic benefit of its own. Almost invariably, the act of communication is an important part of therapy in its widest sense: Occasionally, it is the only constituent. Communication usually requires greater thought and planning than a drug prescription and is unfortunately commonly administered in subtherapeutic doses.

The problem is that very little published material gives busy clinicians simple, practical guidelines. There is no lack of published literature concerning the emotional and psychosocial needs of the dying patient and the important role that communication plays in the delivery of all medical care, particularly palliative care. Some published work is also available on the obstacles to, and the deficiencies in, communication between the dying patient and the health care professional. However, the general medical literature does not provide much detailed practical advice to help improve the communication skills of palliative care practitioners. The major objective of this chapter is to remedy that omission by providing an intelligible and coherent approach to communication between professionals and patients in the palliative care setting. Experienced health care professionals may be familiar with much of this material, but very little of it has been previously published or documented. The objectives of this chapter are therefore practical and pragmatic, and its somewhat unusual structure and style reflect that emphasis.

This chapter has five parts:

1. A brief discussion of the main obstacles to talking about dying, including the factors that make dying a near-taboo subject and an exploration of the origins of those factors (in society, in the patient, and in ourselves)
2. Basic communication skills (the CLASS strategy)
3. A six-point strategy, the SPIKES protocol, for the specific task of breaking bad news
4. A summary of the important elements in therapeutic or supportive dialogue
5. Guidelines for communicating with other people, such as family, physicians, and other professionals

Sources of Difficulty in Communication with Dying Patients

In our society, discussing death and dying can be awkward, perhaps even more so when the discussion takes place between a doctor and a patient. Some of that awkwardness is social and stems from the way in which society currently views death. Some awkwardness originates from the individual patient, but some also originates from the professional. This is because our professional training prepares us to treat sick people but, paradoxically, also leads us to lose touch with our own human skills when the curative treatment of the disease process fails. A conversation with a dying patient also causes some degree of discomfort or awkwardness, even for the most experienced health care provider. It is important to recognize that this discomfort is universal and is not the product of any personal fault or deficiency of the health care professional. The major causes of this sense of unease originate long before the individual patient and the individual doctor begin the conversation. What follows is a broad overview of these issues.

The sources of difficulty can be divided into three groups: first, those related to society (the social causes); second, those related to the individual patients; and third, those related to the health care professional that arise from our own social background and also from our training (e.g., in medical school or nursing college).

THE SOCIAL DENIAL OF DEATH

Contemporary society is going through (and just beginning to emerge from) a phase of virtual denial of death.[1] Such attitudes are probably cyclical, and we may now be seeing this denial phase beginning to fade. However, the current attitude of denial or avoidance carries a price, a price paid by the person whose life is threatened and who faces death, as well as by those who look after and support that person—the family and the professionals. The major social roots of the contemporary fear of dying are discussed in the following subsections.

Lack of Experience of Death in the Family

Most adults today have not witnessed the death of a family member in the home at a time when they themselves were young and still forming their overall view of life. Although the number varies with regional demographics, for the last few decades more than 65% of deaths have occurred in hospitals or institutions. By contrast, a century ago approximately 90% of deaths occurred in the home. This shift is associated with a change in family structure as the norm evolved from that of the extended family to that of the nuclear family. Thus, elderly people are less likely to be living with their grandchildren and usually do not have young, fit relatives available to support them at the time of their last illness. By the same token, in contemporary society, a normal childhood and adolescence do not include the personal experience of a family death that occurs in the home.

Other factors that determine the place of most deaths are the growth and range of modern health services and the increased facilities and treatments they offer. Although these services undoubtedly offer medical and nursing care advantages for the person who is dying in an institution, family support for the patient is disrupted, and surviving relatives are deprived of the experience and understanding of the dying process.

This is not to imply that witnessing a death at home in the past was always a serene or tranquil experience. Although a death at home may not have been a pleasant event, a child who grew up in such a home would be imprinted with a sense of the continuity of life, the process of aging, and the natural inevitability of death ("when you are older you look like dad, when you are much older you look like granddad, when you are very, very old you die"). As the extended family has disappeared, dying has become the province of the health care professional or institution; most people have lost that sense of continuity and now regard the process of dying as intrinsically alien and divorced from the business of living.

High Expectations of Health and Life

Advances in medical sciences are often overreported in the media and hailed as major breakthroughs. The constant bombardment of the public with news of apparently miraculous advances in the fight against disease not only subconsciously raises expectations of health, it also appears to offer tantalizing hopes of immortality. Thus, it becomes even harder for an individual to face the fact that he or she will not be cured despite the many miracles seen on television or in the newspapers.

Materialism

It is beyond the scope of a textbook to assess the materialist values of the modern world, except to point out that our society routinely evaluates a person's worth in terms of material and tangible values. This is our current social system of values, and it is neither good nor bad. However, it is universally accepted in our society that dying means being parted from material possessions. Hence a society that places a high and almost exclusive value on the material possessions of its members implicitly increases the penalty of dying.

The Changing Role of Religion

The role of religion changed in the twentieth century. In North America and in much of Europe the previously near-universal view of a single, exterior God became fragmented and individualized. More individual philosophical stances became possible than in earlier centuries, and it is no longer possible to assume that everyone shares the same idea of a God or of an afterlife. Whereas a Victorian physician in England could have said to a patient, "Your soul will be with its Maker by the ebb-tide" and may have genuinely meant it as a statement of fact and consolation, nowadays we cannot assume that such a statement will bring relief to all, or even most, patients.

For all these reasons, then, our society is passing through a phase of development in which the process of dying is often perceived as alien and fearsome and the dying person is separated and divided from the living. This situation increases the uncertainty that surrounds any conversation about dying.

PATIENTS' FEARS OF DYING

The fear of dying is not a single emotion. It can be composed of any or all of many individual fears, and every human when faced with the prospect of dying probably has a different and unique combination of fears and concerns. Some of these fears are illustrated in Box 3-1. This concept of the patient's fear of dying has important implications for communication in palliative care. First, recognizing that fear of dying is not a single monolithic emotion should prompt the professional to elicit from the patient those particular aspects of terminal illness that are uppermost in his or her mind. Thus, a patient's statement that he or she is afraid of dying should begin dialogue, not end it. Second, an awareness of the many different aspects of dying that cause fear should prompt the professional to initiate a discussion of what triggers the patient's feelings. It is the recognition of and ensuing familiarity with the causes of fear that often enhance the professional's ability to empathize with the patient, thus increasing the value of the professional's support.

FACTORS THAT ORIGINATE IN THE HEALTH CARE PROFESSIONAL

Professionals in any health care discipline are subject to several sources of pressure that add to the discomfort of talking about dying. Some of these factors arise simply because, although we are professionals whose behavior has been ostensibly modified by training, we are human beings in the presence of another person, the patient, who is in distress. Others factors may be the product of our training or experience. The major constituents are noted in the following subsections; fuller discussions are published elsewhere.[2]

> ## Box 3-1. *Common Fears about Dying*
>
> ### FEARS ABOUT PHYSICAL ILLNESS
> Physical symptoms (e.g., pain, nausea)
> Disability (e.g., paralysis or loss of mobility)
>
> ### FEARS ABOUT MENTAL EFFECTS
> Not being able to cope
> "Breakdown" or "losing one's mind"
> Dementia
>
> ### FEARS ABOUT DYING
> Existential issues
> Religious concerns
>
> ### FEARS ABOUT TREATMENT
> Side effects (e.g., baldness, pain)
> Surgery (e.g., pain, mutilation)
> Altered body image (e.g., surgery, colostomy, mastectomy)
>
> ### FEARS ABOUT FAMILY AND FRIENDS
> Loss of sexual relations
> Being a burden
> Loss of family role
>
> ### FEARS ABOUT FINANCES, SOCIAL STATUS, AND JOB
> Loss of job (breadwinner)
> Possible loss of medical insurance
> Expenses of treatment
> Being out of the mainstream

Sympathetic Pain

We are likely to experience considerable discomfort simply by being in the same room as a person who is going through the distress of facing death. This sympathetic pain may seem so patently obvious that it does not need to be stated, but it is often the case that professionals feel distressed by a painful interview and markedly underestimate the intensity of feeling that has originated from the patient. Particularly with trainees and junior staff, the degree of stress experienced by a health care professional is proportional to the intensity of the patient's distress. Until this is openly acknowledged, the professional may not seek the support that he or she needs and may continue to experience feelings of personal inadequacy and guilt, thus creating another set of factors that block good communication.

Fear of Being Blamed

As professionals, our fear of being blamed is partly justified. This fear has two main components. First, as the bearer of bad news, we are likely to be blamed for that news (blaming the messenger for the message). This is probably a basic human reaction to bad news and one with which we are all familiar in daily life (e.g., blaming a traffic warden for writing out a parking ticket), so we are somewhat justified in expecting it when it is our role to bring bad news. Furthermore, many of the trappings of our profession (e.g., uniforms, jargon, ward rounds) help to support the concept that we are in control of the situation. This concept may be valuable when the patient's condition is improving, but the same trappings increase the likelihood that we will become targets of blame when the patient's clinical condition begins to deteriorate.

Second, the notion that someone must be at fault when a patient deteriorates or dies is a concept imbued in us during our training. This attitude is strongly reinforced by medicolegal practice in which monetary sums are attached to a deterioration in health. Medical school training inadvertently reinforces this feeling in physicians. Medical school education prepares doctors (appropriately) to deal with the myriad reversible or treatable conditions, whether common or rare. Until recently, however, there has been little or no teaching on the subject of what to do when the disease cannot be reversed (hence the need for this textbook). Palliative medicine has not previously been included in the undergraduate curriculum of medical school, and, as a result, most medical students evolve into physicians who are keen to treat the curable conditions but who have little training in how to deal with chronic, irreversible diseases. This omission makes it even more difficult for the physician to deal with his or her own sense of therapeutic failure when communicating with a dying patient.[3]

Fear of the Untaught

We also fear talking to a dying patient if we do not know how to do it properly. In all professional training, trainees are rewarded for doing a particular task "properly." In essence, this means following conventional procedures and avoiding deviations from standard practice. Although this is the accepted and justifiable norm for any procedure for which guidelines have been established, if no guidelines exist (as is the case in communicating with the dying), the professional will naturally feel ill at ease and will tend to avoid the area entirely.

Fear of Eliciting a Reaction

In the same way that professionals dislike doing tasks for which they have not been trained, they also avoid the side effects or reactions caused by any intervention unless they have been taught how to cope with them.[4] It is an axiom of medical practice that you "don't do anything unless you know what to do if it goes wrong." If there has been no effective training in talking to patients about dying and death, there will also have been no training in how to deal with complications or side effects of such conversations (e.g., the patient's becoming angry or bursting into tears). Not knowing how to cope with these reactions further increases the aversion an untrained person feels when communicating with a dying patient.

Furthermore, interviews in which patients show emotional reactions may earn discouraging responses from other professionals. Although it is now less common than a few years ago, some senior physicians and senior nurses still think that it is a bad thing to "get the patient all upset." It should be obvious (but it is often ignored) that if a patient bursts into tears during a discussion about the gravity of his or her illness, it is the medical situation, not the discussion, that has caused the tears.

Fear of Saying "I Don't Know"

No matter the training or discipline, health care professionals are never rewarded for saying "I don't know." In all training, and particularly when being tested, we expect that our standing will be diminished if we confess that we do not know all the answers. In everyday clinical practice, by contrast, honesty shown by the professional strengthens the relationship, increases trust, and, in return, encourages honesty from the patient. Conversely, attempts to "flannel" or "snow" the patient, to disguise ignorance, or to pretend greater knowledge or experience weaken the bond between the patient and the doctor or nurse and discourage honest dialogue. Thus, our fears of displaying our ignorance—normal in tests but not appropriate in clinical practice—make communication increasingly difficult when the answers are unknown and, often, unknowable.

Fear of Expressing Emotions

We are also encouraged and trained to hide and suppress our own emotions (this may be truer of medical students than of nursing students or trainees in other disciplines). It is, of course, essential for truly professional behavior that we modulate emotions such as irritation or panic. However, this training inadvertently encourages us to envisage the ideal doctor as one who never shows any emotions and is consistently calm and brave. Although that is not necessarily a bad paradigm for a doctor who is dealing with emergencies or reversible crises, it is unhelpful in the palliative care setting. When a patient is facing death, a professional who expresses no emotions is likely to be perceived as cold or insensitive.

Ambiguity of the Phrase "I'm Sorry"

Even when we want to show human sympathy, the moment we begin do to so, linguistic problems threaten to create further difficulties. Most of us do not realize that the word *sorry* has two quite distinct meanings. It can be a form of sympathy ("I am sorry for you"), and it can also be a form of apology when accepting responsibility for an action ("I am sorry that I did this"). Unfortunately, both meanings are customarily abbreviated to "I am sorry." This reflex abbreviation can commonly lead to misunderstanding. For example:

A. "… and then my mother was brought into hospital as an emergency."
B. "Oh, I am sorry."
A. "You've got nothing to be sorry for."

The first speaker is so used to hearing the word *sorry* as an apology that she or he responds with a reflex reply to an apology before realizing that it was not an apology that was offered but an expression of sympathy. This has relevance to all of us as professionals. Not only is it difficult for us to overcome some of our trained responses to express our own emotions of sympathy and empathy, the moment we try to do so we fall into a linguistic slip and appear to be accepting responsibility (with the associated medicolegal implications) instead of offering support. The solution to this ambiguity lies in paying careful attention to your own speech patterns: Rather than saying "I am sorry," you can use the specific words "I am sorry that happened to you."

Our Own Fears of Illness and Death

As professionals, most of us have some degree of fear about our own deaths, perhaps even more so than the general population. In fact, some psychologists would suggest that the desire to deny one's own mortality and vulnerability to illness is a component of the desire to be a doctor, nurse, or other health care professional. This is sometimes called *counterphobic behavior* and, in real terms, means that each time we have an encounter with a sick person and emerge from the encounter unharmed, we are reinforcing our own illusions of immortality and invulnerability. If this is indeed a major constituent of the desire to be a health care professional, then it may lead to avoidance of those situations in which these illusions are challenged.[5] Hence the professional's own fear of dying can lead to avoidance or blocking of any communication with the dying patient.

Fear of the Medical Hierarchy

Finally, there is the discomforting fact that not all professionals think of these issues as important, perhaps because of their own fears of illness and death, fears of the untaught, and so on. Thus, when trying to have a conversation with a patient about dying, a junior member of a medical team may be under pressure from a senior staff member. In more old-fashioned hierarchical systems (e.g., in the United Kingdom in the 1960s), it was quite possible for a senior physician to state: "No patient of mine is ever to be told that he or she has cancer." Nowadays, for ethical and legal reasons, that stance is less tenable, but occasional instances of this attitude can still make it difficult to respond to the patient's desire for information and support. This problem sometimes has a solution when a hierarchy of care exists in which the patient's questions, reactions, knowledge, or suspicions can be transmitted upward to the senior person concerned.

Basic Communication Skills: The CLASS Protocol

As stated earlier, communication in palliative care is important from the moment that the patient first meets a palliative care professional until the last moment of life. Most significant conversations in palliative care comprise two major elements: one in which medical information is transmitted to the patient (*bearing the news*), and the other in which the dialogue centers on the patient's feelings and emotions and in which the dialogue itself is a therapeutic action (*therapeutic or supportive dialogue*). In practice, most conversations are a mixture of the two, although commonly there is more medical information transmitted in the earlier conversations shortly after starting palliative care, and there is usually a greater need for therapeutic dialogue in the later stages.

Let us start by discussing the basic and central elements of effective communication, particularly as they are important in therapeutic dialogue. Although there are many ways to summarize and simplify medical interviews, few are practical and easy to remember. The five-step basic protocol for medical communication set out here and bearing the acronym CLASS has the virtue of being easy to remember and easy to use. Furthermore, it offers a straightforward technique-directed method for dealing with emotions. This is of crucial importance because a recent study showed that most oncologists (>85%) feel that dealing with emotions is the most difficult part of any clinical interview.[6]

In brief, the CLASS protocol identifies five main components of the medical interview as essential and crucial. They are Context (the physical context or setting), Listening skills, Acknowledgment of the patient's emotions, Strategy for clinical management, and Summary.

C: CONTEXT (OR SETTING)

The context of the interview means the physical context or setting and includes five major components: arranging the space optimally, body language, eye contact, touch, and introductions. A few seconds spent establishing these features of the initial setup of the interview may save many minutes of frustration and misunderstanding later (for both the professional and the patient). These rules are not complex, but they are easy to forget in the heat of the moment.

Spatial Arrangements

Try to ensure privacy. In a hospital setting, draw the curtains around the bed if a side room is not available. In an office setting, shut the door. Next, move any physical objects out of the way. Move any bedside tables, trays, or other impediments out of the line between you and the patient. Ask that any televisions or radios to be turned off for a few minutes. If you are in an office or room, move your chair so you are next to the patient, not across the desk. Evidence indicates that conversations across a corner occur three times more frequently than conversations across the full width of a table. Clear any clutter and papers from the area of desk that is nearest to the patient. If you have the patient's chart open, make sure you look up from it and do not talk to the patient while reading the chart. If you find any of these actions awkward, state what you are doing ("It may be easier for us to talk if I move the table/if you turn the television off for a moment").

Then, arguably the most important component of organizing the physical context, sit down. This is an almost inviolable guideline. It is virtually impossible to assure a patient that she or he has your undivided attention and that you intend to listen seriously if you remain standing. Only if it is absolutely impossible to sit should you try to hold a medical interview while standing. Anecdotal impressions suggest that when the doctor sits down, the patient perceives the period of time spent at the bedside as longer than if the doctor remains standing. Thus, not only does the act of sitting down indicate to the patient that he or she has control and that you are there to listen, but it also saves time and increases efficiency. Before starting the interview, take care to get the patient organized if necessary. If you have just finished examining the patient, allow or help him or her to dress and to restore a sense of personal modesty.

It is also important to be seated at a comfortable distance from the patient. This distance (sometimes called the *body buffer zone*) seems to vary from culture to culture, but a distance of 2 to 3 feet between you will usually serve for the purpose of intimate and personal conversation. This is another reason that the doctor who remains standing at the end of the bed seems remote and aloof.

The height at which you sit can also be important; normally, your eyes should be approximately level with the patient's. If the patient is already upset or angry, a useful technique is to sit so you are below the patient, with your eyes at a lower level. This position often decreases the anger.

Whenever possible, make sure that you are seated closest to the patient and that any friends or relatives are on the other side of the patient. Sometimes relatives try to dominate the interview, and it may be important for you to send a clear signal that the patient has primacy.

In almost all oncology settings, it is important to have a box of tissues nearby. If the patient or a relative begins to cry, it is important to offer tissues. This act not only gives overt permission to cry but also allows the person to feel less vulnerable when crying.

Body Language

Body language makes a difference.[7,8] Try to move and talk in an unhurried fashion to convey that the person to whom you are relating matters. To achieve an air of relaxation, sit down comfortably with both your feet flat on the floor. Let your shoulders relax and drop. Undo your coat or jacket if you are wearing one, and rest your hands on your knees (in psychotherapy this is often termed the *neutral position*).

Eye Contact

Maintain eye contact for most of the time that the patient is talking. If the interview becomes intense or emotionally charged, particularly if the patient is crying or is very angry, it will be helpful to the patient for you to look away (to break eye contact) at that point.

Touching the Patient

Touch may also be helpful during the interview if (a) a nonthreatening area is touched such as a hand or forearm, (b) you are comfortable with touch, and (c) the patient appreciates touch and does not withdraw. Most of us have not been taught specific details of clinical touch at any time in our training.[3,9] We are therefore likely to be ill at ease with touching as an interview technique until we have had some practice. Nevertheless, considerable evidence (although the data are somewhat "soft") suggests that touching the patient (particularly above the patient's waist, to avoid misinterpretation) is of benefit during a medical interview. It seems likely that touching is a significant action at times of distress and should be encouraged, with the proviso that the professional should be sensitive to the patient's reaction. If the patient is comforted by the contact, continue; if the patient is uncomfortable, stop. Touch can mean different things and can be misinterpreted (e.g., as lasciviousness, aggression, or dominance), so be aware that touching is an interviewing skill that requires extra self-regulation.

Commencing the Interview

Ensure that the patient knows who you are and what you do. Many practitioners, including myself, make a point of shaking the patient's hand at the outset, although this is a matter of personal preference. Often the handshake tells you something about the family dynamics as well as about the patient. The patient's spouse will frequently also extend his or her hand. It is worthwhile to make sure that you shake the patient's hand before that of the spouse (even if the spouse is nearer), to demonstrate that the patient comes first and the spouse (although an important member of the team) comes second.

L: LISTENING SKILLS

As dialogue begins, the professional should show that she or he is in *listening mode*. The four most essential points are listed in the following subsections. They are the use of open questions, facilitation techniques, the use of clarification, and the handling of time and interruptions.

Open Questions

Open questions are ones that can be answered in any way or manner. The question does not direct the respondent or require that he or she make a choice from a specific range of answers. In taking the medical history, of course, most of the questions are, appropriately, closed questions (e.g., "Do you have any difficulty with fine hand movements?" "Do you have any areas of numbness or tingling?"). In therapeutic dialogue, when the clinician is trying to be part of the patient's support system, open questions are an essential way of finding out what the patient is experiencing, to tailor support to the patient. Hence open questions ("What did you think the diagnosis was?" "How did you feel when you were told that?" "What did that make you feel?") are a mandatory part of the "nonhistory" therapeutic dialogue.

Silence

The first and most important technique in facilitating dialogue between patient and clinician is the use of silence. If the patient is speaking, do not overlap your speech by talking over her or him. Wait for the patient to stop speaking before you start your next sentence. This, the simplest rule of all, is the most often ignored and is most likely to give the patient the impression that the doctor is not listening.[10]

Silences also have other significance: They can, and often do, reveal the patient's state of mind. Patients often fall silent when they have feelings that are too intense to express in words. A silence therefore means that the patient is thinking or feeling something important, not that he or she has stopped thinking. If the clinician can tolerate a pause or silence, the patient may well express the thought in words a moment later. If you have to break the silence, a helpful way to do so may be to say "What were you thinking about just then?" or "What is it that's making you pause?" or words to that effect.

Evident Hearing

Once you have encouraged the patient to speak, it is valuable to demonstrate that you are hearing what is being said. Hence, in addition to silence, dialogue may be facilitated by using any of these facilitation techniques: nodding, pausing, smiling, and using responses such as "Yes," "Mmm hmm," "Tell me more." In addition, it is often valuable to use repetition as a conscious and deliberate facilitation technique. To demonstrate that you are really hearing what the patient is saying, employ one or two key words from the patient's last sentence in your own first sentence. For instance, if the patient says "I just feel so lousy most of the time," begin your response with "Tell me what you mean by feeling lousy." Reiteration means repeating what the patient has told you, but in your words, not the patient's: "Since I started those new tablets, I've been feeling sleepy" "So you're getting some drowsiness from the new tablets?" Both repetition and reiteration confirm to the patient that you have heard what has been said.

Clarifying

As the patient talks, it is very tempting for the clinician to go along with what the patient is saying, even if the exact meaning or implication is unclear. This may quickly lead to serious obstacles in the dialogue. Hence it is important to be honest when you have not understood what the patient means. Several different phrases can be used ("I'm sorry—I'm not quite sure what you meant when you said… " "When you say … do you mean that …?"). Clarification gives the patient an opportunity to expand on the previous statement and to amplify some aspect of the statement now that the clinician has shown interest in the topic.

Handling Time and Interruptions

Clinicians seem to have a poor reputation for handling interruptions, whether caused by phone, pager, or other people. We may often appear to abruptly ignore the patient we have been speaking with to respond immediately to a phone call, a page, or a colleague. Even though it may be inadvertent, the patient frequently interprets this as a snub or an insult. If it is not possible to hold all calls or to turn off the pager, then it is at least worthwhile to indicate to the patient that you are sorry about the interruption and will resume the interview shortly ("Sorry, this is another doctor I must speak to very briefly. I'll be back in a moment" or "This is something quite urgent about another patient—I won't be more than a few minutes."). The same is true of time constraints ("I'm afraid I have to go to the ER now, but this is an important conversation. We need to continue this tomorrow morning on the ward round.").

A: ACKNOWLEDGMENT (AND EXPLORATION) OF EMOTIONS

The Empathic Response

The empathic response is an extremely useful technique in an emotionally charged interview, yet it is frequently misunderstood by students and trainees. The empathic response need not relate to your own personal feelings: If the patient feels sad, you are not required to feel sad yourself. It can be a technique of acknowledgment, showing the patient that you have observed the emotion he or she is experiencing. Empathic response consists of three steps:

1. Identifying the emotion that the patient is experiencing
2. Identifying the origin and root cause of that emotion
3. Responding in a way that tells the patient that you have made the connection between 1 and 2

Often the most effective empathic responses follow the format of "You seem to be …" or "It must be …"; for example, "It must be very distressing for you to know that all that therapy didn't give you a long remission" or even "This must be awful for you." The objective of the empathic response is to demonstrate that you have identified and acknowledged the emotion that the patient is experiencing and by doing so you are giving it legitimacy as an item on the patient's agenda. In fact, if the patient is experiencing a strong emotion (e.g., rage or crying), you must acknowledge the existence of that emotion or all further attempts at communication will fail. If strong emotions are not acknowledged in some way, you will be perceived as insensitive, and this will render the rest of the interaction useless.

To stress it once more then, the empathic response is your acknowledgment of what the other person is experiencing. It need have nothing to do with your own personal view or judgment of the situation or how you yourself would react if you were facing these circumstances. You do not have to feel the same emotion that the patient is experiencing, nor do you even have to agree with the patient's viewpoint. You are simply observing what the other person is feeling and bringing that emotion into the dialogue between the two of you.

S: MANAGEMENT STRATEGY

Several techniques are useful to help ensure that you construct a management plan that the patient will concur with and will follow. The following are helpful guidelines:

1. Determine what you judge to be the optimal medical strategy. Define the ideal management plan (in your mind or out loud).
2. Assess, in your own mind or by asking the patient, the patient's own expectations of condition, treatment, and outcome. You can summarize this in your mind or clarify and summarize aloud if needed. Be aware of whether there is

a marked mismatch between the patient's view of the situation and the medical facts. You are going to have to work harder to make the plan appear logical and acceptable to the patient if there is significant discordance between the patient's view and reality.

3. Propose a strategy. Bearing in mind your conclusions from steps 1 and 2, propose your strategy. As you explain it to the patient, constantly…

4. Assess the patient's response. For example, make note of the patient's progress in forming an action plan (these stages are often defined as precontemplation, contemplation, and implementation or reinforcement). Acknowledge the patient's emotions as they occur and continue in a contractual fashion until you arrive at a plan that the patient can "buy into" and will follow.

S: SUMMARY

The summary is the closure of the interview. In oncology, the relationship with the patient is likely to be a continuing one and a major component of the patient's treatment. The closure of the interview is an important time to emphasize that point.

It is relatively straightforward to cover three areas in the summary. Provide the following:

1. A précis, or reiteration of the main points covered in the dialogue
2. An invitation for the patient to ask questions
3. A clear arrangement for the next interaction (a clear contract for contact)

This particular part of the interview is not necessarily long, but it does require considerable focus and concentration.

Breaking Bad News: The SPIKES Protocol

In palliative care, there are many occasions when new medical information needs to be discussed. Hence it is essential to have a logical and systematic approach to sharing medical information.[11] The following protocol has been detailed at greater length elsewhere.[2] In practice, it has been found useful in all interviews concerning bad news, whether or not the patient and the professional know each other well. However, formal studies of this protocol (or any other) have not been carried out, and even the design of such investigations poses major difficulties.[12] It consists of six steps or phases.

S: SETTING (PHYSICAL CONTEXT)

The physical context of the interview has already been reviewed. It is of even greater importance for the interview in which bad news will be shared.

P: PERCEPTION (FINDING OUT HOW MUCH THE PATIENT KNOWS OR SUSPECTS)

Before providing further information, it is always important to determine what the patient knows about the medical condition and its effect on the future. In fact, sharing information may be awkward, superfluous, or even impossible without first knowing what the patient already knows. In all cases, you should try to establish what the patient knows about the impact of the illness on his or her future and not focus on the fine details of basic pathology or nomenclature of the diagnosis. This information can be gathered in many ways. Some of the questions that may be useful include the following:

"What have you made of the illness so far?"
"What did the previous doctors tell you about the illness [operation, etc.]?"
"Have you been worried about yourself?"
"When you first had [symptom X], what did you think it might be?"
"What did [Dr. X] tell you when he sent you here?"
"Did you think something serious was going on when [...]?"

As the patient replies, analyze the response. Important information can be obtained from three major features of the reply.

Factual Content of the Patient's Statements

It must be established how much the patient has understood and how close that impression is to the medical reality. At this point, some patients may say that they have been told nothing at all, and this may or may not be true. Even if you know it to be false, accept the patient's statement as a symptom of denial and do not force a confrontation immediately. First, the patient may be about to request information from you and may, in part deliberately, deny previous information to see whether you will tell the same story. Second, if the patient has been given information previously and is in denial, you are unlikely to appear supportive by forcing an immediate confrontation.

In fact, a patient who denies receiving previous information quite often precipitates anger or resentment on the part of the professional (e.g., "My goodness, doesn't Dr. Smythe tell his patients what he found at the operation!"). If you find yourself feeling this, pause and think. You may be seeing a patient in denial, and this may be causing you to suffer from "nobody-ever-tells-their-patients-anything-until-I-do" syndrome. It is very common when patients are sick and the emotional atmosphere is highly charged.

Style of the Patient's Statements

Much can be gleaned from the patient's emotional state, educational level, and articulation skills. Listen to the vocabulary, the kind of words being said, and the kind of words being avoided. Note the style, so when it is your turn to speak, you can start at the right level.

You should, however, ignore the patient's occupation in making this assessment, particularly if he or she happens to be a member of a health care profession, because far too often you will find yourself making assumptions. Even a physician, as a patient, may not be an expert in a particular disease and may not understand a phrase such as "It's only a stage II but I don't like the mitotic index."

Emotional Content of the Patient's Statements

The two major sources of emotional content are verbal and nonverbal. Both may yield information about the patient's state, and discordance between the two may give valuable signals regarding state and motivation. For instance, a patient may speak in a calm manner, but the body language may reveal major anxiety.

I: INVITATION (FINDING OUT HOW MUCH THE PATIENT WANTS TO KNOW)

Invitation is the single most crucial step in any information-giving discussion. It is far easier to proceed with giving the news if there is a clear invitation from the patient to do so. Conversely, although it is universally acknowledged that in contemporary society patients have a right to truth and information, it is often impossible to predict which patients will want to hear the truth and which will not.[13] (For fuller reviews, see Billings and Reiser.[14,15]) The exact proportion of patients who do want full disclosure varies from study to study, but current figures range from 50% to 98.5%, depending on patient demographics and the diagnosis suspected.[13] (For a detailed review, see McIntosh.[16]) Because no characteristics predict whether a patient desires disclosure,[17] it seems logical simply to ask. The way in which this important and sensitive question is phrased is largely a matter of personal style. Some examples are as follows:

"Are you the kind of person who likes to know exactly what's going on?"

"Would you like me to tell you the full details of the diagnosis?"

"Are you the kind of person who likes to have full information on what's wrong or would you prefer just to hear about the treatment plan?"

"Do you like to know exactly what's going on or would you prefer me to give you the outline only?"

"Would you like me to tell you everything relevant about your condition or is there somebody else you'd like me to talk to?"

Note that in all these approaches, if the patient does not want to hear the full details, you have not cut off all lines of communication. You are saying overtly that you will maintain contact and communication (e.g., about the treatment plan) but not about the details of the disease. If the patient does not want to hear the information, you should add that if, at any time in the future, the patient changes her or his mind and wants further information, you will provide it. The phrase "… the sort of person who" is particularly valuable because it suggests to the patient that many patients are like him or her and that if he or she prefers not to discuss the information, this is neither unique nor a sign of extraordinary feebleness or lack of courage.

K: KNOWLEDGE (SHARING MEDICAL INFORMATION)

The process by which medical information is transmitted can be thought of as consisting of two crucial steps.

Aligning

At this point in the interview, you have already heard how much the patient knows about the situation and have learned something of the vocabulary used to express the knowledge. This is the starting point for sharing the information. Reinforce those parts that are correct (using the patient's words if possible) and proceed from there. This gives the patient a great deal of confidence in himself or herself (as well as in you) to realize that his or her view of the situation has been heard and is being taken seriously (even if it is being modified or corrected).

This process has been called *aligning,* a useful term to describe the process by which you line up the information you wish to impart on the baseline of the patient's current knowledge.[11,18] (Maynard uses the word *aligning* to describe one particular style of doctor–patient communication. The meaning has been extended in this schema to describe the first part of the information-sharing process.)

Educating

In the next phase of the interview, having begun from the patient's starting point (i.e., having aligned your information with the patient's original position), you now have to bring the patient's perception of the situation closer to the medical facts as you know them. No word in current usage fully describes this part of the interview, but *educating* is perhaps the closest. The process of sharing information should be a gradual one in which the patient's perception is steadily shifted until it is in close approximation to the medical reality. This part of the interview can usefully be compared with steering an oil tanker. You cannot make sudden lurches and expect the patient's perception to change instantly. You have to apply slow and steady guidance over the direction of the interview and observe the responses as you do so. In the process, you build on those responses from the patient that are bringing him or her closer to the facts and emphasize the relevant medical information if it becomes apparent that the patient is moving away from an accurate perception of the situation. The key ingredients are steady observation and continued gentle guidance of the direction of the interview rather than sudden lurches.

Give Information in Small Amounts: The Warning Shot. Medical information is hard for patients to digest and more so if it concerns a grave prognosis or threat of death. Recall of information is poor at the best of times and is likely to be very poor if medical facts are grim ("The moment you said 'cancer,' doctor, I couldn't remember a thing from then on ..."). The rule is therefore to give the information in small amounts.

One of the most useful principles is the idea of the "warning shot." If there is clearly a large gap between the patient's expectations and the reality of the situation, you can facilitate understanding by giving a warning that things are more serious than they appear ("Well, the situation was more serious than that ...") and then grading the information, gradually introducing the more serious prognostic points and waiting for the patient to respond at each stage.

Use Plain Language. Technical jargon ("medspeak") is an efficient language for transmitting codified information in a short time. Because it takes many years to learn, it is also comforting to the professional. Patients, however, have not learned to speak this language and cannot express their emotions in it. Hence it reinforces the barrier between patient and professional and is most likely to make the patient feel angry, belittled, and isolated. We should avoid jargon if we are trying to support the patient at a difficult time.

Check Reception Frequently. Check that your message is being received, and check frequently. You can use any phrase that feels comfortable, anything to break the monologue. Examples are as follows:

"Am I making sense?"
"Do you follow what I'm saying?"
"This must be a bit bewildering, but do you follow roughly what I'm saying?"
"Do you see what I mean?"

These interjections serve several important functions:

1. They demonstrate that it matters to you if the patient does not understand what you are saying.
2. They allow the patient to speak (many patients feel so bewildered or shocked that their voices seem to seize up and they need encouragement and prompting to speak).
3. They allow the patient to feel an element of control over the interview.

4. They validate the patient's feelings and make them legitimate subjects for discussion between the two of you. You should also check that you are transmitting the information at the same intellectual level as the patient is receiving it by ensuring that your vocabulary and that of the patient are similar.

Reinforce. You can reinforce what you are telling the patient in several ways:
1. Have the patient repeat the general drift of what you have been saying.
2. Repeat important points yourself. Because it is difficult to retain information, particularly if the news is serious, and even more so if denial is operating, you may have to repeat crucial points several times. Accept this as a fact of life when looking after seriously ill patients (you can cover this with a phrase such as "I know it's difficult to remember all this stuff at one go …").
3. Use diagrams and written messages. A few simple scribbles on the back of an envelope or a scrap of paper may serve as a useful aide-mémoire.

Blend Your Agenda with that of the Patient. When transmitting information to the patient, it is important to elicit his or her agenda, or "shopping list" of concerns and anxieties, so further information can be tailored to answer major problems. The following are useful guidelines.

Elicit the "Shopping List. "Quite often the patient's major concerns are not the same as those of the professional. For instance, patients may be more worried about severe pain or loss of mental functioning than about the primary disease itself (see earlier). You do not necessarily have to deal with the items at that particular moment, but you should indicate that you understand what the patient is talking about and will return to it in a moment. ("I know you're very worried about drowsiness, and I'll come to that in a moment, but can I first cover the reasons that we recommend increasing the painkillers in the first place?").

Listen for the Buried Question. Deep personal worries may not emerge easily. Sometimes the patient asks questions while you are talking. These questions ("buried questions") are often highly significant to the patient. When the patient does this, finish your own sentence and then ask the patient what he or she was saying. Be prepared to follow that train of thought from the patient; it is quite likely to be important. Ask another question, such as "Did you have something in mind that triggered that question?"

Be Prepared to Be Led. Quite often you may draw an interview to a close and then find that the patient wants to start part of it again. This is not simply contrary behavior. It often stems from fear and insecurity; by restarting the interview, the patient may be exerting some measure of control, or perhaps he or she has recalled something important. Try to accommodate or at least promise time at the next meeting.

E: EMOTIONS AND EMPATHIC RESPONSES (RESPONDING TO THE PATIENT'S FEELINGS)

In many respects, the patient's reactions to his or her medical condition and the professional's response to those reactions define their relationship and determine whether it offers support for the patient. Hence the professional's ability to understand and respond sensitively to the emotions expressed by the patient is central to all communication in palliative care. In essence, this part of the communication becomes therapeutic (or supportive) dialogue.

In the short space of this chapter, it is not possible to illustrate the wide range of patients' reactions to dying or to bad news in general. However, a detailed analysis has been published elsewhere,[2] together with several options available to the professional in each situation. The central components of the professional's response are (a) assessment of the patient's response and (b) empathic responses from the professional. For the sake of convenience, these two topics are discussed later, in the section on therapeutic dialogue.

S: STRATEGY AND SUMMARY

Organizing and Planning

The sixth and final step in the protocol for breaking bad news is the stage at which the professional summarizes the situation and makes an operational plan and a contract for the future. This process is of great importance to the patient, and it should conclude every interview with a palliative care patient, not just an interview in which bad news is discussed.

Frequently, after hearing news that is new or distressing, the patient may feel bewildered, dispirited, and disorganized. Although the professional should be sensitive to those emotions and be capable of empathy, our responsibilities consist of more than simply reflecting the patient's emotions. The patient is looking to us to make sense of any confusion and to offer plans for the future. At this point in the interview, it is therefore important to try to put together what is known of the patient's agenda, the medical situation, the plan of management, and a contract for the future. This process can be logically divided into six tasks.

Demonstrate an Understanding of the Patient's Problem List. If the interview has been effective so far, you have been achieving an understanding of the patient's problem list since the beginning. From the outset, you have demonstrated that you have heard what most bothers the patient, and a brief "headline" reference to the patient's major concerns will reinforce the fact that you have been listening.

Indicate that You Can Distinguish the Fixable from the Unfixable. With both medical problems and psychosocial problems, some are "fixable" and some are not. This is discussed further in relation to the patient's responses in the next section, but it is a pragmatic step without which your support will appear to be less effective. If the interview becomes stuck or bogged down as the patient explores her or his problems, it is often helpful to try to enumerate the problems in list form by having the patient arrange them in order of priority. You can then begin to set your own agenda by stating which problems you are going to tackle first. This leads logically to the next step.

Make a Plan or Strategy and Explain It. When making a plan for the future, it is quite permissible for that plan to include many uncertainties, "don't knows," and choices (e.g., "If the dizziness doesn't get better, then we'll ..."), acknowledging that uncertainty is often a painful and difficult state with which to cope.[19] What you are actually doing is presenting a decision tree or algorithm. Patients need to know that you have some plan in mind, even if it consists of little more than dealing with each problem as it arises, because it implies that you will not abandon the patient. The act of making a plan and explaining it to the patient is part of what the patient sees as support. It defines the immediate future of your relationship with this particular patient, reinforces the individuality of this person, and explains what you are going to do for him or her.

Identify Coping Strategies of the Patient and Reinforce Them. In our training, strong emphasis is placed on what we do to patients or for patients. Obviously, in acute emergencies, the professionals have to do all the work. However, this attitude of "we will do it all for you" can influence the professional's approach to all patients in every situation, particularly if the patient is feeling overwhelmed and helpless in the presence of bad news. This may be bad for the patient and also bad for us because we may later become overwhelmed by our responsibilities. At this point in the interview, then, it is important to look at the resources available to the patient, both internally and externally.[20] We cannot, and should not, live the patient's life for him or her. Hence, as the problem list and the plan begin to take shape, the professional should begin to help the patient evaluate what he or she can do for himself or herself. This part of the process involves helping the patient identify his or her own coping strategies. It is a continuous process, not usually completed in one interview. It also leads logically to the next component.

Identify Other Sources of Support for the Patient and Incorporate Them. Not only do we tend to forget that the patient has capabilities of his or her own, we also tend to forget that there may be someone outside the professional–patient relationship who can assist. Most people have at least one or two friends or relatives who are close and can offer support. For those patients who have no social supports of their own, it will be necessary to enroll and coordinate the other available services.

Summary and Conclusion. The final part of the interview is the summary and contract for the future. The summary (which also requires a great deal of thought) should show the patient that you have been listening and that you have picked up on the main concerns and issues. It is not a particularly easy task, but you should try to give an overview of the two agendas involved: yours and the patient's. It need not be a long statement and often consists of no more than one or two sentences.

Having summarized the main points, you should then ask: "Are there any (other) questions that you'd like to ask me now?" The patient may have been bottling up concerns over some issue that simply has not arisen or over an aspect of the treatment or the disease that you have merely touched on, so this part of the interview is as important as the question period after a lecture. It is the time when any unresolved issues can be discussed.

Finally, you should make a contract for the future. Even though this may be as simple as a statement (e.g., "I'll see you at the next visit in 2 weeks" or "We'll try the new antisickness medicine and I'll see you tomorrow on the ward rounds"), without it patients may leave the interview feeling that there will be no future contact.

Therapeutic (or Supportive) Dialogue

Many physicians underrate the value of therapeutic dialogue because it is not included in the curricula of most medical schools and thus they are unfamiliar with its use. Supportive communication is obviously central to psychiatric and psychotherapeutic practice, but it is generally not taught to medical or nursing students outside those disciplines.[21] Hence it often seems an alien idea that a doctor or nurse can achieve anything by simply listening to the patient and acknowledging the existence of that individual's emotions.

Nevertheless, supportive dialogue during any stage of palliative care is an exceptionally valuable resource and may be the most important (and sometimes the only) ingredient in a patient's care. The central principle of effective therapeutic dialogue is that the patient should perceive that his or her emotions have been heard and acknowledged by the professional. It may then become apparent that there are problems that can be solved, emotions that can be resolved, and needs that can be met. Even if that is not the case, the simple act of supportive dialogue can reduce distress.

The empathic response is of prime importance in achieving the main objective of acknowledging the patient's emotions, although it cannot be the only component of the professional's side of the dialogue. Obviously, a single technique cannot create an entire relationship. Nevertheless, many professionals are unfairly perceived as insensitive or unsupportive simply because they do not know how to demonstrate their abilities as listeners. The empathic response is one of the most reliable methods of demonstrating effective listening. In addition to responding in this way, the professional should also attempt to assess the nature and value of the patient's coping responses, disentangle the emotions that have been raised by the discussion, and try to resolve any conflicts that may arise.

ASSESSMENT OF THE PATIENT'S RESPONSES

Although this chapter has not detailed all the possible reactions that a patient may experience, it is possible to offer some brief guidelines to assess those emotions so the professional will know which emotions are best reinforced and which require intervention. In essence, three criteria are used to assess a patient's responses.

ACCEPTABILITY

First, a patient's reactions must meet the broadest definitions of socially acceptable behavior. These definitions vary from culture to culture (and some of the gravest misunderstandings arise from misinterpretation because behavior that is normal in one culture may be seen as aberrant in another). In the context of palliative care, however, interpretation of socially acceptable should be very wide. The professional should err on the side of generosity, and assistance should be sought only if extreme behavior is a genuine danger to the patient, staff, other patients, or family members. With the exception of these very rare cases, the professional should accept the behavior, even if he or she does not like it, and assess it on the other two criteria: Does it help the patient, and, if it does not, can it be improved by intervention?

DISTINGUISHING THE ADAPTIVE FROM THE MALADAPTIVE

Second, facing the end of life usually induces major stress and distress: An individual's response to that distress may either help the person to reduce it (an *adaptive response*) or may increase it (a *maladaptive response*). It is frequently difficult to distinguish one from the other at the first interview, and several interviews over a longer period may be required to decide whether a patient is adapting to the medical circumstances.

It is not easy to be dogmatic about which responses are always maladaptive, but some guidelines are shown in Table 3-1. The consensus seems to be, for example, a feeling of guilt is always maladaptive and cannot help a patient. It may be somewhat more controversial, but still helpful, to regard denial in the early stages as an adaptive response that allows the patient to adjust in small "bites" to what would otherwise be an overwhelming threat. Moreover, some responses can buy the patient an immediate short-term decrease in distress, but they can also cause additional problems later. For instance, denial that is prolonged and prevents a patient from making

Table 3-1. Some Adaptive and Maladaptive Responses

Possibly Adaptive	Possibly Maladaptive
Humor	Guilt
Denial	Pathologic denial
Abstract anger	
Anger against disease	Anger against helpers
Crying	Collapse
Fear	Anxiety
Fulfilling an ambition	The impossible quest
Realistic hope	Unrealistic hope
Sexual drive, healthily fulfilled	Despair
Bargaining	Manipulation

decisions with which he or she is comfortable ("We won't even think about that …") may later increase distress. In some cases, only the professional's clinical experience and the passage of time can define the situation.

DISTINGUISHING THE "FIXABLE" FROM THE "UNFIXABLE"

The third criterion by which responses may be assessed is what may be termed *fixability*. If a problem is increasing the patient's distress or obstructing adaptation, can it be remedied? This is largely a matter of clinical experience, and it depends on the professional's confidence and competence in addressing psychosocial problems. Two points, however, are worth stressing. First, the chance of damage is higher when the professional feels that he or she can fix a problem and then perseveres without seeking help than it is when a professional knows his or her own limitations. Second, if a problem appears to be unfixable, it is even more important to seek a second opinion, preferably from a psychologist or psychiatrist. In up to two thirds of cases, problems that the medical team considers to be unfixable can be improved by psychological intervention.[22]

DISTINGUISHING YOUR EMOTIONS FROM THOSE OF THE PATIENT

Another task that must often be undertaken during therapeutic dialogue is the disentangling of the emotions experienced by both the patient and the professional during the interview. We have already seen that strong emotions cannot be ignored without jeopardizing all communication. We should also try to be aware of our own emotions when dealing with an individual person who is dying. We may experience strong emotions because of our own previous experience (countertransference), or we may be moved, attracted, or irritated and intolerant as a result of the patient's behavior patterns. In any event, when emotions arise, it is essential to try to take a step back and ask yourself what you are feeling and where that feeling comes from. If the professional can recognize a strong emotion in himself or herself, that recognition will partly negate the effect of the emotion on judgment and communication. The emotion is far more likely to produce damage if it goes unrecognized.

> **Box 3-2.** *In the Event of Conflict*
>
> 1. Try to take a step back.
> 2. Identify your own emotions and try to describe them, not display them.
> 3. Try to define the area of conflict that is unresolved.
> 4. Try to obtain agreement on that area of difference, even if it cannot be resolved.
> 5. Find a colleague and talk about it.

DEALING WITH CONFLICT

We all want to do our best for the patient, but we also have our limits. Sometimes we simply cannot ease a patient's distress, sometimes a patient does not wish to be relieved, and sometimes the patient appears to have a need for antagonism or conflict to give himself or herself definition or some other gain.

Despite pretences to the contrary, at some time all of us feel exhausted, frustrated, and intolerant. This is unavoidable. However, a few guidelines may reduce the impact of those feelings in our professional life.[23] The most useful are shown in Box 3-2.

In summary, the single most useful tool of therapeutic dialogue is the empathic response that indicates to the patient that the emotional content of his or her reaction is being heard and is legitimized. In addition, the professional should attempt to assess the patient's response, disentangle his or her emotions from those of the patient, and try to resolve conflict. These, then, are some of the most important aspects of communicating with the dying patient. Other parties are almost always involved, however, and the next section deals with communication issues that concern the family and other health care disciplines.

Communication with Other People

All efforts in palliative care are directed at ameliorating the situation of the patient. However, other parties are involved who may assist or hinder efforts at effective communication. (For a major review of communication issues with patients with cancer, their families, and professionals, see Northouse and Northouse.[24]) Only a few broad guidelines can be offered in this limited space, but attention to even these simple issues can noticeably improve quality of care.

COMMUNICATION WITH FRIENDS AND FAMILY

The responses of friends and family to the imminent death of a patient may be as varied as those of the patient. Similarly, they may assist the patient and be of support, or they may be counterproductive and contribute to the patient's problems rather than being part of the solution. Responses from others may resemble the patient's responses, or they may be qualitatively different. Even when they are the same as those of the patient, they may be asynchronous with the patient's responses; for example, the patient may have resolved his or her anger and may have come to accept death while the family is still angry or in denial. Just as the patient's responses may be considered adaptive or maladaptive, so the family's responses may also serve to decrease or increase the patient's distress and to increase or decrease support.

When a patient's treatment is palliative, some effort should always be made to identify the leading members of his or her support systems (friends and family).

When communicating with the family, however, two principles may at first seem mutually exclusive.

The Patient Has Primacy

A mentally competent patient has the ethical and legal right to determine who should be informed about his or her medical condition. All rights of friends or family are subordinate to this. If a patient decides to not share information with anyone else, although that may be an aggressive and vengeful action, it cannot be countermanded by the professional at the family's request. Similarly, however well intentioned, a relative's statement that "the patient is not to be told" does not have primacy over the patient's wishes if the patient wishes full disclosure.

The Family's Feelings Have Validity

Despite the secondary rank of the family's feelings, those feelings have validity and must be acknowledged even if the professional cannot accede to their wishes or instructions. The wishes of the family often arise from a desire to show that they are good and caring sons or daughters (e.g., rationalizing their own feelings, as in "If I cannot stop mother from becoming ill, I can at least stop her from finding out too much about it"). It is important for the professional to identify the family's emotions and to acknowledge them. For this purpose, the empathic response is of great value.

COMMUNICATION BETWEEN PHYSICIANS

Doctors are notoriously bad at communicating with each other. We do not do it frequently enough and, more important, when we do communicate with each other, it is often disorganized and unfocused. Perhaps the most dangerous gaps in doctor–doctor communication occur when a patient moves from one care setting to another, for example from a hospital or home into a palliative care unit.

It is difficult to give useful guidelines about something as ill defined as inter-specialty communication, but perhaps the key principles are that all communication should be task oriented and should clearly define frontiers of responsibility. This means that communications should be related to those aspects of the patient's situation that may have an impact on his or her care. On analysis, much of what is discussed between doctors is simply opinion or conjecture. Although there is nothing wrong with this in and of itself, we often feel that we have thoroughly discussed the case when, in fact, vital management issues have not been discussed at all.

The five-point checklist that follows may be of some value when considering a letter or telephone call to another physician about a palliative care patient.

1. Am I addressing the right person? (For instance, does the patient know the family practitioner well? Have I asked the patient whom he or she wished me to contact?)
2. What do I know about this patient that the other person should know? (And what do I want to know from the other person?)
3. What does this mean for the patient's future care?
4. Who is going to do what? Who is now "the doctor" for this patient?
5. How shall we communicate again if things are not going well?

Even if communications are limited to these five points, they will be more effective than many of the current communications between doctors, not because we are negligent or malevolent, but because we are often too polite and too afraid of stepping on each other's toes in making suggestions for the patient's benefit.

COMMUNICATION BETWEEN PHYSICIANS AND NURSES

By definition, professionals belong to different teams because they have special expertise and training that is identified with that discipline. This is essential for good patient care. However, there is a side effect—namely, that we each speak a different language, and we all tend to believe that our particular language is the only one truly relevant to the patient's care. As a result, different aspects of the patient's problems are often poorly integrated, and large gaps in communication are often apparent between the teams. Because of the way the jobs interrelate, the most common gaps occur between doctors and nurses.

One of the greatest paradoxes (and perhaps one of the greatest losses) in the recent evolution of the nursing profession has been the diminishing of the ward round as the standard method for exchanging information among patient, doctor, and nurse. Although this idea that the ward round is essential in patient care is controversial, it is a view that is now receiving increasing support from all disciplines as well as from patients and families. The days of the 3-hour ward round, during which four patients are reviewed, are over. Nursing time is at a premium, and nursing tasks have increased greatly in number and complexity, However, without the trinity of patient–doctor–nurse present in the same place at the same time, inpatient care is rendered unnecessarily complex and incomplete. In hospitals or hospices where time is limited, it is often possible to agree on time limits (e.g., an average of 10 minutes per patient can enable the team to accomplish almost all the necessary exchanges).

In our own unit, we ensure that the three following points are addressed during the minimum 10-minute period allotted for discussion of each patient:

1. The medical game plan: What is known about the patient's medical status? What measures are planned or being considered? What is the prognosis?
2. Nursing concerns: What are the main difficulties in the day-to-day care of the patient?
3. What does the patient know, and what are the patient's major concerns? For instance, does the patient have strong views about the type of therapy or the location for treatment?

It is surprising how efficient communication can be if all concerned are aware that time is limited and that these three main areas should be covered in the discussion.

PEARLS

- Talking about matters of dying can be difficult for all concerned.
- Take time to consider your own relationship with mortality; you cannot guide others unless you have some maturity in this matter.
- Talk about it with friends, family, colleagues, or a counselor.
- Consider the following common fears among professionals:
  - Discomfort at feeling the patient's suffering
  - Fear of being blamed
  - Fear of the untaught

Continued

PEARLS—con'd

- ○ Fear of eliciting a reaction
- ○ Fear of saying "I don't know"
- ○ Fear of expressing emotions
- ○ Our own fears of illness and death
- ○ Fear of medical hierarchy
- • In general, use CLASS skills in communication:
  - ○ Prepare for the interview (**C**ontext); review the information, determine who will be present, and arrange the setting.
  - ○ Use **L**istening skills; use opening questions, use silence as appropriate; facilitate questions, and clarify understandings.
  - ○ **A**cknowledge the perspectives of the patient and the family.
  - ○ **S**trategically manage the medical care plan, its outcomes, and the expectations of the patient and the family.
  - ○ **S**ummarize the interview, invite the patient to ask questions, and arrange for the next interaction.
- • Specifically, when delivering important information, use the SPIKES protocol:
  - ○ Get the **S**etting right.
  - ○ Make sure you know the patient's **P**erspective.
  - ○ **I**nvite the patient to tell you how he or she wants to receive the information.
  - ○ Share the **K**nowledge.
  - ○ Acknowledge the **E**motions and be empathic.
  - ○ Share the **S**trategy for the next steps.

PITFALLS

- • Avoidance of one's own issues is hazardous. Remember, others can tell when this is the case, so do not imagine that avoidance works.
- • Avoidance of patients who are suffering or dying feels like abandonment to them and their families. Do not do it.
- • Blunt delivery of information without follow-through leaves a patient and family with harsh new realities without offering support or an opportunity to review information. This feels cruel to the patient and family. Allow time for follow-through, and stick to the CLASS and SPIKES protocols or a similar protocol.

Summary

In palliative care, everything starts with the patient, including every aspect of symptom relief and every aspect of communication. There is no doubt that we all want to do our best, but major challenges in palliative care often arise because we do not know how to approach the problem. Nowhere is this truer than in communication. A professional who feels ill equipped and inept at communication will become part of the problem instead of part of the solution. The act of following relatively straightforward guidelines, however simplistic they may appear, will at least give us a feeling of competence and will enhance our ability to learn as we practice.

An expert in palliative care is not a person who gets it right all the time. An expert is someone who gets it wrong less often and is better at concealing or coping with his or her fluster and embarrassment. We are, after all, only human beings.

Resources

1. Parkes CM: Psychological aspects. In Saunders CM, editor: *The Management of Terminal Diseases*, London, 1978, Edward Arnold, pp 55–52.
2. Rando TA: *Grief, Dying and Death*, Chicago, 1984, Research Press Company.
3. Twycross RG, Lack SA: Therapeutics in Terminal Cancer. London, Churchill Livingstone, 1990, pp 209–215.

References

1. Becker E: *The denial of death*, New York, 1973, Free Press.
2. Buckman R: *How to break bad news: a guide for healthcare professionals*, London, 1993, Macmillan Medical.
3. Seravalli EP: The dying patient, the physician and the fear of death, *N Engl J Med* 319:1728–1730, 1988.
4. Gorlin R, Zucker HD: Physicians' reactions to patients, *N Engl J Med* 308:1059–1063, 1983.
5. Radovsky SS: Bearing the news, *N Engl J Med* 513:586–588, 1985.
6. Houts PS, Yasko JM, Harvey HA, et al: Unmet needs of persons with cancer in Pennsylvania during the period of terminal care, *Cancer* 62:627–634, 1988.
7. DiMatteo MR, Taranta A, Friedman HS, Prince LM: Predicting patient satisfaction from physicians' nonverbal communication skills, *Med Care* 18:376–387, 1980.
8. Larsen KM, Smith CK: Assessment of nonverbal communication in the patient-physician interview, *J Fam Pract* 12:481–488, 1981.
9. Older J: Teaching touch at medical school, *JAMA* 252:931–933, 1984.
10. Ley P: *Communicating with patients*, London, 1988, Croom Helm.
11. Maynard D: On clinicians co-implicating recipients' perspectives in the delivery of diagnostic news. In Drew P, Heritage J, editors: *Talk at work: social interaction in institutional settings*, Cambridge, 1990, University Press.
12. Waitzkin H, Stoeckle JD: The communication of information about illness, *Adv Psychosom Med* 8:180–215, 1972.
13. Schulz R: *The psychology of death, dying and bereavement*, Reading, MA, 1978, Addison Wesley.
14. Billings A: Sharing bad news. In *Out-patient management of advanced malignancy*, Philadelphia, 1985, JB Lippincott, pp 236–259.
15. Reiser SJ: Words as scalpels: transmitting evidence in the clinical dialogue, *Ann Intern Med* 92:837–842, 1980.
16. McIntosh J: Patients' awareness and desire for information about diagnosed but undisclosed malignant disease, *Lancet* 2:300–303, 1976.
17. Cassileth BR, Zupkis RV, Sutton-Smith MS, March V: Information and participation preferences among cancer patients, *Ann Intern Med* 92:832–836, 1980.
18. Maynard D: Breaking bad news in clinical settings. In Dervin B, editor: *Progress in communication sciences*, Norwood, NJ, 1989, Ablex, pp 161–163.
19. Maguire P, Faulkner A: Communicate with cancer patients. Part 2: Handling uncertainty, collusion and denial, *BMJ* 297:972–974, 1988.
20. Manuel GM, Roth S, Keefe FJ, Brantley BA: Coping with cancer, *J Human Stress* 13:149–158, 1987.
21. Fallowfield U: Counselling for patients with cancer, *BMJ* 297:727–728, 1988.
22. Buckman R, Doan B: Enhancing communication with the cancer patient: Referrals to the psychologist—who and when? In Ginsburg D, Laidlaw J, editors: *Cancer in Ontario 1991*, Toronto, 1991, Ontario Cancer Treatment and Research Foundation, pp 78–86.
23. Lazare A, Eisenthal S, Frank A: In Lazare A, editor: *Outpatient psychiatry: diagnosis and treatment*, ed 2, Baltimore, 1989, Williams & Wilkins, pp 157–171.
24. Northouse PG, Northouse LU: Communication and cancer: issues confronting patients, health professionals and family members, *J Psychosoc Oncol* 5:17–45, 1987.

CHAPTER 4

Negotiating Goals of Care: Changing Goals Along the Trajectory of Illness

ANNETTE M. VOLLRATH and CHARLES F. VON GUNTEN

"Human dignity, I feel, rests on choice."
MAX FRISCH, SWISS WRITER, 1911–1991

Negotiating goals of care is an example of patient-centered medical decision making, which differs significantly from the problem-oriented method practiced commonly in health care in the United States. A patient-centered approach to medical decisions has proven particularly useful in the setting of advanced or serious illness. This chapter discusses a six-step approach to the goals-of-care discussion, including examples of how the steps can be used and, in a case study, real-world examples of this approach in action. Pearls and common pitfalls are highlighted.

Health care in general aims at preventing or curing disease. When you fracture a bone, you go to the hospital to get it fixed. When you acquire bacterial pneumonia, you take an antibiotic to cure it. However, many diseases cannot be "fixed." Rather, they are managed; examples are hypertension, diabetes, and congestive heart failure. For most diseases that must be managed, increasing longevity, reducing disease-related symptoms, and maintaining function and quality of life for a maximum period of time until the patient's death are the objects of medical care. As a patient's disease progresses, medical decisions are influenced more and more not just by medical information but also by the patient's underlying values and priorities. For patients living with chronic or life-threatening disease, medical decisions are often not as straightforward as they are for simple problems that can be fixed. Rather, these

56

patients face several options that may all be reasonable within the breadth of accepted medical practice.

It is therefore crucial for the health care professional who cares for patients with chronic diseases to be able to elicit underlying values and priorities, to set overall goals for care. Mutually agreed on goals will then lead to appropriate decisions to achieve those goals. It is expected that, as the patient progresses along his or her trajectory of illness, goals may change. For example, for the patient discussed in the case study in this chapter, the initial goal is to cure her cancer, then to shrink it, then to keep it from growing too fast. Another goal may be to be as comfortable and functional as possible regardless of the state of the cancer.

Along the trajectory of illness, several trigger situations invite the patient and health care provider to reflect on and discuss goals of care. These include general advance care planning, a new diagnosis, a change in therapy, the transfer to a new health care provider or institution, and, probably most commonly, the point along the disease trajectory when interventions to cure or control the disease are no longer effective or desired. One reason for this may be that the treatment-associated burden seems to outweigh its benefit.

Patients are open to such discussions. Studies show that between 85% and 95% of patients want to have honest discussions with their health care providers regarding life-threatening diseases.[1] Health care providers do not adequately meet this need. Studies have shown that doctors and nurses underestimate cancer patients' concerns, do not elicit the goals and values of seriously ill patients or include them in treatment decisions, and generally fail to address their patients' emotional concerns.[2-4]

The three chief reasons that doctors do poorly in communicating honestly with patients and families are as follows:

1. Medical education does not devote much time or attention to the development of good communication skills, and medical students see few role models.[5]
2. The culture of medicine in the Western world focuses on organ systems rather than on whole-patient care.
3. The physicians' own attitudes and underlying emotions regarding death and dying also interfere with adequate goals-of-care discussions.[6]

The importance of good communication has been well recognized in the field of palliative medicine. Major educational initiatives such as Education for Physicians on End-of-life Care and End-of-life Nursing Education Consortium (ELNEC) devote significant time to skills training in this area. Communication is a learnable skill that, like many other skills, requires ongoing practice. Brief educational interventions are likely not sufficient to change physician behavior.[7] Intensive communication skills training, however, has been shown in a randomized trial to improve physician communication skills in practice.[8]

For those physicians interested in skills training regarding the negotiation of goals of care, this chapter summarizes a six-step protocol that can be used as a framework anywhere along the disease trajectory, such as advance care planning, discussing treatment options or resuscitation orders, or introducing hospice care. This protocol was adapted from the SPIKES communication protocol for the delivery of bad news, which is discussed in Chapter 3. It is used in the Education for Physicians on End-of-life Care Project.[9]

The protocol uses the general principle of shared decision making. This principle is considered the current standard of care for medical decision making in the United

States.[10] Shared decision making as a process puts great emphasis on patient auton-omy while acknowledging the physician's responsibility to make treatment recom-mendations that are based both on the patient's stated overall goals of care and the physician's medical expertise. The protocol for goals-of-care discussions described here not only reflects common communication styles in the United States but is also strongly influenced by the society's current bioethical value system. Health care professionals balance the underlying ethical principles of autonomy, beneficence, nonmaleficence, and fairness with a strong emphasis on autonomy.

Studies of health care decision making in other parts of the world show that different cultures prioritize these ethical values differently. It seems most common to place less emphasis on autonomy in favor of beneficence and nonmaleficence. For example, although more than 90% of U.S. physicians share a new diagnosis of cancer with their patients, only 44.5% of competent patients were informed of their prog-nosis by their physician in a study from southern France. Studies from China indicate that patients there are rarely informed of a new diagnosis of cancer. In African countries such as Nigeria, Egypt, and South Africa, the type and amount of informa-tion shared seem to depend on patient factors such as level of education or socio-economic status. Bruera and colleagues elicited an additional point when studying attitudes and beliefs of palliative care specialists in Canada, South America, and French-speaking Europe. In this study, all clinicians wanted to be told the truth about their own terminal illnesses, but physician predictions about their patients' wishes differed significantly: Whereas 93% of Canadian physicians thought their patients would wish to know the truth, only 26% of their European and 18% of their South American colleagues thought that most of their patients would want to know about their diagnosis.[11] These results invite the question regarding the degree to which the perceived differences reflect biases of local health care cultures rather than actual differences in patient preferences.

Attitudes toward truth telling also clearly change over time. In 1961, more than 90% of U.S. surgeons did not share a new diagnosis of cancer with their patients. This finding clearly contrasts with today's practice.

These trends demonstrate that medical decision making and information sharing are processes guided by values and underlying ethical principles that are influenced by culture and will change over time. The element of the protocol proposed here that helps to assess this is the step of asking the patient how much he or she wants to know. This permits the professional to adjust the approach for a given individual. Over time and according to the needs of individual patients and health care providers in different parts of the world, overall patterns may also change.

Discussing Goals of Care

Discussing goals is rarely a one-time event; rather, it is a process that develops over the course of multiple visits. The protocol suggested here can be applied at any stage of this process. The protocol relies on common techniques of verbal and nonverbal communication. Great emphasis is placed on empathic listening, a highly underes-timated skill in medical practice. In a patient–doctor interaction, fewer than 25% of patients are provided the opportunity to complete their opening statement of concerns; all others are interrupted in less than 20 seconds. Physicians then tend to focus on closed-ended questions in an attempt to retrieve information as quickly as possible. This approach risks that patients never have the chance to address their major concerns. As a matter of fact, most patients leave the office without ever having their concerns addressed. Because eliciting patient preferences is at the center of goals-of-care discussions, it is especially important to start out the conversation with an open-ended question, followed by active listening. This allows the patient to focus on his or her major concerns and sets the stage for patient-centered care. Active or empathic listening then includes nonverbal communication skills that show full attention such as good eye contact and leaning toward the patient as well as verbal empathic listening techniques such as reflection, paraphrasing, and validation.

When conveying medical information, it is generally recommended that the information be given in small pieces. The physician should use words that the patient can understand and should pause frequently to check for the patient's responses. The higher the emotional impact of the given information on the patient, the less likely the patient is to hear what is being said.[12] It may therefore be necessary to repeat the information at a later time. The use of written information, summary letters, or tape recordings improves patient recall and understanding.[13] In a study of 50 cancer patients, use of an informational videotape after a verbal goals-of-care discussion significantly altered patients' decisions regarding end-of-life care, increasing patients' choice for comfort care from 22% to 91%.[14]

Stone and colleagues suggest always preparing and having difficult conversations at three levels: facts, emotions, and identity issues involved.[15] An example of this triad regarding goals-of-care discussions is to first spend some time discussing the different clinical options such as further chemotherapy versus hospice care; then look for and validate the patient's emotional responses such as fear, worry, and sadness. Last but not least, the physician then reflects on what the discussed options will mean for the patient's and health care provider's identity. Examples of identity issues that influence goals-of-care discussions are as follows: "I have always been a fighter and now you're asking me to give up?" or "I am not someone who just gives up on a patient."

Examples of the communication techniques used in this protocol are given under each step.

Six-Step Protocol

A stepwise approach to goals-of-care discussions helps to remind the clinician to include all major components of the discussion. This is particularly true for those who are inexperienced or early in their training, in whom this skill has generally not been demonstrated.[16] The six steps include preparing and establishing an appropriate setting for the discussion, asking the patient and family what they understand about the patient's health situation, finding out what they expect will happen in the future, discussing overall goals and treatment options, responding to emotions, and establishing and implementing a plan (Box 4-1).

1. PREPARE AND ESTABLISH AN APPROPRIATE SETTING FOR THE DISCUSSION

An important part of preparing for a goals-of-care discussion is to assess the patient's or family member's readiness to have this conversation and to address cultural or

---

Box 4-1. *Six Steps for the Discussion of Goals of Care*

1. Prepare and establish an appropriate setting for the discussion.
2. Ask the patient and family what they understand.
3. Find out what they expect will happen.
4. Discuss overall goals and specific options.
5. Respond to emotions.
6. Establish and implement the plan.

---

personal priorities regarding medical decision making in general. Ask whether your patient would want to have this discussion with you, if someone else should be present, or if your patient would prefer to defer it to someone else such as a family member or designated medical decision maker. A recent study from Australia comparing awareness of treatment goals in patients and their caregivers shows significant discrepancy in nearly half of patient–caregiver pairs, suggesting that you should attempt to include surrogates in as many of these conversations as possible.[17] You can elicit these preferences using the following sentences:

"Some patients like all the information; others like me to speak with someone else in the family. I wonder what is true for you."
"Tell me how you like to receive medical information."
"It there anyone else you would like to have present for our discussion?"

When you enter the actual goals-of-care discussion, do it with a clear understanding of the purpose of the meeting and be prepared to discuss information that the patient and family will need to learn. An example could be the outcomes of different treatment options such as chemotherapy, cardiopulmonary resuscitation survival data, and common treatment side effects. In general, patients are more interested in outcomes ("Life is not worth living if I won't be able to speak") than in the details of interventions ("That means that we would have to put a tube down your throat that is about as thick as your finger").[18]

In addition to medical information, it can be helpful before entering the discussion to reflect on expected emotional responses and possible identity issues as discussed earlier. This approach allows you to gain more insight into the patient's and family's perspective and to feel prepared, especially when their perspective seems "unrealistic."

Arrange to have the meeting itself in a private and comfortable place where everyone participating can sit at eye level. The atmosphere should be unhurried and undisturbed. After general introductions, the purpose of the meeting should be made clear. You can introduce the subject by phrases such as the following:

"I'd like to talk to you about your overall goals of care."
"I'd like to review where we are and make plans for the future."
"I'd like to discuss something today that I discuss with all my patients."

2. ASK THE PATIENT AND FAMILY WHAT THEY UNDERSTAND

Start out with an open-ended question to elicit what the patient understands about his or her current health situation. This is an important question and one that many clinicians skip. If the doctor is doing all the talking, the rest of the conversation is unlikely to go well. You could start with phrases such as the following:

"What do you understand about your current health situation?"
"Tell me how you see your health."
"What do you understand from what the doctors have told you?"

Starting with these questions not only helps to establish trust and set the tone for patient-centered decision making, it also helps to address misconceptions and conflicting or missing information and allows you a quick glimpse into the patient's emotional response to his or her current health state, such as fear, anger, or acceptance. More time may be needed to clarify the current situation before the patient is able to address future medical decisions.

3. FIND OUT WHAT THEY EXPECT WILL HAPPEN

For patients who have a good understanding of the status of their disease, the third step is to ask them to consider their future. Examples of how you could start are as follows:

"What do you expect in the future?"
"Have you ever thought about how you want things to be if you were much more ill?"
"What are you hoping for?"

This step allows you to listen while the patient has the opportunity to contemplate and verbalize his or her goals, hopes, and fears. This step creates an opportunity for you to clarify what is likely or unlikely to happen. You may need to ask follow-up questions to understand the patient's vision of the future as well as his or her values and priorities more clearly. If there is a significant discontinuity between what you expect and what the patient expects from the future, this is the time to discover it.

4. DISCUSS OVERALL GOALS AND SPECIFIC OPTIONS

Now that you have set the stage for a joint understanding of the patient's present and future, you can discuss overall goals of care and specific options. Allowing the patient to reflect on goals that may still be realistic despite reduced functional abilities and a limited life expectancy can be a very effective tool to maintain hope and build trust. Your insight into the patient's values and priorities should then structure the conversation of medical options and should guide your expert opinion. Use language that the patient can understand, and give information in small pieces. As discussed earlier, you should focus the discussion on treatment outcomes rather than on details of medical interventions.[18,19] Stop frequently to check for emotional reactions and to clarify misunderstandings.

It is often helpful to summarize the patient's stated overall goals and priorities as an introduction to the specific options. Following the principle of shared decision making, after the discussion of the available options, you should make clear recommendations that are based both on the patient's stated overall goals of care and on your medical expertise. For example:

> *"You have told me that being at home with your family is your number one priority and that the frequent trips to the hospital have become very bothersome for you. You do have three options at this point (...). Getting hospice care involved seems to be the option that best helps you to realize your goals."*
>
> *"If I heard you correctly, your first priority is to live to participate in your granddaughter's wedding in June. Taking that into account, it may be best to continue the current therapy and try to treat your nausea with a stronger regimen."*
>
> *"I heard you say that you are particularly concerned about being a burden to your children. By getting the hospice team involved, your family could get extra support from the nurse, chaplain, and social worker who would come to see you at the house."*
>
> *"It is clear you want to pursue all options to extend your life as long as possible. That includes being cared for in an intensive care setting with maximal support. However, if you are unable to communicate, and there is no reasonable chance of recovery, you want life support to be stopped."*

A recent Canadian analysis of expert opinion regarding "code status" discussions suggests that clinicians may initiate them at any point during an illness or even when a patient is in good health. The discussion should be framed as an overall goals discussion. It should distinguish between life-sustaining therapies (LST) and cardiopulmonary resuscitation (CPR); describe a cardiac arrest, CPR, LST, and palliative care; explain outcomes of cardiac arrest; offer a prognosis; and make clear recommendations.[20]

A study looking at U.S. patient and caregiver preferences regarding end-of-life care conversations shows that these discussions should include different treatment options, future symptoms, a description of the terminal phase, and patient preferences for place of death. Fears about dying should be addressed, and myths dispelled. The needs of patients and caregivers differed significantly when discussing dying: whereas patients emphasized the importance of reassurance that pain would be controlled and their dignity maintained, caregivers often wanted more detail about the terminal phase and practical information about how to look after a very sick person. Both wanted reassurance that their health care professionals would be available.[21]

5. RESPOND TO EMOTIONS

Patients, families, and health care providers may experience profound emotions in response to an exploration of goals of care. It should not be surprising that patients, when considering the end of their life, may cry. Parents of children with life-threatening diseases are especially likely to be emotional and need extra support from the health care team. In contrast to common worries in the health care community, however, emotional responses tend to be brief. Respond sympathetically. The most profound initial response a provider can make may be silence and offering a facial tissue. Consider using phrases such as the following:

"I can see this makes you sad."
"Tell me more about how you are feeling."
"People in your situation often get angry. I wonder what you are feeling right now."
"I notice you are silent. Will you tell me what you are thinking?"
"Many people experience strong emotions. I wonder whether that is true for you."

A common barrier to this step is the physician's fear to precipitate overwhelming emotional outbursts that they may not be able to handle. Therefore, conversations between physicians and their patients remain in the cognitive realm where emotions are not addressed.[22] The best way to overcome this barrier is to learn how to respond to patient emotions empathically and to learn to be comfortable with silence. Most patients are embarrassed by being emotional and keep their discussions brief. This is because most patients have adequate coping skills and appreciate the presence of a doctor while they work through the experience and their emotions. As with most aspects of being a physician, a sense of competence then leads to a willingness to engage in the challenge.

6. ESTABLISH AND IMPLEMENT THE PLAN

The last step of the goals-of-care discussion protocol involves the establishment and implementation of a plan on which the patient, family members, and physician can agree. You should verbalize a plan that is clear and well understood by everyone involved. Consider using language such as the following:

"You said that it is most important for you to continue to live independently for as long as possible. Because you are doing so well right now and need your current breathing machine only at night, we will continue what we are doing. However, when your breathing becomes worse, you do not want to be placed on a continuous breathing machine. We will then focus on keeping you comfortable with medicines to making sure that you do not feel short of breath."

"The different regimens we have used to fight your cancer are not working. There is no other anticancer therapy that is known to be effective. We discussed your options at this point including getting a second opinion from one of my oncology colleagues or asking a hospice program to get involved in your care. In light of what you told me about your worries about being a burden to your family, you thought that hospice care may be the best option at this point because you would get extra help at home from the hospice team members that come to see you at your house. I am going to call the hospice team today and arrange for them to call you in the morning so they can see you and explain more about what they offer. We can talk more after you see them."

It is often helpful to ask patients or family members to summarize the plan and underlying reasoning in their own words to ensure understanding. Especially for emotionally overwhelmed patients, good continuity of care is important. Ensuring this continuity, for example by arranging for follow-up appointments, speaking to the referring physician, or writing the appropriate orders, is part of the clinician's responsibility. You may want to conclude your conversation with information that gives hope such as a promise of ongoing care.

CASE STUDY

T. S. is a fully independent 53-year-old woman with breast cancer, metastatic to bone. Stage II breast cancer was diagnosed 10 years ago (premenopausal) and was treated with lumpectomy, radiation, and cyclophosphamide-methotrexate–5-fluorouracil chemotherapy. She has received two cycles of doxorubicin (Adriamycin) and paclitaxel chemotherapy. She has multiple bothersome symptoms including neuropathic pain and nausea. During a follow-up visit, T. S. asks you about continuing the chemotherapy. You recognize T. S.'s question as an opportunity to assist her and the health care team to define the goals of care.

After inviting T. S. and her husband into a meeting room, you ask what she understands about her current situation. T. S. is able to describe that her cancer has spread to her bones and wonders whether this means that she will die soon. Her husband knows the cancer cannot be cured. In response to a question about her goals, she says she hopes the cancer will go into "remission." T. S. starts to cry and grabs her husband's hand. "I will be a grandmother soon, I want to see that child grow up, spend time with my family—there is so much we never had time for." Her husband says he does not want her to continue chemotherapy if it is not going to help or if the suffering will be too great. After a moment of silence, you reflect on how difficult all this must be for them and how much you hope that she will be able to reach her goals. T. S. has had several chemotherapy-associated side effects, including persistent delayed nausea and neuropathic pain that is likely related to the chemotherapy. You clarify that it is too soon to know whether this chemotherapy is going to work, but there are things that can be done to help with the nausea and pain. You recommend that continued anticancer treatment is the option most consistent with her goals at this point if the side effects of further chemotherapy are tolerable. You make some suggestions about symptom control and volunteer to telephone her oncologist to confirm your role in the overall plan and to communicate your suggestions. After confirming the patient's understanding of the plan by asking her to repeat it in her own words, you reassure her and her husband that you will revisit goals each time you get together and that you and the oncologist will remain in close touch.

PEARLS

- **Goals are not static and goals-of-care discussions are not a one-time task.**

- **Start with the "big picture."** Many health care providers skip steps 2 and 3 (finding out what the patient understands and expects to happen) and lunge straight into detailed descriptions of medical interventions. These two simple questions set the stage. They show that you are interested in the patient and his or her experience and want to support the patient to achieve his or her goals. Starting from the patient's perspective is not only an invaluable tool to establish trust and a feeling of safety for the patient, but it also makes giving recommendations much easier for you later. When the "big picture" goals are clearly understood, the discussion of specific medical interventions most commonly falls quickly into place.

- **Deferring autonomy is an act of autonomy.** We often come across situations in which a concerned family member asks us not to disclose health care information to our patient. This can make us very uneasy because it interferes with our understanding of patient autonomy; conversely, do we not want to be accused of "truth dumping." You can solve this "dilemma" by first verbalizing understanding for the family member's concern and then conveying that you will need to double check with the patient if this is how he or she would like to proceed (if you have not done that already). When you see the patient alone, ask how he or she would like to handle medical information and decision making. You can use words such as these: "Some people want to know all medical information as we find it and discuss all options with the doctor. Others would rather have their children make decisions and do not want to have to deal with the medical information. Where do you stand?"

- **Cultural competence.** In a multicultural society such as the United States, clinicians are likely to care for patients and families from many different backgrounds. The term *culture* is used here in the broad sense and includes ethnic, religious, social, and professional cultures such as the culture of the local hospital or another specialty. Each of these cultures has its own values and language. Sensitivity to differences in cultural background helps to facilitate communication and understanding. When inquiring about cultural backgrounds, you can use sentences such as this: "People from different backgrounds handle death and dying very differently. Is there anything that we should be aware of regarding your care?"

- **Validate "unrealistic" or conflicting goals.** Physicians are sometimes frustrated by their patients' "unrealistic" goals. "They just don't get it" is a common reason for palliative care consultation requests. Reflecting on our own goals in life, most of us have some hopes that may not be very realistic ("I wish I could win the lottery") but still valid. The great difference lies in how we handle these hopes: Are we leading our life counting on what seems an unrealistic hope? An often cited example of this is a terminally ill parent who is unable to make the necessary arrangements for his or her minor children. A useful strategy to support hope but at the same time assist in making appropriate plans for the future is the "plan B" approach: "Although we hope for plan A, let's also prepare for plan B." Another useful way to validate your patient's hope is the "I wish" statement. An example could sound like this: "I wish this comes true for you. Whatever happens, we will be there for you." Intermittent denial of a terminal prognosis verbalized as unrealistic hopes can be a proficient way of coping and should be accepted as such.

- **Professional translation services rather than hospital staff, family, or volunteers should be used to translate important information.**[13]

PITFALLS

Preparation

- **The goals-of-care discussion happens too late.** We often delay goals-of-care discussions until a catastrophic event makes medical choices no longer meaningful.[23]

- **Patient or family readiness is not assessed.** Pushing this conversation upon a patient and family without evaluating their readiness to consider this profound, often highly emotional topic can lead to significant alienation and suffering.

- **The clinician has an agenda.** If you find yourself entering the room with your own agenda (e.g., to "get the DNR" or to "stop this futile treatment"), you may be headed for trouble. Try to understand the patient's values and priorities first, to assist you in making appropriate medical recommendations that are most likely to achieve the patient's goals. An awareness of the possible agendas of all parties involved in a goals-of-care discussion, such as yourself, patients and families, consultants, or hospital administrators assists in understanding the different perspectives and prevents adversarial outcomes.

- **The stakeholders are not identified.** You may have facilitated a picture-perfect goals-of-care discussion and thought that everyone agreed on a reasonable plan only to find out that the "cousin from out of town" flew in last night and threw over the whole plan. Before starting a goals-of-care discussion, always make sure that all stakeholders are present, over the phone if necessary, or otherwise represented to the extent possible. Stakeholders also include other health care providers involved in the patient's care. Consistency among different clinicians, especially regarding prognostication and when suggesting a plan of care, is of vital importance to maintain trust and avoid suffering.

- **Homework is not done.** Be prepared to answer questions regarding the outcomes and evidence of discussion interventions, such as resuscitation survival data, prognosis, and side effects of treatments. Just as in any other informed consent discussion, patients need accurate information to make good decisions.

Discussion of Overall Goals and Specific Options

- **Information sharing is ineffective.** Each person handles information differently. Although some patients want to understand the numerical probability of success or failure of specific interventions, others do not comprehend statistical information. Many clinicians share an excessive amount of medical details (because it is familiar or interesting to the clinician) using language that the patient cannot understand. Tailor the actual information giving to your patient's needs. It may be helpful to ask the patient to repeat the information back to you using his or her own words. When discussing options, avoid using diffuse language such as "heroic interventions," "comfort care," or "good quality of life" because everyone has a different understanding of what these mean.

- **Care is linked to acceptance of a limited prognosis.** When the clinician unintentionally links the relief of suffering to the demand upon the patient or family to accept a limited prognosis, this may disrupt trust.[23]

Shared Decision Making, Informed Consent, and Decision-Making Capacity

- **The person does not have or is inappropriately denied decision-making capacity.** Before asking someone to make a decision regarding goals of care, ask yourself whether that person has decision-making capacity. This is usually the case if a person can summarize the decision in his or her own words,

PITFALLS—con'd

including appropriate underlying reasoning. Patients with delirium, dementia, depression, or other mental health problems may be able to demonstrate decision-making capacity. This right should not be taken away from them inappropriately. Decision-making capacity is specific for each decision at a specific point in time. A person may be able to make a specific decision at the next visit even if he or she was unable to make it today.

● **The physician offers "restaurant-menu medicine."** The process of shared decision making strongly values patient autonomy, but it also recognizes the duty of the health care provider to make recommendations, based on his or her medical expertise, that are most likely to achieve the patient's stated goals. Many physicians skip this step. It leaves the patient feeling lost and the physician often frustrated as the "waiter" offering different medical options as if they were items on a restaurant menu for the patient to choose.

Summary

Addressing goals of care periodically over the course of a patient's illness is an important part of patient-centered care and has been shown to increase patient satisfaction and to decrease stress and anxiety.[24,25] The outcome of goals-of-care discussions should guide our therapy and will assist us in supporting our patients through stressful life transitions. In this chapter we have discussed a simple, six-step protocol that can be used to facilitate these types of discussions. It is intended as a road map, highlighting the key components of successful negotiations. It is well known that communication is an important part of medical care. As with any other skill, good communication skills are learned with practice over time. The techniques used in this model can be applied to many other fields of patient care and to personal interaction in general.

Resources

Pal Med Connect. Talk to a palliative medicine expert via a free telephone resource hotline for medical professionals. 1-877-PAL-MED4 (1-877-725-6334) or http://www.palmedconnect.org

American Academy on Physician and Patient: AAPP is devoted to the enhancement of physician-patient communication. This organization hosts an annual course on communication skills training. http://www.physicianpatient.org

OncoTalk: A National Cancer Institute–supported biannual retreat for oncology fellows to improve communication skills at the end of life. http://www.oncotalk.info

Bigby J: *Cross-Cultural Medicine*, Philadelphia, 2003, American College of Physicians.

References

1. Jenkins V, Fallowfield L, Saul J: Information needs of patients with cancer: results from a large study in UK cancer centers, *Br J Cancer* 84:48–51, 2001.
2. Goldberg R, Guadagnoli E, Silliman RA, Glicksman A: Cancer patients' concerns: congruence between patients and primary care physicians, *J Cancer Educ* 5:193–199, 1990.
3. Tulsky JA, Fischer GS, Rose MR, Arnold RM: Opening the black box: how do physicians communicate about advance directives? *Ann Intern Med* 129:441–449, 1998.
4. Maguire P, Faulkner A, Booth K, et al: Helping cancer patients disclose their concerns, *Eur J Cancer* 32A:78–81, 1996.
5. Billings JA, Block S: Palliative care in undergraduate medical education: status report and future directions, *JAMA* 278:733–738, 1997.
6. The AM, Hak T, Koeter G, van Der Wal G: Collusion in doctor-patient communication about imminent death: an ethnographic study, *BMJ* 321:1376–1381, 2000.

7. Shorr AF, Niven AS, Katz DE, et al: Regulatory and educational initiatives fail to promote discussions regarding end-of-life care, *J Pain Symptom Manage* 19:168–173, 2000.
8. Fallowfield L, Jenkins V, Farewell V, et al: Efficacy of a Cancer Research UK communication skills training model for oncologists: a randomized controlled trial, *Lancet* 359:650–656, 2002.
9. Education for Physicians on End-of-life Care. Available at http://www.epec.net.
10. Committee on Quality of Health Care in America, Institute of Medicine: *Crossing the quality chasm: a new health system for the 21st century*, Washington, DC, 2001, National Academy Press.
11. Bruera E, Neumann CM, Mazzocato C, et al: Attitudes and beliefs of palliative care physicians regarding communication with terminally ill cancer patients, *Palliat Med* 14:287–298, 2000.
12. Eden OB, Black I, MacKinlay GA, Emery AE: Communication with parents of children with cancer, *Palliat Med* 8:105–114, 1994.
13. Rodin G, Zimmermann C, Mayer C, et al: Clinician-patient communication: evidence-based recommendations to guide practice in cancer, *Curr Oncol* 16:42–49, 2009.
14. El-Jawahri A, Podgurski LM, Eichler AF, et al: Use of video to facilitate end-of-life discussions with patients with cancer: a randomized controlled trial, *J Clin Oncol* 27, 2009. **Online publishment ahead of print.**
15. Stone D, Patton B, Heen S of the Harvard Negotiation Project: *Difficult conversations. How to discuss what matters most*, New York, 2000, Penguin Books.
16. Tulsky JA, Chesney MA, Lo B: See one, do one, teach one? House staff experience discussing do-not-resuscitate orders, *Arch Intern Med* 156:1285–1289, 1996.
17. Burns CM, Brooms DH, Smith WT, et al: Fluctuating awareness of treatment goals among patients and their caregivers: a longitudinal study of a dynamic process, *Support Care Cancer* 15:187–196, 2007.
18. Pfeifer MP, Sidorov JE, Smith AC, et al: The discussion of end-of-life medical care by primary care patients and physicians: a multicenter study using structured qualitative interviews. The EOL Study Group, *J Gen Intern Med* 9:82–88, 1994.
19. Frankl D, Oye RK, Bellamy PE: Attitudes of hospitalized patients toward life support: a survey of 200 medical inpatients, *Am J Med* 86:645–648, 1989.
20. Downar J, Hawryluck L: What should we say when discussing "code status" and life support with a patient? A Delphi analysis, *J Pall Med* 13, 2010. **Online publishment ahead of print.**
21. Clayton JM, Butow PN, Arnold RM, et al: Discussing end-of-life issues with terminally ill cancer patients and their carers: a qualitative study, *Support Care Cancer* 13:589–599, 2005.
22. Levinson W, Gorawara-Bhat R, Lamb J: A study of patient clues and physician responses in primary care and surgical settings, *JAMA* 284:1021–1027, 2000.
23. Weiner JS, Roth J: Avoiding Iatrogenic Harm to patient and family while discussing goals of care near the end of life, *J Pall Med* 9:451–463, 2006.
24. Tierney WM, Dexter PR, Gramelspacher GP, et al: The effect of discussions about advance directives on patients' satisfaction with primary care, *J Gen Intern Med* 16:32–40, 2001.
25. Roter DL, Hall JA, Kern DE, et al: Improving physicians' interviewing skills and reducing patients' emotional distress: a randomized clinical trial, *Arch Intern Med* 155:1877–1884, 1995.

CHAPTER 5

"Who Knows?" 10 Steps to Better Prognostication

G. MICHAEL DOWNING

10 Steps to Improve Prognostication	6. What Is Important to My Patient? To the Family?
1. Start with an Anchor Point	7. Use Probabilistic Planning and Discussion to "Foretell"
2. Assess Performance Status Changes	
3. Review Recent Biological and Laboratory Markers	8. Recognize Limitations of Prognostication
4. Utilize Palliative or End-Stage Prediction Tools	9. Review and Reassess Periodically
	10. Stay Connected
5. Clinician Prediction of Survival: Would I Be Surprised?	**Pearls**
	Pitfalls
	Summary

Although prognostication is most often associated with survival prediction, it is inextricably linked in a triad with diagnosis and treatment. Indeed, there is always the question of the likelihood (prognosis) that a test being ordered will accurately identify the problem. That is, should I put the patient through the investigations, what are the associated burden and costs, and will this likely lead to a diagnosis? Prognosis is also tied to treatment: Will a proposed treatment be successful, when, what would the likely adverse effects be, and how effective will it be in alleviating illness? Both evidence and judgment are required in deciding whether a particular patient will likely benefit from treatment.

So how are we when it comes to prognosis regarding survival prediction? Unfortunately, many patients and family members readily recall how inaccurately and insensitively physicians have given the "blunt" truth, or have avoided the subject altogether, whereas others have found comfort and support from the doctor. Both patients and their bereaved family may have long-lasting anger and difficulty when bad news has been broken badly and incorrectly.[1,2] In addition, prognostic discussion affects timely access to services, decisions about further treatment, funding allocation, and client decision making.[3] At the same time, it is ludicrous to expect that clinicians will be all knowing and will be precise for each individual patient when considering all diseases, all stages, and various treatment responses. So what are the issues, and can anything improve this?

Most physicians tend to overestimate survival by a factor of 1.2 to 5 times,[4] some are fairly accurate, and a few overly pessimistic. Such optimism can be due to limited clinical experience with end-of-life illness trajectories, a lack of skill or reliance on wrong factors to determine prognosis, dependence on selective recall (remembering only the significant and outlier cases from one's experience), the belief in a self-fulfilling prophecy that "positive attitudes" affect outcomes including survival, or even purposeful exaggeration to avoid removing hope.

The concern for hope in the presence of a terminal illness is quite legitimate in that one does not want to inflict harm such as depression or despair by disclosing a poor prognosis, but let's look further. Christakis discusses the value of being optimistic in that it preserves hope, provides encouragement, fosters treatment, and engenders confidence even in the face a terminal illness.[5] He then notes that the "ritualization of optimism" goes beyond this; it is the favorable outlook held by physicians in spite of, or even as a result of, evidence suggesting an unfavorable outcome. Although some physicians have made comments such as, "When in doubt, suspect recovery, and act accordingly," this may in fact be optimism that is out of proportion to the objective reality. This results in false hope and subsequent decision making by the patient and family that likely would have been different if they had known otherwise.

The flip side is "ritualization of pessimism," wherein purposeful disclosure is toward an unfavorable outcome. When both the stakes and degree of uncertainty are high, it can be regarded as a protective no-lose strategy. Christakis notes that some physicians have tried to rationalize this with statements such as, "It may often be better to be pessimistic because if the outcome proves poor, it was not unexpected; and if the outcome proves good, you are a hero." However, neither of these approaches, if intended as so, are helpful to a patient or family who are given information the physician feels should be stretched. These behaviors tend to occur where actual uncertainty of the outcome is higher, because if it is actually known, most will share accordingly. Thus, the skill and accuracy of prognostication come into play as well as the sharing of such information.

10 Steps to Improve Prognostication

As shown in Table 5-1, prognostication involves two overarching concepts: foreseeing and foretelling.[6] The clinician's internal formulation of a prognosis can be improved by linking with emerging evidence of relevant factors and prognostic tools to assist this, and external sharing of bad news by attention to other factors. By paying attention to each of the 10 steps, the prognosis for better prognostication is quite favorable.

1. START WITH AN ANCHOR POINT

It is best to start with what is known and what Quill and Epstein called an anchor point.[7] Most diseases do have general survival statistics that can be found in textbooks, journal articles, or via the web and are usually measured in 1-, 5-, and 10-year survival statistics. They are often based on a staging system, such as tumor-node-metastasis (TNM) staging in cancer, and response rates to first- and second-line

Table 5-1. 10 Steps to Better Prognostication

Concept		10 Steps to Better Prognostication		Action Steps
FORESEE	SCIENCE	Disease	1. Start with an anchor point.	• Obtain details of known survival stats by stage of disease, SEER web, etc.; speak with expert about 1-, 5-, and 10-year survival stats.
		Function	2. Assess changes in performance status (amount; rate of change).	• Use a functional status tool that is part of prognosis (e.g., PPS, KPS, ECOG) to assess illness trajectory.
		Tests	3. Know physical signs and laboratory markers related to prognosis.	• Examples of lab markers include ↑ WBC, ↓ % lymphocytes, ↓ albumin. • Physical signs include delirium, dyspnea, anorexia, weight loss, and dysphagia.
		Tools	4. Utilize palliative or end-stage prognostic tools.	• Tools include PPS, PaP, PPI, SHFM, CCORT, CHESS, nomograms, etc.
	SKILL	Judgment	5. Clinician prediction of survival: Would I be surprised?	• Use your clinical judgment to formulate prediction. • See if it fits with step 4 prognostic factors and adjust accordingly. • Remember common optimistic bias and adjust further.
FORETELL	ART	Center	6. What is important to my patient? To the family?	• Who/what do they want to know/not know? • Is it "how long" or "what will happen"? • What are their goals? What is hoped for?
		Frame it	7. Use probabilistic planning and discussion.	• Offer a ballpark range based on average survival ("Most will live ..."); discuss outliers. Talk in time blocks.
		Cautions	8. Share limitations of your prognosis.	• No one knows for sure; exceptions do occur. • Changes can occur at any time.
		Changes	9. Review and reassess periodically.	• "What is" will change, especially if triggers arise.
		Follow-up	10. Stay connected.	• Discuss advance care planning because things may change further at anytime. • Initiate effective symptom control. • Involve interprofessional and home teams; furthermore, patients want their physician to remain involved, even close to death, and will feel abandoned otherwise.

Modified from Downing M: *10 Steps to Better Prognostication*, Victoria, BC, Victoria Hospice Society, 2009. © 2009 M. Downing. Victoria Hospice Society.

CHESS=Changes in Health End-Stage Signs and Symptoms; CCORT=Canadian Cardiovascular Outcomes Research Team; ECOG=Eastern Cooperative Oncology Group; KPS=Karnofsky Performance Scale; PaP=Palliative Prognostic Score; PPI=Palliative Performance Index; PPS=Palliative Performance Scale; SHFM=Seattle Heart Failure Model.

treatments. For example, the prognosis for stage I melanoma is very different than stage III,[8] and the diagnosis of metastatic brain cancer alters prognosis significantly. Chronic kidney disease and heart failure (New York Heart Association [NYHA] classification) are other examples where staging has prognostic value. They provide a realistic anchor or ballpark from which to begin, as well as a quick review of the illness trajectory and potential future complications. Discussion of one's patient with the relevant specialist is invaluable. Relying solely on personal prior cases is problematic and likely to lead to optimistic or pessimistic bias.

2. ASSESS PERFORMANCE STATUS CHANGES

Continued evidence points toward performance status as one key factor in prognosis for advanced and endstage disease. A common pathway[9] in the last 6 months before death in cancer patients is a steady, almost linear, functional decline that is frequently accompanied by cachexia, anorexia, tiredness, and other symptoms. In the frail elderly with advanced dementia, the decline is very gradual, but final symptoms of dysphagia, development of decubitus skin breakdown, and aspiration pneumonia accompany such frailty and may act as sentinel event flags.

For patients with chronic diseases like congestive heart failure, chronic obstructive pulmonary disease, or end-stage renal disease, it is more difficult to judge, because with acute-on-chronic decompensation and complications rapid decline is often followed by improvement from treatment. Patients may fully regain their previous functional status with initial bouts, but over time, exacerbations requiring hospital admission occur more often and with only partial improvements. The simple question, "Would I be surprised if the patient died within the next 6 months?" can act as a good trigger to reassess the patient and discuss advanced care planning.

One way to visualize the amount and rate of change in functional status is using time blocks,[10] along with a performance status scale such as the Palliative Performance Scale,[11] Eastern Cooperative Oncology Group (ECOG) performance status, the Karnofsky Performance Status in cancer, or other measures such as activities of daily living (ADL). For example, one may assess any functional change in several prior 4-month blocks going back 1 year or possibly more to gauge any differences. When things are changing, move to shorter time blocks such as 4 weeks or 4 days, and vice versa if stable or improving. Sudden change can occur at any time and should be addressed. Using time blocks to show the patient how much and how rapidly change is occurring can assist the clinician to identify and discuss with the patient a number of "what if's" to gauge how much treatment the patient may want if such were to occur.

3. REVIEW RECENT BIOLOGICAL AND LABORATORY MARKERS

Other than accidental or sudden death, a declining trajectory in advanced illness inevitably involves physical and laboratory alterations. Physical decline with delirium, dyspnea, dysphagia, weight loss, persistent tiredness, or development of skin breakdown commonly foreshadows the terminal stage. Laboratory findings that have prognostic significance include leukocytosis in association with lymphocytopenia; elevated C-reactive protein (CRP); low albumin; elevated lactate dehydrogenase (LDH); low sodium; and elevated B-type natriuretic peptide (BNP) in heart disease.[12-15]

Some of these abnormalities may not in and of themselves be prognostic, but they often occur with several diseases and complications. It is perhaps the combined relationship of declining functional status along with changing physical and laboratory findings that should alert the physician.

4. UTILIZE PALLIATIVE OR END-STAGE PREDICTION TOOLS

A systematic review by Lau[16] found several validated prediction scales or tools that could be used to compare with the physician's view of prognosis. Because they use population-based data, they are not exact and so an individual case could fit anywhere in these projections. They do help in figuratively moving from which "ballpark" the patient is in to whether he or she is now in the outfield or infield. Such probability issues are discussed later. Some provide the likelihood of 30-day survival, such as the Palliative Prognostic (PaP) Score,[17] which incorporates performance status (Karonfsky), clinician prediction, laboratory values, and several symptoms; the Palliative Performance Scale (PPS), using performance, intake, and consciousness level; and the Palliative Performance Index (PPI).[18]

Other examples of tools included in Lau's review are for heart failure (Heart Failure Risk Scoring System); dementia (Dementia Prognostic Index); cancer (Intrahospital Cancer Mortality Risk Model, Cancer Prognostic Score); and, for the elderly, Prognostic Index for 1-Year Mortality in Older Adults (PIMOA) and Changes in End-Stage Signs and Symptoms (CHESS).

Survival tables and Kaplan-Meier graphs provide general population sampling, and nomograms and algorithms break down data further by age, gender, disease, and so on and are preferable if available. Examples of the latter in heart failure patients are the Seattle Heart Failure Model[19] and the Canadian Cardiovascular Outcomes Research Team (www.CCORT.ca). Several nomograms for patients with breast, colon, and bladder cancers can be found on the internet.

5. CLINICIAN PREDICTION OF SURVIVAL: WOULD I BE SURPRISED?

The final part of "foreseeing" is clinical skill and judgment. It cannot be expected that medical students or clinicians early in practice will have had the experience of seeing many patients die and noting the manner and timing of these deaths. On the other hand, they are also not clouded by recall bias, and all physicians, including those specializing in palliative medicine, need to be aware of their personal tendency to optimism or pessimism in forecasting survival. It is likely that those who are generally good at prognostication are utilizing many of the factors discussed earlier and have distilled these into skilled judgment. Yet the sudden occurrence of complications, even if not unforeseen, make this more difficult, such as if and when a patient may hemorrhage or develop sepsis, a bowel obstruction, or a fall with resulting hip fracture.

The "surprise" question is not so much about whether one thinks the person will in fact die as it is about the risk of dying and whether it would be perplexing or startling that it occurred. If the answer is no, then one is becoming more attuned to possible demise, and this may alert clinicians to observe the patient more closely for signs such as those noted earlier and also provide opportunity to raise the topic of advanced care planning. A simple but valuable practice point is to jot down in patients' charts your clinician prediction of survival (CPS), or several CPSs over a period of time, and then compare these with the actual survival time. Doing so may help to refine your skill and identify a tendency to overestimate or underestimate survival.

6. WHAT IS IMPORTANT TO MY PATIENT? TO THE FAMILY?

A detailed discussion of communication skills and breaking bad news is beyond the scope of this chapter. The "foretelling" aspect of prognostication is, however, the most important, because one can just as easily harm as help. The approach to discussion and disclosure should always be individualized. Although the physician must be guided by the patients' wants at this point, be aware that patients commonly expect the following of their physician[20]:

- To be realistic
- To listen well
- To communicate in a straightforward and clear manner
- To be sensitive and empathic, especially when delivering a poor prognosis
- To allow time for questions
- To maintain realistic hopes
- To not abandon them

Although it is advocated and indeed helpful to hold a family conference to discuss prognosis, especially if the news is not good, caution is needed in first understanding divergence toward death. This means that the needs and desires for specific information often become different between the patient, who may want less information, and the family, who may need more information.[21] It can sometimes be too much for the patient to hear details of prognosis and expected decline, but this can be quite valuable for the family. Some patients, of course, will want as much information as possible and want the family in attendance, whereas other patients, if asked beforehand by the physician, may decline to attend or leave some discussion with the family until the patient has left.

Culture and religion may also affect what information regarding prognosis is expected and with whom it can be shared. It is imperative that the clinician check with the family and patient regarding how information is to be shared. One should not make assumptions about what is appropriate to share; taking an individualistic approach is imperative.

Before discussing survival information, ascertain the patient's and family members' hopes and goals, because this may help in deciding how to discuss prognosis. When patients ask how long they have to live, it may be preferable to begin with a qualitative prognosis ("You are likely to die from your cancer") rather than quantitative ("You are likely to die in 6 months"). That doesn't mean that is all the information you are prepared to share, but it is a reasonable starting point. In a survey by Kaplowitz, 80% wanted a qualitative prognosis, whereas only 53% wanted a quantitative prognosis.[22] The question of dashing all hope arises here, and a few points can be shared.

7. USE PROBABILISTIC PLANNING AND DISCUSSION TO "FORETELL"

Never give a specific time projection to patients because you will always be wrong, with the patient dying either before or after a stated prognosis. Many patients (and their families) hold anger when they are told they have 3 months or 1 year to live and make life plans and changes based on this information, only to find out such a "temporal" prediction was wrong. At the same time, saying, "No one knows," "I don't play god," or "Could be anytime" is equally unhelpful.

So what can be said and how? Having obtained some insight from the "foresee" section, you can then frame the discussion around the likelihood of death occurring, using facts such as the average survival, the median, or percentages. Patients and families usually prefer that the chances of living be given in lay terms, although some patients (e.g., academics, accountants, or scientists) may want actual numbers. There are exceptions and outliers that may help to frame the conversation. Here are some examples of what might be said:

> "We do not know for sure how long [John] has to live, but given his situation, the average time is about 3 months. That is, about one half of patients live longer than this and one half less. Most people (10%–90%) live somewhere between 1 to 6 months. However, [John] has now developed [complication]; even if we treat it, I feel this may place him on the shorter side of the 3-month time frame."

> "It is impossible to predict for any individual with certainty, but the average person with your condition will live[a few weeks to a few months, 3–6 months]. Treatment, if it works, might extend the time (a month or two). It could be longer and we can do everything possible. Unfortunately, it could also be shorter, so we need to be prepared just in case."[7]

> "It is hard to know for any given patient, but the average person with [Kevin's] illness and the recent changes in his condition will live only a few days or so. It could be longer if we are lucky, but it could also be shorter, so we should talk a little more about what to expect in the next little while, and how we can work to ensure he remains comfortable".[7]

> "[Mary] has changed a lot in the last few weeks, and even more over these past 3 days. It is difficult to know for sure, but if the same amount of change occurs in the next few days, then it is hard for me to see beyond that. She might live longer but I also think it could be quite short, perhaps even by tomorrow, so let's discuss your goals at this point and adjust our plan for what may occur."

These examples are not "guesswork" but illustrate how the reality of uncertainty can be balanced with the knowledge of the real facts of survival, current stage of disease, and expected complications for a given patient. They also provide aspects of hope within reasonable possibility.

8. RECOGNIZE LIMITATIONS OF PROGNOSTICATION

One obvious limitation in prognostication is that these tools and the clinician prediction of survival are based on populations with shared characteristics, not specific individuals. The Kaplan-Meier survival graph, for example, shows the line or curve of survival but does not identify where on that curve any particular patient is. As a palliative nurse noted, the patient at "PPS 30% has many faces".[23] So, will he or she die in a few days, early on the curve, or months later, in the 10th percentile? Second, treatment response may alter survival by controlling progression, causing improvement, and even resulting in cure; alternatively, the decline of treatment may adversely affect prognosis. Third, there is some evidence that psychosocial factors of the patient and family may influence decision making and survival as well as access to care or financial factors. Finally, the personal experience and skill of the clinician, as discussed earlier, affect understanding and accuracy.

In statistical terms, variations are related to the horizon effect (the farther away death is, the harder it is to predict), outliers, exceptions, odds ratios, correlation, precision, and calibration of prognosis. Thus, one's best prediction of prognosis should be modulated and informed by such factors. In doing so, the patient and family receive your best sense of prognosis within the context of its limitations; most will appreciate the attempt, the candor, and the compassion.

9. REVIEW AND REASSESS PERIODICALLY

Toward the end of life, things never stay the same for long. Depending on the disease and comorbidities, and where the patient is in his or her illness trajectory, various sudden or slowly progressive changes occur that will affect prognosis. Some diseases come with well-known complications; in other diseases, particularly when affecting the frail elderly, things may be unclear. In the latter, an interesting term, *ambiguous dying syndrome*,[24] refers to the fact that just a day or so before death, many patients are thought to have several months to live.

Currently, researchers are working to identify sentinel events or triggers that alter prognosis, such as pulmonary embolus, sepsis, and so on. Prognostication is not an event but a process, and therefore clinically one should reassess the patient at regular intervals. Quill and Epstein[7] suggested that the physician review and offer to discuss advanced advance care plans whenever the following occur:

- New diagnosis of serious illness occurs
- A major medical decision with an uncertain outcome must be made.
- The patient or family ask about prognosis.
- The patient or family request treatment not consistent with good clinical judgment.
- You answer no to the question, Would you be surprised if the patient died in 6 to 12 months?
- The patient is actively dying.

10. STAY CONNECTED

There is tremendous value in remaining connected through the final illness trajectory. As discussed earlier, being able to provide some insight on prognosis provides the patient and family opportunity to plan for final visits, share closure issues, and prepare for death. This can only happen with periodic reassessment of prognosis. For those who are at home, there is evidence that the likelihood of a home death is increased when the practitioner remains involved.

Irrespective of location, there is increased safety and reassurance, because nursing and medical visits are times where symptom control can be addressed based on declines in physical status and expected complications. One adage to remember is that toward the end of life, things never stay the same for long, and so plans need to be altered. This leads to valuable discussions and reclarification of goals, hopes, and any change to the advance care plan. Visits do not have to be long; the physician's presence, rather than the amount of time spent on the visit, is what most patients and families find comforting. Finally, personal satisfaction in one's medical career can be enhanced and reinforced when clinicians remain connected through death and bereavement. Therefore, we need to foresee and foretell, but not forego.

PEARLS

○ Using prognostic tools can improve accuracy and reinforce clinical judgment.

○ Prognostication is a process, not a proclamation; use probabilistic ranges, percentages, and caveats.

○ Toward the end of life, things never stay the same for long; thus, it is crucial to review, revise, and refine.

○ Practice assessing your own tendency to overestimate or underestimate prognosis by noting in the chart your estimate and checking the accuracy later.

○ Hope is like dignity and can be crushed in an instant. Unrealistic hope can dash dreams and plans, so empathy and checking with the patient on the desire for information are important.

○ Closer to death, patients often want less information, whereas families need more.

○ Asking "How long do I have?" is partly about prognosis itself but also an opportunity to inquire about fears, misinformation, hopes, and goals. It also offers opportunity to discuss specific plans on how to manage dying, and how the team will assist—that is, it is not just about time but reassurance in how you will care for them when they can't communicate with you.

○ If you are in a hospice palliative program or a facility where death is common, it may be valuable to build a database for the patient profile being cared for and use prognostic tools such as PPS,[25,26] PPI,[18] or PaP[17] to create prediction tables appropriate to the palliative patient profile in that community to assist in formulating a prognostication.

○ The 10 points can also be simplified into 4 Things to Know[10]:

1. Know the disease
   - Current stage and survival statistics (and quartile limits)
   - Prior response to active treatments
   - Available treatments and likelihood of benefit/burden
   - Likely complications in the near future and implications for survival

2. Know your patient
   - Remaining goals, hopes, plans
   - Likelihood of choosing/refusing active treatment in the face of disease progression/complications
   - Possibility that active treatment may alter downward trajectory
   - Actual PPS time-block changes[10] that are unique to patient
   - "Foreseen" survival based on prognostic tools and clinician prediction

3. Know your process for sharing
   - "Foretell" using known "bad news" guidelines (e.g., SPIKES, RELATE, or PREPARE)
   - Be helpful, not hurtful
   - Be honest—including hopefulness, not hopelessness

4. Know yourself
   - Improve prognostication using 10 steps
   - Be present, not absent
   - Disclose, not impose
   - "Practice" prognosticating—record and measure

PITFALLS

- Guessing doesn't work; it more often harms, and your credibility and confidence will suffer.
- Avoiding doesn't help; it simply forestalls effective decision making, and you may appear indifferent.
- Bluntness almost always injures; kindness is more likely to heal.
- Be culturally and individually careful; not all can or want to hear such information.

Summary

The science and art of prognostication should remain as important in medicine as diagnosis and treatment. To do so, clinician predictions of survival, while invaluable, need to be augmented with emerging value of prognostic tools, tables, algorithms, and nomograms. Because one dies only once, it behooves physicians to provide information as accurately and compassionately as possible so that patients and families can make decisions that best fit their time frame, hopes, and goals at the end of life. As a skill and art, assessment and communication do not just occur by happenstance; rather, they take practice and attention to one's tendencies toward optimism or pessimism. By utilizing other prognostic indicators and tools, skill can be honed. These 10 steps may assist clinicians in improving their personal prognostication skills.

Appreciation: These concepts have percolated with me for a while as I have formulated these points. My thanks to Drs. Timothy Quill and Ronald Epstein for several words that became triggers; to Drs. Paul Glare, Paddy Stone, and Chris Todd for supportive feedback; to Dr. Francis Lau for support in prognostic research; and to my wife, Theresa, for her nursing and partner support in completing this material.

References

1. Fallowfield L, Jenkins V: Communicating sad, bad, and difficult news in medicine, *Lancet* 363(9405):312–319, 2004.
2. Parkes CM: The dying adult, *BMJ* 316(7140):1313–1315, 1998.
3. Wright AA, Zhang B, Ray A, et al: Associations between end-of-life discussions, patient mental health, medical care near death, and caregiver bereavement adjustment, *JAMA* 300(14):1665–1673, 2008.
4. Glare P, Virik K, Jones M, et al: A systematic review of physicians' survival predictions in terminally ill cancer patients, *BMJ* 327(7408):195–198, 2003.
5. Christakis NA: The Ritualization of Optimism and Pessimism. In *Death foretold: prophecy and prognosis in medical care*, Chicago, 1999, University of Chicago Press, pp. 163–178.
6. Lamont E: Foreseeing: Formulating an Accurate Prognosis. In Glare P, Christakis NA, editors: *Prognosis in advanced cancer*, New York, 2008, Oxford University Press, pp 25.
7. Quill T, Epstein R: Discussing prognosis with patients and caregivers. Workshop at the American Academy of Hospice and Palliative Medicine Conference, March 25–28, 2009, Austin, Texas.
8. Balch CM, Soong S-J, Gershenwald JE, et al: Prognostic factors analysis of 17,600 melanoma patients: validation of the American Joint Committee on Cancer Melanoma Staging System, *J Clin Oncol* 19(16):3622–3634, 2001.
9. Lunney JR, Lynn J, Foley DJ, Lipson S, Guralnik JM: Patterns of functional decline at the end of life, *JAMA* 289(18):2387–2392, 2003.
10. Downing M, Deb B: Medical Care of the Dying. In Downing M, Wainwright W, editors: *Medical care of dying*, ed 4. Victoria, B. C., Canada, 2006, Victoria Hospice Society, pp. 602–604.

11. Ho F, Lau F, Downing GM, Lesperance M: Reliability and validity of the Palliative Performance Scale (PPS), *BMC Palliat Care* 7(10), 2008. Published online 2008 August 4. doi: 10.1186/1472-684X-7-10. PMCID: PMC2527603
12. Vigano A, Bruera E, Jhangri GS, et al: Clinical survival predictors in patients with advanced cancer, *Arch Intern Med* 160(6):861–868, 2000.
13. Maltoni M, Caraceni A, Brunelli C, et al: Prognostic factors in advanced cancer patients: evidence-based clinical recommendations—a study by the Steering Committee of the European Association for Palliative Care, *J Clin Oncol* 23(25):6240–6248, 2005.
14. Maltoni M, Pirovano M, Nanni O, et al: Biological indices predictive of survival in 519 Italian terminally ill cancer patients. Italian Multicenter Study Group on Palliative Care, *J Pain Symptom Manage* 13(1):1–9, 1997.
15. Berger R, Huelsman M, Strecker K, et al: B-type natriuretic peptide predicts sudden death in patients with chronic heart failure [comment], *Circulation* 105(20):2392–2397, 2002.
16. Lau F, Cloutier-Fisher D, Kuziemsky C, et al: A systematic review of prognostic tools for estimating survival time in palliative care, *J Palliat Care* 23(2):93–112, 2007.
17. Maltoni M, Nanni O, Pirovano M, et al: Successful validation of the palliative prognostic score in terminally ill cancer patients. Italian Multicenter Study Group on Palliative Care, *J Pain Symptom Manage* 17(4):240–247, 1999.
18. Morita T, Tsunoda J, Inoue S, Chihara S: The Palliative Prognostic Index: a scoring system for survival prediction of terminally ill cancer patients, *Support Care Cancer* 7(3):128–133, 1999.
19. Seattle Heart Failure Model [database on the Internet]. University of Washington, 2009 [cited]. Available at http://www.seattleheartfailuremodel.org.
20. Finlay E, Casarett D: Making difficult discussions easier: using prognosis to facilitate transitions to hospice, *CA Cancer J Clin* 59(4):250–263, 2009.
21. Tversky A, Kahneman D: The framing of decisions and the psychology of choice, *Science* 211(4481):453–458, 1981.
22. Kaplowitz S, Campo S, Chiu W: Cancer patients' desires for communication of prognosis information, *Health Commun* 14(2):221–241, 2002.
23. Downing T: *Care through death at home*, Victoria, BC, 2009, Palliative Care: Medical Intensive Course.
24. Bern-Klug M. The ambiguous dying syndrome, *Health Soc Work* 29(1):55–65, 2004.
25. Lau F, Downing M, Lesperance M, et al: Using the Palliative Performance Scale to provide meaningful survival estimates, *J Pain Symptom Manage* 38(1):134–144, 2009.
26. Downing GM, Lau F, Lesperance M, et al: Meta-analysis of survival prediction with the Palliative Performance Scale (PPSv2), *J Palliat Care* 23(4):245–255, 2007.

PART B

Physical and Psychological Symptoms

CHAPTER 6

Multiple Symptoms and Multiple Illnesses

S. LAWRENCE LIBRACH

The term *comorbidity* has been defined as follows:

The presence of coexisting or additional diseases with reference to an initial diagnosis or with reference to the index condition that is the subject of study.

Comorbidity may affect the ability of affected individuals to function and also their survival; it may be used as a prognostic indicator for length of hospital stay, cost factors, and outcome or survival.[1]

In the past, the term was not used to define the interplay of specific diseases and multiple symptoms. Here, the term is used to encompass both.

Patients who have advanced, progressive illness and those who are at the end of life rarely present with just one illness or symptom. Many of us will die with or of two or more chronic illnesses. In 1999, 65% of elderly persons in the United States had two or more types of chronic illnesses.[2] Elderly patients comprise most of those in need of palliative and end-of-life care. In 2002, three fourths of the deaths in the United States occurred in persons aged 65 years and older. Five of the six leading causes of death in this age group were chronic illnesses, including cancer, neurodegenerative diseases such as Alzheimer's disease, and organ (particularly cardiac) or system failure. The frequency and mortality rate of cancer increase with advancing years. The incidence of neurodegenerative diseases and advanced pulmonary, cardiovascular, and renal diseases also increases dramatically with age. Patients with diagnoses other than cancer often have less predictable and longer illness trajectories.[3] As a result, accurate prognostication, goals of care, and therapies are more difficult, and the issues of comorbidity are more prevalent.

Many patients who are at the end of life are also elderly persons who have experienced considerable changes in their function, drug pharmacokinetics, and social situations that also complicate management. Moreover, many clinical research studies exclude patients with significant comorbidities, thus making the application of the results of these studies less effective in the palliative care population. Underreporting of symptoms is a well-documented phenomenon in the elderly that makes symptom management difficult. Concern about being a burden on one's family may be one reason that symptoms are underreported.

Comorbid illnesses and symptoms may make prognosticating that much more difficult, may drastically change the prognosis of an illness such as cancer, may interfere with responses to therapy, and may pose a significant, independent threat to high-quality end-of-life care. Patients with comorbid conditions also have a variety of lifestyles, economic capabilities, families, and other psychosocial and spiritual issues that they bring with them into the terminal phase of their illnesses, and these factors can affect suffering and management of the illnesses.

The cost of care is also considerably affected by comorbid conditions. In one study of congestive heart failure, costs increased with each comorbid condition, especially diabetes and renal failure.[4] In 1999, 65% of the U.S. elderly population had two or more types of chronic medical conditions. Per capita annual expenditures were $1154 for those with one type, $2394 for those with two types, $4701 for those with three, and $13,973 for those with four or more chronic medical conditions.[5]

Superimposed on this multiple illness background and the age factor is the prevalence of many symptoms produced by these illnesses in addition to a superadded terminal illness such as cancer. Pain as a symptom has been the major focus of attention in palliative and end-of-life care. Poor pain treatment continues to be documented. Uncontrolled pain can add to suffering in multiple ways, and compliance with therapeutic regimens may decrease. Depression, loss of function, anxiety, and family problems may result. Pain management that also overlooks the need to manage its common adverse effects such as constipation, sedation, and decreased concentration or cognitive dysfunction can end up adding to suffering rather than reducing it.

Pain is rarely the only symptom, however. Other physical symptoms are common in patients near the end of life and are often not assessed adequately. This deficiency contributes substantially to suffering in terminally ill patients. One recent large study of patients with advanced cancer assessed the prevalence of symptoms.[6] The results are detailed in Table 6-1.

A systematic search of medical databases and textbooks identified 64 original studies reporting the prevalence of 11 common symptoms among patients with end-stage cancer, acquired immunodeficiency syndrome, heart disease, chronic obstructive pulmonary disease, or renal disease. This review consistently showed a high prevalence of almost all considered symptoms: pain, confusion, delirium, cognitive failure, depression, low mood, sadness, anxiety, dyspnea, fatigue, weakness, anorexia, nausea, diarrhea, constipation, insomnia, and poor sleeping.

Table 6-1. Symptom Prevalence in 922 Patients with Advanced Cancer*

Symptom	Number	Percent
Pain	775	84
Easy fatigue	633	69
Weakness	604	66
Anorexia	602	65
Lack of energy	552	60
Dry mouth	519	56
Constipation	475	52
Early satiety	473	51
Dyspnea	457	50
Sleep problems	456	50
Weight loss	447	49
Depression	376	41
Cough	341	37
Nausea	329	36
Edema	262	28
Taste change	255	28
Hoarseness	220	24
Anxiety	218	24
Vomiting	206	22
Confusion	192	21
Dizzy spells	175	19
Dyspepsia	173	19
Belching	170	18
Dysphagia	165	18
Bloating	163	18
Wheezing	124	13
Memory problems	108	12
Headache	103	11
Hiccup	87	9
Sedation	86	9
Aches/pains	84	9
Itch	80	9
Diarrhea	77	8
Dreams	62	7
Hallucinations	52	6
Mucositis	47	5
Tremors	42	5
Blackout	32	4

*From Walsh D, Rybicki L: Symptom clustering in advanced cancer, *Support Care Cancer* 14:831–836, 2006.

Most symptoms were found in one third or more of patients, and multiple symptoms occurred for all five diseases. However, two symptoms, pain and fatigue, were common in all five diseases, occurring in 34% to 96% and 32% to 90%, respectively. Breathlessness was common in most conditions, but it was most consistently found among patients with chronic obstructive pulmonary disease (minimum, 90%) and heart disease (minimum, 60%).[7]

Another recent study reviewed the prevalence of symptoms in 90 older U.S. adults. In this group, 42% had a diagnosis of chronic obstructive pulmonary disease, 37% had a diagnosis of congestive heart failure, and 21% had a diagnosis of cancer. The prevalence of symptoms, as measured by the Edmonton Symptom Assessment Scale, ranged from 13% to 87%. Limited activity, fatigue, physical discomfort, shortness of breath, pain, lack of well-being, and problems with appetite were experienced by the majority (>50%) of participants. Smaller proportions of participants experienced feelings of depression (36%), anxiety (32%), and nausea (13%).[8]

The prevalence of these symptoms in palliative care patients varied widely in other reports and depended on the trajectory of the patients' illnesses, the assessment tools used, and the selection of patients. These symptoms are often either undertreated or not recognized across care settings. More systematic assessments using multiple tools will uncover more symptoms, but options for effective treatment of these symptoms may be limited and often require numerous medications that can pose significant risks and added suffering because of adverse drug effects and interactions.

There is growing literature around the issues of multiple symptoms and clusters of symptoms. Research on symptoms has generally been focused on single symptoms. Patient age, gender, performance status, primary disease, race, symptom severity and distress, and symptom assessment method influence symptom prevalence and epidemiology. Symptom prevalence may also have socioeconomic factors. Symptom clusters such as pain, depression, and fatigue seem to be linked clinically and may have similar interdependent, pathophysiological processes.[9] Patients with cancer who have multiple symptoms have worse outcomes. The synergistic effect of symptoms that constitute a symptom cluster remains to be determined. Palliative care has traditionally understood the need to address multiple issues, but the comorbidities engendered by these multiple symptoms, comorbid illnesses, and multiple care systems provide new challenges in management.

Illustrative Case Studies

CASE STUDY 6-1

Albert is a 62-year-old man with advanced, non–small cell lung cancer with liver and bone metastases. He also has a 30-year history of diabetes mellitus and is insulin dependent. Diabetic complications include increased creatinine (175 mg/L), peripheral neuropathy, hypertension, hyperlipidemia, and mild macular degeneration. He was quite obese (at least 20 kg overweight) until recently and has severe osteoarthritis in one knee. He has developed increased, burning pain in both feet since undergoing chemotherapy. His bone pain and knee pain have been difficult to control with opioids (oxycodone), and he has had two episodes of toxicity from his opioids. Other symptoms include decreased appetite with a weight loss of 10 kg, several hypoglycemic episodes, a sacral ulcer (stage 2), and generalized weakness. He is taking multiple medications, including atorvastatin, ramipril, insulin, sustained-release oxycodone, immediate-release oxycodone, desipramine, sennosides, and lactulose. He was referred to the palliative care service for pain management.

Case Discussion

Even without considering his psychosocial and spiritual issues, this patient's management is made very complex because of the interplay of his diseases, symptoms, and functional disability. Considering his impaired renal function, pain management with oxycodone is a relatively good choice, despite some reports of toxicity in patients with renal failure. Morphine and hydromorphone are not good choices for patients with renal impairment because of the risk of buildup of active metabolites of these drugs. Methadone and transdermal fentanyl may be better choices, but methadone may have significant interactions with some of his other drugs, such as lorazepam and desipramine. The patient's episodes of toxicity occurred when his knee was very painful and he took more than six breakthrough doses over a nighttime period. One episode of toxicity occurred when he used sustained-release oxycodone as breakthrough medication because he was unable to read the label properly at night as a result of his macular degeneration. He had to stop his nonsteroidal anti-inflammatory drug because of his increasing creatinine level. His renal impairment also limits the doses of other neuropathic pain adjuvants such as gabapentin.

This patient's weakness and the limited walking ability caused by his osteoarthritic knee have been cofactors in the development of a painful, stage 2 sacral ulcer. He is not able to monitor his blood glucose very effectively because he is more tired and sleeps for long periods. He is more susceptible to hypoglycemic episodes because of decreased and sporadic food intake. Therefore, his insulin dose should be decreased, and his blood glucose should be allowed to remain in a higher range. Tight blood glucose control leaves him open to significant risk. He should be monitored on a weekly basis by his home care nurses, and control of his diabetes should be supervised by one physician to minimize communication problems.

A medication review is definitely in order. The risk of rhabdomyolysis is greater in patients with renal impairment. Even though he is on a low dose, the hyperlipidemia is the least of his worries at this time. A full medication review should be done on patients with advancing disease. The need for antihypertensive, lipid-lowering drugs (among others) should be assessed regularly, and drugs should be discontinued if benefits are not significant, if multiple drugs complicate care, or if drug discontinuation does not add to patient discomfort.

CASE STUDY 6-2

Antonia is a 54-year-old woman with advanced colon cancer. She was relatively healthy until 5 months ago, when she presented with a bowel obstruction. She was found to have obstructing ascending colon cancer with peritoneal seeding and para-aortic lymph node, sacral, and liver metastases. She had a bowel resection, but she had multiple episodes of partial bowel obstruction over the ensuing months that necessitated multiple hospitalizations. She has a number of persistent symptoms: moderate to severe abdominal pain, severe neuropathic pain in an S1 distribution in the right lower limb, nausea and occasional vomiting, intermittent diarrhea, anorexia, generalized weakness and fatigue, dry and sore mouth, difficulty concentrating, and anxiety panic attacks. This patient is receiving chemotherapy, but each session seems to increase all her symptoms for a few days. She was referred for symptom control. She is currently taking sustained-release morphine, 90 mg twice daily, with 10 mg every hour as necessary for breakthrough. This has helped her abdominal pain a little, but her leg pain is quite severe. She takes some dimenhydrinate for nausea and is taking ondansetron for chemotherapy-related nausea.

Case Discussion

On interviewing the patient, it was obvious that her leg pain was the most distressing symptom. She was not receiving any neuropathic pain adjuvants, and it was decided that she would start one. The question of drug choice for neuropathic pain depends on a number of factors. Tricyclic antidepressants would expose her to adverse effects that could be problematic. She was already experiencing dry mouth, and a tricyclic antidepressant would worsen that symptom. Constipation, another common side effect of tricyclic antidepressants, could be problematic in a person prone to bowel obstruction. Carbamazepine may also be contraindicated because of the common side effects of nausea and sedation and also because of her ongoing liver disease. Gabapentin was determined to be the best choice because its only usual side effect is sedation. She was started on that drug and was titrated to a dose of 900 mg/day. This provided a moderate amount of relief for her neuropathic pain, but attempts to increase the medication further were met with greater and intolerable sedation, as well as an increase in anorexia.

The use of sustained-release morphine tablets in this patient needs some review. This patient's shortened large bowel and the intermittent attacks of diarrhea may interfere with absorption of the morphine because of enhanced transit time through the bowel. She was switched to a transdermal fentanyl patch and was titrated to a dose of 125 mg/hour. The switch to the transdermal route also avoided the need to find alternative routes of morphine administration when she had more severe episodes of nausea and vomiting associated with intermittent bowel obstruction.

The patient was initially prescribed prochlorperazine for her nausea, but this caused too much sedation and some dystonic reaction. Octreotide was started in hospital and seemed to control her symptoms of nausea better, but she could not afford the cost of this medication. She was referred to a palliative home care program that covered her drug costs and the need for twice-daily injections.

CASE STUDY 6-3

George is a 44-year-old man with human immunodeficiency virus (HIV) disease. He has been positive for the virus for 8 years and has been on a regimen of drugs that have been successful in controlling all his disease markers, such as CD4 count and viral load. He had been followed every 3 months by his primary care physician, but he missed the last appointment. He was admitted to hospital with severe pneumonia, and his HIV markers have now worsened significantly. He was admitted to the critical care unit because of respiratory failure and is now on a ventilator. His condition is quite unstable because he is severely hypoxic. His brother is the substitute decision maker and provided more information to the critical care unit team and palliative care consultant in the critical care unit.

His brother stated that he has had some increasing concern about George's health for the last 2 months. George has seemed quite pale and ill, and he has also been quite depressed. His partner of 10 years left him about 4 months ago and moved to another city. George has had to change jobs and take a significant salary cut because of downsizing of the technology company for which he has worked. When George's brother was asked to bring in his brother's current medications, he brought in pill bottles of antiretrovirals that were full and had obviously been untouched for several months. He also brought his brother's journal, in which George had chronicled his decision to withdraw medication and his wish to die.

George's condition began to improve with treatment, and he was taken off the ventilator after 2 weeks. He was able to communicate and said that he just wished to die. An assessment indicated that he was depressed, but he refused treatment for his depression. The psychiatrist felt that George was competent to make such a decision, even in the presence of depression.

Case Discussion

Psychological issues, particularly depression, can be significant complicating features in end-of-life care. This patient had a long-term, chronic illness that was relatively stable until depression and social disruption led to his noncompliance with therapy. Depression can be a significant comorbidity that can lead to diminished quality of life, withdrawal from socialization, and noncompliance with medications and medical surveillance. In this case, the patient's depression was manifested as a wish to die by not complying with treatment.

CASE STUDY 6-4

Brenda is an 86-year-old woman who presented to the emergency department with delirium. Her daughter accompanied her. She was a resident in a senior home. She had a history of congestive heart failure several years ago, atrial fibrillation, hypertension, mild renal failure, and ischemic heart disease. She also had increasing problems with forgetfulness. Her medication list included the following drugs: digoxin, 0.125 mg once daily; furosemide, 20 mg once daily; ramipril, 10 mg once daily; atorvastatin, 20 mg once daily; nitroglycerin spray; paroxetine, 10 mg at bedtime; lorazepam, 1 mg at bedtime; donepezil, 5 mg once daily; acetaminophen with codeine, four to six tablets daily; omeprazole, 20 mg daily; risperidone, 0.5 mg once daily; sennoside tablets, 8.6 mg, two tablets once daily; ginkgo biloba tablets, twice daily; and a multivitamin.

On examination in the emergency department, the patient was quite agitated and confused. Her mucous membranes were dry, and her skin turgor was poor. Her blood pressure was 78/46 mm Hg, and her pulse was 90 and irregularly irregular. She had no edema. She had a loud diastolic murmur, and her liver was quite enlarged and nodular. She had a hard, fixed mass in the left lower quadrant. Her electrocardiogram showed a prolonged QT interval, and her digoxin level was in the toxic range. Her creatinine was 225 mg/L, and her urea was double the normal range. Her hemoglobin was only 90 g/L. All her liver function tests were elevated except for bilirubin, which was normal.

When asked for more information, Brenda's daughter said that her mother lived alone in a seniors' residence. There is a nurse present during the day in this home, but Brenda has rarely needed her assistance. Brenda's daughter had been away on vacation for the last 4 weeks, and when she returned home 2 days ago, she found her mother significantly changed. The doctor on call for the home prescribed risperidone because of Brenda's agitation, but no one examined her. Brenda's appetite had decreased markedly, and therefore her food and fluid intake have been very limited. No one remembers seeing her at meals in the residence for the last 2 days. Brenda had been responsible for administering her own medications, but her daughter found pills all over the small apartment.

Case Discussion

With a background of long-term cardiac disease and some memory problems that may have signaled early Alzheimer's disease, Brenda had become acutely ill. Although imaging had not been done yet, the likelihood that Brenda had cancer was evidenced by her liver findings and by the abdominal mass. In all likelihood, this added to her confusion, weakness, and anorexia.

One of her problems, the prolongation of her QT interval, was potentially life-threatening and was likely the result of a drug interaction between paroxetine and the recently added drug risperidone. Her severely disturbed liver function and its impact on drug metabolism may account for the adverse effects, particularly her confusion. Her confusion has added to her problems, as evidenced by the pills lying around her apartment. Could she have taken too much digoxin, as evidenced by her toxic levels of digoxin? Could her increasing confusion be a result of presumed cancer plus or minus progression of her dementia?

Numerous systems issues have contributed to her problems. No one was designated to keep an eye on Brenda while her daughter was on vacation. The supervision in the residence is limited, and patients in such settings can often go unmonitored for some time. Although dining room staff noted Brenda's absence from the dining room over the last 2 days, it was not reported to the nurse or to the administration. The on-call physician who prescribed the risperidone did not ask about other drugs and was not aware of the number of possible, significant drug interactions.

> **Box 6-1.** *Factors That Affect Morbidity and Suffering*
>
> **DISEASE FACTORS**
> Multiple symptoms: physical
> Multiple symptoms: psychological and spiritual
> Age
> Multiple drugs and drug interactions
> Social factors
> System issues

Factors That Affect Morbidity and Suffering

Factors that affect morbidity and cause suffering are shown in Box 6-1. Each type of factor is then described.

DISEASE FACTORS

Organ failure, especially renal failure, can be a major factor in comorbidity. Poor renal clearance is often seen in elderly patients and can alter the pharmacokinetics of drugs. This may lead to enhanced effects and adverse effects. Examples of drugs used in palliative care include morphine and gabapentin.

Cognitive problems induced by primary brain diseases, such as Alzheimer's disease, or secondary disease, such as brain metastases and metabolic changes, have numerous effects. Patients with some cognitive dysfunction have difficulties in reporting symptoms and in using assessment tools effectively and accurately. Patients who are quite ill often also have poor ability to concentrate. Therefore, their ability to be educated and retain information may be severely impaired, and their decision-making capacity may be quite limited. Examples of this occur frequently in intensive care unit settings. Decision making may be substantially affected, yet substitute decision makers may not have obtained enough information to guide decision making. Reports of symptoms may be inaccurate or impossible to obtain except by indirect means. Confusion may result in poor compliance with drugs and treatment and may lead to inadvertent overdoses.

Physical functioning may be limited by disease and symptom burden. This affects the ability to perform multiple tasks, such as taking medication, visiting offices for appointments, taking food and fluids, and personal care. Occasionally, the symptoms or conditions of one illness exacerbate those of a second illness. For instance, anti-emetic drugs (e.g., prochlorperazine) or major tranquilizers may cause increased symptoms in patients who have preexisting Parkinson's disease.

MULTIPLE PHYSICAL SYMPTOMS

Symptoms do more than cause suffering directly; they complicate other aspects of the patient's condition. For instance, pain often interferes with care in a number of ways. It may be such a focus for the patient and family that reports of other symptoms and issues are suppressed. Pain and other symptoms cause emotional and spiritual distress that may lead to poor compliance, decreased interactions with family and care providers, and poor decision making. Nausea and vomiting interfere with the ability to take medications, food, and fluid and can lead to complications such as dehydration and poor disease control. Dyspnea may interfere with physical functioning to such an extent that it impedes the ability of patients to attend appointments or to participate in any rehabilitation.

MULTIPLE PSYCHOLOGICAL AND SPIRITUAL SYMPTOMS

Anxiety and depression may interfere with patient education and retention of information, and they may contribute to limited communication and compliance. Spiritual angst may lead to poor decision making and disregard of pain.

AGE

Physiologically the very young and the very old handle drugs in different ways, and they may therefore be more susceptible to drug adverse effects and interactions. Adjustment of drug dosing is essential.

MULTIPLE DRUGS AND DRUG INTERACTIONS

The more drugs a patient is prescribed, the greater is the likelihood of major drug interactions. All these can add to suffering. Many patients use alternative treatments, such as herbal remedies. These may cause adverse effects or may promote drug interactions that can lead to toxicity. For example, St. John's wort, which is commonly used for depression, may cause methadone toxicity when these agents are coadministered.

SOCIAL FACTORS

Family support is an important factor in compliance with therapeutic regimens. When support is lacking in dysfunctional families or in families who are not coping, this may cause significant problems that enhance patient suffering.

Patients with limited funding may not be able to afford medications. In this situation, compliance may become an issue, and symptoms such as pain may not be treated effectively. Poor living conditions may affect the delivery of care in the home. The isolated, frail elderly patient is at great risk.

CARE SYSTEM ISSUES

The limited availability of palliative care programs and consultants and late referrals may cause unnecessary suffering related to physical, psychological, and spiritual issues. For patients who are being cared for at home, a lack of home care resources may result in clinicians' unawareness of issues such as compliance, poor living conditions, family problems, and other situations.

An Approach to Management

DO A COMPREHENSIVE ASSESSMENT; LOOK FOR ALL POTENTIAL FACTORS

Whole-patient assessment requires time, input from family and patient, and interdisciplinary collaboration to obtain a complete picture of all the factors and dimensions of comorbidity. Whenever possible, the clinician should use standardized assessment tools such as the Edmonton Symptom Assessment Tool (ESAS) and the Rotterdam Symptom Checklist for symptoms. The Needs at the End of Life Screening Tool (NEST) allows for broad and precise assessment (see Chapter 2),[10] or a broader assessment of spiritual and social needs. These standardized tools can make assessment more systematic and comparable across care settings. None of these assessment

Table 6-2. Common Drug Interactions in Palliative Care Practice

Tricyclic antidepressants and carbamazepine	Cardiac toxicity from tricyclic antidepressants
Methadone and SSRIs and tricyclic antidepressants	Increased methadone levels and potential sedation and cardiac toxicity
Tricyclics and fluconazole and SSRIs	Cardiac toxicity from tricyclic antidepressants, serotonin syndrome
Benzodiazepines and methadone	Increased sedation and risk of respiratory depression

SSRIs, selective serotonin reuptake inhibitors.

tools can define the totality of suffering, however, and they may be difficult to administer as the patient's illness progresses or if there is any cognitive dysfunction. Psychological and social issues or symptoms are the most likely to be assessed on a limited basis, thus leading to unaddressed suffering. If a patient is to be discharged home, an assessment directly in the home will reveal valuable information about the social factors of comorbidity.

The clinician should define for the patient and family the multiple dimensions of suffering that must be addressed to relieve the suffering that is associated with the human experience of dying. This educational process about the relief of suffering should be integrated into the holistic care plan from the time a terminal illness is diagnosed until death. Assessment is a dynamic, not static, process (Table 6-2).

REVIEW MEDICATIONS FREQUENTLY

Many seriously ill patients have long medication lists that need review. Unnecessary medications should be stopped. Examples include lipid-lowering drugs and other drugs that may no longer be a priority in that phase of the illness trajectory. The health care provider should inform the original prescribing physician (if he or she is still involved in that patient's care) which medications are being discontinued.

Drugs Interactions

As a preventive approach, a drug interaction program should always be ordered for patients taking multiple medications before a new medication is added. Online resources for this can be downloaded onto personal digital assistants and are often incorporated into electronic medical records. Many of the medications frequently used for controlling symptoms are very interactive. Some of these are detailed in Table 6-2. Routine screening for drug interactions should be standard for any patient being prescribed methadone or any of the neuropathic pain adjuvants. It is also important to recognize that some common herbal remedies (e.g., St. John's wort) and foods (e.g., grapefruit) can have a major impact on drug pharmacodynamics and pharmacokinetics.

Family involvement in monitoring medications can be very helpful. Dispensing aids such as Dosett containers or blister packs to organize medications should be used in elderly patients. Home care resources should be used to monitor patient compliance and adverse effects. Functional disabilities, such as vision or hearing disabilities and physical handicaps that could impede aspects of management, should be assessed. Chronic family and psychological dysfunction should also be assessed because it may interfere with medication compliance. Local pharmacists should be involved in the monitoring and education of patients and their families.

ACCEPT SOME RISK IN PRESCRIBING

If there is a potential for drug interaction, the clinician should weigh the severity of the risk. If the risk is low to moderate, then the drug should be prescribed but the patient should be monitored frequently for adverse effects. Time trials should be done and ineffective medications stopped as soon as it is clear that they are not helpful. For example, nonsteroidal anti-inflammatory drugs and neuropathic pain adjuvants should show an effect within 2 or 3 weeks. In approaching a particular symptom, such as nausea, one could consider a trial with increasing doses of one drug or using multiple drugs, particularly if the symptom is quite severe. High doses of one drug may be associated with more frequent and more severe adverse effects, whereas smaller doses of multiple drugs with different pharmacodynamics may be preferable. Multiple drugs do expose the patient to increased possibilities of drug interactions. More research is needed on the multiple drug approach to a symptom, and, at this time, the choice is empirical.

EDUCATE AND COUNSEL ABOUT GOALS OF CARE

Priorities in management should be identified for the care team and for the patient and family. Care and compliance will be enhanced if the patient and family understand the goals of care and the way in which multiple issues and factors of comorbidity affect the outcomes of the care plan. This educational process should also include information on how members of the team can be contacted, and it should reassure patients and family about accessibility 24 hours per day. The clinician should recommend Internet resource sites for patient and family education on issues in end-of-life care. Patient and family re-education is necessary when goals of care change. Patient and family education about prognosis should include consideration of how significant comorbid conditions affect outcomes because this may influence treatment choices.

COMMUNICATE WITH OTHERS INVOLVED IN CARE

It is essential to communicate the goals of care and the care plan regularly to family members and other care providers who are still involved in the patient's care. It is hoped that this will minimize conflicting therapeutic regimens, drug interactions, and confusion for the patient and family. Information technology should be used to support decision making and communication. Confidentiality must be ensured.

MONITOR PATIENTS FREQUENTLY WHEN CHANGING THERAPIES

Patient monitoring in this situation is a team responsibility. The care team must be accessible and responsive 24 hours per day for urgent issues.

REFER TO PALLIATIVE CARE TEAMS EARLY FOR COMPLEX CASES

Palliative care professionals are very oriented to dealing with multiple symptom issues and should be consulted for patients with complex cases. Early consultation can limit unnecessary suffering.

ADVOCATE FOR SOCIAL SUPPORTS

Referral for palliative care can be an important component in the ability to address issues of comorbidity. Adequate funding of care support and maximal utilization of community resources may relieve the family of financial burden and may avoid the all too common complications of bankruptcy and job loss.

PEARLS

- Comorbid illnesses and multiple symptoms are common in the population we serve (i.e., the elderly and chronically ill) and affect both prognosis and treatment.
- Medication review is important in managing comorbidity. It is important to discontinue unnecessary medications and perform drug interaction reviews.
- A comprehensive approach that includes patient and family education, communication with other care providers, and regular review may prevent or minimize problems.

PITFALLS

- Failure to consider the impact of multiple comorbid illnesses and symptoms may lead to increased suffering for patients and families.

Summary

It makes sense that suffering increases with multiple disease and symptom burden. By using a biopsychosocial model to address the issues of comorbidity, clinicians are able to understand how suffering, disease, and illness are affected by multiple factors from the physical to system issues and to understand how the patient's subjective experience is an essential contributor to accurate diagnosis, treatment regimens, health outcomes, and humane care.

References

1. On Line Medical Dictionary: Available at http://www.Online-Medical-Dictionary.org/omd. Accessed on November 15, 2010.
2. Wolff JL, Starfield B, Anderson G: Prevalence, expenditures, and complications of multiple chronic conditions in the elderly, *Arch Intern Med* 162:2269–2276, 2002.
3. Murray SA, Boyd K, Sheikh A, et al: Developing primary palliative care: people with terminal conditions should be able to die at home with dignity, *BMJ* 329:1056–1057, 2004.
4. Weintraub WS, Kawabata H, Tran M, et al: Influence of comorbidity on cost of care for heart failure, *Am J Cardiol* 91:1011–1015, 2003.
5. Wolff JL, Starfield B, Anderson G: Prevalence, expenditures, and complications of multiple chronic conditions in the elderly, *Arch Intern Med* 162:2269–2276, 2002.
6. Walsh D, Rybicki L: Symptom clustering in advanced cancer, *Support Care Cancer* 14:831–836, 2006.
7. Solano JP, Gomes B, Higginson IJ: A comparison of symptom prevalence in far advanced cancer, AIDS, heart disease, chronic obstructive pulmonary disease and renal disease, *J Pain Symptom Manage* 31:58–69, 2006.
8. Walke LM, Byers AL, McCorkle R, Fried TR: Symptom assessment in community-dwelling older adults with advanced chronic disease, *J Pain Symptom Manage* 31:31–37, 2006.
9. Miaskowski M, Dodd M, Lee K: Symptom clusters: the new frontier in symptom management research, *J Natl Cancer Inst Monogr* 32:17–21, 2004.
10. Emanuel LL, Alpert HR, Emanuel EE: Concise screening questions for clinical assessments of terminal care: the Needs Near the End of Life Care Screening Tool, *J Palliat Med* 4:465–474, 2001.

CHAPTER 7

Pain

VINCENT THAI and ROBIN L. FAINSINGER

Pain is a complex biopsychosocial event. Studies have shown that all types of pain (acute, chronic, and cancer pain) are undertreated, and poorly controlled pain has been identified consistently as one of the major problems in end-of-life care. In North America, pain is a major reason for referral to palliative care programs. However, adequate pain control can be achieved in most patients at the end of life by using a comprehensive approach that includes analgesics, adjuvants, education, support, and monitoring.

Pain Classification

Pain can generally be classified as nociceptive, neuropathic, or mixed.

NOCICEPTIVE PAIN

Nociceptive pain is caused by the activation of nociceptive nerve fibers by physical tissue destruction or by chemical, pressure, or thermal processes. Nociceptive somatic pain can result from injury to skin, muscle, soft tissue, or bone and can have a strong incident- or movement-related component. It is usually well localized, can be constant or intermittent, and is often described as gnawing or aching pain that may become sharp with movement. Nociceptive visceral pain is typically less well localized, is usually constant, and may be referred (e.g., diaphragmatic pain may be manifested as shoulder pain). It is often described by a variety of terms such as *aching, squeezing,* and *cramping.* Pain arising from liver metastases is an example of nociceptive visceral pain.

NEUROPATHIC PAIN

Neuropathic pain is caused by injury to nerve tissue, including the central or peripheral nervous system and even the autonomic system. Neuropathic pain is frequently described as burning and often radiates along nerves or nerve roots. It can also be associated with dysesthesia (numbness and tingling), hyperalgesia (exaggerated response to a painful stimulus), lancinating pain, and allodynia (pain experienced from a stimulus that does not normally produce pain).

MIXED PAIN

Mixed nociceptive and neuropathic pain is common in illnesses like cancer. As knowledge about pain has advanced, health care professionals have become increasingly aware of the need to develop a more mechanism-based approach to pain control. Pain is often a combination of physical and inflammatory processes. Cancer pain is an example of pain that may result from tissue damage and destruction and stimulation of nerves by inflammatory mediators that are produced by the tumor and also by the body in response to tumors. The clinical usefulness of pain classification relates to the use of certain adjuvant medications for specific pains, particularly for neuropathic pain.

Assessment of Pain

Pain is a subjective sensation, and there is no truly objective method for measuring it. Understanding the multidimensional nature of the physical, psychosocial, and spiritual components of pain is integral to the assessment of pain. Pain assessment should include a detailed history, relevant psychosocial and spiritual evaluation, physical examination, and relevant investigations. It is useful to assess pain in the physical, psychological, and social domains in sequence.

PHYSICAL DOMAIN

A complete assessment of pain includes the following:

- Location
- Pattern of occurrence
- Quality (e.g., sharp, dull, burning)
- Aggravating or relieving factors
- Radiation of the pain
- Severity and variation in severity

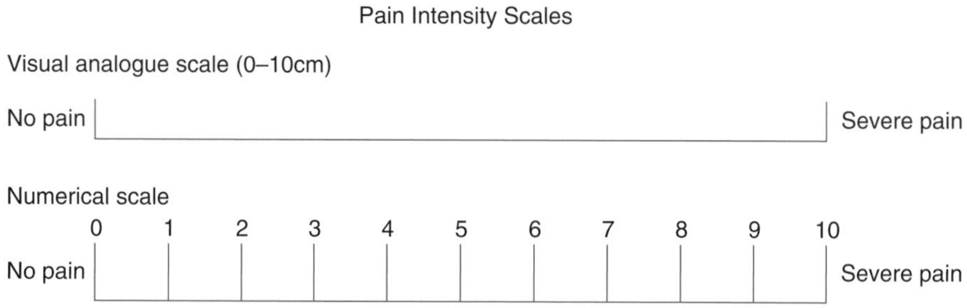

Pain Intensity Scales

Visual analogue scale (0–10cm)

No pain | _____ | Severe pain

Numerical scale

    0   1   2   3   4   5   6   7   8   9   10
No pain | | | | | | | | | | | Severe pain

Figure 7-1. Pain intensity scales.

- Interference with activities of daily living that may reflect the severity of pain
- Report of skin hypersensitivity or numbness, for example, that may suggest an underlying neuropathic component of the pain
- Pain treatment and analgesic history: what worked and what failed, dosage, adverse effects, compliance
- Breakthrough pain (e.g., incident or spontaneous)

The Brief Pain Inventory[1] is a useful tool to quantify pain; alternatively, various types of validated and reliable visual, verbal, or numerical analogue scales can also be used (Figure 7-1).

A history of present and past medical conditions is useful because some conditions complicate pain expression and subsequent management. Inquiry should cover the following:

- Presence of underlying delirium, cognitive failure, or dementia that could alter pain expression and the accuracy of pain history
- Presence of preexisting chronic pain or a history of pain, such as osteoarthritis or diabetic neuropathy
- Previous exposure to neurotoxic antineoplastic agents
- Presence of complicated cancer pain syndromes, such as malignant leptomeningeal spread, plexus involvement, or pathologic fractures
- Location of tumors, such as large retroperitoneal lymph nodes that cause back pain
- Presence of concomitant infection or abscess
- Presence of general medical conditions that could affect management and analgesic dosing, such as significant hepatic or renal impairment
- Current medications that may interact with analgesics or adjuvants

PSYCHOLOGICAL DOMAIN

An assessment of psychological factors adds to the understanding of a patient's suffering and pain expression. Issues in these domains that could affect pain assessment and management include the following:

- Depression and anxiety
- Limited understanding of the illness
- Patient's fears of opioid use
- Anger toward the health care system or health care workers
- Underlying personality disorder or psychiatric disorder

- Loss of body image related to various surgical procedures
- Poor coping mechanisms
- Patient denial
- History of drug abuse or alcohol abuse

SOCIAL DOMAIN

An assessment of the social factors that may have a bearing on the patient's pain expression is also useful. Some factors include the following:

- Fears of opioids
- Family discord and dysfunction
- Guilt within the family
- The family's lack of knowledge and understanding of the disease and prognosis
- Denial or unrealistic expectations of the family
- Financial issues
- Cultural and religious factors
- Drug and alcohol abuse

COMPLICATED CANCER PAIN ASSESSMENT AND CLASSIFICATION

A number of factors may complicate cancer pain assessment and may cause difficulty in achieving stable pain control or require consideration of a referral for the support of a pain specialist. Therefore, assessment of pain should include problems that may complicate pain management or be a poor prognostic factor for pain control. Research to develop an international classification system for cancer pain[2] has highlighted potential poor prognostic factors predictive of increased time to achieve stable pain control, higher opioid doses, and more requirements for adjuvant analgesics:

1. Younger patients
2. Neuropathic pain
3. Incident or episodic pain
4. Psychological distress potentially impacting increased expression of pain intensity
5. Substance abuse disorder potentially predicting inappropriate opioid use or tolerance to opioids
6. Severe pain intensity on initial presentation

For further elaboration and definitions used in the international classification system for cancer pain, see Knudsen and colleagues.[2]

PAIN ASSESSMENT IN THE COGNITIVELY IMPAIRED

Pain in those with cognitive impairment (e.g., dementia patients) can be particularly challenging. Some of the behavioral domains to assess pain in the cognitively impaired include facial expressions (e.g., grimacing, distorted), verbalizations/vocalizations (e.g., moaning, calling out), body movements (e.g., rigid, tense), changes to interpersonal interaction (e.g., aggression), and activity patterns and mentation.[3] None of these behaviors are always indicators of pain. Assessment scales are available, but few of them have been tested widely for validity or reliability. The FACES Scale, which is often used for those who are cognitively impaired, has little proven validity or reliability in this population.

Principles of Pain Management

EDUCATE THE PATIENT AND FAMILY

It is essential to explain to the family and the patient the origin of the pain, the type of pain, the initial management plan (including the role of titration), expected adverse effects and how they will be managed, how the pain will be monitored, and how to access the professional care team. Fears concerning opioid use also need to be addressed.

PREVENT AND MINIMIZE ADVERSE EFFECTS

Common adverse effects such as sedation, constipation, and nausea should be anticipated and prevented through a combination of education and the regular use of drugs that will address these issues. By minimizing adverse effects, additional patient suffering can be avoided, compliance may be enhanced, and anxiety can be reduced.

MATCH PAIN SEVERITY TO ANALGESIC POTENCY

The three-step ladder approach for pain control by the World Health Organization (WHO) remains a useful educational tool, but aspects of clinical application have been questioned. Evidence indicates that for mild to moderate pain, nonopioid analgesics can be effective either alone or in combination with weak opioids. For moderate pain, the recommendation is to consider starting with small doses of a strong opioid. For severe pain, a strong opioid is the initial drug of choice. Adjuvant analgesics can be used for all types of pain if clinically indicated. For a summary of prescribing principles, see Table 7-1.

TITRATE TO PAIN CONTROL

Each patient has different analgesic requirements, depending on the source of the pain and as a result of pharmacokinetic and pharmacodynamic differences among patients and the interplay of other factors, all of which produce the "total pain" experience. Thus, dosages have to be tailored and titrated to the patient's individual pain needs.

Table 7-1. Type of Pain and Analgesics

Type	Typical Analgesics	Adjuvant Analgesics
Nociceptive pain: mild	Nonopioids +/− weak opioids	NSAIDs (brief trial)
Nociceptive pain: moderate to severe	Strong opioids	NSAIDs Radiotherapy Surgery
Neuropathic pain: mild	May not be indicated	Tricyclic antidepressants Typical and atypical anticonvulsants
Neuropathic pain: moderate to severe	Strong opioids	Tricyclic antidepressants Typical and atypical anticonvulsants Radiation Surgery

NSAIDs, non-steroidal anti-inflammatory drugs.

PRESCRIBE AROUND-THE-CLOCK DOSING

Patients with constant pain require around-the-clock dosing at regular intervals to suppress the pain. There is rarely a role for "as necessary" administration of medication for constant pain except as breakthrough dosing.

PRESCRIBE RESCUE OR BREAKTHROUGH DOSES

Pain is rarely completely stable, and extra pain should be treated with breakthrough or rescue doses. Always prescribe rescue dosing.

ALWAYS CONSIDER USING ADJUVANTS

For neuropathic pain, consider starting adjuvant analgesics before opioids for mild pain, or at the same time as opioids for moderate or severe pain. Recommended first-line agents include tricyclic and other antidepressants, anticonvulsants such as gabapentin or pregabalin, and transdermal lidocaine.[4] For bone pain from cancer, the option of radiotherapy must always be explored. For all types of pain, nonopioids such as acetaminophen and nonsteroidal anti-inflammatory drugs (NSAIDs) may be helpful. Brief trials of these nonopioids along with opioids may prove to be beneficial to some patients. Surgery may also be indicated for bone pain or neuropathic pain. These points are summarized in Table 7-1.

MONITOR CONTINUOUSLY

Constant and frequent review of the patient's response to the prescribed regimen of analgesics, adjuvants, and other interventions is important. The patient's medical status must be monitored for conditions that could affect the dose of the analgesic regimen, such as the development of renal failure. Patients, family members, and all health care professionals can be involved in this process.

ASK FOR HELP

Pain specialists and palliative care specialists are available to assist in more complicated cases. Do not hesitate to call and ask them for an opinion.

Addiction, Diversion, Physical Dependence, and Tolerance

Physicians who prescribe opioids need to differentiate the issues of physical dependence, drug abuse and diversion, addiction, and tolerance. However, a history of substance abuse does not exclude someone from having pain. Definitions of *addiction, physical dependence, tolerance,* and *pseudoaddiction* are listed in Table 7-2.[5,6]

Steps the clinician can take to address these issues include adopting a risk management approach that includes universal precautions and using various risk assessment tools.[7]

When prescribing opioids for pain in a person with a history of substance abuse, consider the following:

- Patients who have abused and developed tolerance to opioids may require higher than usual doses of opioids for pain control.
- Patients who are at higher risk of substance abuse can be identified, and questionnaires such as the CAGE substance abuse screening tool may indicate abuse potential.[8]

Table 7-2. Definitions of *Addiction, Physical Dependence, Tolerance,* and *Pseudoaddiction*

Addiction	A primary, chronic, neurobiologic disease with genetic, psychosocial, and environmental factors influencing its development and manifestations Characterized by behaviors that include one or more of the following: • Impaired control over drug use • Compulsive use • Continued use despite harm • Craving
Physical dependence	A state of adaptation manifested by a drug class–specific withdrawal syndrome that can be produced by abrupt cessation, rapid dose reduction, decreasing blood level of the drug, and/or administration of an antagonist
Tolerance	A state of adaptation in which exposure to a drug induces changes that result in a diminution of one or more of the drug's effects over time
Pseudoaddiction	Syndrome of behavioral symptoms that mimic those seen with psychological dependence, including an overwhelming and compulsive interest in the acquisition and use of opioid analgesics An iatrogenic syndrome (unlike true psychological dependence) caused by undermedication of pain; symptoms and aberrant behaviors resolve once pain is effectively controlled

Data from American Academy of Pain Medicine, American Pain Society, and American Society of Addiction Medicine (ASAM): Definitions related to the use of opioids for the treatment of pain. Public Policy Statement, 2001. Available at www.asam.org; and Weissman DE, Hadox DJ: Opioid pseudoaddiction: an iatrogenic syndrome, *Pain* 36:363–366, 1989.

• Common abuse behaviors include reports of "lost" or "stolen" prescriptions, a history of multiple prescribers, obtaining prescription drugs from nonmedical sources, and repeated dose escalations or similar instances of noncompliance despite multiple warnings.[5]
• Emotional, social, and even spiritual issues may complicate and magnify pain expression.
• The patient's behavior may contribute to the difficulty in treating pain, and mistrust between the patient and health care provider can be a barrier.

Simple strategies to prevent abuse may include dispensing a limited amount of opioids at a time, having only one designated prescriber and one designated pharmacy to fill the prescription, and allowing no refills for "lost" or "stolen" prescriptions. Consider using opioids that have less street value (this can vary in different geographic locations). Be aware of analgesic combinations that have potentially hepatotoxic components, such as acetaminophen in drug abusers, who are at high risk of liver damage.

Pharmacologic Options for Pain Management

Analgesics can be classified as nonopioid analgesics, opioid analgesics, and adjuvant drugs.

NONOPIOID ANALGESICS

Nonopioid analgesics are appropriate as single agents for mild pain.

Acetaminophen

Acetaminophen is the most common over-the-counter analgesic drug. Its exact mechanism of action is not completely understood, but it does have peripheral and central actions. Dosage is limited to less than 4 g/day to minimize potential hepatotoxicity. This drug should be used with caution in patients with active hepatitis or hepatic dysfunction, in patients who abuse alcohol, and in those with jaundice. It may also be effective as an adjuvant when added to strong opioids.[9]

Acetaminophen is often combined with codeine or oxycodone. This combination may prove useful in patients who have mild to moderate pain, but the amount of acetaminophen limits the dosages.

Nonsteroidal Anti-Inflammatory Drugs

NSAIDs have peripheral and central actions perhaps related but not totally limited to inhibition of cyclooxygenase enzymes (COX-1 and COX-2). Gastrointestinal and renal toxicity can be a problem with NSAIDs. Some of the newer, specific COX-2 inhibitors may have less severe or fewer gastrointestinal and renal side effects. There are a number of concerns concerning the use of NSAIDs in certain patients.

For patients taking corticosteroids, NSAIDs will increase the risk of gastrointestinal erosion and bleeding. In patients on anticoagulants for deep vein thrombosis or who may even have a coagulopathy secondary to hepatic impairment or platelet problems, the use of NSAIDs puts them at higher risk of upper gastrointestinal bleeding. Clearance of the first-line strong opioids such as morphine and hydromorphone depends on kidney function. NSAIDs may affect renal function and may lead to decreased renal clearance and an increased risk of opioid toxicity. Gastric protection with misoprostol and proton pump inhibitors such as omeprazole can be considered for high-risk patients.

No clear evidence indicates that one NSAID is superior to another. If the patient has no obvious response to an NSAID, the drug should be discontinued. This applies whether the drug is used alone or as an adjuvant.

Tramadol

Tramadol is a unique, synthetic, centrally acting analgesic with both opioid and nonopioid properties. It has some action at the mu opioid receptor, but it also has other actions, including possible anti-inflammatory effects. In addition, it stimulates neuronal serotonin release and inhibits the presynaptic reuptake of both norepinephrine and serotonin at synapses. Naloxone only partially reverses the analgesic effect of tramadol. Its bioavailability is twice that of codeine. It is a pro-drug and relies in part on an active metabolite for its analgesia. It is converted in the liver in the cytochrome P450 system to O-desmethyltramadol, which is itself an active substance, two to four times more potent than tramadol. Further biotransformation results in inactive metabolites that are excreted by the kidneys. Approximately 5% to 10% of the population lacks the isoenzyme to metabolize tramadol, and in such persons tramadol has limited analgesic effect. CYP2D6 inhibitors (e.g., chlorpromazine, delavirdine, fluoxetine, miconazole, paroxetine, pergolide, quinidine, quinine, ritonavir, and ropinirole) may decrease the effects of tramadol. Carbamazepine decreases the half-life of tramadol by 33% to 50%. The concomitant use of monoamine oxidase inhibitors is contraindicated. Tramadol must be used with caution with any central nervous system depressant such as phenothiazines and barbiturates.

By injection, tramadol is one tenth as potent as parenteral morphine. Orally, because of much better bioavailability, it is one fifth as potent. Tramadol can be regarded as double-strength codeine.

Tramadol is available in the United States and Canada as a fixed combination with acetaminophen or in a sustained-release formulation. The ceiling recommended dose is 400 mg/day.

The most common adverse effect is constipation, but this seems to occur less often than with equianalgesic doses of morphine. The risk of seizures is increased with high dose tramadol (e.g. >400 mg/day), and therefore tramadol should probably not be used in patients with a history of seizures.

OPIOIDS

Opioids are the mainstay of pain management in palliative care.

General Properties

Opioids are variably absorbed from the gastrointestinal tract. Morphine and codeine are absorbed relatively poorly (30% to 50%), and methadone has a good oral bioavailability of about 80% (ranges from 41% to 99%). Bioavailability is further reduced by metabolism in the gut wall and the liver (the first-pass effect). Absorption may be genetically determined and may decrease with increasing age.

All opioids are bound to plasma proteins, generally to albumin and alpha-1-acid glycoprotein. However, the extent of binding varies from less than 10% for codeine to 80% to 86% for fentanyl. Morphine is about 20% to 35% protein bound.

Most opioids have a large volume of distribution, depending on the lipophilicity of the parent compound and metabolites. Fentanyl and methadone are the most lipophilic.

Opioids are metabolized to more hydrophilic compounds, predominantly by glucuronidation in the liver, although some extrahepatic metabolism may occur. Most of the metabolites are less active than the parent opioid and may not have much clinically relevant pharmacologic action. However, some metabolites are as potent or more potent opioid agonists than the parent drug (e.g., morphine as a metabolite of codeine, morphine-6-glucuronide derived from morphine). Some metabolic byproducts (particularly morphine-3-glucuronide, hydromorphone-3-glucuronide, and normorphine) may be responsible for the neurotoxic side effects of confusion and myoclonus. Because they are excreted by the kidneys, these metabolites accumulate in patients with renal failure. Methadone and, to some extent, fentanyl are exceptions because they are metabolized in the liver through the cytochrome P450 system and the major route of excretion is fecal. Methadone and fentanyl are therefore more prone to drug interactions with agents that affect that metabolic system. Oxycodone, fentanyl, and methadone have no active final metabolites.

Opioids bind to opioid receptors that are spread throughout the body. In the central nervous system they are concentrated in the thalamus, the periaqueductal gray matter, and the dorsal horn of the spinal cord. Receptors are also present in the lungs, in the myenteric plexuses of the gastrointestinal tract, and in other areas where their exact function remains unclear. The mu receptor is the one most strongly associated with analgesia. Other receptors include kappa and delta receptors. Recent work on opioid receptors suggests that genetic polymorphism may be responsible for the varied interindividual response to the same doses of an opioid.

Opioids can be divided into pure agonists, partial agonists, mixed agonists, and antagonists (Table 7-3) based on their interactions with the various receptor subtypes (mu, kappa, and delta). Partial agonists (e.g., buprenorphine) and the mixed agonists and antagonists (e.g., butorphanol and pentazocine) have the disadvantage of a ceiling effect. The mixed agonist and antagonists are noted to have more psychoto-mimetic side effects, and partial agonists have the potential to cause withdrawal problems when added to pure opioid agonists. Hence, pure agonist opioids are the most useful medications in the management of pain.

Common Adverse Effects

1. *Sedation.* Almost every patient has some sedation from opioids, especially on initial dosing. This sedation often resolves in 3 to 4 days unless the dosage is too high. If mild sedation persists, methylphenidate may be helpful.
2. *Constipation.* This is an almost universal phenomenon with opioids, especially in patients with advanced disease.[10] The effect of opioids on bowel myenteric plexuses results in decreased propulsion of stool and increased transit times, causing increased fluid absorption that results in hard, infrequent stools. Combined with other factors such as weakness, decreased food intake, and other drug effects in patients with advanced illness, constipation can become a major problem. The approach should be preventive, and most patients should be receiving a stimulant laxative such as senna or bisacodyl and may also need an osmotic laxative such as lactulose, polyethylene glycol, or milk of magnesia. Patients should be monitored carefully for constipation.
3. *Nausea and vomiting.* Approximately 70% of the population may develop some nausea with opioids, particularly on initiation of an opioid. Again, the approach should be preventive. Patient education is important because patients who are warned of the possibility of nausea may tolerate the usual, minimal nausea that occurs, and they are less likely to request additional medication for the nausea. Antiemetics (especially those that bind to dopaminergic receptors, such as haloperidol, metoclopramide, and prochlorperazine) are most effective. Antihistamines such as dimenhydrinate are less effective. Prolonged nausea and vomiting is rare and in most patients will stop within a few days, although with titration there is the possibility of some recurrence. Severe nausea and vomiting may occur rarely with even small doses of opioids. Those patients may tolerate transdermal or parenteral administration or a significantly smaller starting dose and gentler titration.

Less Common Adverse Effects

Lesson common adverse effects of opioid use include the following:

1. Urinary retention
2. Pruritus resulting from histamine release in the skin

Table 7-3. Classification of Opioid Analgesics by Receptor Interactions

Agonists	Partial Agonists
Weak	
Codeine	Buprenorphine
Propoxyphene	
Hydrocodone	
Dihydrocodeine	
Strong	
Morphine	**Agonist/Antagonists**
Oxycodone	Pentazocine
Hydromorphone	Butorphanol
Methadone	Nalbuphine
Fentanyl	
Diamorphine (heroin)	
Oxymorphone	
Meperidine	
Levorphanol	
Sufentanil	
Alfentanil	

3. Cognitive problems, including memory impairment (particularly in the presence of an underlying dementia), decreased ability to concentrate, and bad dreams; may progress to delirium
4. Myoclonic jerks

Rare Adverse Effects

Rare adverse effects of opioid use include the following:

1. Allergy to opioids (except for codeine)
2. Respiratory depression (very rare except in circumstances of overdose)

Special Issues

Special issues related to opioid use include the following:

- *Driving while taking opioids.* After an initial period of adjustment to opioids and when sedation is not present, patients may be allowed to drive. However, other factors in their disease process, such as generalized weakness and other symptoms, may preclude driving. Each case should be considered individually.
- *Opioid toxicity.* Some patients may develop opioid toxicity. This is signaled by increasing drowsiness, confusion, hallucinations, and frequent myoclonus. Toxicity may relate to overdosage (with rapid titration, overenthusiastic dosing, medication errors, poor compliance, and other factors), renal failure and other metabolic problems, and sepsis. Patients initially present with increased sedation and then delirium with confusion, hallucinations, agitation, and frequent myoclonus. Severe toxicity may result in coma, respiratory depression, and death, although these are relatively rare with normal opioid use. In the case of

opioid toxicity, the opioid can be withheld, significantly reduced, or rotated to another opioid, and the patient should be monitored carefully.

Practical Tips

Keep in mind the following tips when prescribing opioids:

1. The starting dose for opioid-naive patients can be 5 to 10 mg of morphine equivalent every 4 hours. Dosage can be initiated with sustained-release preparations, but immediate-release preparations allow for more careful titration.
2. Immediate-release and sustained-release opioids should be prescribed regularly around the clock.
3. Initial breakthrough (rescue) doses should be prescribed up to every hour as needed. Breakthrough doses are generally 10% to 15% of the total daily dose of the same opioid.
4. If the patient is very elderly or frail, the initial dose should be smaller, and titration should be done more slowly.
5. The oral and parenteral doses of opioids are not equivalent. The dose of parenteral opioids (subcutaneous or intravenous) is usually one half to one third of the oral dose.
6. Suggested equianalgesic ratios are listed in the formulary. Equianalgesic ratios are guidelines only, and the final doses have to be individualized according to the patient's needs.[11]
7. Patients with acute or poorly controlled pain should be given immediate-release formulations to achieve a quicker response and to allow more rapid titration. Controlled or sustained-release opioid formulations are more appropriate for palliative care patients who have achieved fairly stable pain control and relatively stable dosages and for patients with chronic pain not related to cancer. The initial dose can be titrated or adjusted every 24 to 48 hours. As a general rule, the use of four or more breakthrough doses in a day may warrant a dose increase of the regular opioid. In most cases the breakthrough doses can be added to the total daily dosage, and the new regular daily dosage can be recalculated on a 24-hour basis in divided doses. If this regimen causes sedation or nausea and the patient does not need breakthrough doses, this may indicate the need to decrease the total daily dose.
8. Meperidine should not be used on a long-term basis because of the risk of neurotoxicity (confusion, seizures) from its toxic metabolite, normeperidine, which tends to accumulate with repeated use.
9. The oral route is preferable for all opioids except fentanyl. If the oral route is not suitable, subcutaneous (intermittent or continuous), rectal, and intravenous routes can be considered. Generally, intramuscular administration is not recommended because this route is more painful and is usually unnecessary.
10. Transmucosal fentanyl formulations are available for patients who need a fast-acting medication for incident pain.
11. If the patient is experiencing symptoms of opioid toxicity, check for precipitating factors, such as dehydration, renal failure, and infection. If the pain is well controlled, consider withholding or decreasing the dose of opioid until the patient is more alert or becomes less confused. Consider rotating to another opioid.
12. Augment pain control with adjuvant analgesics.

13. Transdermal fentanyl should be considered for patients who have difficulty swallowing, who experience nausea with the oral route of opioid administration, or who have a preference for this type of analgesic delivery. However, therapeutic levels from the fentanyl transdermal patch are reached only after 6 to 12 hours, and it may take up to 36 to 48 hours to achieve a steady state. Transdermal fentanyl patches should be used cautiously on opioid-naive patients. After the removal of a transdermal fentanyl patch, fentanyl will still be released from the subcutaneous depot for the next 8 to 12 hours. Hence, when switching from transdermal fentanyl to another opioid, it is prudent to wait for about 8 to 12 hours before instituting the new opioid regimen. The patient can use breakthrough doses of another opioid temporarily. If the patient is in severe pain, however, it may be necessary to start the new regimen of opioids, including the transdermal patch, earlier.
14. If the patient is using escalating doses of breakthrough opioids, reassessment is required and other factors should be considered, such as fractures, spinal cord compression, delirium, opioid-induced hyperalgesia, tolerance, and a "total pain syndrome."
15. Most of the time, breakthrough cancer pain can be managed with oral or subcutaneous opioids based on 10% to 15% of the baseline total daily dose. However, for breakthrough pain that is severe and sudden in onset, different routes of medication[12] may have to be considered, such as transmucosal oral or nasal fentanyl. At this time, the availability of some of these preparations in different countries is variable.
16. Opioids are generally not contraindicated in moderate liver disease. In the presence of liver failure, the dose of opioid can be reduced and the frequency of administration decreased.
17. In patients with renal failure, the frequency and dose of opioids that have active, renally excreted metabolites (morphine, hydromorphone) may need adjustment.[13] An alternative is to switch to a drug with no known active metabolites or a cleaner metabolic profile, such as methadone, fentanyl, or oxycodone.

Opioid Rotation

If there are concerns about tolerance (which may be manifested by ever-increasing doses without response) or issues of adverse effects or opioid toxicity, rotation of opioids may be considered.[14] Rotation can be done by taking the morphine equianalgesic dose of the first opioid and reducing it by 20% to 30% for incomplete cross-tolerance and then calculating the equivalent dose for the second opioid.

For example, to rotate from oxycodone to hydromorphone in a patient receiving oral oxycodone 10 mg every 4 hours, the total daily dose is about 90 mg of morphine equivalent (taking an equivalency factor of 1.5). For a dose reduction of about 30%, the new morphine equivalent dose is about 63 mg/day and the oral hydromorphone equivalent dose is about 12.5 mg/day (taking a factor of 5). The final regular dose of oral hydromorphone would be approximately 2 mg every 4 hours. Rotation to transdermal fentanyl is more difficult, and rotation to methadone requires special care.

Methadone

Methadone is a synthetic opioid that has gained renewed interest as an analgesic because of its low cost and potential activity in neuropathic pain syndromes.[15] It is a mu opioid receptor agonist, possibly a delta opioid receptor agonist, and an N-methyl-D-aspartate (NMDA) receptor channel blocker. In general, methadone is recommended for use by experienced prescribers. It is a very lipophilic drug and is well absorbed by the gastrointestinal tract, with a bioavailability of approximately 80%. This is better than the bioavailability of oral morphine and other opioids. Methadone binds extensively to alpha-1-acid glycoprotein. Initial rapid and extensive distribution occurs within 2 to 3 hours, and a subsequent and slower elimination phase lasts for 15 to 60 hours. This half-life does not seem to correlate with the observed duration of analgesia (6 to 12 hours) after steady state is reached.

Methadone is metabolized mainly by type 1 cytochrome P450 enzymes—namely, CYP3A4 (which can be induced or inhibited)—and, to a lesser degree, by CYP1A2 (which can also be induced or inhibited) and CYP2D6 (this level depends on genetic polymorphism). Methadone therefore has more interaction with other drugs than some opioids because of the potential for inhibiting or enhancing these cytochrome P450 pathways. A drug interaction program should be used with every patient considered for methadone therapy and when any new drug is added to the regimen of a patient receiving methadone. Some medications can decrease methadone levels. Among these are some antiretroviral drugs (e.g., nevirapine, ritonavir), phenytoin and carbamazepine, risperidone, rifampicin, and fusidic acid. Long-term alcohol ingestion and cigarette smoking can also reduce serum methadone levels. Some of the medications that can increase methadone levels are tricyclic antidepressants (TCAs), ketoconazole and fluconazole, selective serotonin reuptake inhibitors (SSRIs), erythromycin, and metronidazole. Drug interactions with methadone can lead to prolongation of the QT interval, arrhythmias, and even death.

Approximately 60% of methadone is eliminated by nonrenal routes, primarily fecal, and renal excretion depends on urinary pH. However, methadone does not seem to accumulate significantly in patients with renal failure.

The main concerns when using methadone are the unpredictable half-life and the associated risk of delayed overdose. Hence, careful dose titration and individualized dosing are needed. Equianalgesic dose ratios depend on the patient's opioid requirements, and various guidelines are available for the administration and titration of methadone. The simultaneous use of benzodiazepines and methadone may increase the potential for serious respiratory depression and sedation.

The complex and highly individualized pharmacokinetic properties of methadone dictate the need for experienced physicians to administer methadone and monitor its effects.

ADJUVANT ANALGESICS

Certain drugs can be used as adjuvants in combination with opioids. These include corticosteroids, tricyclic and other antidepressants, anticonvulsants, bisphosphonates, muscle relaxants, anesthetic agents, and antiarrhythmic drugs. These adjuvants may be used with opioids to complement pain relief. However, the problem of polypharmacy with problematic drug interactions and adverse effects has to be considered and weighed against the potential analgesic benefits.

Corticosteroids

Corticosteroids are sometimes used for their anti-inflammatory effects in bone pain, to reduce pain from increased intracranial pressure, and as an adjuvant for recent-onset neuropathic pain from spinal cord compression or peripheral nerve compression or destruction.[16] Adverse effects include immune suppression, hyperglycemia, upper gastrointestinal ulceration, hypertension, accelerating osteoporosis, psychotropic side effects such as depression or overstimulation, fluid retention, proximal myopathy, Cushinoid changes in the face and body, and adrenal suppression.

Dexamethasone is often used because it has less tendency to retain fluids and because of its high potency. Starting doses vary from 4 to 24 mg/day in divided doses. Short-term use and tapering to the lowest effective dose is generally recommended. The drug should be discontinued if pain does not respond quickly.

Tricyclic Antidepressants

TCAs can be used for neuropathic pain.[17] Most of the evidence for their use is in patients with non–cancer-related chronic neuropathic pain; the best evidence available is for the drug amitriptyline, but other drugs in this class are also effective and may have fewer adverse effects. The dosage required is normally in the usual antidepressant dose range. It may take up to 4 weeks for a response, and the drug should be discontinued if there is little response.

Adverse effects are common. The anticholinergic side effects of the drug may worsen or cause urinary retention or glaucoma. Nortriptyline and desipramine (other members of this class of drugs) have fewer of these adverse effects but are not entirely free of them. Coexisting cardiac problems (e.g., heart block, underlying cardiac disease with significant cardiac arrhythmias, significant postural hypotension) are relative contraindications to the use of TCAs. Frail elderly patients are more sensitive to the adverse effects of TCAs.

Other Antidepressants: Selective Serotonin Reuptake Inhibitors and Serotonin-Norepinephrine Reuptake Inhibitors

Serotonin-norepinephrine reuptake inhibitors (SNRIs) can be used for treatment of neuropathic pain,[4] and they may have a better adverse event profile compared with TCAs. Examples of SNRIs include venlafaxine and duloxetine. Some of the adverse events seen with the SNRIs include nausea, vomiting, headache, sweating, increase in blood pressure, dizziness, and insomnia. Duloxetine is metabolized by CYP1A2 and CYP2D6 and has the potential to interact with drugs metabolized by these pathways. At the moment, the role of SSRIs in pain control is unclear and efficacy has yet to be proved.

Anticonvulsant Drugs

Anticonvulsants have been used for many years in the management of neuropathic pain. Numerous drugs are available, including the typical anticonvulsants, such as carbamazepine, phenytoin, valproate, and oxcarbazepine, and atypical anticonvulsants, such as gabapentin, pregabalin, topiramate and lamotrigine, and clonazepam.[18]

Dosages for treatment of pain are generally the same as for typical use as anticonvulsants. Response may take 2 to 4 weeks. In the presence of little or no response, these drugs should be discontinued. Anticonvulsants like carbamazepine and valproate may be contraindicated in patients with bone marrow suppression. The presence of drowsiness, a common side effect of anticonvulsants, may require slower titration of these drugs. Superimposed drug-induced hepatitis from anticonvulsants such as carbamazepine and valproate may worsen liver function in patients with preexisting hepatic impairment.

Bisphosphonates

Bisphosphonates may be of value in treating malignant hypercalcemia and in reducing skeletal events such as pathologic fractures and cancer-associated bone pain. Evidence of a significant effect on bone pain in patients with advanced disease is limited.[19]

Conditions that favor the use of bisphosphonates for bone pain include the following:

- Presence of concomitant hypercalcemia
- Presence of significant osteoporosis with previous fracture
- Diffuse nature of symptomatic bone pain
- Diagnoses of multiple myeloma and breast cancer

A relative contraindication for the use of bisphosphonates is the presence of renal impairment. If use of these drugs is necessary despite renal impairment, patients will require dose adjustment as well as a slower infusion rate. If the subcutaneous route is required, clodronate can be used. Pamidronate and zoledronic acid are given intravenously. If there is no decrease in pain and no other concomitant conditions require bisphosphonates, the drug should be stopped. The high cost of these agents may be an issue.

Cannabinoids

Cannabinoids have a long history of both therapeutic and recreational use. The existence and understanding of the endogenous cannabinoid system is only relatively recent, with the discovery of the *CB1* and *CB2* cannabinoid receptors. The *CB1* receptors are located on the central and peripheral nervous system, where they are involved in many functions, including memory, metabolism, endocrine control, and reproduction. The *CB2* receptor is expressed on the immune cells involved in the modulation of neuroimmune processes, including inflammation and pain. Cannabinioids are lipophilic. Examples of these medications are nabilone and a mixture of cannabidiol and delta-9-tetrahydrocannabinol.

At present, the analgesic properties of cannabinoids are modest but may be of value as useful adjuncts for refractory cancer pain. Some of the side effects include sedation, metal clouding, somnolence, and dizziness, which may limit use.[20]

Muscle Relaxants

Muscle relaxants are commonly used for acute pain from musculoskeletal injuries and for muscle spasm. The disadvantages of these medications are sedation and their anticholinergic side effect profile. Their effect on pain or any significant impact on muscle spasm has not been proven. Some examples of these medications are baclofen, orphenadrine, methocarbamol, and cyclobenzaprine.

Anesthetics

Ketamine can be given orally, subcutaneously,[21] or even as "burst ketamine",[22] in which it is given in incremental doses subcutaneously. The main disadvantage of ketamine is the psychotomimetic adverse effects, with hallucinations and confusion.

Other drugs, such as lidocaine, have been used transdermally, intravenously, and subcutaneously.[23] Oral mexiletine and flecainide have also been tried. However, the prime concerns in the use of these drugs are central nervous system toxicity, which can cause ataxia, tremors, or even confusion, and potential cardiotoxicity, which may induce fatal cardiac arrhythmias.

Nonpharmacologic Options for Pain Management

RADIATION THERAPY

Radiation therapy is often very useful in controlling localized cancer-related bone pain, tumor growth, and infiltration. More than 40% of patients can expect at least a 50% reduction in pain, and slightly fewer than 30% can expect complete pain relief at 1 month.[24] The speed of onset of pain relief is variable. However, because of problematic incident pain associated with bone metastases, radiation therapy is an important adjunct to pain control. Bone metastases can often be treated with a single dose of radiation. Radiation toxicity to the adjacent anatomic structures and radiation-induced fatigue are examples of adverse effects of radiation therapy.

RELAXATION THERAPY

Relaxation and distraction may be useful techniques to help some patients cope with pain and manage psychological factors (particularly anxiety) that could increase the pain experience.

PHYSICAL AND OCCUPATIONAL THERAPY

Physical therapy and occupational therapy are useful adjuncts to the overall management of pain control, especially in patients with contractures and fractures that require various orthopedic devices and supports and in helping patients cope with pain and other disabilities as their disease progresses.

TRANSCUTANEOUS ELECTRICAL NERVE STIMULATION

In experienced hands, transcutaneous electrical nerve stimulation (TENS) can also be considered as an adjuvant for pain, particularly in the limbs and back.

ACUPUNCTURE

The mechanism of action of acupuncture may be through the enhancement of the body's production of endogenous opioids. Acupuncture appears to be more effective in musculoskeletal-related pain, and multiple treatments may be necessary.[25]

Interventional Methods for Pain Management

According to the World Health Organization, only 15% to 20% of patients with cancer require invasive methods of pain relief. In the immediate postinjection period, peripheral nerve blocks can lead to pain relief in about 66% of patients with neurogenic pain and 64% of patients with nociceptive pain.[26] However, long-term pain relief after local anesthetic blocks is usually not observed in palliative care patients. Neuroaxial, epidural, and intrathecal infusions of analgesics can also be used. One survey reported that only 16 of 1205 patients (i.e., 1.33%) with cancer required intraspinal therapy.[27] There is wide variation in the practice patterns for this approach. Opioids and local anesthetics can both be administered. Intrathecal administration of drugs requires less medication than epidural administration. Epidural doses are also smaller compared with parenteral doses. The calculation for intrathecal opioids requires specialized anesthesiology services, and treatment becomes even more complex when intraspinal anesthetics are given together with intraspinal opioids. Intrathecal and epidural medications can be given through a pump. Concerns about infections and the cost-to-benefit ratio must be considered. Some of the devices are very expensive and require specialized expertise.[28] Another consideration is whether enough experienced personnel are available to support this technique at the local institution or home care system. Neuroaxial analgesia should be considered for patients with refractory pain syndromes.

PEARLS

- Pain is a complex biopsychosocial event that requires a comprehensive, interdisciplinary assessment for management to have the most chance of success.
- Pain, particularly cancer pain, is often multifactorial in causation.
- Attention to basic principles of pain management leads to consistent results in pain management.
- Opioids are the mainstay of treatment of pain.
- Every patient should be offered appropriate multiple modes of adjuvant therapy.
- Adverse effects of opioids, particularly constipation, which is the most common adverse effect, can be prevented for the most part.

PITFALLS

- Although the World Health Organization ladder can be very helpful, remember to begin with the analgesic whose potency best matches the severity of the pain.
- Failure to deal with the fears of patients and families about opioids may impede good pain control.
- Failure to prevent or minimize adverse effects of opioids will also inhibit the achievement of good pain control.
- Failure to monitor pain and the patient's response to treatment adequately may lead to delays in achieving good pain control.

Summary

Pain is a complex phenomenon. Adequate pain control can be achieved in most, but not all, patients at the end of life. The approach to management involves comprehensive, interdisciplinary assessment, the effective use of opioids and adjuvants, and constant monitoring. In some situations, the average physician will require the expertise and support of palliative or pain management specialists[29] and multidisciplinary pain management programs.

Pain is a multidimensional, complex symptom expression that requires careful evaluation. The use of opioids and nonopioids requires thorough consideration, and the risk-to-benefit ratio must be taken into account. Improper titration leads to poor pain control and frustration for health care professionals, patients, and families.

Resources
Internet Resources
AIDS Info
U.S. Department of Health and Human Services human immunodeficiency virus treatment guidelines, updated as new data become available. Available at www.aidsinfo.nih.gov/
American Academy of Pain Medicine (AAPM)
Promotes quality of care for patients with pain through research, education, and advocacy. Available at www.painmed.org/
American College of Physicians Home Care Guide for Advanced Cancer
Guide for family members, hospice workers, and caregivers who are caring for patients with advanced cancer. Information is offered on respite, pain management, symptoms, helping younger people, and grieving. Available at www.acponline.org/public/h_care/index.html
Edmonton Palliative Care Program
Available at www.palliative.org
Medical College of Wisconsin
Fast Facts at End of Life/Palliative Education Resource Center. Available at www.eperc.mcw.edu
International AIDS Society USA
Not-for-profit continuing medical education organization offering up-to-date information for physicians who are actively involved in the care of people living with human immunodeficiency virus/acquired immunodeficiency syndrome. Information is disseminated through continuing medical education courses around the United States, the publication *Topics in HIV Medicine,* and the development of treatment guidelines. Available at www.iasusa.org/
International Association for the Study of Pain
Available at www.iasp-pain.org
National Cancer Institute, National Institutes of Health Physician Data Query
Available at www.nci.nih.gov/cancertopics/pdq
World Health *Organization (WHO): WHO Cancer Pain Relief,* ed 2, Geneva, Switzerland, 1996, WHO.
Provides a proposed method for pain relief and includes information on how pain medications are available internationally. Available at www.who.int/ncd/cancer/publications/en

Print Resources
Pereira J: *The Pallium Palliative Pocketbook, Canadian* ed 1, Edmonton, 2008, The Pallium Project.
Walsh D, Caraceni AT, Fainsinger R, et al, editors: *Palliative medicine,* Philadelphia, 2008, WB Saunders.
Bruera E, Higginson IJ, Ripamonti C, Von Gunten C: *Textbook of palliative medicine,* Hodder Arnold, 2006, Oxford University Press, USA.

Guidelines
Joint Commission on Accreditation of Healthcare Organizations: Pain Management Standards for Accreditation of Healthcare Organizations
Available at www.jcaho.org/standard/pm_hap.html
National Guideline Clearinghouse: Clinical Practice Guidelines for Chronic Non-Malignant Pain Syndrome Patients: An Evidence Based Approach
Available at www.guideline.gov
American Pain Society: Guideline for the Management of Cancer Pain in Adults and Children
Available at www.ampainsoc.org/pub/cancer.htm
Cancer-related Pain Management: A Report of Evidence-Based Recommendations to Guide Practice
Cancer-related Pain Management Working Panel—A Quality Initiative of the Program in Evidence-Based Care (PEBC), Cancer Care Ontario (CCO)
Available at www.cancercare.on.ca/pdf/pebc16-2f.pdf
Canadian Pain Society. Pain—Consensus Statement and Guidelines from the Canadian Pain Society
Available at www.canadianpainsociety.ca/indexenglish.html

References
1. Keller S, Bann CM, Dodd SL, et al: Validity of the brief pain inventory for use in documenting the outcomes of patients with noncancer pain, *Clin J Pain* 20(5):309–318, 2004.
2. Knudsen AK, Aass N, Fainsinger R, et al: Classification of pain in cancer patients—a systematic literature review, *Palliat Med* 23(4):295–308, 2009.

3. Buffum MD, Hutt E, Chang VT, et al: Cognitive impairment and pain management: review of issues and challenges, *J Rehabil Res Dev* 44(2):315–330, 2007.
4. Dworkin RH, O'Connor AB, Backonja M, et al: Pharmacologic management of neuropathic pain: evidence-based recommendations, *Pain* 132(3):237–251, 2007 5.
5. Passik SD, Kirsh KL: The need to identify predictors of aberrant drug-related behavior and addiction in patients being treated with opioids for pain, *Pain Med* 4(2):186–189, 2003.
6. Weissman DE: Pseudoaddiction #69, *J Palliat Med* 8(6):1283–1284, 2005.
7. McCarberg B, Stanos S: Key patient assessment tools and treatment strategies for pain management, *Pain Pract* 8(6):423–432, 2008.
8. Steinweg DL, Worth H: Alcoholism: the keys to the CAGE, *Am J Med* 94(5):520–523, 1993.
9. Stockler M, Vardy J, Pillai A, Warr D: Acetaminophen (paracetamol) improves pain and well-being in people with advanced cancer already receiving a strong opioid regimen: a randomized, double-blind, placebo-controlled cross-over trial, *J Clin Oncol* 22(16):3389–3394, 15, 2004.
10. Clemens KE, Klaschik E: Management of constipation in palliative care patients, *Curr Opin Support Palliat Care* 2(1):22–27, 2008.
11. Pereira J, Lawlor P, Vigano A, et al: Equianalgesic dose ratios for opioids. a critical review and proposals for long-term dosing, *J Pain Symptom Manage* 22(2):672–687, 2001.
12. Hagen NA, Biondo P, Stiles C: Assessment and management of breakthrough pain in cancer patients: current approaches and emerging research, *Curr Pain Headache Rep* 12(4):241–248, 2008.
13. Dean M: Opioids in renal failure and dialysis patients, *J Pain Symptom Manage* 28(5):497–504, 2004.
14. Indelicato RA, Portenoy RK: Opioid rotation in the management of refractory cancer pain, *J Clin Oncol* 21(9 Suppl):87s–91s, 2003.
15. Nicholson AB: Methadone for cancer pain, *Cochrane Database System Rev* 3, 2009.
16. Watanabe S, Bruera E: Corticosteroids as adjuvant analgesics, *J Pain Symptom Manage* 9(7):442–445, 1994.
17. Saarto T, Wiffen PJ: Antidepressants for neuropathic pain, *Cochrane Database System Rev* 3, 2009.
18. Wiffen PJ, Collins S, McQuay HJ, et al: Anticonvulsant drugs for acute and chronic pain, *Cochrane Database System Rev* 3, 2009.
19. Wong RKS, Wiffen PJ: Bisphosphonates for the relief of pain secondary to bone metastases, *Cochrane Database System Rev* 3, 2009.
20. Farquhar-Smith WP: Do cannabinoids have a role in cancer pain management? *Curr Opin Support Palliat Care* 3(1):7–13, 2009.
21. Bell RF, Eccleston C, Kalso EA: Ketamine as an adjuvant to opioids for cancer pain, *Cochrane Database System Rev* 3, 2009.
22. Jackson K, Ashby M, Martin P, et al: "Burst" ketamine for refractory cancer pain: an open-label audit of 39 patients, *J Pain Symptom Manage* 22(4):834–842, 2001.
23. Brose WG, Cousins MJ: Subcutaneous lidocaine for treatment of neuropathic cancer pain, *Pain* 45(2):145–148, 1991.
24. McQuay HJ, Collins SL, Carroll D, Moore RA: Radiotherapy for the palliation of painful bone metastases, *Cochrane Database Syst Rev* (2)(2):CD001793, 2000.
25. White P, Lewith G, Prescott P, Conway J: Acupuncture versus placebo for the treatment of chronic mechanical neck pain: a randomized, controlled trial, *Ann Intern Med* 141(12):911–919, 21, 2004.
26. Johansson A, Sjolund B: Nerve blocks with local anesthetics and corticosteroids in chronic pain: a clinical follow-up study, *J Pain Symptom Manage* 11(3):181–187, 1996.
27. Hogan Q, Haddox JD, Abram S, et al: Epidural opiates and local anesthetics for the management of cancer pain, *Pain* 46(3):271–279, 1991.
28. Bedder MD, Burchiel K, Larson A: Cost analysis of two implantable narcotic delivery systems, *J Pain Symptom Manage* 6(6):368–373, 1991.
29. Fainsinger RL, Nekolaichuk CL: Cancer pain assessment—can we predict the need for specialist input? *Eur J Cancer* 44(8):1072–1077, 2008.

CHAPTER 8

Nausea and Vomiting

ELIEZER SOTO and ANN M. BERGER

Nausea and vomiting are two of the most common and feared symptoms experienced by palliative care patients. It is reasonable to distinguish two different forms of nausea and vomiting in cancer patients: that associated with chemotherapy and other oncologic treatments, and the chronic, multifactorial nausea and vomiting associated with the illness itself. It occurs in 40% to 70% of people with advanced cancer.[1] The evidence for treatment-related causes of nausea and vomiting is more robust than for disease-related causes. Most of the relevant research concerns chemotherapy-induced nausea and vomiting (CINV) in patients with cancer. However, despite major advances in antiemetic regimens, the incidence and severity of these symptoms is still significantly high. These symptoms are also common in other chronic, advanced progressive illnesses such as hepatitis C, renal failure, inflammatory bowel disease, and neurologic diseases.

These interrelated symptoms of nausea and vomiting can be associated with a broad spectrum of physical, psychological, social, and spiritual distress, including decreased physical activity, mood and sleep disturbances, changes in social roles, and existential questions about the meaning of life. Several observational studies have shown that CINV induces a decrease in health-related quality of life compared with patients without nausea and vomiting.[2] In addition, CINV can potentially interfere with the treatment process and hasten the course of the primary illness. Although research on these symptoms is ongoing, enough is known for assessment and development of a comprehensive, individualized plan that will improve quality of life for the patient and family.

Many specialists now favor a mechanism-based approach to nausea and vomiting management, which takes into account the cause of the symptoms, the likely mechanisms of action, and the central emetogenic pathway involved.

Definitions

A complete understanding of the terminology is essential for a more reliable assessment of the symptoms. Emesis comprises three different phases: *Retching* is the attempt to vomit without actually expelling stomach contents, characterized by repetitive diaphragmatic and abdominal musculature movements with a closed glottis. *Nausea* is the patient-defined sensation of wanting to vomit, associated with autonomic signs such as pallor, diaphoresis, and tachycardia, involving a subjective component unique to the individual. *Vomiting* is defined as forcefully regurgitating ingested food. It involves a constellation of actions, including contraction of the abdominal wall musculature, pylorus, and antrum; rise of the gastric cardia; decreased lower esophageal sphincter pressure; and esophageal dilation. The emetic syndromes are physically and psychosocially distressing to the patient and can lead to metabolic disturbances and changes in the treatment of the underlying disorder.

Pathophysiology

VOMITING CENTER

The pathophysiology of nausea and vomiting is complex and involves several different mechanisms of action. Current knowledge of the pathophysiology is based on previous studies on chemotherapy-induced, radiotherapy-induced, and postoperative nausea and vomiting. Despite the wide variety of clinical presentations, all cases of emesis share similar general pathophysiologic features. A physiologic or psychological trigger activates the central nervous system's innate pathways for emesis, culminating in the so-called *vomiting center* (VC), which is located in the lateral reticular formation of the medulla. It has been described as a physiologic control center without a discrete anatomical site consisting of neuronal networks that coordinate the act of vomiting. This center includes the nucleus tractus solitarius (NTS) and the dorsal motor nucleus of the vagus nerve (DMV). Impulses are transmitted to the VC by one of the following pathways: the chemoreceptor trigger zone (CTZ), in the area postrema of the medulla oblongata, which responds to chemical stimuli in the cerebrospinal fluid and blood; the cerebral cortex and limbic system, which are stimulated by the senses and learned associations; the vestibular apparatus of the middle ear; a peripheral pathway that involve neurotransmitter receptors in the gastrointestinal tract; and/or vagal and spinal sympathetic nerves respond to chemical and physical stimuli.

CHEMORECEPTOR TRIGGER ZONE

A chemoreceptor trigger zone (CTZ) located in area postrema of the medulla directly detects toxins in the blood and cerebrospinal fluid and relays that information to the VC. The CTZ is primarily activated by chemotherapeutic agents in CINV, by toxins from food poisoning, by metabolic products (e.g., uremia in renal failure, hypercalcemia, and liver failure), and by a wide spectrum of medications. It also receives input from the vestibular apparatus and vagus nerve. However, it cannot initiate emesis independently and does so only through stimulation of the NTS localized in the deeper layers of the area postrema. The CTZ contains numerous receptor sites for neurotransmitters such as serotonin 5-hydroxytryptamine type 3 (5-HT$_3$), dopamine (D$_2$), histamine, and neurokinin-1 (NK-1), all of which may be involved in vomiting.

CEREBRAL CORTEX

Cortical signals can also activate the VC. The cerebral cortex is largely responsible for nausea and vomiting associated with increased intracranial pressure, such as that caused by tumor or closed head injury, as well as that associated with central nervous infection such as meningitis and encephalitis. It is also seen in anticipatory nausea and vomiting associated with the memory of a past trigger such as chemotherapy and radiation, in anxiety and other emotional triggers, and in the recognition of certain tastes, sights, or smells.

VESTIBULAR SYSTEM

The vestibular center is responsible largely for nausea and vomiting caused by motion sickness. It integrates and interprets information on balance from the inner ear, peripheral receptors (e.g., nociceptors), and the visual system. After receiving this information, it sends signals to the VC to activate emesis associated with dizziness, loss of balance, motion sickness, and other vestibular disorders. Drugs such as opioids directly stimulate the vestibular apparatus and may cause nausea and vomiting by the same pathway.

GASTROINTESTINAL TRACT

Peripheral emesis is associated with a complex system of afferent nerves that induce or inhibit the response in the CTZ or VC. Chemoreceptors and mechanoreceptors in the gastrointestinal tract send signals to the brain through the vagus nerve and autonomic nervous system in response to irritation of the tissues of the gut, including intestinal smooth muscle and the peritoneum. These tissues may be irritated by drugs, toxins, or viral or bacterial infections. Additionally, complete or partial bowel obstruction and tumor growths in the gastrointestinal tract, celiac plexus, and liver often trigger emesis. When the clinician is making a diagnosis in cases of peripheral emesis, constipation should also be considered along with the emetic symptoms.

NEUROTRANSMITTERS AND RECEPTORS

Chemotherapy-induced nausea and vomiting has been the prototype in trying to understand the pathophysiology of nausea and vomiting and the neurotransmitters involved. Dopamine appears to play an important role in CINV, whereas serotonin, substance P, histamine, acetylcholine, and other neurotransmitters have been found in the gastrointestinal tract. Many effective antiemetics, such as phenothiazines and butyrophenones, are dopamine antagonists that may bind specifically to the D$_2$ receptor. These were among the first agents with demonstrated antiemetic efficacy.[3] However, there is a high degree of variation in dopamine receptor binding affinity by these drugs. It is known that not all the receptors in the CTZ are dopaminergic because the effect of dopamine antagonists is not equal to surgical ablation of the

CTZ. Studies on high-dose metoclopramide, a central and peripheral dopamine antagonist, have shown that the degree of antiemetic activity cannot be explained solely on the basis of dopamine blockade. Metoclopramide is also a weak antagonist of peripheral 5-HT$_3$ receptors and can stimulate gastrointestinal motility by increasing acetylcholine release from the cholinergic nerves of the gastrointestinal tract.

During the past two decades, multiple studies have demonstrated that 5-HT$_3$ and substance P–natural killer-1 (NK-1) receptor pathways play major roles in the modulation of CINV and perhaps in other conditions, such as opiate-induced and postoperative nausea and vomiting.[4] The 5-HT$_3$ receptors are located in both central and peripheral locations. Antagonism of 5-HT$_3$ receptors on vagal afferents likely causes or significantly contributes to the antiemetic effect.[5] The introduction of 5-HT$_3$ receptor antagonists offered an improved treatment option for prevention of acute CINV.

Substance P (mediated by NK-1 receptors) is known to modulate nociception. High-density NK-1 receptors are located in the regions of the brain implicated in the emetic reflex, such as the area postrema and NTS, as well as in peripheral sites such as the gastrointestinal tract. The primary mechanism of the NK-1 receptor blockade appears to be central, and antagonists of these receptors are effective for both acute and delayed events in CINV. NK-1 antagonists augment the antiemetic activity of 5-HT$_3$ receptor antagonists and corticosteroids in the prevention and treatment of CINV.

The vestibular system may also play a role in nausea and vomiting by stimulating the VC via histamine and muscarinic cholinergic receptors stimulation. Conditions such as acoustic neuroma and metastasis affecting the vestibular apparatus at the base of the skull can influence the vestibular system. Histamine (H$_1$ and H$_2$) receptors are found in abundance in the CTZ; however, H$_2$ antagonists do not work well as antiemetics. H$_1$ antagonists mostly help to alleviate nausea and vomiting induced by vestibular disorders and motion sickness.

Chemotherapeutic agents and many other types of medications such as aspirin and opioids directly stimulate the vestibular apparatus. Opioids can alter the sensitivity of the vestibular center, resulting in nausea associated with movement. Motion can stimulate receptors in the labyrinth, which transmits impulses to the vestibular nucleus, cerebellum, CTZ, and VC. Opioid receptors are also found in the CTZ. It is known that opioids have mixed emetic and antiemetic effects that are blocked by naloxone, removing inhibitory input into the CTZ. These facts have led to the proposal to use certain opioids and enkephalins as antiemetics.[6]

Cannabinoid receptors are located throughout the central and peripheral nervous systems. They are especially localized in the brainstem, basal ganglia, amygdala, and several cortical regions. Although the mechanism of action is not entirely clear, it has been shown that most cannabinoid receptors have an inhibitory effect on neurotransmission and may inhibit emesis. Cannabinoids and cannabinoid agonists (including dronabinol and nabilone, synthetic tetrahydrocannabinols) may be indicated for some patients who are receiving mildly emetogenic chemotherapy and likely helpful in nausea and vomiting in other advanced illnesses states.

The importance of taste and odor perception in relation to enhancement of gagging, nausea, and vomiting is well appreciated, although the exact mechanism is unknown. There are corticobulbar afferents to the VC that mediate vomiting in response to smells, sights, and tastes, playing a role in psychogenic vomiting. Women who have suffered from hyperemesis during pregnancy show taste damage.[7] In addition to indirect effects on taste, some chemotherapeutic agents can be tasted. Clearly, changes in taste secondary to infection or medications may contribute to both nausea and vomiting, as well as to anorexia.

Etiology

DRUG-INDUCED NAUSEA AND VOMITING

Palliative care patients are often on medication regimens including drugs with known emetogenic potential, such as opioids and nonsteroidal anti-inflammatory drugs (NSAIDS). These drugs can cause nausea and vomiting through different mechanisms. Opioids bind to their receptors in the gastrointestinal tract, decreasing peristalsis and increasing the risk for constipation. High levels of opioids in the blood can stimulate the CTZ, which responds to perceived toxins by sending an impulse to the VC. Impaired liver and kidney functions adversely affect the excretion of opioids and their metabolites, resulting in toxic levels in the blood, brain, and liver, causing nausea and vomiting. Opioids can also increase the sensitivity of the vestibular center by an unknown mechanism. In addition to opioids, many other drugs, such as NSAIDS, steroids, iron supplements, and antibiotics, have been associated with nausea and vomiting secondary to irritation of the gastric lining. Antibiotics may also cause nausea by a direct effect on the CTZ.

ANTICIPATORY NAUSEA AND VOMITING

Anticipatory nausea and vomiting (ANV) has been referred to as conditioned, learned, or psychological nausea and vomiting. It develops in up to a third of patients undergoing chemotherapy, usually occurring several hours before the expected chemotherapy, triggered by talking or thinking about the medication. Classical conditioning plays an important role in the development of ANV in patients receiving chemotherapy.[8] This phenomenon, where the conditioned stimulus is the thought of chemotherapy or of conditioned elements associated with it, has been called a Pavlovian conditioned reflex.[9] Studies on AVN have shown that the intensity of anticipatory nausea is also a significant predictor of the severity of the posttreatment nausea patients experience during the 24-hour period after the chemotherapy infusion.[10] Probably this is also true in nonchemotherapy states.

CHEMOTHERAPY-INDUCED NAUSEA AND VOMITING

Two of the most feared symptoms experienced by palliative care patients are nausea and vomiting secondary to a chemotherapeutic regimen. Up to 80% of cancer patients receiving chemotherapy will develop CINV.[11] The formulation of better medication regimens to target different mechanisms of action and improved treatment guidelines have played central roles in CINV research. These symptoms can have a significant impact on patients' quality of life, performance status, and daily functioning. The duration, more than severity, seems to be responsible for the impact of CINV on patients' daily lives. This leads to poor compliance with the chemotherapy regimen and interruptions in treatment, complicating disease management and leading to poor outcomes and increased overall health care costs.

CENTRAL NERVOUS SYSTEM DISORDERS

An increase in intracranial pressure resulting from space-occupying lesions in metastatic or primary cancer, infections such as meningitis and encephalitis, and cerebral edema secondary to cerebrovascular accidents directly trigger pressure receptors in the brain, which transmit the information to the VC, inducing nausea and vomiting. On the other hand, several primary central nervous system diseases, such as multiple sclerosis, Parkinson's disease, amyotrophic lateral sclerosis, and myasthenia gravis, may also produce a disturbance in central control of gastrointestinal motility through different mechanisms. Some of these conditions may cause gastroparesis, gastrointestinal dysmotility, gastric atony, or dysphagia, resulting in gastrointestinal syndromes that cause vomiting or intestinal pseudo-obstruction.

GASTROINTESTINAL PROBLEMS

Constipation is one of the most common causes of nausea and vomiting in patients with end-stage cancer and other chronic conditions such as renal failure. A combination of decreased oral intake, immobility, hypercalcemia, hyponatremia, decreased bowel transit secondary to tumor compression or metabolic disturbances, neurologic diseases, and use of medications such as opioids may cause constipation. As intestinal transit slows down, abdominal pressure and bowel distension increase, activating neurotransmitters throughout the gut. These stimulate the peripheral pathway along the vagus nerve, which then communicates with the VC.

Bowel obstruction is also a common problem among patients with advanced cancer, particularly abdominal pathologies such as peritoneal carcinomatosis from metastatic colon or ovarian carcinoma. The onset is usually slow, as the tumor compresses the bowel extrinsically or grows intraluminally. It often manifests in pain with severe nausea and vomiting. For patients who are not surgical candidates, these symptoms can be controlled by a combination of medications.

Assessment

The most important consideration when assessing nausea and vomiting is to ascertain its cause or causes. Nausea can be caused by the disease process itself, side effects of medications, complication of treatments, or psychogenic factors. Patients with life-threatening palliative care illnesses can have nausea and vomiting for many different reasons (Table 8-1).

A detailed history and physical examination are essential for an adequate assessment of patients' symptoms. In the evaluation of nausea and vomiting, each symptom should be assessed separately. The clinician must ask specific questions about the symptoms, including both qualitative and quantitative measures that may be useful for diagnosis and treatment. When assessing nausea, the patient should be questioned about the intensity, frequency, duration of the episodes, time of day when they occur, the presence of emesis, and other possible triggers such as movement, smells, tastes, memories, or medications. When assessing emesis it is important to obtain detailed information on the number and duration of episodes; volume, contents, and color of the vomitus (e.g., undigested food, bile); and associated symptoms such as dizziness, altered mental status, syncopal episodes, abdominal pain, constipation, and emotional response. Several validated multidimensional assessment tools, such as the Edmonton Symptom Assessment System, are available to aid in better assessment and formulation of the therapeutic plan.[12] These are used for the initial assessment to establish a baseline, as well as for monitoring the same symptoms, allowing the clinician to have a better sense of therapy effectiveness.

Table 8-1. Causes of Nausea and Vomiting

Cause	Examples
Medications	Chemotherapy
	Opioids
	Antibiotics
	Antifungals
	Anticholinergic drugs
Metabolic causes	Uremia
	Liver failure
	Hypercalcemia
Gastrointestinal causes	Gastritis
	Gastric or duodenal ulcers
	Bowel obstruction
	Constipation
	Motility problems
Infections: bacterial or viral	Sepsis
	Hepatitis
Vestibular problems	Auditory nerve tumors
	Motion sickness
	Increased intracranial pressure
	Brain tumors
	Infections
Psychological conditions	Anxiety
	Fear
	Grief
Radiation therapy	

A detailed medical history also benefits the clinician in making a better assessment. Several comorbidities have been associated with nausea and vomiting, including anxiety disorder, peptic ulcer disease, and diabetic neuropathy causing gastroparesis and autonomic failure and chronic renal failure, among others. A thorough physical examination in combination with imaging studies and basic laboratory investigations may be helpful to rule out certain conditions associated with nausea and vomiting, such as constipation, bowel obstruction, liver failure, uremia, hypercalcemia, and hyponatremia. Some physical examination findings for specific conditions include abdominal tenderness, distension, and abnormal bowel sounds in bowel obstruction or ileus; abdominal fullness, decreased bowel sounds, and fecal impaction in constipation; abdominal ascites or masses in abdominal malignancy; papilledema associated with increased intracranial pressure; and orthostatic hypotension in several neurologic conditions, such as diabetic neuropathy secondary to autonomic insufficiency. A detailed medication history (past and current) is also important to rule out easily correctable causes of nausea and vomiting as well as prevent future episodes.

Patient Risk Factors

An understanding of the risk factors for CINV and ANV is of great value because they can predict chronic nausea and vomiting caused by other medications. They are the same for all patients with nausea and vomiting in the palliative care setting. Risk factors for developing CINV include those that are patient specific and treatment specific.

Patient-specific risk factors include age (younger than 50) and female gender, which can predict a patient's response to CINV. Aging is usually attributed to a combination of decreasing receptor sensitivity and greater familiarity with nausea and vomiting because of more experience with illness. Anxiety associated with treatment and expectations of posttreatment nausea are also strong predictors of severe nausea after chemotherapy.[13] Previous experience with chemotherapy very often sets the stage for success or failure in controlling emesis with future chemotherapy cycles. There is also a role for susceptibility to motion sickness, history of morning sickness or hyperemesis during pregnancy, food intake and amount of sleep before chemotherapy, roommate experiencing nausea and vomiting, motivational level, and performance status as prognostic indicators.[14]

The only patient-specific risk factor that has been shown to exert a protective role in the control of emesis is a history of heavy alcohol consumption, defined as intake greater than 100 g of ethanol, or five mixed drinks per day. This implies that someone who is sensitive to the effects of alcohol and has a history of relatively minimum intake may have a higher chance of CINV.[15]

Treatment-specific factors include the chemotherapy drug, its dose, and the infusion rate. Clearly, the chemotherapy agents are the primary determinants of subsequent episodes of nausea and vomiting. Almost all patients receiving highly emetogenic chemotherapy regimens, such as those that are platinum based or cyclophosphamide based, will develop both acute and delayed nausea and vomiting if not treated appropriately. Higher doses and faster infusion rate have also been associated with worsening nausea and vomiting.

Anticipatory nausea and vomiting is a learned response that usually occurs before, during, or after the exposure to chemotherapy or other emetogenic medications. Risk factors associated with an increased incidence of ANV are similar to the ones associated with CINV and include age (younger than 50), severe or intolerable nausea and vomiting after the last chemotherapy, sweating and generalized weakness after the last treatment, schedule of chemotherapy, numerous cycles, prior exposure to tastes and odors, history of motion sickness, depression, and anxiety.[14,16]

Treatment

The goals of therapy in the management of nausea and vomiting are to enhance the patient's quality of life, to prevent or eliminate nausea and vomiting, and to reduce hospital and clinic length of stay and treatment costs. Management includes two different aspects, prevention and treatment, pharmacologic and nonpharmacologic.

PREVENTIVE MANAGEMENT

The goal of prevention is to reduce distressful symptoms, morbidity, and complications from treatment; shorten hospital stays; and lower overall costs. The following guidelines are used in the prevention of nausea and vomiting in palliative care patients:

- Know the patient's individual risk factors and prior symptoms before starting emetogenic medications.
- Give the appropriate antiemetic medication when it is known that emesis is likely to occur.
- Ensure that patients have antiemetics available when they start emetogenic medications such as opioids or chemotherapy.
- Prevent medication-induced constipation.
- Respond rapidly to nausea and vomiting.

PHARMACOLOGIC MANAGEMENT

It is important to be aware of the antiemetic agents, their mechanism of action, and potential causes in individual patients to adequately prevent and treat nausea and vomiting. There is a growing diversity of antiemetic classes. Most pharmacologic management of emesis is based on interference with the neurotransmitters associated with the syndrome (Table 8-2). Because the precise mechanism of emesis may be very difficult to assess in some patients and because multiple medications can target several neurotransmitters or receptors, the empirical approach is usually the most effective. Adjusting medications and dosages over time should help the patient reach at least a tolerable level of symptoms, if not a total palliation.

General principles of pharmacologic management include the following:

- Take into consideration the available routes of administration and side effect profile.
- Ensure that antiemetics are given regularly, rather than on an as-needed basis.
- Use one antiemetic first and go to maximum doses or intolerable side effects before switching or adding a second medication. If the first agent is only partially effective at maximum doses, try a different class of antiemetic.
- A combination of antiemetics may be necessary to help relieve the nausea and vomiting targeting different neurotransmitters pathways.

Dopamine and 5-HT$_3$ are the two neurotransmitters most commonly involved in eliciting an emetic response. Dopamine antagonists (e.g., metoclopramide, haloperidol, chlorpromazine, and prochlorperazine) and 5-HT$_3$ antagonists (e.g., ondansetron, granisetron, dolasetron, tropisetron, and palonosetron) are highly effective at blocking these receptors and relieving symptoms. Metoclopramide, also a prokinetic agent, which sensitizes tissues to acetylcholine, stimulating upper gastrointestinal tract motility, is often useful because it combines central and gastric-emptying effects.

The NK-1 receptor antagonists are a new class of antiemetics for CINV. Aprepitant was the first available agent within the class, approved by the Food and Drug Administration in 2003. Several clinical trials in cancer patients on highly emetogenic chemotherapy regimens have shown that aprepitant may provide superior efficacy in prevention of CINV.[17] Its use in other types of nausea and vomiting requires more study.

Certain antihistamines, including meclizine and dimenhydrinate, are indicated for vestibular-induced nausea. Scopolamine, an M$_1$-muscarinic (cholinergic) receptor antagonist, is also indicated for vestibular-induced emesis. Cortical-associated emesis is generally associated with the neurotransmitters 5-HT$_3$ and GABA. Therefore, 5-HT$_3$ antagonists, as well as GABA agonists such as lorazepam, may be helpful. Lorazepam and other benzodiazepines are also particularly helpful in anxiety-induced emesis.

Table 8-2. General Antiemetic Dosing Chart*

Medication	Suggested Dose and Route	Adverse Effects	Comments
Serotonin Antagonists			
Ondansetron	8 mg IV or 0.15 mg/kg IV q3h × 3 12–24 mg PO qd or 8 mg PO bid	Mild headache Constipation Lightheadedness Diarrhea Mild sedation Asymptomatic liver Transaminase elevation Rarely EPS	First dose 30 min before chemotherapy; no renal adjustment
Granisetron	2 mg PO qd or 1 mg PO q12h 0.01 mg/kg IV over 5 min	See above; taste changes	PO first dose <1 hr before chemotherapy; IV first Dose <30 min before chemotherapy; no renal adjustment
Dolasetron	100 mg PO or IV 1.8 mg/kg IV	See above	See above
Palonosetron	No oral form; 0.25 mg IV	Headache Constipation QT prolongation	Give 30 min before chemotherapy; 40-hr half-life; no renal adjustment
Dopamine Antagonists			
Metoclopramide	5–20 mg PO/IV q6h 4–8 mg PO bid	EPS (greater risk if younger)	Pretreat with diphenhydramine to decrease EPS when using to prevent/treat CINV; prolonged half-life with renal failure; >10-mg dose should be given IVPB; avoid in bowel obstruction
Chlorpromazine	10–25 mg PO q4h 25–50 mg IV/IM q4h 50–100 mg PR q6h	Sedation Tardive dyskinesia Hypotension NMS	May use for intractable hiccups
Haloperidol	0.5–5 mg PO, SC, IV q 8h (max 100 mg in 24 hr)	NMS EPS Tardive dyskinesia Drowsiness Anticholinergic effects Gynecomastia	Half-life ~20 hr; usual max 30 mg/day

Table 8-2. General Antiemetic Dosing Chart* (Continued)

Medication	Suggested Dose and Route	Adverse Effects	Comments
Prochlorperazine	5–10 mg PO/IM q6h 2.5–10 mg IV q3h 25 mg PR bid	Drowsiness NMS Tardive dyskinesia Dry mouth Constipation Urinary retention	Multiple adverse reaction risks; max 40 mg/day
Neurokinin Antagonists			
Aprepitant	See specific CINV prevention and treatment guidelines	Diarrhea Fatigue Hiccups Constipation Rarely neutropenia	Contraindicated with cisapride and pimozide (for QT prolongation risk)
Steroid (1)			
Dexamethasone	4–8 mg PO bid 8–20 mg IV qd 0.5–0.6 mg/kg divided q12h	Mood swings Insomnia Peptic ulcer Appetite increase	Increase dose as needed; often dosed empirically
Methylprednisolone	See CINV guideline for dosing	See above	Used as a substitute for dexamethasone in CINV prevention and treatment
Antihistamine			
Diphenhydramine	25–50 mg PO q4h 10–50 mg IV q2h	Drowsiness Dry mouth Urinary retention Confusion See above: for Diphenhydramine	Max 400 mg/day; EPS treatment dose is 50 mg
Hydroxyzine	25–100 mg PO/IM q6h	Bitter taste Headache	Max 600 mg/day
Meclizine	25–50 mg PO q2h	Drowsiness Dry mouth Confusion Nausea/vomiting Tachycardia	
Anticholinergic			
Scopolamine	1.5-mg patch q72 hr 0.6–1 mg IV/SC q4h	Dry mouth Blurred vision Urinary retention Tachycardia	In palliative care, used for excess secretions and with intestinal obstruction
Glycopyrrolate	1–2 mg PO bid 0.1–0.2 mg IM/IV q6h	Constipation Dry mouth Urinary retention	In palliative care, used for excess secretions and with intestinal obstruction

Continued on following page

Table 8-2. General Antiemetic Dosing Chart* (Continued)

Medication	Suggested Dose and Route	Adverse Effects	Comments
Cannabinoid			
Dronabinol	2.5–5 mg PO q6h (max 20 mg/day)	Dysphoria Somnolence Difficulty concentrating	Generally better tolerated in younger patients
Benzodiazepine			
Lorazepam	0.5–2 mg PO, SL, IV q6h	Sedation Amnesia	Not intrinsically an antiemetic; Very useful as an adjunct; See CINV guidelines
Miscellaneous			
Octreotide	50–300 g SC bid; (max 1500 g/day)	Diarrhea Dizziness Biliary tract abnormalities Fatigue Fever	Start at 50 and titrate up based on response; used in palliative medicine for nausea/vomiting resulting from complete bowel obstruction; Decreases secretions

*These dosing guidelines are not meant to replace US Food and Drug Administration guidelines or clinical judgment.

bid, twice daily; EPS, extrapyramidal symptoms; CINV, chemotherapy-induced nausea and vomiting; IM, intramuscularly; IV, intravenously; IVPB, by intravenous piggyback; NMS, neuroleptic malignant syndrome; PO, orally; PR, rectally, qd, once daily; SC, subcutaneously; SL, sublingually.

From Berger A, Berger S: Introduction. In Berger A (ed): *Prevention of chemotherapy-induced nausea and vomiting*, New York, 2004, CMP Healthcare Media, pp ix–xii.

Other medications, such as cannabinoids (e.g., dronabinol and nabilone) and corticosteroids (e.g., dexamethasone), may also be effective in treating cortical-associated emesis, emesis secondary to increased intracranial pressure, and CINV.[18]

NONPHARMACOLOGIC MANAGEMENT

Nonpharmacologic techniques are important as a complementary approach for the management of emetic syndromes. Acupuncture, electroacupuncture, and acupressure may relieve some of the symptoms of nausea. Several studies have shown that acupressure at the P6 point is a value-added technique in addition to pharmacologic management for patients undergoing chemotherapy or radiation to reduce the amount and intensity of delayed CINV.[19,20] Acupressure bands are safe, low-cost, nonintrusive, well-accepted adjuncts to standard antiemetic medications. However, a recent Cochrane review on acupuncture-point stimulation for CINV has shown that stimulation of all methods combined reduced the incidence of acute vomiting. By modality, electroacupuncture reduced the proportion of acute vomiting but manual acupuncture did not. Acupressure reduced first-day nausea but had no benefit on vomiting.[21]

Relaxation therapy, guided imagery, and hypnosis are especially effective for CINV, ANV, and other cortical emetic syndromes.[22,23] Group psychotherapy has been shown to reduce the incidence of vomiting in advanced-stage cancer patients treated with chemotherapy.[24] Studies on the use of ginger for CINV have shown that it reduces nausea and the amount of antiemetic medications used, which holds the potential of representing a novel, nutrition-based treatment for emesis.[25] Regulating the patient's food intake and working with a nutritionist to discover and avoid trigger foods or smells are also recommended, especially for patients with chronic nausea and vomiting.

PEARLS AND PITFALLS

- It is important to determine whether nausea and vomiting are related to central, vestibular, taste/smell, peripheral, or psychological causes.

- The key aspect of treating nausea and vomiting is prevention rather than interventional or salvage therapy.

Summary

The management of nausea and vomiting is a commonly encountered issue in palliative care practice. These symptoms have a great impact on quality of life for the patient and family and are often detrimental to the treatment of the underlying disease. The multifactorial origin of these symptoms presents a challenge for the patient, the family, and the clinician and requires careful assessment and a personalized treatment plan. Emerging pharmacologic and nonpharmacologic approaches, combined with improved understanding of the complex pathophysiology of these disorders, will aid the clinician in their alleviation.

Resources

American Academy of Hospice and Palliative Medicine (USA)
    West Lake Avenue, Glenview, IL 60025; (847) 375–4712. Available at www.aahpm.org
National Hospice and Palliative Care Organization (USA)
    Diagonal Road, Suite 625, Alexandria, VA 22314; (703) 837–1500. Available at www.nhpco.org
World Health Organization
    Avenue Appia 20, 1211 Geneva 27, Switzerland; (+ 41 22) 791 21 11. Available at www.who.int

References

1. Grond S, Zech D, Diefenbach C, et al: Prevalence and pattern of symptoms in patients with cancer pain: A prospective evaluation of 1635 cancer patients referred to a pain clinic, *J Pain Symptom Manag* 9:372–382, 1994.
2. Osoba D, Zee B, Warr D, et al: Effect of postchemotherapy nausea and vomiting on health-related quality of life, *Support Care Cancer* 5:307–313, 1997.
3. Moertel CG, Reitemeier RJ, Gage RP: A controlled clinical evaluation of antiemetic drugs, *JAMA* 186:116–118, 1963.
4. Miner WD, Sanger GJ, Turner DH: Evidence that 5-hydroxytryptamine3 receptors mediate cytotoxic drug and radiation-evoked emesis, *Br J Cancer* 56:159–162, 1987.

5. Endo T, Minami M, Hirafuji M, et al: Neurochemistry and neuropharmacology of emesis—the role of serotonin, *Toxicology* 153:189–201, 2000.
6. Wiser W, Berger AM: Practical management of chemotherapy-induced nausea and vomiting, *Oncology* 19:637–645, 2005.
7. Sipiora ML, Murtaugh MA, Gregoire MB, et al: Bitter taste perception and severe vomiting during pregnancy, *Physiol Behav* 69:259–267, 2000.
8. Stockhorst U, Hans-Joachim S, Enck P: Pavlovian conditioning of nausea and vomiting, *Auton Neurosci Basic* 129:50–57, 2006.
9. Carey MP, Burish TG: Etiology and treatment of the psychological side effects associated with cancer chemotherapy: a critical review and discussion, *Psychol Bull* 104:307–325, 1988.
10. Bovbjerg D: The continuing problem of postchemotherapy nausea and vomiting: contributions of classical conditioning, *Auton Neurosci Basic* 129:92–98, 2006.
11. Moran C, Smith DC, Anderson DA, et al: Incidence of nausea and vomiting with cytotoxic chemotherapy: a prospective randomized trial of antiemetics, *Br Med J* 1:1323–1324, 1979.
12. Bruera E, Kuehn N, Miller MJ, et al: The Edmonton Symptom Assessment System (ESAS): a simple method for the assessment of palliative care patients, *J Palliat Care* 7:6–9, 1991.
13. Roscoe J, Bushunow P, Morrow G, et al: Patient expectation is a strong predictor of severe nausea after chemotherapy, *Cancer* 101(11):2701–2708, 2004.
14. Berger AM, Clark-Snow RA: Adverse effects of treatment. In DeVita VT Jr, Hellman S, Rosenberg SA, editors: *Cancer: principles and practice of oncology*, ed 6, Philadephia, 2001, Lippincott Williams & Wilkins.
15. D'Acuisto RW, Tyson LB, Gralla RJ, et al: Antiemetic trials to control delayed vomiting following high-dose cisplatin, *Proc Am Soc Clin Oncol* 5:257, 1986.
16. Morrow GR, Rosenthal SN: Models, mechanisms and management of anticipatory nausea and emesis, *Oncology* 53:4–7, 1996.
17. Rapoport BL, Jordan K, Boice JA, et al: Aprepitant for the prevention of chemotherapy-induced nausea and vomiting associated with a broad range of moderately emetogenic chemotherapies and tumor types: a randomized, double-blind study, *Support Care Cancer* 2009 (online publication ahead of print).
18. Mieri E, Jhangiani H, Vredenburgh JJ, et al: Efficacy of dronabinol alone and in combination with ondansetron versus ondansetron alone for delayed chemotherapy-induced nausea and vomiting, *Curr Med Res Opin* 23(3):533–543, 2007.
19. NIH Consensus Conference: Acupuncture, *JAMA* 280:1518–1524, 1998.
20. Roscoe JA, Bushunow P, Jean-Pierre P, et al: Acupressure bands are effective in reducing radiation therapy-related nausea, *J Pain Symptom Manage* 38(3):381–389, 2009.
21. Ezzo J, Richardson MA, Vickers A, et al: Acupuncture-point stimulation for chemotherapy-induced nausea or vomiting, *Cochrane Database of Systematic Reviews* 2006, Issue 2. Art. No.: CD002285. DOI: 10.1002/14651858.CD002285.pub2.
22. Lyles JN, Burish TG, Krozely MG, et al: Efficacy of relaxation training and guided imagery in reducing the aversiveness of cancer chemotherapy, *J Consult Clin Psych* 50:509–524, 1982.
23. Marchioro G, Azzarello G, Viviani F, et al: Hypnosis in the treatment of anticipatory nausea and vomiting in patients receiving cancer chemotherapy, *Oncology* 59:100–104, 2000.
24. Parvez T, Moteab-Alharbi T, Dong-Mein F: Impact of group psychotherapy in chemotherapy induced vomiting for treatment of advanced breast and lungs cancer, *Journal of College of Physicians and Surgeons Pakistan* 17(2):89–93, 2007.
25. Levine ME, Gillis MG, Yanchis-Koch S, et al: Protein and ginger for the treatment of chemotherapy-induced delayed nausea, *J Altern Complem Med* 14(5):545–551, 2008.

CHAPTER 9

PART A: *Cachexia*

AMNA F. HUSAIN

Pathophysiology	Pearls
Assessment	Pitfalls
Management	Summary
Future Directions	

Cachexia is a complex syndrome with loss of muscle mass as its prominent feature. It occurs in many disease states, such as cancer, chronic infections (human immunodeficiency virus [HIV], tuberculosis), and other chronic illnesses (rheumatoid arthritis; chronic obstructive pulmonary disease; renal, heart, and liver failure). Although anorexia and decreased intake often accompany cachexia, nutritional supplementation in oral or parenteral form does not reverse cachexia. Beyond this, there is inconsistency in the definition, which poses significant challenges to research and clinical care. For example, some claim that loss of fat tissue is invariably present in cachexia, whereas a recent consensus meeting of experts reported that loss of fat tissue may or may not be present. Recent attempts at standardizing the definition of cachexia have included cutoff levels of weight loss and calculations that include biologic markers for inflammation.[1–3]

As challenging as the clinical definition appears to be, the meaning and impact of cachexia for patients, families, and caregivers is even more complex and layered.[4] The fact that cachexia is not reversed by improved intake is confusing to patients, their caregivers, and some health care professionals. It is counter to the very human instinct that a good diet is disease fighting and life maintaining. In addition, feeding is an essential component of nurturing and perceived as a sign of competent caregiving. In some instances, these perceptions are reinforced by health care professionals who may say to patients that if they are able to gain weight and strength, they may be offered further chemotherapy. This message is particularly damaging, considering that our evolving understanding of cachexia tells us that gaining weight is often not in the patient's or caregiver's control. However, what is evident is that cachexia is associated with poor response to cancer therapy, decreased survival,[5] and poor quality of life.[6–7] One study showed that in a sample of 3047 patients with metastatic cancer, weight loss greater than 5% before chemotherapy was associated with decreased survival in a multivariate analysis that controlled for performance status, tumor type, and stage.[5] Beyond survival, enjoyment of food and maintaining normal levels of activity are important to patients' quality of life. Decreased levels of activity and altered body image may lead to social isolation.[8,9] In many cultures with high prevalence of HIV disease, cachexia is stigmatized regardless of etiology. In images

129

that are ubiquitous in society, cachexia is frequently mirrored in the skeletal forms used to depict the dead and dying and is therefore perceived as a metaphor for death itself.

Pathophysiology

The fundamental problem in cachexia syndrome is the combination of anabolic blockade and increased catabolism, which results in accelerated weight loss.[10] This is where cachexia differs from a starvation state, in which decreased intake results in adaptive mechanisms of decreased metabolic rate and increased efficiency of energy utilization. Although our understanding of the underlying mechanisms that result in the metabolic disturbances of cachexia is incomplete, systemic inflammation has been consistently found to be a factor across many disease states, including cancer, heart failure, chronic obstructive pulmonary disease, and cachexia in the elderly.[11] In cancer, cachexia is generally thought to be due to a varied and complex set of interactions between tumor and host that triggers a chronic inflammatory state (Figure 9-1). Proinflammatory cytokines are mediators implicated in this process.[12,13] This chronic inflammatory state, together with procachectic factors secreted by the tumor,[14] results in protein and fat breakdown.[10] It also causes a chain of related abnormalities in neuroendocrine function that result in an increased catabolic drive as a result of insulin resistance and elevated cortisol levels.[15,16] Further compounding these

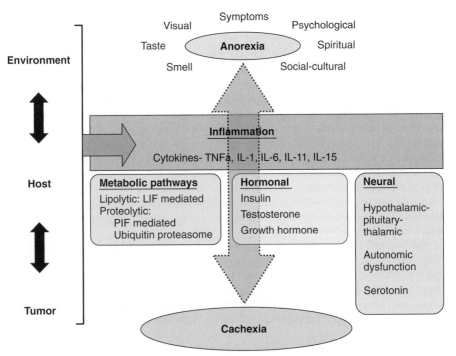

Figure 9-1. Pathophysiologic mechanisms involved in cachexia.

metabolic defects are the upregulation of protein degradation pathways, such as the ubiquitin-proteosome system (UPS), and the disturbance of the dystrophin glycoprotein complex (DGC), which selectively consume muscle protein.[17,18]

Assessment

The assessment of cachexia and its often related symptom of anorexia should begin with a detailed history and systematic search for potentially reversible causes. A scan of the social, cultural, economic, and emotional context of the patient and the family is a crucial step. Understanding the supports available for shopping, meal preparation, and social interaction at meal times may lead to practical strategies such as employing a personal support worker to assist with shopping or meal preparation. In home palliative care, a look in the kitchen and fridge of a socially isolated patient may reveal much about the adequacy of their home supports and financial resources to meet nutritional needs.

A comprehensive assessment of symptoms is required because symptoms like altered taste, mouth sores, difficulty swallowing, early satiety, nausea, and vomiting impact appetite and the patient's overall nutritional state. Distress related to symptoms like pain, dyspnea, anxiety, and depression also affect appetite. The objective of this part of the assessment is to optimize the conditions that are needed for eating rather than to push the patient to eat more. Gauging the patient's, family's, or caregiver's perspectives, anxieties, and fears about eating and feeding is important at this stage too. Depending on where the patient is during the trajectory of disease and in terms of their goals of care, it may be appropriate not to investigate cachexia further and to focus instead on improving the patient's and family's understanding of cachexia and teaching ways of nurturing other than feeding.

If, on the other hand, a patient has a longer prognosis and the expectation that the disease may stabilize for a time, some further assessment may be appropriate for early recognition, to monitor effectiveness of management in the clinical setting, or as an endpoint for trials. As part of the history and physical examination, a bedside assessment of the extent and rate of weight loss is possible. Weight loss alone is a meaningful endpoint for assessing effectiveness of interventions for cachexia because it is related to quality of life. From the history or interval measurement of weight, the percent of weight loss in proportion to weight can be obtained. This serves as a baseline to compare subsequent rates of weight loss. In many instances, a favorable response to an intervention may be measured in a decreased rate of weight loss rather than a reversal of the cachexia.

Although rarely done in routine clinical practice, simple and inexpensive measures of nutritional status, body composition, and function exist. Hand dynamometry is a portable device that measures grip strength and has been shown to correlate to other nutritional parameters and function. Bedside anthropometry measures mid-arm muscle circumference and triceps skinfold thickness in comparison to age-adjusted reference values.[19] Bioimpedance analysis (BIA) is a technique that measures total body resistance at different frequencies and calculates total body water, extracellular fluid, lean body mass, and fat mass. Although this requires specialized equipment, the equipment is portable and the test is safe and quick.[19]

Impairment in physical functioning is closely related to cachexia and is another endpoint that is gaining favor. Performance status measurement using the Karnofsky Performance Status or the Palliative Performance Scale is one component of functional status that is familiar and easy to assess. There are more extensive assessments of physical activity, such as the Simmonds Functional Assessment, which includes a patient-reported questionnaire and nine physical tasks. Because the tasks include dressing and walking tests, the tool may preclude the participation of a significant number of palliative patients.

In addition, standardized tools for nutritional status are available that combine objective measures and patient-reported information. An example is the Subjective Global Assessment (SGA) tool, which generates categories of nutritional state and was found to be effective in identifying cancer patients at risk for cachexia.[20] The Mini Nutritional Assessment (MNA) was originally developed to identify elderly patients at risk for malnutrition. It has been subsequently found to correlate with initial weight loss and C-reactive protein (CRP), a biomarker of inflammation, in advanced cancer patients receiving palliative chemotherapy.[21] Admittedly these tools are difficult to implement without the resources of a fully staffed multidisciplinary clinic or research team; however, they appear to have a role in early identification of cachexia and as endpoints in clinical trials.

Biomarkers are being studied for both clinical and research applications. The evidence is most robust for CRP, a hepatic acute-phase reactant that is a marker for systemic inflammation. CRP has been associated with anorexia, accelerated weight loss, and decreased survival. A plasma CRP level greater than 10 mg/L, along with weight loss of greater than 10% and reduced food intake of less than 1500 kcal/day, has been proposed as criteria for diagnosis of cachexia.[10] Although a variety of pro-inflammatory cytokines have been implicated in cancer cachexia, the findings across numerous studies are inconsistent. Cytokines that have been studied are tumor necrosis factor-alpha (TNF-α), interleukin-1 (IL-1), interleukin-6 (IL-6), and interferon-gamma (IFN-γ). Other potential biomarkers being studied include angiotensin II (involved in muscle catabolism) and leptin and ghrelin (peptides involved in control of food intake).

Management

In the majority of palliative patients, the main principle of management of cachexia is communication with the patient and family geared to listening to their fears, educating them about cachexia in the context of their advanced disease, helping them to come to terms with declining intake, and teaching them new ways of nurturing and caring.[22] It is of course important to treat what is potentially reversible so that symptoms and factors that may interfere with eating and activity are minimized.

A 1989 position paper of the American College of Physicians, summarizing the results of a number of nutrition trials performed in the 1980s, stated that "parenteral nutritional support was associated with net harm, and no conditions could be defined in which such treatment appeared to be of benefit"[23] in patients receiving chemotherapy. These studies may have had design flaws and were based on nutrition as the sole intervention, with regimens that may not meet current nutritional standards. However, there is still no evidence that either nutritional supplementation or artificial nutrition alone reverses cachexia.

More recently, a few studies have identified subsets of patients that may benefit from nutritional intervention. This has given rise to several guidelines regarding oral nutritional supplementation, enteral feeding, and parenteral nutrition, but the recommendations are inconsistent and difficult to apply in practice.[24–26] The guidelines propose that a subset of patients with medical indications such as intestinal obstruction, high-output fistula, short-gut syndrome, combined with relatively good performance status (>50 on the Palliative Performance Scale) and longer prognosis (>3 months), may benefit from parenteral nutrition. Because prognostication is often inaccurate, identifying this subgroup may be challenging. In addition, parenteral nutrition is invasive, costly, and requires a high burden of care from families. Therefore, applying the proposed guidelines is fraught with problems.[27]

An exploratory study by Bozzetti et al. enrolled 69 advanced cancer patients, the majority of whom had intestinal obstruction or "were almost aphagic",[28] to receive parenteral nutrition. The results suggest some stabilization of nutritional parameters but are limited by not having a control group. Another study, by Lundholm et al., involved 309 patients with solid tumors and prognoses longer than 6 months as estimated by the clinician. Patients were randomized to receive multimodal treatment consisting of indomethacin, erythropoietin (when indicated by hemoglobin cutoffs), and nutritional support (when indicated by study targets) or base treatment consisting of indomethacin and erythropoietin (when indicated by hemoglobin cutoffs). Of interest, patients did not have the typical medical indications for parenteral nutrition but were being provided parenteral support to maintain target intakes. Initially the nutritional intervention consisted of dietetic consultation and oral supplements to achieve a target intake of 30 kcal/kg body weight/day. If voluntary intake fell below 70% of these targets, parenteral nutrition was instituted. The results of this study suggest improvements in survival and total body fat and greater maximum power output during exercise.[29]

Our current knowledge of cachexia suggests that providing increased substrate alone is ineffective because cachexia is a disturbance in both the use of substrate to build new tissue as well as an accelerated breakdown of existing muscle and tissue. Nutritional interventions are likely to be important in combination with therapies to correct the metabolic disturbances underlying the cachexia. It is clear that the management of cachexia involves a complex set of decisions that requires a multidisciplinary team to implement effectively. Within this team, the role of a nutritionist is important in optimizing the presentation, texture, taste, nutritional quality, and enjoyment of food.

Cachexia has inspired a flurry of research activity with a remarkable number of high-quality clinical trials in the last two decades. Despite this, few agents have shown benefit. In cancer patients, megesterol acetate, a progestational agent, has shown modest improvement in appetite and increase in weight as a result of increases in fat stores but not lean body mass. These gains do not seem to translate to improved survival, and no overall conclusion about improvement in quality of life could be drawn because of statistical heterogeneity.[30,31] The 2009 Cochrane Review search yielded studies that tested doses ranging from 100 mg to 1600 mg daily of megestrol acetate. The evidence is lacking to make any specific recommendations regarding optimal dosing; however, ranges of 400 mg to 800 mg daily of the standard oral formulation of megestrol acetate are commonly used in clinical practice. The recommended duration of treatment is 6 weeks or more. Corticosteroids have shown modest benefit in improving appetite and well-being, but they are limited by side effects in prolonged use.[32] Both megestrol and steroids appear to provide transient benefit.[33] The concern with steroids, in particular, is the potential for steroid-induced myopathy and for a net catabolic effect.

Eicosapentanoic acid (EPA), an N-3 fatty acid, thought in preliminary trials to have beneficial effects on appetite and on underlying metabolic abnormalities, has not proven efficacious in phase III clinical trials.[34,35] Cannabinoids are another class of agents hypothesized to have an appetite-stimulating effect, but a well-conducted three-arm trial of oral cannabis extract versus delta-9-tetrahydrocannabinol (dronabinol) versus placebo showed no statistical difference in appetite or quality of life in any of the treatment arms.[36] Anabolic androgens, such as the synthetic oxandrolone, have been tested in preliminary trials, but their efficacy in cachexia is unknown. Etanercept, which belongs to yet another class of agents, one that blocks tumor necrosis factor-alpha, was tested in a phase III trial after preclinical and clinical studies showed promise. This was a study of etanercept versus placebo in 63 cancer patients. There were no significant differences in appetite and weight gain across both groups.[37]

Future Directions

Further work is needed in developing a standardized definition of cachexia that is useful clinically and for research. The development of robust biomarkers for precachexia will lead to earlier targeted and individualized interventions. Models of multimodal therapy that include nutritional support, exercise, best supportive care, correction of secondary factors, and combination therapy are being proposed.[10] Some preliminary trials of combinations of agents that target multiple mechanisms in cachexia are showing promise. Such trials have tested megesterol acetate in combination with ibuprofen, high-protein oral nutritional supplementation with eicosapentanoic acid, oral nutritional supplements with indomethacin and erythropoietin. These early results await confirmatory clinical trials. Such multimodal therapy requires the collaborative and coordinated efforts of a multidisciplinary care team. Notwithstanding the disappointing results of agents tested to date, research in cachexia has been invaluable in elucidating underlying metabolic pathways, many that have informed research in the area of fatigue as well.

PEARLS
- Cachexia shortens survival and quality of life.
- Early recognition and early treatment may reduce suffering.
- As a multifactorial syndrome, cachexia requires an individualized, multimodal approach to treatment.

PITFALLS
- Confusion about definition and classification hinders treatment and research.
- Isolated nutritional intervention does not reverse cachexia.
- Cachexia has no predictable course or outcomes.

Summary

Cachexia significantly impacts survival and quality of life. Early identification and education are likely to reduce suffering. Cachexia is a complex, multifactorial syndrome that requires individualized, multimodal management. This, in turn, requires the work of a coordinated multidisciplinary team.

Resources

A. CH Regional Palliative Care Program: Clinical Practice Guidelines: Home parenteral nutrition and cancer selection criteria for patients with advanced cancer. Available at www.palliative.org

References

1. Evans WJ, Morley JE, Argiles J, et al: Cachexia: a new definition, *Clin Nutr* 27(6):793–799, 2008.
2. Fearon KC, Voss AC, Hustead DS: Definition of cancer cachexia: effect of weight loss, reduced food intake, and systemic inflammation on functional status and prognosis, *Am J Clin Nutr* 83(6):1345–1350, 2006.
3. Lainscak M, Filippatos GS, Gheorghiade M, et al: Cachexia: common, deadly, with an urgent need for precise definition and new therapies, *Am J Cardiol* 101(11A):8E–10E, 2008.
4. Reid J, McKenna H, Fitzsimons D, McCance T: The experience of cancer cachexia: a qualitative study of advanced cancer patients and their family members, *Int J Nurs Stud* 46(5):606–616, 2009.
5. Dewys WD, Begg C, Lavin PT, et al: Prognostic effect of weight loss prior to chemotherapy in cancer patients. Eastern Cooperative Oncology Group, *Am J Med* 69(4):491–497, 1980.
6. Fouladiun M, Korner U, Gunnebo L, et al: Daily physical-rest activities in relation to nutritional state, metabolism, and quality of life in cancer patients with progressive cachexia, *Clin Cancer Res* 13(21):6379–6385, 2007.
7. Persson C, Glimelius B: The relevance of weight loss for survival and quality of life in patients with advanced gastrointestinal cancer treated with palliative chemotherapy, *Anticancer Res* 22(6B):3661–3668, 2002.
8. Hinsley R, Hughes R: "The reflections you get": an exploration of body image and cachexia, *Int J Palliat Nurs* 13(2):84–89, 2007.
9. McClement SE, Woodgate RL: Care of the terminally ill cachectic cancer patient: interface between nursing and psychological anthropology, *Eur J Cancer Care (Engl)* 6(4):295–303, 1997.
10. Fearon KC: Cancer cachexia: Developing multimodal therapy for a multidimensional problem, *Eur J Cancer* 44(8):1124–1132, 2008.
11. Baracos VE: Cancer-associated cachexia and underlying biological mechanisms, *Annu Rev Nutr* 26:435–461, 2006.
12. Argiles JM, Busquets S, Lopez-Soriano FJ: Cytokines in the pathogenesis of cancer cachexia, *Curr Opin Clin Nutr Metab Care* 6(4):401–406, 2003.
13. Johnen H, Lin S, Kuffner T, et al: Tumor-induced anorexia and weight loss are mediated by the TGF-beta superfamily cytokine MIC-1, *Nat Med* 13(11):1333–1340, 2007.
14. Todorov P, Cariuk P, McDevitt T, et al: Characterization of a cancer cachectic factor, *Nature* 379(6567):739–742, 1996.
15. Pisters PW, Cersosimo E, Rogatko A, Brennan MF: Insulin action on glucose and branched-chain amino acid metabolism in cancer cachexia: differential effects of insulin, *Surgery* 111(3):301–310, 1992.
16. Schaur RJ, Fellier H, Gleispach H: Tumor host relations. I. increased plasma cortisol in tumor-bearing humans compared with patients with benign surgical diseases, *J Cancer Res Clin Oncol* 93(3):281–285, 1979.
17. Acharyya S, Butchbach ME, Sahenk Z, et al: Dystrophin glycoprotein complex dysfunction: a regulatory link between muscular dystrophy and cancer cachexia, *Cancer Cell* 8(5):421–432, 2005.
18. Attaix D, Combaret L, Tilignac T, Taillandier D: Adaptation of the ubiquitin-proteasome proteolytic pathway in cancer cachexia, *Mol Biol Rep* 26(1–2):77–82, 1999.
19. Dahele M, Fearon KC: Research methodology: cancer cachexia syndrome, *Palliat Med* 18(5):409–417, 2004.
20. Ravasco P, Monteiro-Grillo I, Vidal PM, Camilo ME: Nutritional deterioration in cancer: the role of disease and diet, *Clin Oncol (R Coll Radiol)* 15(8):443–450, 2003.
21. Slaviero KA, Read JA, Clarke SJ, Rivory LP: Baseline nutritional assessment in advanced cancer patients receiving palliative chemotherapy, *Nutr Cancer* 46(2):148–157, 2003.
22. Moynihan T, Kelly DG, Fisch MJ: To feed or not to feed: is that the right question? *J Clin Oncol* 23(25):6256–6259, 2005.
23. American College of Physicians: Parenteral nutrition in patients receiving cancer chemotherapy, *Ann Intern Med* 110(9):734–736, 1989.
24. Easson AM, Hinshaw DB, Johnson DL: The role of tube feeding and total parenteral nutrition in advanced illness, *J Am Coll Surg* 194(2):225–228, 2002.
25. Fainsinger RL, Bruera E: A practical approach to the management of the cachexia/anorexia syndrome in advanced cancer patients, *South Am J Cancer* 1:173–179, 1997.

26. Sitzmann JV, Pitt HA: Statement on guidelines for total parenteral nutrition. The Patient Care Committee of the American Gastroenterological Association, *Dig Dis Sci* 34(4):489–496, 1989.

27. Mirhosseini N, Fainsinger RL, Baracos V: Parenteral nutrition in advanced cancer: indications and clinical practice guidelines, *J Palliat Med* 8(5):914–918, 2005.

28. Bozzetti F, Cozzaglio L, Biganzoli E, et al: Quality of life and length of survival in advanced cancer patients on home parenteral nutrition, *Clin Nutr* 21(4):281–288, 2002.

29. Lundholm K, Daneryd P, Bosaeus I, et al: Palliative nutritional intervention in addition to cyclooxygenase and erythropoietin treatment for patients with malignant disease: effects on survival, metabolism, and function, *Cancer* 100(9):1967–1977, 2004.

30. Loprinzi CL, Ellison NM, Schaid DJ, et al: Controlled trial of megestrol acetate for the treatment of cancer anorexia and cachexia, *J Natl Cancer Inst* 82(13):1127–1132, 1990.

31. Berenstein EG, Ortiz Z: Megestrol acetate for the treatment of anorexia-cachexia syndrome, *Cochrane Database Syst Rev* (2):CD004310, 2005.

32. Willox JC, Corr J, Shaw J, et al: Prednisolone as an appetite stimulant in patients with cancer, *Br Med J (Clin Res Ed)* 288(6410):27, 1984.

33. Behl D, Jatoi A: Pharmacological options for advanced cancer patients with loss of appetite and weight, *Expert Opin Pharmacother* 8(8):1085–1090, 2007.

34. Dewey A, Baughan C, Dean T, et al: Eicosapentaenoic acid (EPA, an omega-3 fatty acid from fish oils) for the treatment of cancer cachexia, *Cochrane Database Syst Rev* (1):CD004597, 2007.

35. Fearon KC, Barber MD, Moses AG, et al: Double-blind, placebo-controlled, randomized study of eicosapentaenoic acid diester in patients with cancer cachexia, *J Clin Oncol* 24(21):3401–3407, 2006.

36. Strasser F, Luftner D, Possinger K, et al: Comparison of orally administered cannabis extract and delta-9-tetrahydrocannabinol in treating patients with cancer-related anorexia-cachexia syndrome: a multicenter, phase III, randomized, double-blind, placebo-controlled clinical trial from the Cannabis-In-Cachexia-Study-Group, *J Clin Oncol* 24(21):3394–3400, 2006.

37. Jatoi A, Dakhil SR, Nguyen PL, et al: A placebo-controlled double blind trial of etanercept for the cancer anorexia/weight loss syndrome: results from N00C1 from the North Central Cancer Treatment Group, *Cancer* 110(6):1396–1403, 2007.

PART B: *Fatigue*

AMNA F. HUSAIN

In studies, fatigue is consistently found to be the most prevalent symptom in palliative patients, and yet in practice it is underreported and undertreated.[1] This may stem from the sense of futility that often pervades the approach of both patients and health care providers to this symptom.[2] Fatigue is often viewed as the inevitable consequence of advanced disease and the processes involved in cell death and organ failure. Although this is true at one stage in a patient's illness, recognizing and acknowledging fatigue and teaching ways of responding to it are important at all stages. In addition, there are many secondary causes of fatigue that need to be explored and can be addressed. Once other causes have been considered, there is emerging evidence that psychosocial, exercise, and a few pharmacologic interventions may improve fatigue.

Prevalence rates of 70% or more indicate the scope of the problem of fatigue in palliative care, across cancer and noncancer diagnoses. Equally important is that the impact of fatigue on patients can be devastating. The following case study illustrates the meaning and impact of fatigue in a palliative patient.

CASE STUDY

Mr. C. is a 68-year-old Portuguese-speaking man with locally advanced rectal cancer. He is a husband, a father of three daughters, and grandfather of two granddaughters. As a result of an injury, he retired from construction work some years ago. Before he became ill with cancer, Mr. C. took care of his wife's sister when she was dying of cancer. He also babysat his 2- and 3-year-old granddaughters while his daughters and wife were at work. Despite his cancer being stable and his other symptoms being adequately treated, he has an unrelenting fatigue that pervades all aspects of his life. Most troubling to Mr. C. is his inability to spend time with his family and in

137

particular his granddaughters. His 4-year-old granddaughter jumps on his bed, hugs him, and wants to talk to him about her day. He is devastated that he cannot muster the mental and emotional energy to be with her for more than a few minutes. Even brief social interaction exhausts him. He feels acutely that time is short and helpless that he cannot spend it with his family in a way that is meaningful to him.

Assessment

DEFINITION

Assessment of fatigue is challenging in part because there continues to be confusion about its definition. Broadly, there is consensus among experts that fatigue is multi-dimensional and that it has physical and cognitive domains. More specifically, the National Comprehensive Cancer Network (NCCN) defines cancer-related fatigue as "a distressing, persistent, subjective sense of physical, emotional and/or cognitive tiredness or exhaustion related to cancer or cancer treatment that is not proportional to recent activity and interferes with usual functioning".[8] The second edition of the *Oxford Textbook of Palliative Medicine* uses an altogether different conceptual approach, describing fatigue as only one aspect of asthenia. Asthenia is described as having three major dimensions: fatigue or easy tiring, generalized weakness, and mental fatigue. Yet another definition of fatigue is that proposed by the Fatigue Coalition, defining it as a clinical syndrome and using the International Classification of Diseases-10 (ICD-10) criteria. The diagnosis of the syndrome of cancer-related fatigue requires the presence of "significant fatigue, diminished energy or increased need to rest, disproportionate to any recent change in activity level" along with the presence of 5 out 10 additional symptoms over a two-week period.[3] The 10 additional symptoms include the following:

1. Generalized weakness
2. Diminished concentration
3. Decreased motivation or interest to engage in usual activities
4. Insomnia or hypersomnia
5. Experience of sleep as unrefreshing
6. Perceived need to struggle to overcome inactivity
7. Marked emotional reactivity (sadness, irritability) to being fatigued
8. Difficulty completing tasks
9. Perceived problem of short-term memory
10. Postexertional malaise lasting several hours

Employing this definition of fatigue requires excluding fatigue that is assessed to be "the primary consequence of comorbid psychiatric disorders such as major depression, somatization or somatoform disorder or delirium."[3] This definition was intended to identify fatigue that is more specifically related to cancer or its treatment, but the Fatigue Coalition's findings indicate that it excludes a significant portion of cancer patients who reported debilitating fatigue that required assessment and treatment. An additional limitation may be that this definition, although feasible for research settings and well-resourced centers of care, may not be practical for many community clinical settings. A more workable definition may be the one proposed by the European Association for Palliative Care (EAPC) expert working group: "Fatigue is a subjective sensation of tiredness, weakness or lack of energy".[4]

The difficulty in arriving at a consistent definition is due to several factors. In order to focus research on elucidating mechanisms and proposing interventions, there is a need to distinguish fatigue related to disease and its treatment from the significant background prevalence of fatigue in the general population. Controversy remains about the nature of the fatigue itself. Several studies have shown that the fatigue experienced by chronically ill individuals is qualitatively different from the fatigue in healthy individuals. However, the EAPC consensus group is of the opinion that cancer-related fatigue simply represents one end of the continuum of intensity of fatigue that includes fatigue in healthy persons.[4] Additionally, there is some overlap between fatigue and other syndromes such as cachexia and depression. However, fatigue is distinct from either of these presentations.[5-7]

MEASUREMENT

A single-item question such as "Do you feel unusually tired or weak?" or a single item 0 to 10 numeric rating scale may be used as a simple effective screen. Both the NCCN Fatigue Guidelines and the EAPC consensus group agree that the key is to apply the screening question or tool at all initial and follow-up assessments.[4,8] Fatigue rarely occurs as an isolated symptom. It is frequently related to pain, distress, anemia, and sleep disturbances. Therefore, measuring fatigue as part of an inventory of symptoms checklist or instrument such as the Edmonton Symptom Assessment Scale (ESAS) is a reasonable approach. Those who report significant levels of fatigue should then be evaluated with a comprehensive history and physical and a systematic search for treatable contributing factors. If appropriate for the patient's context and feasible for the health care provider, a focused survey of fatigue such as the Brief Fatigue Inventory[9] or the fatigue subscale of the Functional Assessment of Cancer Therapy[10] may be useful as part of the overall assessment to monitor response to management. However, in practice these surveys have a role primarily in interventional research as they are shown to detect clinically meaningful differences in response to treatment. In addition, because fatigue is multifactorial, there are multidimensional surveys, such as the Piper Fatigue Scale[11] and the Multidimensional Fatigue Inventory,[12] that capture more fully the different aspects of fatigue. The length of these surveys limits their usefulness clinically, but once again these surveys may supplement information obtained in a clinical interview and are useful for research purposes.

The patient's subjective report of fatigue is the principal marker because objective measures such as ergometric testing are of limited value in palliative care and robust biologic markers are not yet available. The advent of physical activity meters,[13] which are devices that record changes in position throughout the day, may move assessment of fatigue in the direction of using a combination of both subjective and objective measures.

Pathophysiology

Because fatigue can be the end result of many, if not all, comorbid conditions and concurrent syndromes, it is useful to distinguish between primary fatigue and secondary fatigue when considering causal mechanisms.[4] However, it is also important to remember that in patients with advanced disease, fatigue will not lend itself to be neatly categorized. At any given point in the patient's course of illness, multiple factors will likely contribute to the patient's fatigue, and the relative contribution of each factor will vary.[4]

Secondary fatigue may result from anemia, depression, sleep-related disorders, cachexia, dehydration, electrolyte abnormalities, infection, and medication-related sedation. From clinical experience, fatigue is known to be a symptom of anemia. The experience from research is that a significant but modest correlation exists between hematocrit and fatigue severity.[14,15] Cancer patients with anemia are more fatigued than those without.[16] A small study further investigated the nature of this relationship by examining fatigue severity and oxygen binding. It found no difference in the oxygen saturation curves of cancer patients and healthy controls and no association with fatigue.[17] Depression and psychological distress have also been associated with fatigue in the chronically ill and the general population. However, several studies show that depression does not account for all the fatigue experienced by cancer patients. In a randomized controlled trial of patients undergoing chemotherapy, mood improved in the intervention arms while fatigue did not.[18] Similarly, Andrykowski and colleagues demonstrated that even after strictly excluding patients with comorbid psychiatric disorders, 26% of patients receiving adjuvant chemotherapy were fatigued.[19] Cancer patients commonly suffer from insomnia,[20] a symptom related to both depression and fatigue. However, the relationship between sleep disorders and fatigue is not a simple causal one. This is suggested by a study that found cognitive behavioral therapy effective in improving sleep but not fatigue in breast cancer patients.[20] An important iatrogenic cause for fatigue is the sedative properties of many of the medications commonly used in palliative care, such as opioids, benzodiazepines, and anticonvulsants. Combinations of these medications may have additive effects that further exacerbate fatigue.

Although the mechanisms for primary fatigue are likely to be multiple, there is some preliminary, albeit inconsistent, evidence that pro-inflammatory cytokines studied in cachexia may play a role in fatigue too. A recent systematic review of the role of biological mediators in cancer-related fatigue concluded that interleukin-6 (IL-6), interleukin-1 receptor antibody (IL-1ra), and neopterin have been found to be consistently related to fatigue; however, other pro-inflammatory cytokines such as IL-1β or tumor necrosis factor-alpha (TNF-α) have not.[21] In persons with human immunodeficiency virus (HIV), increased levels of IL-1 and TNF have been associated with fatigue and sleep disturbances.[22] Therefore, chronic inflammation is one proposed mechanism for fatigue. In patients with heart failure, disorders of anabolism and catabolism may lead to reduced muscle strength and endurance.[23] The basis of this metabolic disturbance is unclear. Other pathways for fatigue that are being studied in animal models include a mechanism that decreases somatic muscle tone through vagal stimulation. This results in rats that exhibit decreased activity, and vagotomy corrects or partially corrects the response. Another overlapping pathway involving the dysregulation of the hypothalamic-pituitary-adrenal axis has been suggested. Disturbance of the diurnal cortisol rhythm and blunting of the cortisol response to stress was found in fatigued breast cancer survivors when compared with nonfatigued survivors.[24,25] Similar findings were seen in metastatic breast cancer patients.[26,27] In patients with HIV, dysregulation of growth hormone[28] and hypothyroidism[29] have also been implicated in the pathophysiology of fatigue.

Management

TREATMENT OF COMORBID CONDITIONS AND CONCURRENT SYNDROMES

A systematic assessment for causes of secondary fatigue will lead to an optimal approach to the management of the patient's total burden of fatigue. For patients who are fatigued and anemic, consideration should be given to correction of the anemia. For patients with hemoglobin levels less than 12 g/dL (120 mmol/L), treatment is recommended with erythropoietic agents such as erythropoietin or darbepoetin, which have been shown in randomized control trials to reduce fatigue with increases in hemoglobin.[30,31] However, erythropoietic agents are expensive and carry the risk of thrombosis and the rare complication of pure red cell aplasia. These agents have been tested in cancer patients receiving chemotherapy, so the risk-benefit profile of these agents for palliative patients is not known. Use of these agents in palliative care is also limited by the duration of effect, which is typically 12 weeks. Blood transfusions are another approach to correcting anemia. Although there are no clinical trials to support blood transfusions, there may be a role in some palliative patients with fatigue and anemia. The effect of blood transfusions, although quick in onset, is short in duration, sometimes requiring repeated transfusions within days. Except for palliative patients with severe drops in hemoglobin, the burden of a repeated hospital-based intervention and potential for complications often make the risk-benefit analysis of this approach less than ideal. Although there is no clinical trial–level evidence of efficacy in reversing fatigue, consensus guidelines all stress the importance of addressing causes of secondary anemia, such as infection, cachexia, dehydration, electrolyte abnormalities, hypercalcemia, hypomagnesemia, sleep disorders, depression, and medications.[4]

PSYCHOSOCIAL INTERVENTIONS

Psychosocial interventions include psychological, educational, and support group interventions. A review of psychosocial interventions for cancer-related fatigue by Jacobsen and colleagues reported a small but significant positive effect.[32] A just-published Cochrane review on the same topic concludes that there is limited evidence to suggest that psychosocial interventions specifically focused on fatigue are effective. The interventions in this category were brief, provided by nurses and consisted of education about fatigue, self-care or coping techniques, and learned activity management.[33]

EXERCISE INTERVENTIONS

Many studies have examined the role of exercise in fatigue. A 2009 Cochrane review of exercise for fatigue in adult cancer patients reports significant improvement in fatigue in the intervention groups compared with controls.[34] This supports the findings of previous meta-analyses. The type or frequency of exercise is unclear and needs to be adjusted to patient's phase of illness and performance status. Most of these studies have involved breast cancer patients, either at the time of receiving chemotherapy or disease-free survivors. Therefore, it is questionable that the exercise regimens apply to palliative patients. However, recent findings suggest that the benefit of exercise may translate to palliative patients. A preliminary study in a population with advanced disease showed the benefit of a twice weekly, 50-minute exercise program in patients with limited prognosis.[35]

DRUG INTERVENTIONS

In a recent Cochrane review of drug interventions for fatigue, Minton and colleagues reviewed the evidence for the following pharmacologic agents: hematopoietic agents, psychostimulants, bisphosphonates, anti-TNFα antibodies, antidepressants, and progestational steroids.[36] They found some evidence that treatment of cancer-related fatigue with methylphenidate appears to be effective. There was more robust evidence for treatment with hematopoietic agents in fatigued patients, but it was limited to those with chemotherapy-induced anemia. They found insufficient evidence to recommend any of the other agents reviewed.

The EAPC consensus working group states that modafinil, which has been used in trials for the treatment of fatigue in multiple sclerosis, amyotrophic lateral sclerosis, and HIV, may have some role to play in treating fatigue in palliative patients. Although the evidence for steroids is scant, the EAPC working group based their recommendation for the use of corticosteroids on experiences in clinical practice suggesting that prednisone or dexamethasone are effective in relieving fatigue for short periods.[4]

PEARLS

- Fatigue is the most prevalent symptom in cancer and other chronic diseases, particularly in the palliative phase.
- A subjective report of fatigue is the current standard for diagnosis.
- Fatigue is a multidimensional symptom or syndrome

PITFALLS

- Confusion exists about the definition and classification of fatigue.
- It is important to distinguish the fatigue of palliative care patients from the fatigue common in the general population.
- The sense of futility surrounding this symptom may prevent a search for treatable causes.

Summary

Fatigue is the most prevalent symptom in palliative patients. Despite this, management of fatigue is hindered by a lack of consistency in the definition and a sense of futility about effective treatments. However, it is important to not lose sight of the goal of systematic and standardized assessment for fatigue.

A number of pharmacologic and nonpharmacologic strategies show promise in the management of fatigue, led by the core principle in palliative care of excellent communication, which consists of listening, acknowledging, and helping patients understand their fatigue.

Resources

National Comprehensive Cancer Network: Clinical Practice Guidelines. Available at http://www.nccn.org/professionals/physician_gls/f_guidelines.asp.

References

1. Vogelzang NJ, Breitbart W, Cella D, et al: Patient, caregiver, and oncologist perceptions of cancer-related fatigue: Results of a tripart assessment survey. The Fatigue Coalition, *Semin Hematol* 34 (3 Suppl 2):4–12, 1997.

2. Passik SD, Kirsh KL, Donaghy K, et al: Patient-related barriers to fatigue communication: initial validation of the fatigue management barriers questionnaire, *J Pain Symptom Manage* 24(5):481–493, 2002.

3. Cella D, Davis K, Breitbart W, Curt G: Cancer-related fatigue: prevalence of proposed diagnostic criteria in a United States sample of cancer survivors, *J Clin Oncol* 19(14):3385–3391, 2001.

4. Radbruch L, Strasser F, Elsner F, et al: Fatigue in palliative care patients—an EAPC approach, *Palliat Med* 22(1):13–32, 2008.

5. Stewart GD, Skipworth RJ, Fearon KC: Cancer cachexia and fatigue, *Clin Med* 6(2):140–143, 2006.

6. Morrow GR, Hickok JT, Roscoe JA, et al: Differential effects of paroxetine on fatigue and depression: a randomized, double-blind trial from the University of Rochester Cancer Center Community Clinical Oncology Program, *J Clin Oncol* 21(24):4635–4641, 2003.

7. Husain AF, Stewart K, Arseneault R, et al: Women experience higher levels of fatigue than men at the end of life: a longitudinal home palliative care study, *J Pain Symptom Manage* 33(4):389–397, 2007.

8. National Comprehensive Cancer Network: Clinical Practice Guidelines, 2009. Available at http://www.nccn.org/professionals/physician_gls/f_guidelines.asp.

9. Mendoza TR, Wang XS, Cleeland CS, et al: The rapid assessment of fatigue severity in cancer patients: use of the Brief Fatigue Inventory, *Cancer* 85(5):1186–1196, 1999.

10. Yellen SB, Cella DF, Webster K, et al: Measuring fatigue and other anemia-related symptoms with the Functional Assessment of Cancer Therapy (FACT) measurement system, *J Pain Symptom Manage* 13(2):63–74, 1997.

11. Piper BF, Dibble SL, Dodd MJ, et al: The revised Piper Fatigue Scale: psychometric evaluation in women with breast cancer, *Oncol Nurs Forum* 25(4):677–684, 1998.

12. Smets EM, Garssen B, Bonke B, De Haes JC: The Multidimensional Fatigue Inventory (MFI) psychometric qualities of an instrument to assess fatigue, *J Psychosom Res* 39(3):315–325, 1995.

13. Dahele M, Fearon KC: Research methodology: cancer cachexia syndrome, *Palliat Med* 18(5):409–417, 2004.

14. Stone PC, Minton O: Cancer-related fatigue, *Eur J Cancer* 44(8):1097–1104, 2008.

15. Prue G, Rankin J, Allen J, et al: Cancer-related fatigue: a critical appraisal, *Eur J Cancer* 42(7):846–863, 2006.

16. Cella D, Lai JS, Chang CH, et al: Fatigue in cancer patients compared with fatigue in the general United States population, *Cancer* 94(2):528–538, 2002.

17. Stone PC, Abdul-Wahab A, Gibson JS, et al: Fatigue in cancer patients is not related to changes in oxyhaemoglobin dissociation, *Support Care Cancer* 13(10):854–888, 2005.

18. Roscoe JA, Morrow GR, Hickok JT, et al: Effect of paroxetine hydrochloride (Paxil) on fatigue and depression in breast cancer patients receiving chemotherapy, *Breast Cancer Res Treat* 89(3):243–249, 2005.

19. Andrykowski MA, Schmidt JE, Salsman JM, et al: Use of a case definition approach to identify cancer-related fatigue in women undergoing adjuvant therapy for breast cancer, *J Clin Oncol* 23(27): 6613–6622, 2005.

20. Savard J, Morin CM: Insomnia in the context of cancer: a review of a neglected problem, *J Clin Oncol* 19(3):895–908, 2001.

21. Schubert C, Hong S, Natarajan L, et al: The association between fatigue and inflammatory marker levels in cancer patients: a quantitative review, *Brain Behav Immun* 21(4):413–427, 2007.

22. Darko DF, Mitler MM, Henriksen SJ: Lentiviral infection, immune response peptides and sleep, *Adv Neuroimmunol* 5(1):57–77, 1995.

23. Clark AL: Origin of symptoms in chronic heart failure, *Heart* 92(1):12–16, 2006.

24. Bower JE, Ganz PA, Dickerson SS, et al: Diurnal cortisol rhythm and fatigue in breast cancer survivors, *Psychoneuroendocrinology* 30(1):92–100, 2005.

25. Bower JE, Ganz PA, Aziz N: Altered cortisol response to psychologic stress in breast cancer survivors with persistent fatigue, *Psychosom Med* 67(2):277–280, 2005.

26. van der PG, Antoni MH, Heijnen CJ: Elevated basal cortisol levels and attenuated ACTH and cortisol responses to a behavioral challenge in women with metastatic breast cancer, *Psychoneuroendocrinology* 21(4):361–374, 1996.

27. Spiegel D, Giese-Davis J, Taylor CB, Kraemer H: Stress sensitivity in metastatic breast cancer: analysis of hypothalamic-pituitary-adrenal axis function, *Psychoneuroendocrinology* 31(10):1231–1244, 2006.

28. Darko DF, Mitler MM, Miller JC: Growth hormone, fatigue, poor sleep, and disability in HIV infection, *Neuroendocrinology* 67(5):317–324, 1998.
29. Derry DM: Thyroid therapy in HIV-infected patients, *Med Hypotheses* 45(2):121–124, 1995.
30. Jones M, Schenkel B, Just J, Fallowfield L: Epoetin alfa improves quality of life in patients with cancer: results of metaanalysis, *Cancer* 101(8):1720–1732, 2004.
31. Rodgers GM III, Cella D, Chanan-Khan A, et al: Cancer- and treatment-related anemia, *J Natl Compr Canc Netw* 3(6):772–789, 2005.
32. Jacobsen PB, Donovan KA, Vadaparampil ST, Small BJ: Systematic review and meta-analysis of psychological and activity-based interventions for cancer-related fatigue, *Health Psychol* 26(6): 660–667, 2007.
33. Goedendorp MM, Gielissen MF, Verhagen CA, Bleijenberg G: Psychosocial interventions for reducing fatigue during cancer treatment in adults, *Cochrane Database Syst Rev* (1):CD006953, 2009.
34. Cramp F, Daniel J: Exercise for the management of cancer-related fatigue in adults, *Cochrane Database Syst Rev* (2):CD006145, 2008.
35. Oldervoll LM, Loge JH, Paltiel H, et al: The effect of a physical exercise program in palliative care: a phase II study, *J Pain Symptom Manage* 31(5):421–430, 2006.
36. Minton O, Richardson A, Sharpe M, et al: A systematic review and meta-analysis of the pharmacological treatment of cancer-related fatigue, *J Natl Cancer Inst* 100(16):1155–1166, 2008.

CHAPTER 10

Depression and Anxiety

BILL MAH

CASE STUDY

Mrs. A. is a 61-year-old, married woman diagnosed approximately 1 year ago with small cell carcinoma of the lung. She has undergone multiple treatments, including several chemotherapy regimens.

She presents to hospital with some mild confusion and inability to cope at home. She has become virtually immobile and complains of severe weakness and fatigue. She has lost a significant amount of weight over the months just before hospitalization. On investigation, she is found to have diffuse bilateral brain metastases, for which she receives palliative radiotherapy. After this, Mrs. A. is told that there are no longer any curative treatments available. She becomes quite withdrawn, and staff and family note her spontaneously crying on several occasions. Her appetite diminishes significantly, and she refuses to take oral nutrition. Occasionally, she refuses her oral medications, believing that they are causing her to see things. Her energy level declines as the hospital admission progresses. She is noted to be sleeping most of the time. When she is able to converse, she has some difficulty retaining information over the short term. She wishes for the cancer to "take her quickly" but denies any intent to harm herself. She is noted to be fidgety and frequently pulls at her hair when speaking to physicians.

She has a history of anxiety treated with alprazolam for more than 20 years. Notably, 6 months before this admission she was started on bupropion 150 mg, which had reportedly lessened her crying episodes. In the past she cared for a sister who had bowel cancer.

She is seen by the Psychiatry Consultation Liaison service for assessment of her cognition and for possible depression.

145

As the clinical case highlights, the physical and psychological aspects of illness occur in tandem and are linked by a complex interplay of cause and effect. It frequently becomes difficult to separate the two. In fact, the act of trying to do so may result in missing some important links in treating the spectrum of suffering a person may experience when facing a life-threatening illness or the end of life.

A psychological response to the presence of stressors is the norm. We think about what is happening, and we draw on our past experience to direct us how to cope.

A discussion of what is meant by *stress, distress,* and *coping* is a necessary but often underappreciated and misunderstood step in understanding the possible genesis of clinical syndromes involving depression and anxiety.

"Psychological stress is a particular relationship between the person and the environment that is *appraised* by the person as taxing or exceeding his or her resources and endangering his or her well-being".[1] That is to say, distress occurs when the situation is thought by the person to exceed his or her ability to cope.

Cognitive appraisal is the process of "categorizing an encounter, and its various facets, with respect to its significance for well-being".[1] Appraisal in turn is affected by a person's associations (real or imagined), which have been formed by their own history of contact with illness, death, and dying. For instance, in the clinical vignette, Mrs. A had watched her sister become more fatigued and withdrawn before her death, which Mrs. A described as "dreadful"; Mrs. A's fears about her own death became amplified as she projected what was in store for her. In this case, the outcome of the appraisal process was anxiety, worry, and tension.

Anxiety may precede the appraisal process just as much as follow it. In the former case, anxiety serves as a signal of the presence of a stressor in the environment, such as being told that no further treatment is available. In the latter case, the presence of excessive amounts of anxiety is a sign of incomplete or maladaptive coping.

Coping is defined as a series of "constantly changing cognitive and behavioral efforts to manage specific external and/or internal demands that are appraised as taxing or exceeding the resources of the person".[1] Coping, then, is a *process* whereby a person manages stress, and thereby manages anxiety. Coping is the response to restore homeostasis—that is, to reduce or contain the feeling of anxiety.

Adaptation, or coping, can be categorized into three main streams:

1. *Problem-based coping:* In this type of coping, a problem is identified and a solution is sought to ease the distress. For example, "I am in pain, so I will take some morphine."
2. *Emotion-focused coping:* Here the focus is not on solving the problem at hand; rather, it is to modulate the feelings that are caused by the problem; for example, "I am nervous about the results of the MRI scan, so I will distract myself by watching television."
3. *Meaning-based coping:* In this method of coping, the focus is finding a meaning in the events that have taken place, to see things in a larger context. The meaning that one assigns to an event will be a reflection of one's core beliefs about the world. For example, "I will put up with the pain so that I can attend my daughter's wedding in 2 weeks."

People may have developed any combination of these methods of coping. Typically people try to use what has worked in the past as their primary and first response. Difficulties may arise when, for example, a person typically utilizes a problem-solving approach and is told there is no further treatment available. Thus, there is no solution of curing the disease. The result may be a crisis because the person's primary coping method has been taken away.

The awareness and articulation of underlying psychological processes is quite variable in different people. It is readily apparent that pain can consist of various dimensions, encompassing the physical, the psychological, and the spiritual. It is possible for psychological symptoms to be interpreted in the physical domain, resulting in complaints of increased physical pain.

Patients may be under the impression that psychological pain is always normal, that it must be endured, and that there is no method of addressing it. By believing that their suffering is normal, they may be afraid to bring up their psychological distress for fear of being labeled as weak. It is necessary for the clinician to broach these subjects, to explore and normalize the presence of psychological reactions, and to assess for the presence of distress as a result of incomplete coping, whether this takes the form of demoralization or as symptoms or syndromes of depression or anxiety.

This discussion now turns to the clinical syndromes of depression and anxiety. They are discussed together because their symptomatology often overlap; in fact, some see them as existing on the same emotional spectrum.

Depression

Depression is a commonly used word that has multiple meanings, frequently resulting in miscommunication and misunderstanding. Colloquially, it is often used a synonym for a feeling of sadness, the presence of tears, or to describe a multitude of more nuanced emotions for which the person has no vocabulary.

It is a common belief that sadness or "depression" is the natural reaction to the distressing events at the end of life, such as learning that one's disease is progressing or that there is no longer any curative treatment; when one is suffering significant physical impairment or pain; or when one is reflecting on facing the end of life. "Who wouldn't be depressed?" is the common phrase heard from the affected individual, from his or her support network, or even from within the interdisciplinary treatment team.

As previously discussed, the presence of distress, as manifested by sadness or anxiety, over the course of any chronic life-threatening illness *is* likely to be one of the normal reactions to either external or internal cues. Mrs. A, for example, cried more after the news of the absence of any further curative treatment. Her internal cue was the thought that she was going to die. The presence of distress needs to be differentiated from clinical depression, which has a much more precise definition.

The accurate and timely diagnosis of depression is critical. A recent meta-analysis has demonstrated that both depressive symptoms and clinical depression are small but statistically significant predictors of mortality in cancer patients, although not of disease progression.[2]

Depression may lead to a lowered functional status. For instance, concentration problems may hamper adherence with treatments. Depression results in a lower ability to cope with either physical or psychological issues that arise as illness progresses, resulting in increased dysfunction and, ultimately, in increased suffering.

> **Box 10-1.** *DSM-IV Major Depressive Episode Symptoms*
>
> Depressed mood most of the day, nearly every day
> Markedly diminished interest or pleasure in all, or almost all, activities of the day
> Significant weight loss or gain
> Insomnia or hypersomnia
> Psychomotor agitation or retardation
> Fatigue or loss of energy
> Feelings of worthlessness or excessive or inappropriate guilt
> Diminished ability to think or concentrate, or indecisiveness
> Recurrent thoughts of death (not just fear of dying), suicidal ideation, suicide attempt,
>   or a specific plan for committing suicide

Modified from American Psychiatric Association: *Diagnostic and statistical manual of mental disorders,*
  ed 4, Washington, D.C., 2000, American Psychiatric Association.

DIAGNOSIS

Clinical depression is a syndrome consisting of the presence of five of nine possible symptoms, according to the *Diagnostic and Statistical Manual of Mental Disorders,* edition IV-TR (DSM IV-TR), the diagnostic manual of the American Psychiatric Association (Box 10-1).[3]

With respect to specific symptoms, there must be the presence of a depressed mood *and/or* markedly diminished interest or pleasure in all or almost all daily activities. These symptoms must cause clinically significant distress or impairment in the person's function, and the symptoms must not be due to the direct physiologic effects of a substance or a general medical condition. Notably, these are usually assessed on the basis of self-report but also can be assessed by external observation.

In the physically ill person, there may be marked overlap between the symptoms of illness or side effects from medications and the physical manifestations of depression. Indeed, it may be very difficult or impossible to distinguish them. For instance, in the case of Mrs. A, her weakness, fatigue, sleep disturbance, change in appetite leading to weight loss, and cognitive difficulties may be symptoms of advanced disease and/or depression.

Therefore, there are multiple approaches one can take to try to solve this dilemma, each with its own implications. In an inclusive approach, the physical symptoms are taken as indicators of depression regardless of the cause. This will yield a higher rate of diagnosis of depression and potentially more false positives. One could exclude any physical symptoms from the diagnosis; however, the result would be many fewer diagnoses of depression and one would run the risk of missing a clinically significant issue.

Others have suggested a substitutive approach, where the physical symptoms have psychological analogues (Table 10-1).[4]

There is some evidence that asking the single question "Are you depressed?" may provide an accurate assessment of the presence of the clinical syndrome of depression.[5]

Depression is not a categorical diagnosis. That is, one does not either have or not have depression. More realistically, depression is experienced along a continuum, ranging from mild to extremely severe. It is important to rate the severity, as it affects

Table 10-1. Endicott Substitution Criteria

Symptom	Substitution
Significant weight loss or gain	Depressed appearance
Insomnia or hypersomnia	Social withdrawal or decreased talkativeness
Fatigue or loss of energy	Brooding, self-pity, or pessimism
Diminished ability to think or concentrate, or indecisiveness	Lack of reactivity, cannot be cheered up

Modified from Endicott J: Measurement of depression in patients with cancer, *Cancer* 53:2243–2248, 1984.

the choice and efficacy of treatment. It has been shown that mild depression may respond to psychotherapeutic techniques alone, whereas moderate to severe depressive disorders respond best to a combination of psychotherapeutic and medication management strategies.

Depression, especially in severe cases, may present with psychotic symptoms. This may involve the presence of hallucinations in any sensory modality, although auditory and visual hallucinations are most likely. There may be the presence of delusions: fixed beliefs about something despite incontrovertible evidence to the contrary.

The differential diagnosis of depression can include other psychological/psychiatric illnesses such as bipolar disorder, substance abuse, anxiety disorders, schizophrenia, or delirium. One must rule out a bipolar disorder because starting an antidepressant medication may induce a manic episode. Ask about a previous history of mania or times when the mood has been elevated, expansive, or very irritable. Other symptoms of the manic phase of a bipolar disorder include the following:

- Inflated self-esteem or grandiosity
- Markedly decreased need for sleep
- More talkative than usual
- Flight of ideas or racing thoughts
- Distractibility
- Increase in goal-directed activity
- Excessive involvement in pleasurable activities that have high potential for painful consequences

From a medical perspective, one should be aware of common medical problems leading to depressive symptoms, such as hypothyroidism, low vitamin B_{12} or folate levels, anemia, low testosterone levels in men, and substance abuse. The alleviation of physical pain is critical because uncontrolled pain may lead to feelings of helplessness and/or hopelessness around the future, resulting in poorer coping, and ultimately accelerate the onset of or worsen an already present depression. Conversely, the presence of depression may worsen existing physical pain.

Delirium may mimic the symptoms of depression. The major differentiation lies in the fluctuating level of consciousness seen in delirium (see Delirium for a more complete discussion). The connection between depression and anxiety is a strong one; each can fuel or cause the other. This connection is discussed in greater detail later in this chapter in the section on anxiety disorders.

Consideration must be given to the cultural context in which depression occurs. Some cultures do not have a word for depression, or it may be considered a weakness to have or show any such emotion. Cultural norms can greatly affect the expression of emotions, and knowledge of these norms aids in understanding the genesis and "normality" of a person's reactions.

Clarke and Kissane[6] have proposed a demoralization syndrome consisting of the core features of hopelessness, loss of meaning, and existential distress, but not necessarily accompanied by a feeling of sadness or anhedonia. There may exist the ability to enjoy a pleasurable experience, so-called consummatory pleasure, but it is difficult for the demoralized person to anticipate pleasure. Depression is thought to lack both consummatory and anticipatory pleasure. At the present, there is a lack of clinical data demonstrating the uniqueness of this syndrome from depression.

SCREENING TOOLS

Screening tools are not meant to make the diagnosis of depression, but they can be applied to rapidly assess for the likelihood of a clinically significant syndrome of depression, aid in assessing severity of depression, and be administered sequentially over time to monitor treatment response. Following are two commonly used scales:

- The Beck Depression Inventory-short form (BDI-sf)[7]
- Hospital and Anxiety and Depression Scale (HADS)[8]

The BDI-sf is a 13-item scale (compared with the standard BDI, which has 21 items) designed to screen for depression in medical patients. The HADS is a 14-item scale with the subscales of depression and anxiety. It places greater emphasis on cognitive symptoms than somatic symptoms.

PREVALENCE

Given the aforementioned issues in the diagnosis of depression, it is not surprising that the prevalence rates in individuals with cancer range anywhere from 3% to just under 50%. These studies are inconsistent with regard to stage of disease and prognosis; it is not completely clear if the risk of depression increases with disease progression. Certainly, there are points in the disease process that place the individual at greater risk of emotional distress, such as failing a specific treatment or therapy, learning that no further curative or disease-controlling treatments are available, and losses in functional status.

RISK FACTORS

The robust risk factors in depression include the following:

- Gender: Females have approximately a two times higher risk than males.
- History of depression: Individuals with previous episodes of depression are at higher risk for subsequent depression.
- Family history of depression: There is good evidence to indicate a genetic component to the transmission of depression.
- Lack of social support: The presence of a supportive network is a strong positive factor that helps bolster resilience to distress.
- Functional status: Declining functional status is associated with higher incidence of depression.
- Poorly controlled pain: Individuals with pain are at higher risk for depression than those whose pain is adequately controlled.

- Type of malignancy: Depression is more prevalent in those with pancreatic cancers than other intra-abdominal malignancies.
- Substance abuse: Be wary of abuse of painkillers, alcohol, or illicit substances.
- Poor adaptation to past life crisis: This will be discussed in detail in the anxiety section of this chapter.

MANAGEMENT

The biopsychosocial model provides a comprehensive, multidimensional way to think about treatment that considers the biological sphere, the persons' inner psychology, and the social milieu.

PHARMACOLOGIC TREATMENT

In the biological sphere, the first action is to rule out physical causes and to correct them if possible. For instance, simple blood tests to check levels of vitamin B_{12}, folate, thyroid-stimulating hormone, and hemoglobin can rule out correctable causes of fatigue. The treatment of fatigue can subjectively improve a person's outlook tremendously. Steroids may cause depression or mood lability. Antineoplastic agents may do the same. Although it may not be possible to discontinue the medications that cause or contribute to depression, the simple act of informing patients of these effects may help them to cope by allowing them to attribute their symptoms to an external source instead of to themselves.

Because they are readily available and relatively easy to apply, pharmacologic agents are the mainstay in treating depression. They comprise antidepressants, psychostimulants, and mood stabilizers (Table 10-2).

Medication is chosen on the basis of desired effects, possible interactions, and side effects. If there is a history of successful treatment of a previous episode of depression, restarting the same agent is sensible. As a general principle when starting any antidepressant in any medically compromised person, the rule is to "start low and go slow." It can take up to 4 to 6 weeks before their full clinical effect is seen, which presents a problem in individuals with a poor prognosis. Remember that side effects can be used to advantage. For instance, a very sedating antidepressant can be used as a sleep aid.

If a person has a short expected lifespan, the use of psychostimulants is advised. Although not antidepressants in their own right, they can alleviate some symptoms of depression. They can be highly effective in counteracting fatigue or the drowsiness caused by opiates or disease progression and tend to be effective almost immediately, given the right dose. Preference is given to short-acting medications, such as methylphenidate. The usual starting dose of methylphenidate is 2.5 mg in the morning (7 to 8 AM) and at noon, titrated in 2.5- to 5-mg increments per dose to reach the desired effect. Doses are not given after 4 PM because this can interfere with sleep. Side effects include tremor, increase in blood pressure, agitation, and confusion. A psychostimulant can be combined with an antidepressant as an augmenting strategy; however, care is necessary to not overstimulate the patient.

Among antidepressants, selective serotonin reuptake inhibitors (SSRIs) tend to be the best tolerated because they have fewer side effects than older medications such as tricyclic antidepressants (TCAs) or monoamine oxidase inhibitors (MAOIs). As a class, the most common side effects are gastrointestinal upset, sexual dysfunction, nausea, agitation or restlessness, and insomnia. Escitalopram and citalopram are the

Table 10-2. Antidepressants

Class and Generic Name	Dose Range (mg)
Selective Serotonin Reuptake Inhibitors (SSRIs)	
Sertraline	25–200
Citalopram	10–40
Escitalopram	5–20
Fluoxetine	5–60
Paroxetine	10–60
Fluvoxamine	50–300
Tricyclics (TCAs)	
Amitriptylline	25–125
Nortriptyline	10–125
Desipramine	25–150
Clomipramine	25–150
Imipramine	25–150
Serotonin-Norepinephrine Reuptake Inhibitors (SNRIs)	
Venlafaxine	37.5–225
Duloxetine	30–60
Mirtazepine	15–45
Norepinephrine-Dopamine Reuptake Inhibitor (NDRI)	
Bupropion	100–300
Other	
Trazadone	25–300
Monoamine Oxidase Inhibitors (MAOIs)	
Phenelzine	45–90
Tranylcypromine	20–60
Moclobemide (Canada only)	300–600
Psychostimulants	
Methylphenidate	2.5–20 bid (AM + noon)
Dextroamphetamine	5–30 bid (AM + noon)
Modafanil	50–200 bid (AM + noon)
Mood Stabilizers	
Lithium	300–1200
Valproic acid	250–1500
Olanzapine	2.5–20

Dosages listed are common ranges. Patients may respond to less.

least likely to interact with the cytochrome P450 system and therefore have the fewest drug interactions. Both have the effect of increasing energy in most people, although paradoxical sleepiness can occur. Sertraline is generally well tolerated. Paroxetine is a potent inhibitor of the cytochrome P450 2D6 system and is generally not recommended because of its numerous interactions. It is contraindicated with tamoxifen.

Fluoxetine has an extremely long half-life and an active metabolite; it may be active for as long as 14 days. SSRIs carry an increased risk of bleeding, possibly caused by platelet dysfunction.[9]

Because venlafaxine is a highly stimulating drug, it can be effective in treating fatigue. However, common side effects are anxiety, irritability, and overstimulation. Increases in blood pressure are also possible.

Duloxetine has efficacy as an antidepressant and also in the treatment of neuropathic pain. This is also true of nortriptyline, desipramine, and amitriptyline; however, their effectiveness may be limited by the side effect of sedation.

Mirtazapine has the very useful side effect of sedation, which can aid in the induction of sleep. Some experience a hangover and tiredness upon waking and possibly throughout the day. Stimulation of appetite is a favorable side effect in patients with anorexia, and weight gain is possible. It should be given at nighttime. Trazadone is not used clinically as an antidepressant but has utility as sleep-inducing agent at doses of 25 to 150 mg.

TCAs are useful agents because they have efficacy in the treatment of neuropathic pain. They can also be used to aid in sleep because most will cause a degree of sedation. Unfortunately, they may have significant anticholinergic side effects.

Bupropion is generally well tolerated and is quite activating. Unfortunately, this is sometimes experienced as agitation and anger, which are common side effects. Bupropion is known to lower the seizure threshold.

All antidepressants may be rarely associated with the onset of suicidal thoughts. The mechanism of this is unclear; however, it may be related to agitation caused by the medications. The treatment is immediate cessation of the antidepressant and careful assessment of suicidality; inpatient admission to ensure safety may be warranted.

Although generally not contraindicated, care must be taken when combining classes of medications because it increases the risk of serotonin syndrome, which can be life threatening. Symptoms of this syndrome are autonomic instability, abdominal pain, and a fluctuating level of consciousness. Hospitalization with supportive care is the main treatment.

MAOIs are generally not recommended because of their numerous drug interactions and long washout period. They *cannot* be combined with any other antidepressant. Additionally, they have very strict dietary requirements. Moclobemide is a reversible inhibitor of monoamine oxidase (RIMA); thus, it has a shorter washout period of a few days, compared with 2 weeks for MAOIs. Typically it is only used when other treatments have failed.

Lithium can be used when the person has a history of or current bipolar disorder or when there is reason to suspect a risk of a manic episode, such as steroid-induced mood instability. Care must be taken to monitor renal function and state of hydration, as lithium has a very narrow therapeutic window. Lithium levels should be monitored regularly. Lithium is one of the only mood stabilizers with proven efficacy in the treatment of the depressive phase of a bipolar illness.

Valproic acid is a mood stabilizer that is useful if there is history of seizures or in the case of intracranial lesions. Blood levels may be drawn, but be wary that the levels for effective seizure control may not be the same as those for mood control.

Olanzapine is an antipsychotic with mood-stabilizing properties. It also is very effective in controlling symptoms of delirium.

PSYCHOSOCIAL TREATMENTS

Psychotherapy

A multitude of individual or group psychotherapies are available for the treatment of depression. The choice of therapy is determined by the needs and goals of the patient, discussed in concert with the psychotherapist. Multiple factors must be considered, such as the ability of the patient to engage in therapy, the ability to reflect on oneself and one's life situation, awareness of the emotions that are present, and the ability to communicate those thoughts and feelings. People are highly variable in these domains, and keeping this in mind may help to mitigate some of the counter-transference (e.g., feelings of frustration, blaming, anger, helplessness) of the treatment team.

An additional consideration in deciding on therapy is the person's mental status, which might be compromised as a result of physical factors such as the disease process itself, pain, medications, or, more likely, any combination thereof.

Mild depression can respond to treatment by psychotherapy alone, whereas moderate to severe depression is best treated with a combination of psychotherapy and medication management.

The general goals and principles of psychosocial treatment include the following[10]:

- Reduce fears and distress as much as possible
- Maintain personal sense of identity
- Enhance or maintain critical relationships
- Set and attempt to reach realistic goals

An open discussion about a topic of concern, free of judgments, is often the most therapeutic measure that a clinician can offer. Indeed, active listening is a powerful tool that strengthens the therapeutic relationship. Awareness of one's own attitudes and reactions to death, dying, depression, and anxiety is critical to allow for a discussion without the application of one's own agenda to the patient's situation. Indeed, just acknowledging the challenges being faced and normalizing these feelings can be helpful. Premature normalization of fears and sadness before fully exploring the underlying thoughts and feeling associated with the situation carries the danger of the patient closing down as a result of feeling unheard or misunderstood. Alternatively, asking and educating around the symptoms of depression (or anxiety) can alleviate a person's sense of shame for having these feelings.

Dignity therapy[11] is a means of addressing the aforementioned goals of Weisman. Although it is not an empirically validated treatment for depression, it can certainly ameliorate the distress that contributes to depressive symptoms. It takes into consideration three domains that can affect a person's sense of dignity in response to disease: illness-related concerns, the dignity-conserving repertoire, and the social dignity inventory. Each of these is further composed of subdomains with associated diagnostic questions and therapeutic interventions (Table 10-3).

Supportive psychotherapy is designed to help the person recover and bolster preexisting coping mechanisms that are overwhelmed by current circumstances.

Narrative therapy is based around the person writing a narrative of his or her experiences and sharing them with either a clinician alone or with a group, who then use the narrative as a basis for further exploration.

Cognitive behavioral therapy (CBT)[12] can be utilized to help uncover ways in which the person's underlying thoughts contribute to feelings of depression and to

Table 10-3. Dignity Therapy: Domains and Subdomains

Illness-Related Concerns	Dignity-Conserving Repertoire	Social Dignity Inventory
Symptom distress	Dignity-conserving perspectives	Privacy boundaries
Physical distress	Continuity of self	Social support
Medical uncertainty	Maintenance of pride	Care tenor
Death anxiety	Role preservation	Burden to others
Level of independence	Hopefulness	Aftermath concerns
Cognitive acuity	Generativity/legacy	
Functional capacity	Autonomy/control	
	Acceptance	
	Resilience of fighting spirit	
	Dignity-conserving practices	
	Living in the moment	
	Maintaining normalcy	
	Finding spiritual comfort	

learn how to reconceptualize one's appraisal and response to the situation. Behavioral interventions may include relaxation training or breathing techniques to help lessen symptoms of depression, anxiety, and pain. Guided imagery has utility in symptom management. Hypnotherapy has some efficacy in treating anxiety and pain.

Group psychotherapy encourages recovery through social support, emotional expression, education, and cognitive restructuring.[13] Group therapy reduces social isolation, normalizes experiences and emotions, and fosters improvements in communication between the person, his or her primary support group, and the treating team. Improving communication is an essential component of recovery from an interpersonal psychotherapeutic point of view. For instance, making sure that the person understands the symptoms of depression and that treatment is available can relieve a great burden of guilt over why the person feels the way he or she does and also offer hope.

SUICIDE

No discussion of depression is complete without mentioning suicide. It is of utmost importance to assess for the presence of suicidal thoughts because they can be a symptom of depression. However, the presence of suicidal thoughts is not pathognomonic of depression. In fact, the desire for a hastened death can be present with no current or past psychopathology. The most important task for the clinician is to ascertain the thought process underlying the desire. Is the person trying to avoid perceived or real physical or mental suffering? Is the person in pain? Why is he or she considering it at this time? In what context does the thought occur? Hopelessness has been found to have a higher correlation with suicidality than depression.[14] Suicidal thoughts are twice as likely in patients with cancer than in the general population.

The mere presence of suicidal thoughts does not indicate intent. *Passive suicidal ideation* refers to having only thoughts or wishes that life were over. This is in contrast to *active suicidal ideation,* when the person is in the process of or has formulated a plan to kill himself or herself and has the intent to actively put that plan into action.

Psychiatric consultation is highly recommended in these cases where suicidal ideation is deemed as moderate to high risk, or whenever the clinician feels uncomfortable in the assessment process.

Passive suicidal ideation may serve as an escape valve for the person; it may give him or her a way out if the person believes that other options have run out; however, the person will continue to entertain any other options. Indeed, in the absence of options, whether perceived or real, loss of hope can occur.

For a more comprehensive overview of the desire for hastened death from a psychiatric perspective, see Olden, Pessin, Lichthenthal, and Breitbart.[15]

Anxiety

In considering the feeling of anxiety, recall the previous discussion on stress, appraisal, and coping. The presence of a stressor experienced as taxing or exceeding the coping ability of the person, whether it is the result of disease or individual or social factors, will result in anxiety. For instance, in the case study, Mrs. A's anxiety spiked enormously when she was informed that she would not receive any further palliative radiotherapy to her brain. This meant to her that she would now surely die of the cancer she had fought for so long. She fretted about her own demise, which she predicted would take the same difficult course as her sister's dying process.

Anxiety is a common feeling when faced with a life-threatening illness. Prevalence rates of symptomatic anxiety vary between 10% and 30% in patients with cancer.

As illness progresses, the patient will likely experience increased physical and psychological challenges and burden, resulting in more distress. The fears that a person experiences are the result of that person's associations to the stressor. They are, therefore, unique; attunement to the individual's personal struggle, through the process of active listening and careful exploration, enhances the therapeutic alliance and helps guide further treatment strategies. The concept of a biopsychosocial model aids in understanding the multiple etiologies of anxiety.

Common physical causes of anxiety include medications, abnormal metabolic states (electrolyte imbalances, B_{12} deficiency, hypoxia), endocrine disturbance, poor pain control, substance withdrawal (alcohol, benzodiazepines, hypnotics, antidepressants), substance toxicity, and structural lesions in brain.

The symptoms of anxiety can be both somatic and psychological in nature. Physical symptoms may include increased heart rate, shortness of breath, headaches, muscle tension, tremors, difficulty falling or staying asleep, loss of appetite, loose bowel movements, and heightened pain. Psychological manifestations may include any number of fears, worries, difficulty making decisions, poor concentration, poor memory, irritability, and denial. Contrary to the use of denial in other circumstances, it can be a useful coping mechanism in palliative patients because it allows the focus to remain on the here and now and to keep more intrusive and anxiety-provoking thoughts at bay.

Common worries revolve around the fear of uncontrolled pain and suffering; financial issues; separation from friends and family; loss of bodily function and integrity, resulting in loss of independence; being a burden; disintegration of self; and loss of meaning in one's life. Loss of dignity, as explored earlier, may encompass several of these factors. *Existential anxiety* is a term encompassing many of the aforementioned fears, especially loss of meaning, helplessness, and hopelessness in the context of disintegration of self and ultimately of "not being."

Anticipatory anxiety is common. It is formed when a person has a certain experience, usually accompanied by negative feelings and memories. When this event recurs, the negative associations are recalled, resulting in an expectation of the same feelings and the feeling of anxiety. For instance, the patient may remember nausea induced by receiving a certain medication intravenously; the starting of an intravenous line can trigger anticipation of experiencing nausea again, resulting in anticipatory anxiety. People may become afraid to move a certain way because a previous movement caused great discomfort; they anticipate the same result and feel nervous trying again. The patient may be aware (conscious) or unconscious of this conditioning process.

Given the multitude of manifestations of anxiety, careful history taking is necessary to explore fears and to rule out other entities that mimic anxiety. For example, poorly controlled pain has the same physical manifestations as anxiety, and anxiety can occur secondary to pain. Treatment of the underlying cause is most helpful, although treating the anxiety may prevent the formation of a secondary anticipatory anxiety.

As with depression, the diagnosis of an anxiety *disorder* is based on the presence of certain criteria (Table 10-4). However, in the absence of a disorder, treatment should still be considered because the symptoms of anxiety can still cause great distress and suffering. Preexisting symptoms that did not reach the threshold for diagnosis as a disorder may worsen in the face of the increasing illness factors. Additionally, preexisting disorders may worsen in the presence of the distress of ongoing illness factors.

TREATMENT OVERVIEW

The goal of treatment should not be to render a person anxiety free. The lack of any anxiety response means that the person loses a critical signaling mechanism. The goal is to keep the anxiety at a manageable level, which allows for a more realistic appraisal process and coping response. In other words, one strives for symptomatic control of the anxiety.

PSYCHOTHERAPEUTIC APPROACHES

Psychoeducation is the first step in assuaging anxiety. Conveying medical information involves providing *enough* information in an *understandable* way *at the right time.* These factors depend on the clinician actively assessing the person's reactions in real time and adjusting his or her behavior accordingly. Giving information about the side effects of a painkiller when the patient has just received bad news is likely to be fruitless. On the other hand, the simple act of explaining what a radiation therapy room looks like, while explaining palliative radiation, can help to contain anxiety. Learning can be facilitated by providing information in multiple modalities, such as speaking and encouraging the person to take notes or providing written information. Repetition and consistency are very helpful. The presence of family members during education/feedback is helpful because a "second set of ears" allows for more complete processing of information.

As with depression, having an open discussion about one's fears and acknowledging their reality (i.e., normalizing them) is often helpful. Again, premature normalization without adequate exploration may serve to shut down further discussion. The first task is to explore in an open-ended way the potential causes of the anxiety. Questions such as "Are you in pain?" "What are you most worried about?" and "What

Table 10-4. DSM-IV-TR–Defined Anxiety Disorders*

Disorder	Main Symptoms
Adjustment disorder with predominately anxious mood	Development of emotional or behavioral symptoms in response to an identified stressor Marked distress that is in excess of what would be expected from exposure to the stressor
Anxiety disorder due to a general medical condition	Prominent anxiety, panic attacks, or obsessions/compulsions A direct physiologic consequence of a general medical condition, not occurring in the presence of other mental disorders or delirium
Phobia(s)	Marked and persistent fear that is excessive or unreasonable queued by the presence of anticipation of a specific object or situation
Panic disorder	Presence of panic attacks characterized by: palpitations, sweating, trembling, shortness of breath, choking, chest pain, nausea, dizziness, derealization, or depersonalization, fear of losing control, fear of dying, paresthesias, chills, or hot flashes Concern about having additional attacks and consequences of having one, resulting in a significant behavior change
Generalized anxiety disorder	Excessive anxiety and worry for at least 6 months that is difficult to control, associated with restlessness, easy fatigue, difficulty concentrating, irritability, muscle tension, or sleep disturbance
Obsessive compulsive disorder	Obsessions: Recurrent thoughts, impulses, or images that are intrusive and are not simply excessive worries about real-life problems, which the person attempts to ignore or suppress and recognizes as a product of his or her own mind Compulsions: Repetitive behaviors in response to the obsession that are aimed at preventing or reducing the stress
Posttraumatic stress disorder	Exposure to a traumatic event that involves actual threat of death or serious injury Reexperiencing the traumatic event through flashbacks, nightmares, or recurrent intrusive thoughts Persistent avoidance of stimuli associated with the trauma Persistent symptoms of increased arousal (difficulties sleeping, anger, hypervigilance, difficulty concentrating, exaggerated startle response)

*Adapted from DSM-IV-TR, American Psychiatric Association, Washington, D.C., 2000.

is your biggest concern right now?" are helpful in uncovering fears. Recognize that you can't know for sure what a person's question will be, or what his or her fears are about, but that simply letting the person speak will prevent your assumptions from misleading you and frustrating your patient.

Relaxation training, deep breathing, visualization, and guided imagery are effective behavioral methods for treating mild to moderate anxiety. Cognitive behavioral therapy tries to uncover underlying thoughts and processes that are distorted or unrealistic and attempts to restructure them in a realistic way. Common ways of thinking that contribute to anxiety are catastrophizing, all-or-nothing thinking, overgeneralization, and/or emotional reasoning (thinking something is true because one feels it so strongly, while ignoring or discounting evidence to the contrary). Restructuring one's thoughts and expectations about the remainder of one's life can be an effective intervention.

Mindfulness-based stress reduction may help reduce depressive symptoms and anxiety.[16] Consultation with a spiritual counselor can be helpful to contain anxiety in the context of a religious belief system. Group psychotherapy has demonstrated efficacy in the treatment of distress in patients with cancer.

MEDICATIONS

If the anxiety is deemed to be a side effect of medication, consider discontinuing the medication or decreasing the dose of the offending drug. If this is not possible, the addition of an anxiolytic is recommended.

The mainstay of drug treatment is the benzodiazepines. Lorazepam, oxazepam, and temazepam are recommended because they do not rely on the cytochrome p450 system to be cleared; instead they are conjugated in the liver and are removed by renal excretion, thereby avoiding metabolic interactions with other drugs. (See Table 10-4 for dosages and half-lives.) Lorazepam is particularly useful when anxiety is acute; its effects are usually noticeable within 5 to 10 minutes of sublingual or intravenous administration. Another useful alternative is clonazepam, 0.25 to 2 mg in either twice daily or three times daily dosing. Dosing should be increased in 0.25- or 0.5-mg increments. Its half-life is typically 8 to 12 hours, which is longer than that of lorazepam (approximately a 6-hour half-life). Note that the dose may be varied with the amount of anxiety that is experienced; patients are aided by the knowledge that if the first dose is ineffective, the drug may still bring benefits if taken at higher dosages.

With all benzodiazepines, side effects include sedation and possible respiratory depression. Their effects are additive to other drugs with the same effects, such as opioids. Other mental status changes to monitor for include impaired concentration, confusion, difficulty registering new information or memory loss, and delirium. The elderly and more medically compromised person is at greater risk of side effects.

Patients already taking a benzodiazepine for a preexisting anxiety issue, unless there is a good enough reason to switch, should continue it. Abrupt withdrawal of a longstanding medication may induce symptoms of withdrawal, including increased anxiety, tremors, confusion, sleep disruption, irritability, and even delirium.

For treatment over the longer term, serotonergic antidepressants can be considered (see Table 10-3). They are typically not used for immediate and short-term symptom relief because it takes 2 to 6 weeks to realize an effect. However, if the person has several months or longer to live, they represent a good treatment option. A benzodiazepine and an antidepressant can be used concurrently; the former will provide immediate relief until the latter becomes effective, at which point the benzodiazepine may be withdrawn.

Depression

PEARLS

- Depression is a well-defined psychiatric syndrome characterized chiefly by low mood and anhedonia.
- The biopsychosocial model is most helpful in considering the factors influencing the etiology of depression.
- Mild to moderate depression is responsive to psychotherapeutic intervention.
- SSRIs (especially escitalopram, citalopram, and sertraline) are the antidepressants of choice.
- Stimulant medications are recommended for symptomatic relief, especially when time is limited.
- The presence of suicidal thoughts is variable throughout the illness process. The context of the thoughts is vital to understanding them.

PITFALLS

- It is a common misperception that "depression" is a normal response to illness and the dying process.
- Undiagnosed and untreated depression contributes significantly to overall suffering.
- Treatment with SSRIs may require 2 to 6 weeks before a clinical effect is seen.
- Be aware that antidepressants, stimulants, and mood stabilizers may interact with other medications.

Anxiety

PEARLS

- Anxiety is a normal response to a threat.
- Physical symptoms of anxiety include increased heart rate, shortness of breath, headaches, muscle tension, tremors, difficulty falling or staying asleep, loss of appetite, loose bowel movements, and heightened pain.
- Psychological manifestations may include any number of fears, worries, difficulty making decisions, poor concentration, poor memory, irritability, and denial.
- Benzodiazepines are the drugs of choice in treatment: lorazepam, oxazepam, temazepam, and clonazepam are most recommended.
- Muscle relaxation, deep breathing, and cognitive behavioral therapy are effective treatments for anxiety.

PITFALLS

- Don't assume that you know what a person's fears will be. They are unique to each person.
- Benzodiazepines can contribute to sedation and confusion, especially in the elderly.
- Abrupt withdrawal of benzodiazepines may produce withdrawal syndrome.

Summary

Both depressive and anxious symptoms can be conceptualized as occurring along a spectrum. Each person has different coping mechanisms to deal with distress; consequently, their psychological reactions will also be unique. A biopsychosocial framework is a useful way both to conceptualize etiology and to guide treatments. The recognition, diagnosis, and appropriate treatment of depression and anxiety can aid in diminishing the suffering that can occur in the palliative population.

Resources

1. Chochinov HM, Breitbart W, editors: *Handbook of psychiatry in palliative medicine*, Oxford, UK, 2009, Oxford University Press.

References

1. Lazarus RS, Folkman S: *Stress, appraisal and coping*, New York, NY, 1984, Springer Publishing.
2. Satin JR, Linden W, Phillips MJ: Depression as a predictor of disease progression and mortality in cancer, *Cancer* 115:5349–5361, 2009.
3. American Psychiatric Association: *Diagnostic and statistical manual of mental disorders*, ed 4, Washington, DC, 2000, American Psychiatric Association.
4. Endicott J: Measurement of depression in patients with cancer, *Cancer* 53:2243–2248, 1984.
5. Chochinov HM, Wilson K, Enns M, Lander S: "Are you depressed?" Screening for depression in the terminally ill, *Am J Psychiatry* 154:674–676, 1997.
6. Clarke DM, Kissane DW: Demoralization: its phenomenology and importance, *ANZ J Psychiatry* 36:733–742, 2002.
7. Furlanetto LM, Mendlowicz MV, Romildo Bueno J: The validity of the Beck Depression Inventory—Short Form as a screening and diagnostic instrument for moderate and severe depression, *J Affect Dis* 86(1):87–91, 2005.
8. Snaith RP, Zigmond AS: The Hospital Anxiety and Depression Scale, *Acta Psychiatrica Scandinavia* 67:361–370, 1983.
9. Gärtner R, Cronin-Fenton D, Hundborg HH, et al: Use of selective serotonin reuptake inhibitors and risk of re-operation due to post-surgical bleeding in breast cancer patients: a Danish population-based cohort study, *BMC Surg* 10:3, 2010.
10. Weisman AD: *On dying and denying: a psychiatric study on terminality*, New York, 1972, Behavioral Publications.
11. Chochinov HM: Dying, dignity and new horizons in palliative end-of-life care, *CA Cancer J Clin* 56:84–103, 2006.
12. Beck JS: *Cognitive therapy: basics and beyond*, New York, NY, 1995, Guilford Press.
13. Spiegel D, Leszcz M: Group Psychotherapy and the Terminally Ill. In Chochinov HM, Breitbart W, editors: *Handbook of psychiatry in palliative medicine*, Oxford, UK, 2009, Oxford University Press, pp 490–503.
14. Chochinov HM, Wilson KG, Enns M, Lander S: Depression, hopelessness, and suicidal ideation in the terminally ill, *Psychosomatics* 39:366–370, 1998.
15. Olden M, Pessin H, Lichtenthal WG, Breitbart W: Suicide and Desire for Hastened Death in the Terminally Ill. In Chochinov HM, Breitbart W, editors: *Handbook of psychiatry in palliative medicine*, Oxford, UK, 2009, Oxford University Press, pp 101–112.
16. Carlson LE, Garland SN: Impact of mindfulness-based stress reduction (MBSR) on sleep, mood, stress and fatigue symptoms in cancer outputients, *Int J Behav Med* 12(4):278–285, 2005.

CHAPTER 11

Delirium

BILL MAH

Diagnosis and Assessment	**Pearls**
Risk Factors	**Pitfalls**
Etiology	**Summary**
Management	
Behavioral Management	
Medication Management	

Delirium goes by many names, such as *acute confusion, metabolic encephalopathy,* and *acute brain syndrome,* which adds to the confusion around diagnosis. Delirium is not a distinct disease state, and it has multiple etiologies. This wide range of symptoms and etiologies leads to difficulties in diagnosis.

The prevalence is variable and appears to be related to severity of illness. Estimates range from 20% to as high as 80% in patients with cancer or acquired immunodeficiency syndrome (AIDS). A recent prospective study found a 47% prevalence rate in inpatients with terminal cancer.[1] The prevalence can be as high as 85% in the final hours before death.

Clinically, presenting symptoms can include the following:

- Restlessness
- Disturbances in the sleep-wake cycle
- Confusion
- Distractibility
- Disorientation to time or place or person
- Illusory experiences (misinterpreting stimuli that is perceived)
- Hallucinations (no external stimuli present) in any perceptual modality, although auditory and visual are the most common
- Delusions
- Disorganized thinking and incoherent or inappropriate speech
- Emotional dysregulation (including lability, contextually inappropriate emotions, inappropriate fear, sadness, anger, irritability, and euphoria)

Neurologic symptoms can include asterixis, tremor, myoclonus, incoordination, and urinary and fecal incontinence.

The presence of delirium adds significantly to morbidity. It can hinder communication with both health professionals and family. As a result, evaluation of other symptoms, especially pain, can be compromised. Family members are distressed that they are not able to communicate with their loved one. Disorientation can lead to dangerous behaviors, such as pulling out lines, trying to get out of bed and falling,

> **Box 11-1. *DSM-IV Major Depressive Episode Symptoms*** *
>
> Depressed mood most of the day, nearly every day
> Markedly diminished interest or pleasure in all, or almost all, activities of the day
> Significant weight loss or gain
> Insomnia or hypersomnia
> Psychomotor agitation or retardation
> Fatigue or loss of energy
> Feelings of worthlessness or excessive or inappropriate guilt
> Diminished ability to think or concentrate, or indecisiveness
> Recurrent thoughts of death (not just fear of dying), suicidal ideation, suicide attempt, or a specific plan for committing suicide

*DSM-IV-TR, American Psychiatric Association, Washington, D.C., 2000.

or acting aggressively to those in close proximity. It is difficult to understand the wishes of the delirious patient because they can be communicative one moment and nonsensical the next. Given the fluctuating nature of delirium, it is critical to be vigilant regarding the competence of the patient to make decisions around his or her own care and to assess this on a continuous basis. Collateral information from allied health professionals and family is an important element of this appraisal. The continuous assessment of competence is a requirement in delirious states; this is frequently overlooked by health care professionals.

Diagnosis and Assessment

Given the multitude of possible presentations, a structured approach to the diagnosis is most helpful. The diagnostic criteria of the American Psychiatric Association, as stated in the *Diagnostic and Statistical Manual of Mental Disorders,* revised fourth edition (DSM-IV-TR),[2] narrows the focus to disturbances of consciousness and cognition and emphasizes the fluctuating nature of the illness (Box 11-1). This fluctuating nature is a critical and pathognomonic feature of delirium. Indeed, one of the more common presentations is "sundowning," in which the symptoms present or worsen near twilight. Therefore, serial assessments at different times of the day are mandatory to ensure accurate diagnosis.

Assessment tools for delirium and cognitive status are listed in Box 11-2. They can be used to quantitatively measure changes in cognitive status. Devlin and colleagues[3] reviewed the advantages and disadvantages of various assessment tools for intensive care unit use.

> **Box 11-2. *Assessment Tools***
>
> Memorial Delirium Assessment Scale (MDAS)[4]
> Confusion Assessment Method (CAM)[5]
> Delirium Rating Scale (DRS)[6]
> Mini-Mental State Examination (MMSE)[7]
> Montreal Cognitive Assessment (MOCA)[8]

Delirium is classified into two subtypes: hyperactive and hypoactive. In the former, agitation and increased activity is the hallmark. The presence of hallucinations, delusions, and illusions is frequent. In contrast, hypoactive delirium is frequently missed because patients do not present with overt behavioral issues. Instead, they are often lethargic, confused, and have a decreased level of alertness; they are the "quiet" patients. Delirium exists on a continuum from hypoactive to hyperactive; the symptoms may also be mixed. Hypoactive delirium may appear similar to depression. Careful assessment of mood states when the patient is oriented is helpful. If the patient is not able to communicate in a goal-directed fashion, an electroencephalogram (EEG) can help differentiate them. The EEG show diffuse slowing in delirium.[4]

Delirium and dementia can present with similar symptoms. They can be differentiated by careful history taking and review of the chart (if available), looking specifically for the time of onset. Dementia will have a much more insidious onset than the rapid onset of delirium. Dementia itself is a risk factor for delirium; certainly, it is possible to have the acute onset of delirium on a background of chronic cognitive changes of dementia.

RISK FACTORS

Risk factors include older age (>65), preexisting brain injury, dementia or cognitive impairment, history of delirium, sensory impairment, malnutrition, alcohol or other substance dependence (from withdrawal), cancer, and AIDS.

ETIOLOGY

As previously stated, there are multiple causes of delirium, which may act alone or in concert with other etiologies (Box 11-3).

Management

The first principle of management is always to try to determine and treat the underlying cause. The search for an underlying cause should not delay treatment, because untreated delirium can present physical danger and cause suffering to the patient and those around him or her.

BEHAVIORAL MANAGEMENT

Behavioral management is a relatively simple and cost-effective strategy to implement. Orientation strategies include provision of the following:

- A quiet, destimulating room
- Good room lighting that approximates a day–night cycle
- Visible reminders of time and date such as a clock and calendar
- Verbal orientation for the person

Generally approach the person in a nonthreatening manner. Communicate in a clear and simple manner. Minimize sensory impairments with hearing aids or glasses. Avoid the use of physical restraints unless absolutely necessary.

Family and other caregivers should be educated about the presentation of possible symptoms, because their presence can be quite distressing to witness. People are quite surprised at the fluctuating nature of the delirium. Informed caregivers can serve as a second set of eyes and ears to monitor the course of the delirium throughout the day, because they frequently are the ones who spend the most time with the patient and are familiar with the patient's baseline level of behavior.

Box 11-3. *Causes of Delirium*

DRUGS
Anticholinergics
Antineoplastic agents
Benzodiazepines
Opiates
Sedative/hypnotics
Steroids

DISEASE STATES
Hepatic encephalopathy
Uremic encephalopathy
Hypoxia
Cardiac failure

INFECTIOUS
Sepsis
Meningitis
Encephalitis

METABOLIC IMBALANCES
Electrolyte balance
Glucose levels
Thyroid imbalance
Parathyroid imbalance
Adrenal imbalance
Pituitary imbalance
Thiamine deficiency
Vitamin B_{12} deficiency
Folic acid deficiency

STRUCTURAL
Metastases
Brain lesions
Head trauma (e.g., from falls)

MEDICATION MANAGEMENT

In addition to the measures above, medications can also be used to regulate behavior. Antipsychotic medications are the mainstay in treating delirium (Table 11-1). Haloperidol is the most used and versatile, given its routes of administration. It is usually started at 0.5 mg bid and can be titrated up in 0.5-mg to 1-mg increments to a maximum of 5 mg/dose. Breakthrough doses are helpful to control agitation and can be given every 1 to 2 hours. Haloperidol has a higher incidence of extrapyramidal side effects than atypical antipsychotics.

Both risperidone and olanzapine have a formulation that dissolves rapidly in the mouth, which is useful in patients who cannot swallow and have no parenteral access. Risperidone is usually started at 0.5 mg bid and titrated in 0.5-mg to 1-mg doses to maximum of 6 to 8 mg total daily. Olanzapine is also administered as a twice daily dose, starting at 2.5 mg and increasing in 2.5-mg to 5-mg increments to a maximum of 20 mg daily.

Table 11-1. Medications for Treatment of Delirium

Name	Dose (mg)	Schedule (hr)	Route
Antipsychotics			
Haloperidol	0.5–5	2–12	PO, IM, IV, SC
Loxapine	12.5–25	2–12	PO, IM
Olanzapine	2.5–20	2–12	PO, SL
Risperidone	0.5–3	2–12	PO, SL
Quetiapine	12.5–200	2–12	PO
Ziprasidone	10–80	2–12	PO
Methotrimeprazine	5–25	4–8	PO, IV, SC
Benzodiazepines			
Lorazepam	0.5–2		PO, SL, IM, IV
Midazolam	30–100	1–6	IV, SC

IM, Intramuscular; IV, intravenous; PO, oral; SC, subcutaneous; SL, sublingual.

Atypical antipsychotics may increase the likelihood of cardiac arrhythmias in the elderly; a baseline EEG is helpful to minimize risk. All antipsychotics may lower the seizure threshold.

Atypical antipsychotics have been associated with a small increased mortality in the elderly[5] and carry a black box warning from the U.S. Food and Drug Administration. A retrospective study of typical antipsychotics revealed that they have at least the same, if not greater, risk of death than the atypical agents.[6] These risks must be weighed against the potential risks of not treating delirium. It is recommended that any antipsychotic be given at the lowest dose possible for the shortest period possible.

Benzodiazepines should be avoided in the delirious patient because they frequently result in greater cognitive slowing and the worsening of symptoms. Any benzodiazepines regularly taken for a prolonged period before the onset of delirium need to be evaluated carefully because their rapid or sudden cessation can precipitate a withdrawal reaction and worsen delirium. The role of benzodiazepines may be to aid in sedation, but they must be used judiciously in this case, in conjunction with an antipsychotic (see Table 11-1).

PEARLS

- Delirium is characterized by rapid fluctuations in the level of consciousness.
- Delirium can be present in up to 85% of patients with terminal illness.
- Behavioral measures such as reorientation and destimulation are always first-line treatments.
- Delirium is best treated by diagnosing and treating the underlying cause (when possible).
- Antipsychotics, particularly haldol, are the medication treatments of choice in managing delirium.
- Avoid the use of benzodiazepines in delirium because it can worsen the condition, especially in the elderly and medically compromised patient.

PITFALLS

- Be cognizant that competency can be compromised by the presence of delirium. Repeated assessments of competence are a requirement.

- Be aware of the acute on chronic presentation when delirium occurs on the background of dementia. Assess baseline levels of cognitive function with collateral information when possible.

- Terminal delirium may not respond to any pharmacologic treatments.

- Untreated delirium can be associated with significant morbidity and mortality.

Summary

Delirium is a common syndrome in terminally ill patients. The appropriate diagnosis and treatment of delirium can decrease the significant morbidity and mortality associated with it. Behavioral management and antipsychotic medications are effective treatments.

Resources

1. Chochinov HM, Breitbart W, editors: *Handbook of Psychiatry in Palliative Medicine*, Oxford, UK, 2009, Oxford University Press.
2. Breitbart W, Rosenfeld B, Roth A, et al: The Memorial Delirium Assessment Scale, *J Pain Symptom Manage* 13(3):128–137, 1997.
3. Inouye SK, van Dyck CH, Alessi CA, et al: Clarifying confusion: The Confusion asssessment method for detection of delirium, *Ann Intern Med* 113:941–948, 1990.
4. Trepacz PT, Mittal D, Torres R, et al: Validation of the Delirium Rating Scale–Revised–98: Comparison with the Delirium Rating Scale and the Cognitive Test for Delirium, *J Neuropsychiatry Clin Neurosci* 13:229–242, 2001.

References

1. Fang CK, Chen HW, Liu SI, et al: Prevalence, detection and treatment of delirium in terminal cancer inpatients: a prospective survey, *Jap J Clin Oncol* 38(1):57–63, 2008.
2. American Psychiatric Association: *Diagnostic and statistical manual of mental disorders*, ed 4, Washington DC, 2000, American Psychiatric Association.
3. Devlin JW, Fong JJ, Fraser GL, et al: Delirium assessment in the critically ill, *J Intensive Care Med* 33:929–940, 2007.
4. Brenner RP: Utility of EEG in delirium: Past views and current practice, *Int Psychogeriatr* 3(2):211–229, 1991.
5. Schneider LS, Dagerman KS, Insel P: Risk of death with atypical antipsychotic drug treatment for dementia: meta-analysis of randomized placebo-controlled trials, *J Am Med Assoc* 294(15):1935–1943, 2005.
6. Wan PS, Schneeweiss S, Avorn J, et al: Risk of death in elderly users of conventional vs. atypical antipsychotic medications, *N Engl J Med* 353(22):2335–2341, 2005.
7. Folstein MF, Folstein SE, McHugh PR: "Mini-mental state." A practical method for grading the cognitive state of patients for the clinician, *J Psychiatr Res* 12(3):189–199, 1975.
8. Nasreddine ZS, Phillips NA, Bédirian V, et al: The Montreal Cognitive Assessment (MoCA): a brief screening tool for mild cognitive impairment, *J Am Geriatr Soc* 53:695–699, 2005.

CHAPTER 12

Constipation

S. LAWRENCE LIBRACH

Constipation is sometimes regarded as a minor symptom by care providers. However, this is not the case with palliative care patients. The prevalence of constipation in the overall population varies from 2% to 28% in population surveys, and it is more prevalent in elderly patients. It is a very prevalent symptom in patients who have advanced, progressive illnesses and is a significant source of suffering. Prevalence rates for constipation are approximately 25% to 50% for those with any type of terminal illnesses.[1,2] One study indicated that laxatives were administered to 87% of terminally ill patients with cancer.[3] From my personal, on-call experience in a large, home-based palliative care practice, constipation ranks as one of the major reasons for accessing the on-call service after hours. The approach to managing constipation is similar to that of other symptoms: Start with a comprehensive assessment, consider pharmacologic and nonpharmacologic management, follow through with careful monitoring, and be sure to educate the patient, family, and other care providers about the issues and the management.

Definition

Infrequent defecation (fewer than three bowel movements per week) has generally been regarded as the most important marker of constipation. However, other symptoms, such as excessive straining, hard stools, and a feeling of incomplete evacuation, have recently been recognized as equally important and perhaps more common.[4] More formal definitions like the Rome III are used in research studies, but they are not very useful in the clinical situation. A number of scales have been developed to assess the symptom of constipation. The Victoria Hospice Society Bowel Performance Scale is one of several scales currently used in Canada. Other scales include the Bristol Stool Form Scale and the Sykes DISH (Difficulties, Infrequent, Smaller,

Straining, Harder) scale.[5-7] Constipation may be associated with other symptoms and may be the major cause of nausea and vomiting, confusion, agitation, intermittent diarrhea, bloating, and abdominal pain. Rarely, severe constipation can be associated with bowel perforation and sepsis.

Etiology

Constipation has a multifactorial origin, as do other symptoms commonly seen near the end of life. The normal physiology of defecation is complex and involves the central and peripheral nervous system, hormones, and reflexes that are unique to the gastrointestinal system. The peripheral sympathetic and parasympathetic nervous system controls colonic motility, colonic reflexes such as the gastrocolic reflex, and relaxation and contraction of the anal sphincter. The urge to defecate and the process of defecation itself are mediated by the central nervous system and require contraction of skeletal muscles to increase abdominal pressure to facilitate evacuation. Adrenergic, opioid, muscarinic, and dopaminergic receptors all have a role in gut motility. Gastrointestinal hormone physiology is controlled by the endocrine and paracrine systems, as well as by neural pathways.[8] Problems in any one or a number of these systems may lead to constipation.

Opioid-induced constipation is one of the more common problems seen in palliative care. It results from decreased intestinal motility; poor propulsive action leads to prolonged intestinal transit time, increased fluid absorption in the colon, and hard stools. Opioids may also increase anal sphincter tone and may reduce awareness of a full rectum.

Contributing factors, both reversible and irreversible, to constipation in palliative care patients include the following:

1. *Preexisting constipation.* Elderly patients, in particular, have decreased bowel motility for various reasons. Long-term constipation is a problem seen in the general population, especially in women.[8] These patients may also suffer from having taken laxatives for many years, a practice that can result in constipation.
2. *Neurologic abnormalities.* These conditions include spinal cord lesions and autonomic dysfunction or neuropathy seen in diabetes and in cancer.
3. *Metabolic causes.* Conditions include dehydration, uremia, hypokalemia, hypercalcemia, hypothyroidism, and diabetes mellitus.
4. *Structural obstruction.* Conditions include fibrosis from radiation, adhesions, and bowel obstruction from tumors.
5. *Decreased food, fiber, and fluid intake.* Anorexia is a common symptom in many terminally ill patients. It is important to realize that 50% of stool weight is derived from cells, mucus, and bacteria, so even patients who eat very little will produce significant amounts of stool.
6. *Uncontrolled pain.* Uncontrolled pain may limit mobility and the patient's ability to strain at stool.
7. *Medications frequently used in palliative care patients, such as certain chemotherapy drugs, opioids, antidepressants, nonsteroidal anti-inflammatory drugs, and others.* Even vitamins and minerals commonly taken by patients can add to constipation. All opioids are associated with constipation.
8. *Limited mobility.*

9. *Generalized weakness.* Patients may not be able to sit or develop the increased abdominal pressure needed to evacuate the rectum.
10. *Hypomotility disorders secondary to diabetes, advanced age, and paraneoplastic problems.* These disorders cause increased transit time and ineffective propulsion of stool in the colon.
11. *Environmental issues.* These issues include lack of privacy, change in care setting, the use of bedpans, and inconveniently located washrooms.
12. *Care provider neglect.* Unfortunately, in the hustle and bustle of care, constipation may be overlooked, and protocols to address assessment and management may not be in place. Constipation may be seen as a minor problem and may not be addressed by physicians in particular.
13. *Patient issues.* Patients may be too embarrassed to discuss constipation or may feel that it is a minor symptom. Cultural issues may also hinder a discussion of constipation.

Assessment

A history of decreased frequency and description of hard bowel movements are often the key indicators of constipation. Color, odor, and size of stools should be determined. Patients may report associated symptoms, such as the inability to defecate at will, pain and discomfort when defecating, straining, unproductive urges, flatulence or bloating, or a sensation of incomplete evacuation.[9] However, other symptoms that result from constipation (e.g., nausea or vomiting, generalized malaise, headache, intermittent diarrhea, stool and urine incontinence, abdominal pain, and bloating) may be presenting problems.

Constipation should still be considered even in patients who are anorexic and have limited oral intake, because stools continue to be produced even in the absence of good oral intake (fecal content also consists of unabsorbed gastrointestinal secretions, shed epithelial cells, and bacteria).

Nursing records in institutions often indicate the frequency of bowel movements. A thorough medication history uncovers factors in constipation, including inappropriate or inadequate laxative regimens. A long history of recurring problems of constipation refractory to dietary measures or laxatives often suggests a functional colorectal disorder. An assessment of physical functioning may reveal significant weakness and inability to access washroom facilities. Physical examination may reveal abdominal distention and palpable abdominal masses, fecal and other. Neurologic examination may be required if a spinal cord lesion or brain lesion is suspected.

A gentle rectal examination is essential. Privacy and cultural sensitivities should be taken into consideration before performing a rectal examination. Perineal sensation can be checked. Assess anal sphincter tone, the presence of hemorrhoids and anal fissures, the presence and consistency of stool in the rectum, and the absence of stool and rectal dilation. A lack of stool in the rectum associated with rectal dilation may indicate constipation higher in the left side of the colon or colonic obstruction.

Plain upright radiographic films of the abdomen may be needed when the diagnosis is not evident. A classification system can be used by the radiologist to quantify the degree of constipation, but this is rarely reported or used.[10] However, it can be quite helpful in the patient with difficult-to-control constipation.

Management

GENERAL MANAGEMENT ISSUES

Preventive management is always better than responsive management. For palliative care patients, who tend to be sedentary and often on opioids, a bowel regimen to prevent constipation should be a routine consideration. Other considerations in the management of constipation include the following:

1. *Correct reversible causes when possible.* In most patients, the cause of constipation is multifactorial, so simple changes rarely produce significant change in the problem of constipation. Stopping opioids may, in fact, leave the patient in severe pain. Alternatives to opioids in patients with moderate to severe pain are very limited.
2. *Prevent constipation.* For instance, opioids almost always cause constipation. When opioids are prescribed, a laxative regimen using bowel stimulants and osmotic laxatives should be started immediately, before serious constipation develops. Constipation is one of the most feared adverse effects of opioids. A preventive approach should also be taken with other drugs that commonly cause constipation, such as tricyclic antidepressants.
3. *Educate the patient, family, and other care providers about the cause of and management plan for constipation.* Stress the importance of preventing constipation, thereby avoiding other symptoms and unnecessary suffering. Inquiry about constipation and frank discussions may not be possible in certain cultures. Avoid the cycles of alternating constipation and diarrhea by setting clear protocols for patients and their care providers.
4. *Create realistic expectations.* Although some patients would prefer to have a daily bowel movement, a soft, easy-to-pass movement every 2 days may be the best result.
5. *Monitor the patient frequently.* Pain diaries should also chart bowel movements. Protocols should be in place in all care settings to monitor patients at high risk of developing constipation—that is, most palliative care patients.

NONPHARMACOLOGIC MEASURES

Increase fluid intake if possible. Intake of 2 to 3 L/day is recommended. Too much coffee or tea should be avoided, however, because of the diuretic properties of these fluids. Increase physical activity if possible. Patients may maintain higher levels of function early in the course of a progressive illness. Exercise, even in small amounts, improves bowel motility. A high-fiber diet increases stool weight and accelerates colonic transit time. Daily fiber intake must increase by 450% to increase stool frequency by 50%.[11] A high-fiber diet does not benefit all patients with constipation. Increasing dietary fiber in the palliative care population is often not possible or practical in light of the high prevalence of anorexia, food preferences, and poor intestinal motility, and to do so may actually cause more constipation. Use wheeled bedside commodes to bring patients into washrooms. Ensure adequate privacy for patients. Use of drapes and screens is recommended for patients who cannot be wheeled in a bedside commode to toilet facilities. Avoid the use of bedpans for bowel movements because they are uncomfortable for many patients. Try to ease patients into a regular routine of having a bowel movement at a certain time of the day, usually following some food intake.

LAXATIVES

A recent evidence-based review[12] of constipation in palliative care patients found that all laxatives demonstrated a limited level of efficacy, and a significant number of participants required rescue laxatives in each of the studies. The authors concluded that "treatment of constipation in palliative care is based on inadequate evidence, such that there are insufficient RCT data. Recommendations for laxative use can be related to costs as much as to efficacy. There have been few comparative studies. Equally there have been few direct comparisons between different classes of laxative and between different combinations of laxatives. There persists an uncertainty about the 'best' management of constipation in this group of patients." The authors also noted that the prescribing preferences of the individual health care provider often prevailed over evidence-based practice.

Two systematic reviews of laxatives have been published. The only clear evidence for laxative efficacy rests with two osmotic laxatives: lactulose and polyethylene glycol (PEG-3350). There is only limited evidence for the efficacy of many commonly used laxatives, including docusate preparations and stimulant laxatives.[13,14]

For palliative care patients, program algorithms without much evidence base are used with reasonable success, although adverse effects of these regimens are rarely reported.[12] The use of laxatives, often in combination, is a common way to manage constipation.[15] There is reasonable evidence to exclude docusate from most regimens and instead to use lactulose or PEG to soften stools. Many palliative care patients are also put on stimulant laxatives, often in large doses, such as six to eight tablets of sennosides (Senokot) per day, much more than the usual recommended doses. (See Tables 12-1 and 12-2 for specifics; see also the formulary in the Appendix, available online at www.expertconsult.com.) Titrate laxatives to effect. Set up effective protocols that give day-by-day instructions for the family caregiver or nurse. A sample protocol is shown in Table 12-1.

Table 12-1. Sample Protocol

Set up regular dosing of laxatives:	Sennosides or bisacodyl: 2–4 tablets at bedtime to begin *plus* Lactulose 30 mL at bedtime *or* PEG 3350 powder 17 g once or twice daily
Monitor daily.	
If no bowel movement by day 2:	Increase sennosides by 2 tablets (can be given in two doses) and increase lactulose or PEG 3350 to 30 mL twice daily
If no bowel movement by day 3:	Perform rectal examination
If stool in rectum:	Use phosphate enema or bisacodyl suppository
If no stool in rectum and no contraindication:	Give oil enema followed by saline or tap water enema to clear Increase regular laxatives
If problems continue:	Do flat-plate radiograph of abdomen Switch stimulant laxative Use regular enemas

Table 12-2. Laxatives

Laxative Class	Examples	Mechanisms of Action	Special Issues
Bulk forming	Psyllium Increase dietary fiber Soluble fiber	Increase bowel motility, soften stool	Do not use if severely constipated or dehydrated; may increase bloating
Lubricant	Mineral oil orally	Soften & lubricate stool passage	*Do not use* Risk of aspiration & lipoid pneumonia, vitamin deficiency with long-term use
Osmotic laxatives	PEG-3350 Lactulose Sorbitol	Pull water into stool	May cause bloating
Stimulants	Bisacodyl Sennosides	Increase colonic motility	May cause cramps
Detergent	Docusate	Initially thought to soften stools	No evidence for use
Peripheral opioid receptor antagonist	Methylnaltrexone	For opioid-induced constipation	May cause some cramping

PERIPHERAL OPIOID RECEPTOR ANTAGONISTS

Opioid-induced constipation is predominantly mediated by gastrointestinal mu opioid receptors. Selective blockade of these peripheral receptors might relieve constipation without compromising centrally mediated effects of opioid analgesia or precipitating withdrawal. Two of these types of drugs have been developed: alvimopan and methylnaltrexone (MNTX). Only one specific peripheral opioid receptor antagonist, methylnaltrexone (MNTX), is available for use in opioid-induced constipation in Canada and the United States at the present time.

In randomized controlled trials conducted in patients with advanced illnesses, the median time to laxation was significantly shorter in the methylnaltrexone group than in the placebo group, with most patients having a bowel movement within the first 2 hours after administration. No evidence of withdrawal or changes in pain scores were observed. The incidence of adverse events with MNTX was similar to placebo and generally reported as mild to moderate. Abdominal pain and flatulence were the most common adverse events.[16]

MNTX is an option for patients who have failed to respond to optimal laxative therapy, recognizing that there is not enough information to make firm conclusions about the safety or effectiveness of MNTX; however, the drug does show promise.

ENEMAS

Enemas can be used for fecal impaction. They induce bowel movements by softening hard stool and by stimulating colonic muscle contraction in response to rectal and colonic distention. An oil retention enema (120 mL vegetable oil), followed by a tap water enema (500 mL/day), is generally preferable to salt-containing enemas (phosphate and soapsuds enemas) because oil and water are less irritating to the rectal mucosa. Bisacodyl suppositories or phosphate enemas may also be used to empty the rectum if the stool is relatively soft. If the stool is very hard, then a small-volume (60 mL) rectal oil enema may be used first. Gentle, low-volume enemas can be used through colostomies by experienced nurses. Enemas should be used cautiously in patients with a history of bowel stricture or recent lower bowel surgery and in immunocompromised patients.

MANUAL DISIMPACTION

Manual disimpaction may occasionally be necessary for low rectal impaction. Use a rectal oil enema in small volume to soften and lubricate the stools first. Appropriate sedation and analgesics are usually required to make the procedure comfortable. Manual disimpaction should not be needed often. Regular enemas should be sufficient to manage cases of recurrent, severe constipation.

THE PARAPLEGIC PATIENT

Constipation is a frequent issue for paraplegic patients and may be associated with stool incontinence. Setting up a regular regimen of enemas is essential and often avoids incontinence.

PEARLS

- Constipation is a highly prevalent problem for palliative care patients and may manifest as a variety of other problems.
- A rectal examination is essential in assessing problematic constipation.
- Education of patients, families, and health care providers is important in addressing the problem of constipation.
- Constipation protocols are necessary, although a clear evidence base does not exist for these.
- Use lactulose or PEG as osmotic laxatives to soften stool.
- Avoid the use of docusate.

PITFALLS

- Failure to address constipation vigorously can lead to significant suffering.
- Prescription of opioids without a bowel regimen is almost always a mistake.

Summary

Constipation is one of the most common symptoms in palliative care. If it is not addressed carefully, it can lead to more suffering. Constipation is multifactorial, and not all factors can be addressed in all patients. Careful history and physical examination provide important clues to the cause and to appropriate management. Combinations of laxatives and careful monitoring are key ingredients in the care plan.

References

1. Solano JP, Gomes B, Higginson IJ: A comparison of symptom prevalence in far advanced cancer, AIDS, heart disease, chronic obstructive pulmonary disease and renal disease, *J Pain Symptom Manage* 31:58–69, 2006.
2. Curtis EB, Krech R, Walsh TD: Common symptoms in patients with advanced cancer, *Palliat Care* 7:25–29, 1991.
3. Sykes N: The relationship between opioid use and laxative use in terminally ill cancer patients, *Palliat Med* 12:375–382, 1998.
4. Pare P, Ferrazzi S, Thompson WG, et al: An epidemiological survey of constipation in Canada: definitions, rates, demographics and predictors of health care seeking, *Am J Gastroenterol* 96:3130–3137, 2001.
5. Downing M: Victoria Bowel Performance Scale. In *Medical care of the dying*, ed 4, Victoria, B.C., 2006, Victoria Hospice Society, p. 343.
6. Thompson WG, Longstreth GF, Drossman DA, et al: Functional bowel disorders and functional abdominal pain, *Gut* 45(Suppl 2):1143–1147, 1999.
7. Lewis SJ, Heaton KW: Stool form scale as a useful guide to intestinal transit time, *Scand J Gastroenterol* 32(9):920–924, 1997.
8. McMillan S: Assessing and managing opiate-induced constipation in adults with cancer, *Cancer Control* 11(3):S3–S9, 2004.
9. Larkin PJ, Skyes NP, Centeno C, et al: The management of constipation in palliative care: clinical practice recommendations, *Palliat Med* 22:796–807, 2008.
10. Starreveld JS, Pols MA, van Wijk HJ, et al: The plain abdominal radiograph in the assessment of constipation, *Gastroenterology* 28:335–338, 1990.
11. Everhart JE, Go VLW, Hohannes RS, et al: A longitudinal study of self-reported bowel habits in the United States, *Dig Dis Sci* 34:1153–1162, 1989.
12. Miles C, Fellowes D, Goodman ML, Wilkinson SSM: *Laxatives for the management of constipation in palliative care patients*, London, United Kingdom, 2009, The Cochrane Collaboration.
13. Ramkumar D, Rao SS: Efficacy and safety of traditional medical therapies for chronic constipation: Systematic review, *Am J Gastroenterol* 100:936–971, 2005.
14. American College of Gastroenterology Chronic Constipation Task Force: an evidence-based approach to the management of chronic constipation in North America, *Am J Gastroenterol* 100:S1–S22, 2005.
15. Sykes N: Constipation management in palliative care, *Geriatr Med* 27:55–57, 1997.
16. McNicol ED, Boyce D, Schumann R, Carr DB: Mu-opioid antagonists for opioid-induced bowel dysfunction, *Cochrane Database Syst Rev* 2, 2008.

CHAPTER 13

Urinary Incontinence

S. LAWRENCE LIBRACH

Urinary incontinence is a relatively common problem seen in patients at the end of life, but the exact prevalence is not clear. Studies of symptom prevalence at the end of life often do not mention urinary incontinence at all,[1,2] yet most patients who receive palliative care are also elderly, and this population is often affected by urinary incontinence. In fact, urinary incontinence affects 15% to 35% of community-dwelling older adults and more than 50% of nursing home residents.[3] There is a general reluctance for patients and families to discuss urinary incontinence. It may be that care providers assume that urinary incontinence is not a symptom in the ordinary sense, but rather a common, although less serious, problem at the end of life.

Urinary incontinence can have a significant impact on quality of life. In its various forms, urinary incontinence may limit patients' mobility and social interactions. Elderly patients with urinary incontinence are more likely to be placed in a nursing home. Those with limited economic resources struggle to cope with the costs of investigations and treatment. Urinary incontinence may also lead to depression. The impact of urinary incontinence on the place of care or on other aspects palliative care is not reported. If not properly managed, however, urinary incontinence may add to the suffering of these patients. Neglected urinary incontinence may lead to systemic infections, skin problems, and skin wounds, thus introducing other significant physical morbidity to patients who are already dealing with numerous symptoms at the end of life.

One study showed that men are more likely than women to develop sexual dysfunction in association with urinary incontinence.[4] Another study indicated that, among heterosexual couples, urinary incontinence correlates with interference of sexual satisfaction.[5]

176

Cultural attitudes toward urinary incontinence vary significantly. In North American culture, urinary incontinence is gaining recognition as a medical illness and is discussed more openly, even in television commercials. In other societies, however, urinary incontinence is still traditionally viewed as evidence of self-neglect, being unclean, having poor self-discipline, or being socially incompetent. Patients with urinary incontinence who live in such societies may manage their symptoms in isolation and secrecy.[6] The onset of urinary incontinence may adversely affect self-esteem.

Physiology and Pathophysiology

Micturition, the process of voiding urine from the bladder, is a complex process that involves the interplay of involuntary smooth muscle, voluntary striated muscle, the autonomic and somatic nervous systems, and the brain, as well as a cognitive aspect. The components of the system include the following[7]:

- The bladder wall is composed of a mesh of smooth muscle fibers.
- An internal, involuntary sphincter is composed of layers of smooth muscle at the bladder neck that surrounds the urethral orifice, known as the detrusor muscle.
- The outer layer of this smooth muscle continues in a circular fashion along the full length of the urethra in girls and women and to the distal prostate in boys and men, forming the involuntary urethral sphincter.
- An external, voluntary sphincter made up of striated muscle interdigitating with smooth muscle is located between the layers of the urogenital diaphragm. In boys and men, these fibers are concentrated at the distal aspect of the prostate; in girls and women, they are found mainly in relation to the middle third of the urethra.
- The innervation of the system is complex. The bladder receives its principal nerve supply from one paired somatic and two paired autonomic nerves. The hypogastric nerves (arising from lumbar spinal segments L1 and L2) mediate sympathetic activity, whereas the pelvic nerves (derived from S2–S4) contain parasympathetic fibers. The pudendal nerves (S2–S4) are primarily somatic fibers innervating the striated, voluntary sphincter. With distention of the bladder wall, stretch receptors trigger parasympathetic pelvic nerve fibers that, unless inhibited by higher centers, lead to a parasympathetic motor response and bladder contraction. In micturition, the detrusor muscle contracts, thus drawing the bladder downward, and the external sphincter, under voluntary control, relaxes. Micturition is inhibited by sympathetic nervous system stimulation. All are coordinated by higher centers to initiate or inhibit bladder emptying. Therefore, problems can arise at one or more levels: the physical structure of the bladder, the enervation of the bladder and urethra, and the cognitive function of the patient. Each may result in or may be a factor in urinary incontinence.

Other factors may be involved in producing urinary incontinence. Estrogens may be associated with increased prevalence of urinary incontinence. Benzodiazepines and selective serotonin reuptake inhibitors are also associated with an increase in the frequency of urinary incontinence. Another factor in urinary incontinence needs to be mentioned here: Urinary incontinence may result from failure by the care provider to manage reversible causes, such as urinary tract infections.

Types of Urinary Incontinence

OVERACTIVE BLADDER SYNDROME

Overactive bladder (OAB) is characterized by urgency, a sudden compelling desire to pass urine that is difficult to defer. It is usually accompanied by frequency and nocturia, and it may occur with urge urinary incontinence. The exact cause of OAB is not entirely known, but it is both myogenic and neurogenic. OAB affects about 16% of the adult population, and the prevalence increases with age. OAB can have a negative impact on health, ability to function, and quality of life. Elderly patients with urge urinary incontinence are also more likely to be admitted to nursing homes.[8] Patients, families, and physicians may treat OAB as a normal consequence of aging, an attitude that results in underdiagnosis and undertreatment of this condition. In the typical population requiring palliative care—namely, elderly patients—preexisting OAB can lead to urinary incontinence. As palliative care patients become weaker or have significant pain, it is more difficult for them to reach the washroom in time, and the result is urgency urinary incontinence.

OTHER FORMS OF URGENCY INCONTINENCE

Inflammation of the bladder, tumors at or near the internal urethral orifice, urinary infections, inflammation secondary to radiation, and some neurologic disorders may also result in an urgency type of urinary incontinence.

Stress Incontinence

Stress urinary incontinence consists of involuntary urethral loss of urine associated with increased intra-abdominal pressure from coughing, sneezing, jumping, laughing, or, in severe cases, even walking. It is associated with faulty urethral support that results in abnormal sphincter function and an inability to resist increased bladder pressure. It is more common in women, but it can be present in men, especially those who have had prostate or bladder neck surgery. In female patients, parity, pelvic surgery, obesity, menopause, and smoking are also cofactors in the development of stress urinary incontinence. In palliative care, preexisting stress urinary incontinence may be made worse by symptoms such as poorly controlled coughing or nausea. New stress urinary incontinence may be caused by surgery to the bladder neck, radiation-induced inflammation and fibrosis, tumors external to the bladder that cause increased intravesical pressure, and spinal cord damage.

Overflow Incontinence

The continuous urinary leakage seen with overflow urinary incontinence is mostly the result of overflow with chronic urinary retention secondary to urethral stricture or blockage. The bladder remains palpable and percussible, considerable residual urine is present, and the condition is nonpainful. Benign or malignant prostatic disease, spinal nerve damage, and urethral obstruction from tumors are common causes of this problem in palliative care patients.

Incontinence Secondary to Neurologic Dysfunction

Spinal cord damage from any cause, sacral tumors, pelvic surgery, and pelvic tumors that invade the nerve supply to the bladder may result in partial or total urinary incontinence.

Incontinence Associated with Cognitive Failure

Patients who suffer from significant dementia or delirium are almost always incontinent.

Assessment

An initial evaluation should include the following:

1. *A good history.* Ask about the following:
   - Urinary frequency
   - Presence of the sensation of urgency
   - Leakage
   - Influence of activities that increase intra-abdominal pressure
   - Pattern of urinary incontinence (occasional, continual)
   - Neurogenic symptoms such as paresthesia, dysesthesia, anesthesia, motor weakness, or lack of sensation of bladder fullness or of bladder emptying
   - Pain
   - Presence of hematuria or dysuria
   - How often does the patient void during the day and night and how long can she or he wait comfortably between urinations?
   - Why does voiding occur as often as it does (urgency, convenience, attempt to prevent incontinence)?
   - How severe is incontinence (e.g., a few drops, saturate outer clothing)?
   - Are protective pads worn?
2. *A review of the patient's disease process and treatments.*
3. *A review of previous imaging to look for sources of neurogenic urinary incontinence and pelvic masses.* New imaging may be required, depending on the stage of the patient's illness and whether this will change management.
4. *Patient, caregiver, or care provider monitoring for at least 2 days.* Ask for a voiding diary, which should record urinary frequency, urgency, volume of urine, relation to other symptoms (if any), and the presence of pain on urination.
5. *A targeted physical examination.* Ask for the following:
   - Abdominal examination to exclude a distended bladder
   - Neurologic assessment of the perineum and lower extremities
   - Pelvic examination in women, if warranted
   - Genital and prostate examination in men, if warranted
   - Rectal examination to assess for pelvic masses and anal sphincter tone

The rectal examination may include a bulbocavernosus reflex. Both are tests of nerve function to the area.

6. *Urinalysis.* Reagent strip testing of urine is a sensitive and inexpensive screening method that can be supplemented with urine microscopy and culture.
7. *Further testing as needed.* Depending on the patient's illness stage, further investigations such as residual urine determination, urodynamic studies, and cystoscopy may be indicated if they can help with the management of urinary incontinence. Consultation with a urologist can be very helpful.

Management

The management of urinary incontinence starts with evaluation for and treatment of reversible causes. Infections should be treated after urine has been obtained for a culture. Some change may need to be made once the organism's sensitivity to antibiotics is determined. Prostatic obstruction may require surgical intervention, again depending on the stage of the illness. Urethral stricture may require dilation. Obviously, spinal cord compression must be dealt with in the usual fashion. For most palliative care patients, however, the conditions leading to urinary incontinence are not reversible, and a palliative approach must be taken.

One of the most important steps in managing patients with nonreversible urinary incontinence is to educate the patient (when possible) and the family about the cause of the urinary incontinence and the various aspects of the treatment. Patients may need counseling to deal with their grief over this particular issue because it is often equated with the need for institutional care. The benefits of appropriate treatment should be emphasized.

BEHAVIORAL THERAPY

Behavioral therapy includes techniques such as bladder training, timed or prompted voiding, pelvic muscle exercises, and biofeedback. Behavioral therapy may improve bladder control by changing the incontinent patient's voiding habits and teaching skills for preventing urine loss.[9] However, because of the multitude of issues facing palliative care patients, these techniques may be applicable only in the early palliative stages.

It may be possible to prevent urgency urinary incontinence by prompting the patient to void frequently and to suppress the urge initially by tightening the voluntary sphincter. In institutions, the patient must be brought to toileting facilities before the urge becomes too great. If the patient is bed bound, ready access to urine bottles for men or to slipper-type bedpans for women may avoid embarrassing urinary incontinence. Reduced cognitive abilities may, however, make these interventions ineffective.

PHARMACOLOGIC THERAPY

Overactive Bladder

First-line therapy of OAB involves the use of anticholinergic drugs aimed at decreasing the urgency from detrusor muscle contractions. Commonly used agents include oral oxybutynin hydrochloride, tolterodine tartrate, and flavoxate hydrochloride. Controlled-release oxybutynin and transdermal oxybutynin are clearly effective in reducing episodes of urinary incontinence and are superior to placebo. Tolterodine, at a dose of at least 2 mg, is similarly effective in reducing episodes of urinary incontinence. Direct comparisons between oxybutynin and tolterodine show little treatment effect difference between the two drugs.[10]

Newer drugs have been marketed for the treatment of OAB. Trospium chloride has efficacy equivalent to twice-daily immediate-release oxybutynin and a lower incidence of dry mouth. Both darifenacin and solifenacin have proven efficacy and are available in once-daily formulations. Whether these agents have a distinct advantage over other anticholinergic drugs has yet to be determined, although they are marketed as having fewer side effects. Tricyclic antidepressant agents, often used as adjuvants for neuropathic pain, may be used for their anticholinergic effects (Table 13-1).

Table 13-1. Antimuscarinic Agents Available Worldwide for Treatment of Incontinence Secondary to Detrusor Overactivity

Antimuscarinic Drugs	Level of Evidence
Darifenacin	A
Oxybutynin	A
Propiverine	A
Tolterodine	A
Trospium	A
Solifenacin	A
Propantheline	B
Hyoscyamine	C

Modified from Anderson KE, Appell R, Cardozo L, et al: Pharmacological Treatment of Urinary Incontinence. In Abrams P, Cardozo L, Khoury S, Wein A, editors: *Incontinence*, 3rd International Consultation on Incontinence. London, United Kingdom, 2005, Health Publications, pp 809–854.

Pharmacologic treatment is problematic, however. Many patients do not improve much and may experience only a small reduction in episodes of urinary incontinence, and many experience no improvement. Complete continence is rarely achieved. Although this may be important for some patients, if urinary incontinence continues despite treatment, it produces a continued burden and frustration with quality of life. Because the benefits are unpredictable and have not been studied well in the palliative care patient (in whom OAB may be related to tumors and treatments), patients should be offered a brief trial of these anticholinergic agents.

The most difficult part of taking these drugs may be the significant adverse effects associated with their anticholinergic properties. Dry mouth is common, occurring in the majority of patients. Palliative care patients often already have dry mouth because of oral candidiasis, chemotherapy and radiation treatments, and other medications, particularly opioids. The addition of further xerostomia from these agents may be intolerable to these patients. Constipation, already a very common problem in palliative care patients, may also be increased. These drugs should be used cautiously in patients with gastric or intestinal hypomotility because they enhance those problems. Anticholinergic drugs should also be avoided in patients with significantly impaired renal or hepatic function. Patients with cardiac arrhythmias cannot take these drugs. Major side effects, such as ventricular arrhythmias or sudden death, are not associated with anticholinergic drugs. Few central nervous system effects are observed in clinical trials of the specific agents, but these drugs may be associated with sedation, hallucinations, and confusion, particularly in elderly patients. Again, palliative care patient populations have not been studied.

Stress Incontinence

Alpha-adrenergic and beta-adrenergic agonists, such as phenylpropanolamine hydrochloride, midodrine, and pseudoephedrine, increase the internal sphincter tone and bladder outflow resistance. Beta-adrenergic agonists may also have some effect. Alpha-adrenergic receptors are widespread in the cardiovascular system, however, which is the mechanism for systemic cardiovascular side effects such as arrhythmia and hypertension. A meta-analysis of the effects of the adrenergic agonist drugs phenylpropanolamine and midodrine suggests that an adrenergic agonist drug is more effective than placebo in reducing the number of pad changes and episodes of urinary incontinence and in improving subjective symptoms.[11] Patients who use adrenergic agonists usually experience minor side effects that rarely result in discontinuation of treatment. These include dizziness, palpitations, excitability, and sleep disturbance. Rare but serious side effects, such as cardiac arrhythmias and hypertension, may occur.

Overflow Incontinence

For the overflow urinary incontinence that results from benign prostatic hypertrophy, the relief of outflow obstruction using alpha-blocker therapy is based on the hypothesis that clinical prostatic hypertrophy is caused partly by alpha-1-adrenergic–mediated contraction of prostatic smooth muscle that results in bladder outlet obstruction. Treatment options for symptomatic patients include alpha-adrenergic antagonists such as alfuzosin, doxazosin, tamsulosin, and terazosin. The data suggest that these agents are equally effective. Data are insufficient to support a recommendation for the use of prazosin hydrochloride. Adverse effects of these drugs include nasal congestion, hypotension, fatigue, ejaculatory problems, cardiac arrhythmias, headaches, and edema.[12]

The 5-alpha-reductase inhibitors finasteride and dutasteride are effective for patients who have demonstrable prostatic enlargement, but these are long-term treatments. Patients who have symptomatic prostatic enlargement but no symptoms of OAB or incontinence can be offered a 5-alpha-reductase inhibitor to retard progression of the disease, but response is limited. The benefit of these drugs in palliative care patients is not clear.

USE OF DIAPERS

Diaper or pad technology has advanced rapidly. Diapers are now more absorbent, suppress odors better, and are more fitted, thus reducing the possibility of leakage. The cost may be significant, but it is offset by reductions in care provider time, reduced needs to launder bedding, the better ability to keep someone at home, and reduced stress on family caregivers. Diapers must be changed frequently. Family members who are caring for the patient at home should be educated about how to apply the diapers so minimal lifting is required. Patients can be dressed and still wear a diaper. Diapers may be problematic in the patient with severe incident pain, however, so urinary catheters should be considered in these patients. Incontinence pads are probably overused and are not very effective in absorbing large quantities of urine.

SKIN CARE

Urinary incontinence that is not adequately treated can lead to skin problems. Skin maceration and irritation can be minimized by frequent diaper changes, the treatment of skin candidiasis and intertrigo, and the use of barrier creams that usually contain silicone or zinc oxide to protect the skin. Skin that is irritated is much more likely to develop wounds, and wound prevention strategies must be employed.

URINARY URETHRAL CATHETERS

Urinary catheters are often seen as a last resort for patients with urinary incontinence. The major problem with catheters relates to the development of infections with long-term use. Although urinary catheters are used with relative frequency in palliative care settings, few reviews have been done.

A urinary catheter should be considered for incontinent patients if behavioral changes, nursing care, special clothes, special bed clothes, and medication changes are unsuccessful. Indications for the use of a urinary catheter in palliative care patients include the following[13]:

1. Management or prevention of decubitus ulcers and other skin wounds
2. Painful, physical movements that preclude frequent changes of clothes and bed linen
3. A decision by the patient and family that dryness and comfort outweigh the risks of catheterization
4. Overflow urinary incontinence associated with obstruction
5. Urine retention that is not surgically correctable
6. Continuous bladder irrigation in patients with hemorrhage from bladder tumors
7. An explicit request from the patient or family (primarily for patients at the end of life)

External condom catheters have been used for a long time in men. They are poorly accepted by patients, are often difficult to apply and maintain in place, and are uncomfortable. They are associated with skin irritation and ulceration, urinary infections, and (rarely) penile gangrene from inappropriate fitting and neglect. Unless they are preferred by patients, it is probably best to avoid the use of these devices in palliative care.

Indwelling urinary catheters can be made of material such as rubber or silicone and may be impregnated with antibacterial chemicals. Complications of indwelling catheters include bladder and urethral infections, pyelonephritis, septicemia, bladder spasm, and hemorrhage from the bladder. It has not been determined whether palliative care patients are more susceptible to these problems because of their cachexia and reduced immune function.

Most patients with catheters and asymptomatic bacteriuria should not receive antimicrobial therapy.[14] The rationale for this recommendation includes the following:

1. The risk of complications from asymptomatic bacteriuria is low.
2. Treatment does not prevent bacteriuria from recurring.
3. Treatment may lead to the presence of antimicrobial-resistant bacteria that are more challenging to treat.

Most experts recommend against using antimicrobial agents to eradicate bacteriuria in asymptomatic patients unless the patient has an abnormal urinary tract or will soon undergo genitourinary tract manipulation or instrumentation.

The introduction of the closed-drainage indwelling catheter system is an extremely important advance in the prevention of urinary catheter-related infections. The use of a presealed urinary catheter junction (as delivered in most catheter sets these days) is important. Aseptic insertion techniques and careful maintenance of the catheter and drainage bag are essential. The collection bag should remain below the level of the bladder to prevent reflux of urine into the bladder, and the drainage tube should be checked for kinking. The drainage bag should be emptied at least twice daily. Finally, glove use and proper hand hygiene practices are important in preventing the acquisition of pathogens.

Several different types of urethral catheters with anti-infective properties have been developed and evaluated. One such anti-infective catheter uses silver, an effective antibacterial substance, in the form of silver alloy. Results of one meta-analysis indicate that silver alloy catheters are likely to prevent bacteriuria,[15] but the effect of these catheters on the more important clinical outcomes (e.g., bacteremia) remains to be determined. Although silver alloy catheters are more expensive, they seem economically efficient when they are used in patients who receive indwelling catheterization for 2 to 10 days.[16] Catheters impregnated with antibiotics are now being evaluated, although they may be problematic because of the induction of antibiotic-resistant organisms.

Intermittent catheterization is a common method of urinary collection in patients with overflow urinary incontinence, especially from spinal cord damage. Inserting and removing a sterile or clean urinary catheter several times daily may reduce the risk of bacteriuria (compared with an indwelling catheter), and the technique can be taught to patients and family members. Suprapubic catheters may be required in patients with urethral obstruction from tumors.

PEARLS

- Urinary incontinence has important negative effects on quality of life.
- Careful assessment to determine the type of urinary incontinence may lead to specific but limited pharmacologic treatment.
- Indwelling urinary catheters can be used effectively in palliative care patients when indicated.

PITFALLS

- Ignoring urinary incontinence will increase patients' suffering and will decrease quality of life.
- Unless managed properly with aseptic technique, indwelling catheters can become a source of infection.

Summary

Urinary incontinence is a relatively frequent occurrence in palliative care patients, and it is a sensitive issue for patients and family. Management requires careful assessment, education and counseling, and a variety of medications. It often requires instrumentation such as catheters, especially in the last few days of life.

References

1. Kutner JS, Kassner CT, Nowels DE: Symptom burden at the end of life: hospice providers perceptions, *J Pain Symptom Manage* 21:473–480, 2001.
2. Solano JP, Gomes B, Higginson IJ: A comparison of symptom prevalence in far advanced cancer, AIDS, heart disease, chronic obstructive pulmonary disease and renal disease, *J Pain Symptom Manage* 31:58–69, 2006.
3. Diokno AC: The epidemiology of urinary incontinence, *J Gerontol Med Sci* 56:3–4, 2001.
4. Temml C, Haidinger G, Schmidbauer J, et al: Urinary incontinence in both sexes: prevalence rates and impact on quality of life and sexual life, *Neurourol Urodynam* 19:259–271, 2000.
5. Barber MD, Visco AG, Wyman JF, et al: Continence Program for Women Research Group: Sexual function in women with urinary incontinence and pelvic organ prolapse, *Obstet Gynecol* 99:281–289, 2002.

6. Wilson MG: Urinary incontinence: a treatise on gender, sexuality, and culture, *Clin Geriatr Med* 20:565–570, 2004.
7. Madersbacher H, Madersbacher S: Men's bladder health: Part I. urinary incontinence in the elderly, *J Mens Health Gender* 2:31–37, 2005.
8. Thom DH, Haan MN, Van Den Eeden SK: Medically recognized urinary incontinence and risks of hospitalization, nursing home admission and mortality, *Age Ageing* 26:367–374, 1997.
9. Lavelle JP, Karam M, Chu FM, et al: Management of incontinence for family practice physicians, *Am J Med* 119(Suppl 3A):37–40, 2006.
10. Thomas DR: Pharmacologic management of urinary incontinence, *Clin Geriatr Med* 20:511–523, 2004.
11. Alhasso A, Glazener CM, Pickard R, N'Dow J: Adrenergic drugs for urinary incontinence in adults, *Cochrane Database Syst Rev* 2003;2CD001842.
12. American Urological Association Practice Guidelines Committee: AUA guideline on management of benign prostatic hyperplasia (2003). Chapter 1: diagnosis and treatment recommendations, *J Urol* 170:530–547, 2003.
13. Fainsinger R, Bruera E: Urinary catheters in palliative care, *J Pain Symptom Manage* 6:449–451, 1991.
14. Saint S, Chenoweth CE: Biofilms and catheter-associated urinary tract infections, *Infect Dis Clin North Am* 17:411–432, 2003.
15. Saint S, Elmore JG, Sullivan SD, et al: The efficacy of silver alloy coated urinary catheters in preventing urinary tract infection: a meta-analysis, *Am J Med* 105:236–241, 1998.
16. Plowman R, Graves N, Esquivel J, Roberts JA: An economic model to assess the cost and benefits of the routine use of silver alloy coated urinary catheters to reduce the risk of urinary tract infections in catheterized patients, *J Hosp Infect* 48:33–42, 2001.

CHAPTER 14

Sexuality

S. LAWRENCE LIBRACH and TIMOTHY J. MOYNIHAN

Sexuality is a universal human phenomenon. It is an integral part of the lives of most people and is a fundamental aspect of their quality of life. A terminal illness does not and should not preclude all sexual activity. Although much has been written on human sexuality in the last 50 years, little has been written about sexuality in end-of-life care.

Sexual dysfunction at the end of life has not been studied. The exact incidence and prevalence are not known and are likely to be highly dependent on the illness, the disabilities incurred, the side effects of treatment, and comorbid medical conditions. Cancer or treatments that directly affect the sexual organs (e.g., prostate, testes, cervix, ovaries, vagina, bladder, or rectum) can lead to significant hormonal, local, and mechanical problems. Other malignant diseases and advanced, progressive illnesses of any type may also greatly impair sexual function because of symptoms and disabilities such as fatigue, pain, dyspnea, altered body image (e.g., head and neck disfigurement or mastectomies), the presence of ostomies, lack of flexibility related to limitation of movement, chronic wounds, lack of desire, or other physical and psychological distress. For men with cancer, it appears that the major problems with sexual dysfunction are erectile dysfunction, diminished desire, and fatigue. For women, dyspareunia, lack of desire, vaginal dryness, the inability to achieve an orgasm, fatigue, and altered body image are the predominant concerns.

The taboos of sexuality have been eroding slowly; many health care providers still feel uncomfortable assessing this area. Patient surveys suggest that many would appreciate a discussion of sexuality from their health care providers.[1,2] One study suggested that cancer patients were significantly more eager to discuss their sexual lives than were control participants, and even though cancer patients had lower

Table 14-1. Patient Factors that Interfere with Sexual Function of the Expression of Sexuality

Physical	Symptoms such as pain, fatigue, dyspnea, and nausea
	Ostomies of various types
	Erectile dysfunction secondary to pelvic or prostate surgery
	Surgery on genital areas leading to problems such as vaginal fibrosis or stenosis
	Open wounds
	Amputations
	Lumpectomy or mastectomy for breast cancer
	Paralysis
	Brain tumors
	Previous erectile dysfunction
	Arthritis and diminished flexibility
Medications	Hormonal or antihormonal therapy
	Erectile dysfunction secondary to medications
Radiation therapy	Skin reactions or burns
	Destruction of neurovascular pathways and arterial vascular beds
	Fatigue, nausea, vomiting, and diarrhea
	Vaginal dryness, stenosis, and fibrosis
	Erectile dysfunction
Psychological issues	Anxiety and depression
	Couple or family dysfunction
	Body image issues
	Partner aversion to sex
	Grief
	Hopelessness and loss of meaning

strength and frequency of sexual activity, they reported no less sexual satisfaction than did control participants.[3]

Another small, qualitative study investigated the meaning of sexuality to patients in a palliative care program.[4] Several themes emerged. First, sexuality continues to be important at the end of life, and all patients in this study felt that their health care providers should have discussed sexuality as part of their assessment, yet only 1 in 10 did so. Second, emotional connection to others was reported to be an integral component of sexuality, taking precedence over physical expressions. Finally, lack of privacy, shared rooms, staff intrusion, and single beds were considered barriers to expressing sexuality in hospital and hospice settings. The whole-person approach to providing high-quality end-of-life care must therefore address issues of sexuality as part of the assessment and care plan (Table 14-1).

Definition

Sexuality can be defined as the quality or state of being sexual. Sexuality can be expressed in ways other than sexual intercourse. It may quite often be expressed through close physical contact, caressing, and other touching. A patient at the end of life needs and often seeks physical and emotional closeness with others; sexuality with a partner can be part of this closeness. As with other needs at the end of life, sexuality has a number of components: biological, physical, psychological, social, cultural, and moral. Understanding sexuality in palliative care patients involves comprehensive assessment of each of these components and recognizing how they interact.

Sexuality and Palliative Care

The issues that arise in sexuality in palliative care patients represent the complex interaction of all the components of sexuality as described earlier.

PATIENT AND FAMILY ISSUES

When people develop a serious, life-limiting illness, they may appear to lose interest in sex as they adjust to dealing with the illness and its treatment. Many patients have a poor understanding of their own sexual needs and ways of expressing those needs in the setting of illness. They may be very reluctant to raise the issue of sexual function or to discuss issues of sexuality with their physicians because many patients expect their physician to initiate the discussion. Some cultures may not allow patients to discuss sexual concerns, even with professional health care providers.

A patient's physical disabilities, symptoms, medications, surgery, treatment regimens, and associated psychological issues (e.g., anxiety and depression) may affect the desire for sexual expression and the physical ability to have such contact. Patients may worry that their partner may no longer be sexually attracted to them because of the changes in their body and the fact that they have cancer or another serious illness. Serious illness puts a great strain on partner and family relationships. This stress may cause problems in the relationship between partners and may disturb usual sexual function. The partner may feel guilty for having sexual feelings at a time when the patient is coping with the illness and associated problems. Similarly, the sexual partner may also be affected by the illness and may feel that sexual expression is not possible or even appropriate or may even be less attracted to his or her partner because of changes in appearance. This may be manifested by sexual dysfunction in the partner, such as erectile dysfunction or lack of arousal in either partner.

AGING PATIENTS

Many patients who need palliative care are elderly. The Masters and Johnson's four stages of human sexual response (excitement/arousal, plateau, orgasm, and resolution) are all affected by the aging process. Nonetheless, elderly men and women can continue to enjoy fulfilling sexual experiences.[5] Therefore, elderly patients should also have sexual assessments as part of their comprehensive assessment. The clinician should also be cognizant of the possibility of preexisting sexual dysfunction that often has never been addressed.

Physiologic changes that should be taken into account include the following:

- More and longer direct stimulation of the penis may be required to achieve erection in older men.
- Erections are usually not as full and may occur less frequently.

- The plateau phase is prolonged, resulting in better control of ejaculation compared with that of younger men.
- During orgasm, both the force of ejaculation and the number of contractions with each ejaculation are reduced, but the subjective feeling of pleasure is not diminished.
- Older men who lose an erection before orgasm may not be able to achieve another because they experience a longer refractory period before another erection can begin.

Women also experience changes in sexual functioning with age. Most of these changes probably result from the decline in estrogen production that occurs with the onset of menopause. The reduced estrogen stimulation causes many changes in anatomy, including thinning of the vaginal mucosa, shrinking of the uterus, and replacement of breast glandular tissue by fat. Sexual arousal in older women requires more and longer direct stimulation. Vaginal lubrication is reduced, and the vaginal opening expands less fully. During the succeeding plateau phase, older women experience less vasocongestion and tenting of the vagina. With orgasm, fewer uterine contractions occur and, during resolution, clitoral tumescence is lost more rapidly than in younger women.

Dying individuals often are elderly, and their sexual needs may not include intercourse. They may have found that their sensuality can be expressed by hugging and cuddling.

HEALTH CARE PROVIDER ISSUES

Poor knowledge and attitudes about sexual function and dysfunction are still issues with many health care providers. Curricula in this area and clinical teaching experience in assessing and managing sexuality may be lacking. This means that skills in assessing and managing issues of sexuality are likely to be suboptimal among most clinicians.

The health care provider's reluctance to assess a patient's sexuality and to deal with related issues often stems from the provider's own sensitivity to discussing this very intimate function. This reticence can occur even if the patient wishes to discuss the issue of sexuality. Health care providers may be reluctant to ask questions about their patients' sexual functioning because they themselves are embarrassed and not comfortable with their own sexuality, they may not believe that sexuality is part of the presenting problem, or they may feel that they are not trained adequately to deal with sexual concerns.[6]

In considering all the issues for patients at the end of life, health care providers may feel that sexuality must have a low priority. Health care providers often wait for the patient to initiate discussion, yet most patients want and expect the physician to initiate the conversation.[7-9] The cultural and religious background of the health care provider may also inhibit such discussion of sexuality, especially if there is a significant difference between the health care provider's beliefs and those of the patient. Some health care providers have significant difficulties dealing with patients whose sexual orientation and practices may be very different from their own, and these difficulties provide yet another barrier for effective patient care and evaluation. In such cases, clinicians must recognize and acknowledge their own beliefs and be willing to refer their patients to others who are better equipped to help.

SYSTEM ISSUES

The structure of health care institutions presents another barrier to sexuality for those patients who reside in the facility. Simple items, such as the use of single beds, inhibit the ability of partners to experience sexual relations. Privacy is in short supply in most health care settings. Multipatient rooms are not conducive to intimate exchanges between a patient and his or her partner. Even private rooms may not have doors or locks, so anyone can enter without notice, and this creates an environment that is not conducive to sexual intimacy.[10] In addition, patient's lives are often discussed freely among the staff, a situation that leaves no sense of privacy. Many institutions still are reluctant to endorse a policy in which sexual contact or activity is allowed on site. Patients may be confined to the facility and may not have access to items such as condoms that would allow for safe sex practices. Institutions must develop policies that will allow patients access to such items and must develop systems that allow for the private and safe conduct of sexual activity for its residents.

Assessment

The best way to assess issues in sexuality is to address them through direct and frank communication with the patient and/or partner. The process of acquiring information about sexual needs and function requires some careful consideration in light of the sensitivities around this subject:

1. Written assessment forms that are filled in by patients or health care providers seem ubiquitous in palliative care. However, they are not a good way to collect information about sexuality. Patients rarely want to write this information down and may be a little suspicious if they see a health care provider check off boxes or write down comments as the subject is discussed. This is not an appropriate situation for the use of visual analogue scales!
2. Privacy and confidentiality must be ensured both in discussions and in recording information in the medical record. It may be best to share limited information in the written medical record, especially if that information is sensitive (e.g., sexual preferences, sexual orientation, practices, dysfunction, or sexual abuse).

If one senses that patients are reluctant to discuss psychosocial issues, it may be wise to build up a relationship of trust before beginning to probe the area of sexuality. It may take several interviews before patients, particularly men, are willing to explore this area. The clinician should explore the patient's background, culture, and religion because the patient's beliefs may preclude the discussion of sexual function. It may be possible to learn culturally sensitive and appropriate methods to broach the subject from a spiritual leader in the community. The health care provider who is not confident in his or her own ability to take a history in this area should bring in someone who is knowledgeable and who can provide feedback on the process of obtaining information.

The health care provider should begin with open-ended questions in the third person such as the following:

"For many people with your condition, sexual function is an important part of the quality of life. Is this something you would be willing to discuss with me or another member of the team?"

"Many people who are ill have difficulty finding time alone with the ones closest to them. Have you been able to find time to be close and intimate with your partner? Is this something that would be important for you?"

"Sometimes people who have had this type of surgery find it difficult to be intimate with their partner. Is this something you would like to discuss? Can we talk about how things are going so far?"

If the patient gives a positive response, the health care provider can begin the process of obtaining a more detailed history of sexual function. A sexual history may include topics and questions such as the following:

- How important is sexual intimacy to the patient? To the partner?
- What are the partner's issues and attitudes?
- Has the patient experienced problems with sexual function in the past? Is the patient experiencing any current changes in pattern and abilities?
- Have the patient and partner discussed their feelings and changes in sexual function?
- Have they discussed or thought about any alternative ways to express intimacy?
- Are there any interfering or inhibiting issues?
- If there has been dysfunction, what has been tried?
- Can the patient provide details on previous sexual dysfunction and causes, if known?
- What are the patient's perceived wishes in this area of sexuality?

At some point, if the patient consents, it is important to take information from the partner.

Counseling

The PLISSIT model of sexual counseling presents an easily remembered framework for addressing the needs of a patient and his or her partner.[11] Box 14-1 details the model and possibilities for counseling the palliative care patient.

Surgical Techniques

In recent years, modification of certain surgical procedures (particularly pelvic surgery) has led to better preservation of sexual function. For men with prostate cancer, nerve sparing at the time of complete prostatectomy has led to less impotence.[13] Similar results have been seen in nerve-sparing cystectomy.[14] Preservation of the neurovascular bundles has retained clitoral arousal and has preserved better sexual function in women who have undergone pelvic surgery for cancer.[15] These techniques are not infallible, however, and sexual dysfunction may still occur.

Other Interventions

TREATMENTS FOR MALE IMPOTENCE

Multiple forms of treatment for male impotence now exist. These include vacuum constriction devices, intracorporeal injections, intraurethral alprostadil, and oral medications (sildenafil and others). Vacuum constriction devices are effective for impotence that results from many different etiologies. Success rates vary from 60%

Box 14-1. *PLISSIT Model of Sexual Counseling*

PERMISSION

Get permission for determining the patient's or couple's interest in discussing sexual intimacy and permission to ask questions and discuss the issues openly without fear of being judged in any way.

Transmit a perception of the normalcy of sexual needs even at the end of life.

First, determine the patient's or couple's interest in talking about sexual intimacy. Get permission to ask questions, and encourage an open discussion of issues of sexuality without fear of being judged.

Reassure the patient or couple regarding the normalcy of sexual needs even at the end of life.

LIMITED INFORMATION

Describe how the specific illness and its treatment may limit sexual activity, and offer ideas for adapting or facilitating sexual activity.

Discuss the impact of illness on self-image and self-esteem, and emphasize the need to be honest with each other.

Provide an opportunity to educate the patient and partner about sexuality and other possibilities for intimacy if intercourse is not possible. Discuss the importance of touching and fondling.

Issues around safe sex need to be addressed, particularly in light of potential serious infections such as human immunodeficiency virus.

Offer to provide names of specific health care providers for more detailed discussion. Recommend available literature.

SPECIFIC SUGGESTIONS

Specific suggestions may include pacing activity to accommodate tolerance, positions that facilitate comfort, and medications that may enhance comfort or sexual performance.[12]

Intimacy can be achieved through cuddling, fondling, and kissing if intercourse is not physically possible or if there is too much pain.

Privacy can be requested, even in institutions.

Specific suggestions for aids and medications can be given.

INTENSIVE THERAPY

This is rarely appropriate for patients close to the end of life. However, it may be relevant early in the course of the illness.

It may be necessary to refer partners with major problems to qualified sexual counselors before or after the patient's death.

In addition, sexual practices that seem quite "abnormal" may require consultation with sexual counseling experts.

to 80%, with the majority able to achieve vaginal penetration and intercourse. Compliance does tend to decrease with time, and the device can be somewhat difficult to use.

Intracorporeal injections have the advantage of bypassing neural pathways and are thus effective in patients who have nerve damage or a vascular cause of erectile dysfunction. Papaverine, phentolamine, and alprostadil are each individually effective, but combinations tend to work better and can decrease the side effects. A commercial preparation of all three drugs known as Tri-mix is available. Although intracorporeal injections can be highly effective (85%), many men discontinue their use because of pain, penile fibrosis, corporal plaque, or unsatisfactory erections.

Intraurethral prostaglandin places a pellet of alprostadil into the urethra that is subsequently absorbed by the corpus cavernosa. Low success rates, coupled with local discomfort, significantly limit the usability of this therapy, but it remains one viable option for some patients.

Oral phosphodiesterase-5 inhibitors have recently become the treatment of choice for most cases of erectile dysfunction. Three drugs are now commercially available: sildenafil, vardenafil, and tadalafil. Phosphodiesterase-5 inhibitors work by increasing intracavernosal cyclic guanosine monophosphate levels, thereby restoring erectile function. These drugs should be used with caution or not at all in patients with cardiac disease or hypotension, in men who are using nitrates, or in patients who are concurrently taking CYP 3A4–inducing drugs such as rifampin and phenytoin. Although all three drugs are effective in men after radical prostatectomy, side effects can vary; a randomized trial[16] showed that 60% of men chose a drug based on side effects, but only 40% chose a drug based on efficacy.

FEMALE SEXUAL DYSFUNCTION

Early intervention and education can be very helpful for women who undergo therapy for pelvic cancer. Early education in sexual rehabilitation can decrease the negative impact of gynecologic operations.[17] Newer, nerve-sparing operations (analogous to those in prostate operations) may help to decrease female sexual side effects further. Otherwise, current treatment options for improving female sexual function after cancer therapy are limited by a lack of systematic studies and concerns about side effects of certain treatments.

Hormonal therapy is often contraindicated in many women with breast or other hormonally sensitive tumors. Estrogens can improve clitoral and vaginal sensitivity, lubrication, and sexual desire.[18] Androgens can also improve sexual arousal and clitoral sensitivity,[19] but many women do not tolerate the masculinizing side effects. Randomized, controlled trials of testosterone therapy have been done in postmenopausal women with decreased libido. These trials showed that the use of testosterone increased libido, but all trials excluded women with cancer, and all trials maintained women on estrogen replacement therapy.[20,21] A randomized, placebo-controlled trial of testosterone alone, without concomitant estrogen therapy, in 132 women with a history of breast cancer and diminished libido showed that, contrary to the previously noted trials in postmenopausal women, there was no effect of testosterone on libido in these women.[22] Thus, it may be that testosterone alone is insufficient to improve libido, and because estrogen replacement therapy may be contraindicated in women with certain cancer types, this strategy may not be beneficial.

Phosphodiesterase-5 inhibitors are being studied in female sexual function, but their exact role remains undefined at this time. Early data suggest that these agents do improve clitoral sensation and vaginal lubrication.[23] If lubrication is an issue, the use of vaginal lubricants is indicated.

ENVIRONMENTAL CHANGES

Institutions should allow conjugal visits and should provide double beds if necessary. "Do Not Disturb" signs on doors to bedrooms at home or in institutions may be needed. The staff should be educated about the sexual needs of patients.

Condoms should be provided. Institutions and community agencies should try to provide cosmetic and hair styling opportunities for patients who feel physically unattractive. It may be possible to obtain these services through volunteers.

PEARLS
Sexuality is important to patients and their partners at the end of life.
Patients expect physicians to address sexuality.
Discussions of sexuality must be sensitive and culturally appropriate.
The PLISSIT model of sexual counseling is an easy and effective way to initiate counseling.
Sexuality can be expressed in ways other than intercourse.
Education of other health care providers about patients' sexual needs is advised.
Specific interventions are possible for male and female sexual dysfunction.

PITFALLS
Ignoring sexual needs of patients may enhance their suffering.
Not providing privacy for patients and partners can add to sexual dysfunction.
Lack of education in taking a sexual history increases physicians' distress and decreases the likelihood that the topic will be addressed.

Summary

Sexuality in palliative care patients is an issue that needs to be raised with sensitivity, approached in a matter-of-fact manner without being judgmental, and attended to with the goal of optimizing quality of life for patients and their families. Methods that include counseling, medical, and technical techniques, as well as environmental arrangements, can provide effective intervention. Policies and procedures must be developed in chronic care facilities that will allow patients to express their sexuality in a private and safe environment to maximize quality of life at the end of life.

Resources

About.Com Health and Fitness Section
    Available at sexuality.about.com/od/seniorsexuality
Sexual Information and Education Council of Canada
    Available at www.sieccan.org
Sexual Information and Education Council of the United States
    Available at www.siecus.org
Shibley Hyde JS, DeLamater J: *Understanding Human Sexuality*, 8th ed. New York, 2003, McGraw-Hill.
Society for Human Sexuality
    Available at www.sexuality.org

References

1. Waterhouse J: Nursing practice related to sexuality: a review and recommendations, *NTRes* 1:412–418, 1996.
2. Kirby R, Watson A, Newling D: Prostate cancer and sexual functioning, *Prostate Cancer Prostatic Dis* 1:179–184, 1998.

3. Ananth H, Jones L, King M, Tookman A: The impact of cancer on sexual function: a controlled study, *Palliat Med* 17:202–205, 2003.
4. Lemieux L, Kaiser S, Pereira J, Meadows LM: Sexuality in palliative care: patient perspectives, *Palliat Med* 18:630–637, 2004.
5. Richardson JP: Sexuality in the nursing home patient, *Am Fam Physician* 51:121–124, 1995.
6. Katz A: The sounds of silence: sexuality information for cancer patients, *J Clin Oncol* 23:238–241, 2005.
7. Matchota L, Waterhouse J: Current nursing practice related to sexuality, *Res Nurs Health* 16:371–378, 1993.
8. Kirby R, Watson A, Newling D: Prostate cancer and sexual functioning, *Prostate Cancer Prostatic Dis* 1:179–184, 1998.
9. Matchota L, Waterhouse J: Current nursing practice related to sexuality, *Res Nurs Health* 16:371–378, 1993.
10. Bauer M: Their only privacy is between their sheets: privacy and the sexuality of elderly nursing home residents, *J Gerontol Nurs* 25:37–41, 1999.
11. Annon J: The PLISSIT model: a proposed conceptual scheme for the behavioral treatment of sexual problems, *J Sex Educ Ther* 2:1–15, 1976.
12. Stausmire JM: Sexuality at the end of life, *Am J Hosp Palliat Care* 2:33–39, 2004.
13. Walsh PC, Marschke P, Ricker D, Burnett AL: Patient-reported urinary continence and sexual function after anatomic radical prostatectomy, *Urology* 55:58–61, 2000.
14. Vallancien G, Abou El Fettouh H, Cathelineau X, et al: Cystectomy with prostate sparing for bladder cancer in 100 patients: 10-year experience, *J Urol* 168:2413–2417, 2002.
15. Stenzl A, Colleselli K, Poisel S, et al: Anterior exenteration with subsequent ureteroileal urethrostomy in females: anatomy, risk of urethral recurrence, surgical technique, and results, *Eur Urol* 33(Suppl 4):18–20, 1998.
16. Nandipati KC, Raina R, Agarwal A, Zippe CD: Efficacy and treatment satisfaction of PDE-5 inhibitors in management of erectile dysfunction following radical prostatectomy: SHIM analysis. In 30th Annual Meeting of the American Society of Andrology. Seattle, American Society of Andrology, 2005, abstract 99.
17. Capone M, Good R, Westie K, et al: Psychosocial rehabilitation of the gynaecologic oncology patients, *Arch Phys Med Rehabil* 61:128–132, 1980.
18. Collins A, Landgren BM: Reproductive health, use of estrogen and experience of symptoms in peri-menopausal women: a population-based study, *Maturitas* 20:101–111, 1994.
19. Basson R: Female sexual response: the role of drugs in the management of sexual dysfunction, *Obstet Gynecol* 98:350–353, 2001.
20. Buster JE, Kingsberg SA, Aguirre O, et al: Testosterone patch for low sexual desire in surgically meno-pausal women: a randomized trial, *Obstet Gynecol* 105:938–940, 2005.
21. Braunstein GD, Sundwall DA, Katz M, et al: Safety and efficacy of a testosterone patch for the treatment of hypoactive sexual desire disorder in surgically menopausal women: a randomized, placebo-controlled trial, *Arch Intern Med* 165:1582–1589, 2005.
22. Barton DL, Loprinzi CL, Wender D, et al: Transdermal testosterone in female cancer survivors with decreased libido: NCCTG N02C3. In *Proceedings of the American Society of Clinical Oncology*. Alexandria, VA, 2006, p. 8507.
23. Kaplan SA, Reis RB, Kohn IJ, et al: Safety and efficacy of sildenafil in postmenopausal women with sexual dysfunction, *Urology* 53:481–486, 1999.

CHAPTER 15

Dyspnea

CORINNE D. SCHRODER and DEBORAH J. DUDGEON

Dyspnea, an uncomfortable awareness of breathing, is a common symptom in people with advanced disease who are approaching the end of life. The presence of dyspnea is associated with significant functional and social limitations and psychological distress that impair quality of life and contribute to suffering. Good palliative care requires knowledge and skill in the management of dyspnea.

Definition

Dyspnea has been defined by the American Thoracic Society as "a subjective experience of breathing discomfort that consists of qualitatively distinct sensations that vary in intensity".[1] This subjective experience of dyspnea, like pain, involves many factors that modulate both the quality and the intensity of its perception. Distinct sensations of breathing are produced by stimulation of various neurophysiologic pathways, the conscious perception of the stimuli, and interpretation of the stimuli in the context of lifelong previous experience and learning (Figure 15-1).

Prevalence and Impact

The prevalence of dyspnea varies depending on the stage and type of underlying disease. In a general outpatient population of patients with cancer, approximately 50% of patients describe some dyspnea,[2] and the prevalence rises to 70% in the terminal phases of cancer.[3] Dyspnea is more common in patients with lung cancer, approaching 90% just before death.[4] A systematic review reporting studies of the prevalence of dyspnea in patients with chronic and progressive conditions noted ranges of 90% to 95% in those with chronic obstructive pulmonary disease (COPD),

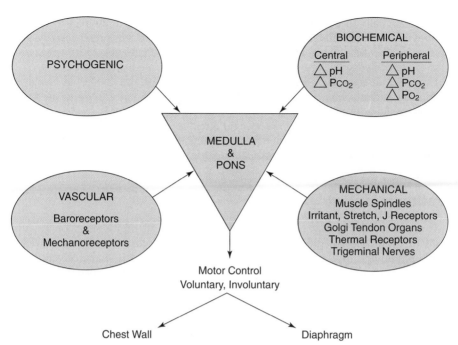

Figure 15-1. The psychogenic, vascular, biochemical, and mechanical pathways of breathing. Distinct sensations of breathing are produced by stimulation of various neurophysiologic pathways, the conscious perception of the stimuli, and interpretation of the stimuli in the context of lifelong previous experience and learning.

10% to 70% in cancer patients, 60% to 88% in patients with heart disease, 11% to 62% in those with renal disease, and 11% to 62% in patients with acquired immunodeficiency syndrome (AIDS).[5] Patients with end-stage COPD[6] and those with incurable lung cancer[7] have reported difficulties in breathing as their most distressing symptom. Dyspnea is often present for prolonged periods, frequently exceeding 3 months in patients with late-stage cancer,[8] thus compounding suffering.

Patients with advanced disease typically experience chronic shortness of breath with intermittent acute episodes. The acute attacks of breathlessness frequently contribute to feelings of anxiety, fear, and panic for both the patient and family members and, when severe enough, a sensation of impending death for the patient. Dyspnea severely impairs quality of life by limiting functional ability and interfering with mood, relationships, and enjoyment of life. In a study of patients living with end-stage COPD, 98% were unable to perform strenuous activities, 87% were unable to take a short walk around the house, and 57% required help with washing, dressing, and reaching the toilet.[6] In patients with advanced cancer, dyspnea was intensified with climbing stairs (95.6%), walking slowly (47.8%), getting dressed (52.2%), and talking or eating (56.5%); approximately 26% of the patients were dyspneic even at rest.[8] Patients universally respond by decreasing their activity to whatever degree relieves the breathlessness. Patients also socially isolate themselves from friends and outside contacts to cope with dyspnea.[6] As a result, depression, fatigue, generalized dissatisfaction with life, and a high degree of emotional distress are very common.

In terminally ill patients with cancer, as death approached, the will to live was found to be directly related to the severity of breathlessness.[9] The presence of dyspnea prompted the use of terminal sedation in 25% to 53% of patients requiring sedation for uncontrolled symptoms.[10] Dyspnea has been associated with increased severity of spiritual distress and weakness in patients, and with more distress in caregivers and staff. Patients who experience breathlessness are also more likely to die in the hospital than at home.

Unfortunately, patients often receive no direct medical or nursing assistance with dyspnea and are left to cope with this debilitating symptom in isolation.[8] They need health care providers who will anticipate their fears and provide symptomatic relief of their breathlessness and anxiety as death approaches.

Pathophysiology

Management of dyspnea requires an understanding of its multidimensional nature and the pathophysiologic mechanisms that cause this distressing symptom. The pathophysiologic mechanisms of dyspnea can be categorized as increased ventilatory demand, impaired mechanical responses, or a combination of these two mechanisms. The effects of abnormalities of these mechanisms can also be additive.

INCREASED VENTILATORY DEMAND

Ventilatory demand is increased because of increased physiologic dead space resulting from reduction in the vascular bed, hypoxemia and severe deconditioning with early metabolic acidosis (with excessive hydrogen ion stimulation), alterations in carbon dioxide output (Vco_2) or in the arterial partial pressure of carbon dioxide (Pco_2) set point, and nonmetabolic sources such as increased neural reflex activity or psychological factors such as anxiety and depression.

IMPAIRED VENTILATION

Impaired mechanical responses result in restrictive and obstructive ventilatory deficits. A *restrictive ventilatory defect* is caused by decreased distensibility of the lung parenchyma, pleura, or chest wall (parenchymal disease or reduced chest compliance) or by a reduction in the maximum force exerted by the respiratory muscles (muscle weakness). An *obstructive ventilatory deficit* refers to impedance of the flow of air. Both structural changes (external compression or internal obstruction) and functional changes (bronchoconstriction) can lead to progressive narrowing of the airways. Patients may also have a mixed restrictive and obstructive disorder. Box 15-1 outlines the pathophysiologic mechanisms of dyspnea with potential clinical causes in persons with advanced cancer and other end-stage diseases.

SPECIAL END-OF-LIFE CONSIDERATIONS

Asthenia and generalized muscle weakness are common in patients with advanced COPD and other end-stage diseases. Exercise capacity is limited by abnormalities in either endurance or weakness of the skeletal muscles in patients with chronic heart failure, COPD, and cancer.[11] Both peripheral muscle and respiratory muscle strength are reduced in patients with cardiorespiratory diseases and cancer, and muscle strength is a significant contributor to the intensity of exercise-induced dyspnea.[11] Patients with chronic heart failure have abnormal skeletal muscle metabolism during

Box 15-1. *Pathophysiologic Mechanisms and Clinical Causes of Dyspnea in Patients with End-Stage Disease*

INCREASED VENTILATORY DEMAND

Increased physiologic dead space
- Thromboemboli
- Tumor emboli
- Vascular obstruction
- Radiation therapy
- Chemotherapy
- Emphysema

Severe deconditioning
Hypoxemia
- Anemia

Change in Vco_2 or $Paco_2$ set point
Increased neural reflex activity
Psychological factors
- Anxiety
- Depression

IMPAIRED VENTILATION

Restrictive ventilatory deficit

Pleural or parenchymal disease
- Primary or metastatic cancer
- Pleural effusion
- Pulmonary fibrosis
- Congestive heart failure
- Pneumonia

Reduced movement of diaphragm
- Ascites
- Hepatomegaly

Reduced chest wall compliance
- Pain
- Hilar/mediastinal involvement
- Chest wall invasion with tumor
- Deconditioning
- Neuromuscular factors
- Neurohumoral factors

Respiratory muscle weakness
- Phrenic nerve paralysis
- Cachexia
- Electrolyte abnormalities
- Steroid use
- Deconditioning
- Asthenia
- Neuromuscular factors
- Paraneoplastic conditions

Continued

> **Box 15-1.** *Pathophysiologic Mechanisms and Clinical Causes of Dyspnea in Patients with End-Stage Disease—cont'd*
>
> ### Obstructive ventilatory deficit
> External or internal
> * Primary or metastatic cancer
>   Functional
> * Asthma
> * Chronic obstructive pulmonary disease
>
> ### MIXED OBSTRUCTIVE/RESTRICTIVE DISEASE
> Any combination of factors

exercise and significant ultrastructural skeletal muscle abnormalities that affect both the respiratory and the peripheral muscles.[11]

Cachexia is a common final presentation of several chronic conditions, including cancer, COPD, chronic heart failure, acquired immunodeficiency syndrome, and renal failure.[11] Cachexia differs from simple nutritional imbalance because there are modifications in the metabolism of proteins, lipids, and carbohydrates, with a preferential loss of muscle tissue over fat, enhanced protein degradation, and unresponsiveness to nutritional interventions. Weakness of both respiratory and peripheral muscles can result from impaired nutritional status.[11]

Neurologic paraneoplastic syndromes can contribute to the development of dyspnea in patients with cancer. Thirty percent of patients with malignant thymoma have myasthenia gravis that can weaken respiratory muscles and cause respiratory failure.[11] Eaton-Lambert syndrome, associated with lung, rectal, kidney, breast, stomach, skin, and thymus cancers, can also produce respiratory muscle weakness and result in dyspnea.[11]

For patients with advanced cancer and other end-stage diseases, there is an interrelationship between psychological factors and dyspnea. Breathlessness may evoke anxiety or fear, and emotions may contribute to dyspnea either by increasing respiratory drive or altering the perceptions of breathlessness. Anxiety, depression, fatigue, and psychological ability to cope with disease have been noted as predictors of dyspnea in patients with advanced lung cancer.[12] In general, anxious, obsessive, depressed, and dependent persons appear to experience dyspnea that is disproportionately severe relative to the extent of the pulmonary disease.

Multidimensional Assessment

PATIENT REPORTS

Because dyspnea is a subjective experience, the key to assessment is the patient's report of breathlessness through the use of unidimensional instruments and descriptions related to its effect on level of activity. Individuals with comparable degrees of functional lung impairment may experience considerable differences in how they perceive the intensity of dyspnea. Factors such as adaptation, differing physical characteristics, and psychological conditions can modulate both the quality and the intensity of the person's perception of breathlessness. Therefore, medical personnel must ask for and accept the patient's assessment, often without measurable physical correlates.

To determine the presence of dyspnea, it is important to ask more than "Are you short of breath?" Patients often respond in the negative to this simple question either because the activity that they are performing at that moment is not causing dyspnea or because they have limited their physical activity to ensure that they do not experience breathlessness. It is therefore important to ask about shortness of breath in relation to specific activities (e.g., walking at the same speed as someone else of your age, walking upstairs, or eating).

QUALITATIVE ASPECTS OF DYSPNEA

Dyspnea is also not a single sensation. Clinical investigations suggest that the sensation of breathlessness encompasses several qualities that may, as in the assessment of pain, allow discrimination among the various causes. For example, in assessing pain, descriptors such as "burning" or "shooting" suggest a neuropathic etiology. Similarly, the descriptor "My chest feels tight" has been associated with asthma and "My breathing requires effort/work" with lymphangitic carcinomatosis.[13] Although studies have noted association of specific sets of descriptor clusters with different pathologies, there is significant overlap across chronic medical conditions and a lack of consistency within medical conditions.[14] Research to date does not support the use of descriptors as a tool for delineating differential diagnosis or targeting treatment, but the language used by breathless patients may provide another dimension to understand and evaluate their experience.[14]

CLINICAL ASSESSMENT

Clinical assessment of dyspnea includes the patient's report and history of the symptom and a focused physical examination. The assessment directs management and provides a baseline on which to evaluate the patient's response to treatment. Table 15-1 outlines a general approach to the clinical assessment of dyspnea in palliative care patients.

The history includes the temporal onset (acute or chronic), pattern, severity and qualities of dyspnea, associated symptoms, precipitating and relieving events or activities, and response to medications. A history of smoking, underlying lung or cardiac disease, concurrent medical conditions, allergy history, and details of previous medications or treatments should be elicited. The physical, social, and emotional impact of dyspnea on the patient and family members and the coping strategies used are also important components of the history. The use of unidimensional or multidimensional tools to measure the quality and severity of dyspnea and its effect on functional ability can assist in assessment and monitoring the effects of treatment.

The Visual Analog Scale (VAS) is commonly used to measure perceived intensity of the dyspnea. This scale is usually a 100-mm vertical or horizontal line, anchored at either end with words such as "not at all breathless" and "very breathless".[15] Patients are asked to mark the line at the point that best describes the intensity of their breathlessness. The Edmonton Symptom Assessment Scale (ESAS) can also be used to measure perceived intensity of dyspnea. It uses a numeric 0 to 10 scale where 0 means no breathlessness and 10 means the worst possible breathlessness. Patients are asked to indicate the number that corresponds to their present intensity of breathlessness. The Modified Borg Scale (mBORG) has a 0 to 10 scale with nonlinear spacing of verbal descriptors of severity of breathlessness.[15] Patients are asked to pick

Table 15-1. Clinical Assessment of Dyspnea in Palliative Care Patients

Patient report	• Presence in relationship to daily activities • Qualities/descriptors • Severity (use clinical tools)
History	• Temporal onset: chronic/acute • Pattern (e.g., acute exacerbations) • Precipitating factors (e.g., activities, pets, scents, smoking, anxiety) • Relieving factors (e.g., positioning, medication) • Associated symptoms (e.g., pain) • History underlying /concurrent conditions • Smoking history • Allergy history • Medication use and effect: prescribed, over the counter • Other treatment use and effect (e.g., oxygen, complementary, continuous positive airway pressure, bilevel positive airway pressure) • Impact: emotional, sleep, activities • Coping strategies
Physical examination	• Vital signs • Cyanosis, skin tone and color • Use of accessory muscles, pursed lips, ability to speak • Positioning (e.g., bed, chair, seated leaning forward) • Chest auscultation • Specific system examination based on history • Cognitive assessment: mood, affect, ability to concentrate and solve problems • Behavioral changes (e.g., agitation, restlessness)
Diagnostic tests*	• Chest radiograph • Electrocardiogram • Pulmonary function tests • Oxygen saturation • Arterial blood gases • Complete blood cell count • Biochemistry (e.g., potassium, magnesium, phosphate) • Other specific tests (e.g., echocardiography, computed tomography angiogram)

*Appropriate to stage of disease, prognosis, risk-to-benefit ratio, and the wishes of the patient and family.

the verbal descriptor that best represents their perceived exertion. Conceived as a ratio scale (e.g., 4 is twice as severe as 2), the mBORG has theoretical advantages over numeric rating scales.

The Oxygen Cost Diagram is a visual analog scale that consists of a 100-mm vertical line used to measure the functional impact of breathlessness.[15] Everyday activities such as walking, shopping, and bed-making are listed in proportion to their oxygen cost. Patients are asked to identify the level of activity that they cannot perform because it causes too much breathlessness. As dyspnea worsens, the score decreases. The Cancer Dyspnea Scale (CDS) is a 12-item questionnaire addressing sensations of effort (5 items), anxiety (4 items), and discomfort (3 items).[15] Patients rate the severity of each item from 1 (not at all) to 5 (very much). It requires more time and effort to complete but can provide an understanding of the quality of breathlessness.

The physical examination should be performed with focus on possible underlying causes of dyspnea and the details obtained from the history. Particular attention should be directed at signs linked with certain clinical syndromes associated with common causes of dyspnea in people who have the patient's particular underlying disease. For example, dullness to percussion, decreased tactile fremitus, and absent breath sounds are associated with pleural effusion in a person with lung cancer; elevated jugular venous pressure, an audible third heart sound, and bilateral crackles audible on chest examination are associated with congestive heart failure.

Accessory muscle use has been suggested as a physical finding that may reflect the intensity of dyspnea. Patients with COPD who were experiencing high levels of dyspnea were found to have significant differences in the use of accessory muscles as compared with patients with low levels of dyspnea, although there were no significant differences in respiratory rate, depth of respiration, or peak expiratory flow rates.[16]

The choice of appropriate diagnostic tests should be guided by the stage of the disease, the prognosis, the risk-to-benefit ratios of any proposed tests or interventions, and the desire of the patient and family. If the person is actively dying or wants no further investigations or invasive or disease-oriented interventions, it is appropriate to palliate the symptom without further testing. If, however, the patient is at an earlier phase of illness, diagnostic tests helpful in determining the origin of dyspnea could include chest radiography; electrocardiography; pulmonary function tests; arterial blood gases; complete blood cell count; serum potassium, magnesium, and phosphate levels; cardiopulmonary exercise testing; and tests specific for underlying pathologic conditions (e.g., computed tomography angiogram for pulmonary embolism).

Management

The optimal management of dyspnea is to treat the underlying disease and any reversible causes. For persons with advanced disease, this is often no longer possible or desirable, and palliation becomes the goal. As with choosing appropriate diagnostic tests, the choice of treating or not treating a particular underlying cause of breathlessness should be guided by the stage of disease, the prognosis, the burden and benefit to the patient, and the desire of the patient and family. Both nonpharmacologic and pharmacologic interventions can be helpful in alleviating breathlessness without addressing the underlying cause, and, whenever possible, a team approach to management should be utilized. Social services, nursing, and family input will need to be increased as the patient's ability to care for himself or herself decreases.

Box 15-2 and Tables 15-2 and 15-3 provide guidelines for the management of dyspnea in palliative care patients. In applying the guidelines, clinical judgment should be used to determine the appropriateness for a specific patient.

Table 15-2. Management of Dyspnea in Palliative Care Patients

Activity	• Plan for and pace activities
	• Encourage rest periods as needed
	• Assistance with feeding, hygiene, toileting, and ambulation as needed
	• Use assistive devices as needed (e.g., wheelchair, walker)
Environment	• Provide a calm, clean, and orderly environment
	• Avoid triggers (e.g., perfume, flowers, pets)
	• Caution against smoking in patient's room/house
	• Check with patient about opening of windows, curtains, doors
	• Have essential supplies available at all times (e.g., medications, oxygen if needed)
	• Have resource/contact numbers readily available
	• Encourage short visits from people other than immediate family and caregivers
Patient/family education	• Educate/inform regarding progression of symptoms and disease
	• Inform about signs and symptoms requiring medical assistance
	• Identify and address patient/family fear and anxiety
	• Ensure patient/family at home have resource and contact numbers and an emergency plan in place
	• Provide information on medications and oxygen therapy
	• Inform about importance of remaining calm
	• Teach coping techniques (e.g., positioning, fan, relaxation)
	• Identify triggers, control environmental irritants, smoking, pets
Treatment	• Treat underlying conditions and reversible causes considering stage of disease, risk-to-benefit to patient, patient/family wishes
	• Use fan or open window, door
	• Use positioning techniques (e.g., reclining chair with foot rest, over-bed table, pillows)
	• Use breathing strategies (e.g., pursed-lip breathing)
	• Use complementary therapies (e.g., acupuncture, imagery, massage, music, relaxation techniques)
Medications	• See Table 15-3

NONPHARMACOLOGIC INTERVENTIONS

Although evidence to recommend specific nonpharmacologic interventions for relief of dyspnea in patients with advanced malignant and nonmalignant disease is limited, until studies with sufficient sample size and power calculations are conducted, a number of single and multiple component strategies have been found of benefit.

Patients can obtain relief of dyspnea with positioning techniques such as leaning forward while sitting and supporting the upper body and arms on a table. This position has demonstrated efficacy in patients with emphysema, probably because of increased efficiency of the diaphragm resulting from an improved length-tension state.[17]

Breathing strategies such as pursed-lip or diaphragmatic breathing are beneficial in the management of acute shortness of breath.[17] Pursed-lip breathing slows the respiratory rate and increases intra-airway pressures, thus decreasing small airway collapse during periods of increased dyspnea.

Box 15-2. *Dyspnea Management Guidelines for Palliative Care Patients**

GENERAL CONSIDERATIONS

- Assess dyspnea using patient reports, standardized tools, and focused physical examination.
- Identify and treat common exacerbating medical conditions underlying dyspnea (e.g., COPD, congestive heart failure, pneumonia) as appropriate.
- Implement nonpharmacologic interventions (e.g., fan, positioning techniques, breathing strategies) as appropriate, and provide patient/family education and support.
- Initiate pharmacologic interventions as suggested in Treatment section of this table.
- Use the Edmonton Symptom Assessment Scale (ESAS) to choose treatment options and measure outcome.

OXYGEN

Hypoxemic patients (O_2 saturation $\leq$ 88% at rest or on exertion):

- Start humidified supplemental oxygen by nasal prongs either continuously or on an as-needed basis (flow rates 1–7 L/min) to maintain oxygen saturation > 90%. Continue if effective and tolerated.
- If dyspnea and low oxygen saturation persist despite maximum tolerated flow of humidified oxygen, consider a trial of supplemental oxygen by oxymizer (nasal cannulae with reservoir), ventimask or non-rebreathing mask, or face tent. If not tolerated, the patient can return to the best tolerated flow of humidified oxygen by nasal prong or discontinue supplemental oxygen.

Nonhypoxemic patient (O_2 saturation > 88%):

- If a fan or humidified ambient air via nasal prongs (if available) are not effective or tolerated, consider a trial of supplemental oxygen via nasal prong. Assess benefits and discontinue if not effective in relieving dyspnea.

*These are meant as guidelines. Clinicians need to use their own clinical judgment regarding the appropriateness of the intervention in an individual patient.

People who are short of breath often obtain relief by sitting near an open window or in front of a fan. Cold directed against the cheek and through the nose can alter ventilation patterns and can reduce the perception of breathlessness, perhaps by affecting receptors in the distribution of the trigeminal nerve that are responsive to both thermal and mechanical stimuli.[17]

Planning for and pacing of activities, together with some reduction in level of activity, help to reduce the intensity of breathlessness. Walking aids such as wheeled walkers can help to reduce dyspnea. Some patients find that isolation from others helps them to gain control of their breathing and diminishes the social impact.[17] Other patients use structured relaxation techniques, conscious attempts to calm down, and prayer and meditation.[18] Avoidance of triggers and aggravating factors and self-adjustment of medication can also be beneficial.[17]

Nursing actions thought to be helpful include a friendly attitude, empathy, providing physical support, presence at the bedside, and providing information about the possible cause of the breathlessness and interventions.

Table 15-3. Dyspnea Management Guidelines for Palliative Care Patients

Level of Dyspnea	Treatment
Mild Dyspnea (ESAS 1–3) • Usually can sit and lie quietly • May be intermittent or persistent • Worsens with exertion • No anxiety or mild anxiety during shortness of breath • Breathing not observed as labored • No cyanosis	Consider a trial of systemic (oral or parenteral) opioids,[†] weighing potential risks and benefits, for patients with mild continuous dyspnea if nonpharmacologic interventions have not provided adequate relief. Discontinue if not effective in relieving dyspnea.
Moderate Dyspnea (ESAS 4–6) • Usually persistent • May be new or chronic • Shortness of breath worsens if walking or with exertion; settles partially with rest • Pauses while talking every 30 seconds • Breathing mildly labored	**Systemic Opioids** Opioid-naive patient: • Initiate immediate-release opioids (e.g., morphine 5 mg PO q4h regularly & 2.5 mg PO q2h prn for breakthrough *or* hydromorphone 1 mg PO q4h regularly & 0.5 mg PO q2h prn for breakthrough). If the subcutaneous route is needed, divide oral dose by half. Patient currently using opioids: • Increase the patient's regular dose by 25%, guided by the total breakthrough doses used in the previous 24 hours. • The breakthrough dose is 10% of the total 24-hour regular opioid dose, using the same opioid and route. Dose adjustment: • If dyspnea remains inadequately controlled, consider increasing the regular opioid dose every 24 hours when using immediate-release opioids and after 48 hours when using sustained-release opioids. • Increase the regular dose by 25% as guided by the total breakthrough doses used in the previous 24 hours. • Increase the breakthrough dose in accordance with the total 24-hour regular opioid dose. • Once the effective regular dose is determined, consider converting the regular opioid to an oral sustained-release formulation for patient convenience. • Monitor for opioid side effects (e.g., nausea, drowsiness, myoclonus); if significant, either consider a reduction in dose or switch to an alternative opioid and re-titrate. **Other Medications** • If patient has known or suspected COPD or lung involvement with cancer, consider a 5-day trial of corticosteroids, such as dexamethasone 8 mg or prednisone 50 mg per day. Discontinue if no obvious benefits are seen after 5 days. Add prophylactic gastric mucosal protection therapy if the corticosteroid is continued after the trial; monitor for side effects and manage appropriately.

Table 15-3. Dyspnea Management Guidelines for Palliative Care Patients (Continued)

Level of Dyspnea	Treatment
	• If opioids provide only a limited effect, consider a trial of phenothiazines, such as methotrimeprazine 2.5–10 mg PO/SC q6–8h or chlorpromazine 12.5–25 mg PO q4–6h regularly or as needed. Monitor for side effects and manage appropriately.
Severe Dyspnea (ESAS 7–10)	Refer to the Moderate Dyspnea section of this table, along with the following additional options.
• Often acute on chronic	***Systemic Opioids***
• Worsening over days/weeks	Opioid-naive patient:
• Anxiety present	• Give a subcutaneous bolus of morphine 2.5 mg or an equivalent dose of an alternative opioid. If tolerated, repeat every 30 minutes as needed. If tolerated but 2 doses fail to produce adequate relief, consider doubling the dose; monitor respiratory rate.
• Patient often wakes suddenly with shortness of breath	
• Cyanosis may or may not be present	• If intravenous access is available, consider giving a bolus of morphine 2.5 mg or an equivalent dose of an alternative opioid to achieve more rapid effect. If tolerated, repeat every 15 minutes as needed. If tolerated but 2 doses fail to produce adequate relief, consider doubling the dose; monitor respiratory rate.
• Confusion may or may not occur	
• Labored breathing present when awake and asleep	
• Patient pauses every 5–15 seconds while talking	• When patient's dyspnea has improved, start a regular dose of immediate-release opioid as outlined in the Moderate Dyspnea section, guided by the bolus doses used.
	Patient currently using opioids:
	• Give a subcutaneous bolus of the patient's current opioid using a dose equal to 10% of the regular 24-hour parenteral dose equivalent.
	• If intravenous access is available, consider giving a bolus of the patient's current opioid using a dose equal to 10% of the regular 24-hour parenteral dose equivalent.
	• Increase the regular dose by 25%, guided by the total breakthrough doses used.
	Other Medications
	• If the patient has significant anxiety, consider a trial of benzodiazepines (e.g., lorazepam 0.5–1 mg PO/IV/SC/SL or midazolam 0.5–1 mg SC/IV regularly or as needed; if the patient is currently on a higher dose of benzodiapzepine, dose accordingly). Monitor for paradoxical agitation and excessive drowsiness.
	If dyspnea remains unrelieved despite these approaches, request the assistance of a palliative care consultation team.

[†]For details, refer to Systemic Opioids in the Moderate Dyspnea section of this table.

IV, Intravenously; PO, by mouth; SC, subcutaneously; SL, sublingually.

Adapted with permission from © KFL&A Palliative Care Integration Project. Dyspnea Management Guidelines for Palliative Care. In Symptom Management Guidelines. Kingston, Ontario, Canada, 2003, pp. 41–46.

Patient and Family Education

The goals of patient and family education are maintenance of patient comfort and reduction of the frequency and severity of acute episodes. Health care providers should offer information and address questions and concerns regarding disease, expected progression of symptoms, and management plan. The patient and family should be taught how to identify and control environmental and psychological triggers, conserve energy, and prioritize activities. They should also be instructed to consider the use of a fan or open window. Medications should be reviewed to ensure that the patient and family understand their use and know how to maximize the effectiveness of the agents. The patient and family should be taught the signs and symptoms of an impending exacerbation and how to manage the situation. They should learn problem-solving techniques to prevent panic, positioning techniques, and breathing strategies. An emergency plan that details step-by-step interventions and lists contact numbers should be discussed.

Complementary Treatment

Acupuncture and acupressure have been found to relieve dyspnea in patients with moderate to severe COPD.[17] Acupuncture has also provided marked symptomatic benefit in patients with cancer-related breathlessness.[17] Patients with COPD noted a reduction in breathlessness when muscle relaxation was used with breathing retraining.[17] In patients with advanced lung cancer, a combined approach with breathing retraining, exercise counseling, relaxation, and coping and adaptation strategies significantly improved breathlessness and the ability to perform activities of daily living.[17] Guided imagery and therapeutic touch have resulted in significant improvements in quality of life and sense of well-being in patients with COPD and terminal cancer, respectively, without any significant improvement in breathlessness.[17]

Oxygen

Palliative oxygen for the management of breathlessness is commonly prescribed, although there is still no conclusive evidence as to whether all patients with advanced disease benefit from its use. Recent systematic reviews in patients with COPD concluded that short-term oxygen provided significant clinical improvement in dyspnea for patients with variable Pao_2 levels (52 to 85 mm Hg),[18] and supplemental continuous oxygen demonstrated clinically and statistically significant benefit in mildly hypoxemic (Pao_2 55 to 59 mm Hg) or nonhypoxemic (Pao_2 > 59 mm Hg) patients.[19] "Short burst" oxygen did not show a benefit in this patient population.[19] Supplemental oxygen was noted to provide neither a clinically or statistically significant improvement in dyspnea in patients with cancer and refractory dyspnea who would not normally qualify for home oxygen ($Pao_2 \geq 55$ mm Hg).[20] Data to support the use of oxygen for symptom relief are growing, but larger trials are needed to conclusively answer the question as to the role of oxygen in palliation of dyspnea. In the interim, a trial of oxygen, monitoring its effects on dyspnea, could be considered based on goals of care, cost, and the psychological and social effect on the patient and family.

Noninvasive Ventilation

Noninvasive ventilation (NIV) uses a mask or other device to provide intermittent ventilatory support through the patient's upper airway without an endotracheal or tracheostomy tube. It includes ventilator modalities such as bilevel positive airway pressure (BiPAP) and continuous positive airway pressure (CPAP). Unlike invasive ventilation, NIV allows patients to eat and drink, to communicate verbally, and to maintain some mobility. Studies, predominantly in patients with COPD and congestive heart failure, have shown that NIV reduces the need for intubation, decreases in-hospital mortality, and improves arterial blood gases, respiratory rate, and dyspnea. As such, it has become an integral tool in the management of both acute and chronic respiratory failure, but its role in terminal breathlessness is unclear. NIV may be appropriate in the management of dyspneic patients with end-stage disease to provide time to clarify the diagnosis or response to treatment, to enable patients to get well enough to return home, or to give patients and families extra time to come to terms with dying and achieve "closure."

PHARMACOLOGIC INTERVENTIONS

Opioids

Opioids remain the class of medications with the best level of evidence of benefit in refractory breathlessness. A Cochrane review that focused on opioids for palliation of breathlessness in terminal illness reported statistically strong evidence for the use of oral and parenteral opioids but no support for the use of nebulized opioids because they appeared no more effective than nebulized saline for the relief of breathlessness.[21] These recommendations were supported in a recent systematic review of the management of dyspnea in cancer patients.[22] The proposed mechanisms for the effect of opioids on dyspnea include an alteration in the perception of breathlessness, a decrease in the ventilatory drive and response to stimuli such as hypoxemia and hypercapnia, and a decrease in oxygen consumption at any level of exercise. Some health care professionals fear that the respiratory depressant effects of opioids will induce respiratory failure and hasten death. However, of the 11 studies identified that contained information on oxygen saturation or blood gases after intervention with systemic opioids, none noted a significant effect on oxygen saturation, and in the 3 studies reporting statistically significant effects in respiratory rate and carbon dioxide levels, differences were clinically small.[22] Development of clinically significant hypoventilation and respiratory depression with opioid therapy appears to depend on the history of previous exposure to opioids, on the rate of change of the opioid dose, and possibly on the route of administration. The early use of opioids can improve quality of life and can allow the use of lower doses while tolerance to the respiratory depressant effects develops. It has also been suggested that early use of morphine or another opioid, rather than hastening death in dyspneic patients, may actually prolong survival by reducing physical and psychological distress and exhaustion.

Opioids for dyspnea are given in doses similar to those used for pain relief. Patients should be started on an oral immediate-release formulation on a regular basis, with breakthrough doses as needed. Titrate the dose upward according to need. Once dyspnea is well controlled on a stable dose, a sustained-release opioid formulation can be substituted, with an immediate-release opioid maintained for breakthrough distress. Systemic adverse effects of opioid use, such as constipation, drowsiness, and nausea and vomiting, should be anticipated and managed expectantly.

Anxiolytics and Phenothiazines

Current evidence supports the use of oral promethazine, alone or in combination with systemic opioids, as a second-line agent for dyspnea.[22] There are no comparative trials available to recommend or not recommend the use of chlorpromazine and methotrimeprazine, but a trial of either may be considered in a patient with persistent dyspnea despite other therapies. For patients who have difficulty taking oral medication, methotrimeprazine can be given subcutaneously.

Although anxiolytics, such as diazepam and midazolam, potentially relieve dyspnea by reducing hypoxemic or hypercapnic ventilatory responses as well as altering the emotional response to dyspnea, studies to date have failed to demonstrate consistent improvement in dyspnea.[22] Their widespread use for the management of breathlessness is not recommended. However, in patients with excessive anxiety in addition to breathlessness, a trial of anxiolytic therapy may be warranted. Preliminary reports with buspirone, a serotonin agonist and nonbenzodiazepine anxiolytic, and sertraline, a selective serotonin reuptake inhibitor, postulate improvement in dyspnea through serotonergic modulation of breathing and its sensation.[23] Further research may determine whether anxiolytics help to relieve dyspnea in patients who are not experiencing significant anxiety.

Other Medications

The use of systemic corticosteroids may benefit patients with COPD or other underlying causes of dyspnea by decreasing airway inflammation and edema, but to date there are no comparative trials available to support or refute their use for managing dyspnea in advanced cancer patients.[22] Long-term use of systemic corticosteroids has significant adverse effects, including steroid myopathy, which can worsen dyspnea. Therefore, corticosteroids should be used with caution when treating breathlessness. It has been postulated that nebulized furosemide may have effects on breathlessness independent of diuresis. The strongest evidence has been in patients with asthma and other reversible airway diseases,[23] but further research is needed to determine its role in the palliative care population.

END-STAGE MANAGEMENT

Withdrawal from Ventilation

Withdrawal of mechanical ventilation is viewed as more problematic than withdrawal of other interventions. It is recommended that the health care team discuss the procedure, strategies for assessing and ensuring comfort, and the patient's expected length of survival with the family and patient (if possible).

Once the decision has been made to discontinue ventilation, the patient can be extubated immediately or ventilation can be reduced slowly, weaning the patient, before extubation. In either case, the patient's comfort and family support are essential. Protocols for ventilator withdrawal include the use of intravenous bolus doses and continuous infusions of medications such as opioids, benzodiazepines, barbiturates, and propofol.[24] The intravenous route for administration of medications is preferred because subcutaneous and enteral medications require longer periods of time to be effective. Clinicians should be present at the bedside during the process to ensure good symptom control is maintained.

Severe Escalating Dyspnea

Patients may experience a severe escalation of dyspnea at the end of life. This often causes high anxiety and fear in both the patient and family. The goal is to control breathlessness rapidly while maintaining a calm and reassuring environment.

High-flow oxygen along with administration of parenteral opioid bolus doses until dyspnea settles is recommended. The preferred route of administration is intravenous, but if the patient has no intravenous access, the subcutaneous route can be used. In patients with significant anxiety, a benzodiazepine, such as midazolam, can be considered, and for patients with agitation, methotrimeprazine is recommended.

PEARLS AND PITFALLS

- Dyspnea is a subjective experience, and the patient's report is key to its assessment.
- Tachypnea is not dyspnea.
- Unidimensional tools and instruments based on function assist in measuring the severity of breathlessness and should be used to guide management.
- Nonpharmacologic strategies are essential components in controlling dyspnea.
- Opioids are the mainstay of pharmacologic management and should be commenced early.
- Health care providers can improve the quality of life and can reduce suffering in dyspneic palliative care patients.

Summary

Dyspnea is a common symptom in patients with advanced disease. Studies have demonstrated that dyspnea severely impairs the quality of life and contributes significantly to patient and caregiver stress. Management of breathlessness in patients at the end of life requires expertise that includes an understanding and assessment of the multidimensional components of the symptom, knowledge of the pathophysiologic mechanisms and clinical syndromes that are common in people with advanced disease, and recognition of the indications for and limitations of available therapeutic approaches.

Resources

Bausewein C, Booth S, Gysels M, Higginson IJ: Non-pharmacological interventions for breathlessness in advanced stages of malignant and non-malignant diseases, *Cochrane Database Syst Rev* 2008;2:CD005623. DOI:10.1002/14651858.CD005623.pub2.

Booth S, Dudgeon D, editors: *Dyspnoea in advanced disease: a guide to clinical management*, Oxford, UK, 2006, Oxford University Press.

Mahler DA, O'Donnell DE, editors: *Dyspnea: mechanisms, measurement, and management*, Boca Raton, FL, 2005, Taylor & Francis Group.

References

1. American Thoracic Society: Dyspnea: mechanisms, assessment, and management: a consensus statement, *Am J Respir Crit Care Med* 159:321–340, 1999.
2. Dudgeon DJ, Kristjanson L, Sloan JA, et al: Dyspnea in cancer patients: prevalence and associated factors, *J Pain Symptom Manage* 21:95–102, 2001.
3. Reuben DB, Mor V: Dyspnea in terminally ill cancer patients, *Chest* 89:234–236, 1986.
4. Muers MF, Round CE: Palliation of symptoms in non-small cell lung cancer: a study by the Yorkshire Regional Cancer Organisation thoracic group, *Thorax* 48:339–343, 1993.
5. Solano JP, Gomes B, Higginson IJ: A comparison of symptom prevalence in far advanced cancer, AIDS, heart disease, chronic obstructive pulmonary disease and renal disease, *J Pain Symptom Manage* 31:58–69, 2006.

6. Skilbeck J, Mott L, Page H, et al: Palliative care in chronic obstructive airways disease: a needs assessment, *Palliat Med* 12:245–254, 1998.
7. Tishelman C, Petersson LM, Degner L, et al: Symptom prevalence, intensity, and distress in patients with inoperable lung cancer in relation to time of death, *J Clin Oncol* 25:5381–5389, 2007.
8. Roberts DK, Thorne SE, Pearson C: The experience of dyspnea in late-stage cancer: patients' and nurses' perspectives, *Cancer Nurs* 16:310–320, 1993.
9. Chochinov MH, Tataryn D, Clinch JJ, Dudgeon D: Will to live in the terminally ill, *Lancet* 354:816–819, 1999.
10. Fainsinger R, Waller A, Bercovici M, et al: A multicentre international study of sedation for uncontrolled symptoms in terminally ill patients, *Palliat Med* 14:257–265, 2000.
11. Dudgeon D: Measurement of dyspnea at the end of life. In Mahler DA, O'Donnell DE, editors: *Lung biology in health and disease*, Boca Raton, FL, 2005, Taylor & Francis Group, pp. 429–461.
12. Henoch I, Bergman B, Gustafsson M, et al: Dyspnea experience in patients with lung cancer in palliative care, *Eur J Oncol Nurs* 12:86–96, 2008.
13. Wilcock A, Crosby V, Hughes A, et al: Descriptors of breathlessness in patients with cancer and other cardiorespiratory diseases, *J Pain Symptom Manage* 23:182–189, 2002.
14. Garrard AK, Williams M: The language of dyspnea: a systematic review. Internet, *J Applied Health Sci Pract* 6:1–14, 2008.
15. Dorman S, Byrne A, Edwards E: Which measurement scales should we use to measure breathlessness in palliative care? A systematic review, *Palliat Med* 21:177–191, 2007.
16. Gift AG, Plaut SM, Jacox A: Psychologic and physiologic factors related to dyspnea in subjects with chronic obstructive pulmonary disease, *Heart Lung* 15:595–601, 1986.
17. Carrieri-Kohlman V: Non-Pharmacological Approaches. In Booth S, Dudgeon D, editors: *Dyspnea in advanced disease*, Oxford, UK, 2005, Oxford University Press, pp. 71–203.
18. Bradley JM, Lasserson T, Elborn S, et al: A systematic review of randomized controlled trials examining the short-term benefit of ambulatory oxygen in COPD, *Chest* 131:278–285, 2007.
19. Uronis HE, Currow DC, McCrory DC, et al: *Oxygen for relief of dyspnea in mildly or nonhypoxemic patients with chronic obstructive pulmonary disease (COPD): a systematic review and meta-analysis*, San Francisco, 2007, American Thoracic Society.
20. Uronis HE, Currow DC, McCrory DC, et al: Oxygen for relief of dyspnea in mildly or nonhypoxemic patients with cancer: a systematic review and meta-analysis, *Br J Cancer* 98:294–299, 2008.
21. Jennings AL, Davies AN, Higgins JPT, et al: Opioids for the palliative of breathlessness in terminal illness. Non-pharmacological interventions for breathlessness in advanced stages of malignant and non-malignant diseases, *Cochrane Database Syst Rev* 2001; 3:CD002066. DOI:10.1002/14651858.CD002066.
22. Viola R, Kiteley C, Lloyd NS, et al: Supportive Care Guidelines Group of the Cancer Care Ontario Program in Evidence-Based Care: The management of dyspnea in cancer patients. A systematic review, *Support Care Cancer* 16:329–337, 2008. DOI 10.1007/s00520-007-0389-6.
23. Currow DC, Abernathy AP: Pharmacological management of dyspnea, *Curr Opin Support Palliat Care* 1:96–101, 2007.
24. von Gunten C, Weissman DE: Ventilator withdrawal in the dying patient. Parts 1–3: Fast Facts and Concepts #33-35, 2nd ed. End-of-Life Physician Education Resource Center, 2005. Available at www.eperc.mcw.edu/fastfact.

CHAPTER 16

Supporting the Family in Palliative Care

SUSAN BLACKER

As an individual's illness progresses, family members play an increased role in caregiving and decision making. In the effort to manage changing care needs and maximize their loved one's quality of life, specific crises and challenges can arise for the family's members. The caregiving experience has potentially profound short- and long-term effects on the family member's physical, psychological, and economic well-being.[1,2,3] The degree of support received in caregiving is an important factor in the bereavement experience of family caregivers.[4] This underscores the importance of palliative care's philosophical approach to the family as "the unit of care." For those without training in working with families, this can be daunting, but some guiding principles are helpful to consider.

Caring for the Family: The Psychosocial Dimension of Care

The psychosocial dimension of palliative care involves addressing the practical, psychological, and social challenges and losses that affect a patient and those close to them.[5] As Jeffrey[5] has noted, psychosocial care "involves the spiritual beliefs, culture and values of those concerned and the social factors that influence the experience." Interventions are aimed at improving the well-being of the patient and their family members. Often these are entwined with ensuring that physical and practical needs are met—that symptoms are well controlled, for example, or supports are put in place to help manage a patient's physical caregiving needs. Hence, all members of the team provide aspects of psychosocial care, and those with specialized skill (such as social work or others trained to provided psychological interventions) focus on specific problems and approaches to helping the patient and family to respond to needs.

213

Adjustment to a family member's illness and increasing care needs requires the family to reestablish patterns and integrate this reality into their functioning as a family unit. When a member is dying, it is imperative to remember that family members' caregiving roles typically intensify while at the same time they are bearing the effects of grief. As King and Quill have noted, "the task of the health care team is to support the family's positive adaptive capabilities so that systemic equilibrium is eventually reestablished in a manner that supports the health and well-being of all surviving members."[6] Strategies for doing this are discussed later in this chapter.

FAMILY FACTORS TO CONSIDER IN ASSESSMENT

Considering the following areas as part of the assessment of a family's needs can be very helpful to identifying how the palliative care team can optimally form a collaborative relationship with the family and avoid common reasons for conflict.

Structure of the Family: Roles Assumed by its Members

Roles and responsibilities for tasks in the family may shift, and those related to caregiving become a greater focus of energy as a member's illness progresses. Levine and Zuckerman[7] have highlighted that family members may play a number of distinct roles: care providers, advocates, trusted companions, surrogate decision makers, and second-order patients (with their own distress response to the circumstances). When engaging a patient's family, it is imperative to determine who the patient wants to have involved and share information with and who will be involved in decision making. It should never be assumed. Establishing this early on will avoid challenging situations and ensure that patient privacy is not breached later.[1]

Assessment of the burden of caregiving responsibilities, and the degree of impact experienced by the individual, is paramount. There may be strain, as well as positive aspects, related to this role.

As any or all these roles intensify, family members may find themselves interacting in significantly different ways with the health care team than earlier in the disease continuum (i.e., seeking information as opposed to relying on the patient for it, bringing their perception of the patient's needs to the attention of care providers). Taking on a new role may not always be an easy adjustment for family members, and hence the team needs to be aware of this and support them as needed.[8,9] If they feel unsuccessful, or that the health care professionals are reacting negatively or critically to their efforts, conflict may result.

History of Loss Related to Illness (Current and Other Family Members)

Many patients and families the palliative care team meets have already met a number of other health care providers during the course of the patient's illness. Their experiences often shape their expectations and perceptions of the health care providers who become involved in their care. They may bring with them experiences of chronic illness, dying, and death of other family members or friends, which may not have been positive. It is important to consider this as part of the family's story because it may very much shape their approach to decision making or understanding of options and care, as well as degree of engagement with and trust in the care team.

Coping Strengths and Challenges

Palliative care providers should consider that a family must deal with crises and losses at multiple points along the illness trajectory and try to understand their history with the disease. Understanding how, as a family, they have been coping and managing the challenges they have encountered up to this point can be valuable in identifying and building on the family's strengths.[7]

Coping with progressing disease and increasing caregiving needs can result in intense emotional responses and new problems in the family. Family members, like patients, may be experiencing psychosocial distress, including depression and anxiety. This may affect their ability to be involved in the patient's care at present or in future. Preexisting problems in the family, such as long-standing disagreements and fragmented communication, strained relationships, and history of abuse (substance, physical, or emotional), are often magnified and may require special attention and referral to those with appropriate expertise.[8]

Values and Belief Systems

A family's needs and decisions are shaped by their culture and established ways of managing problems and challenges in the family.[10] This might include beliefs and values about the following[8]:

- Roles in caregiving
- Approaches to decision making and communication with the health care team
- Socially acceptable expression of grief in response to associated losses
- Perceptions about accepting help from outside the family or cultural community

The team may also find that members within the same family have differing beliefs or values about specific issues.

Information Needs

Families living with life-threatening illness experience significant information and support needs.[9] In the earlier phase of the illness, this is related primarily to understanding the disease and its effects, its treatment, and the immediate adjustments they need to make in their family life. Over time, they must adjust to additional demands in terms of time involved, type of care—from practical and emotional support to hands-on care—and psychological impact to themselves. Families often are unsure how to get help with their questions and concerns and may, as a result, be struggling with unmet needs.[11] The information and other support needs of each family (and sometimes each family member) vary. The team may need to consider the following:

- Family's readiness for information or assistance
- Amount of detailed desired
- Amount of information they can process if emotional distressed (e.g., coping style)
- Degree of involvement in care of the patient they are able or willing to have

Lack of needed information can negatively affect the patient's care, as well as the physical, psychological, and social well-being of family members.[12] As a general rule, families wish for specific kinds of information and interactions with the care team. According to Levine,[7] these interactions should include a focus on providing the following:

- Understandable, timely information about what to expect
- Preparation and training for the technical and emotional aspects of their roles

- Guidance in defining their roles and responsibilities in patient care and decision making
- Support for setting fair limits on their sacrifices

Prompting with questions such as "What do you understand to be happening?" and "What changes you have noticed?" is useful to elicit the perception of the illness and current treatment. Asking "What is most important to you now?" or "What is most troubling to you now?" helps to engage in a discussion regarding values and goals of care, as well as specific stressors that the individual or family is facing. "How are you feeling about things?" or "How are those closest to you coping with your illness?" can be valuable to elicit perceptions of how the individual and others involved in the family are coping. Responses will help the physician and the interprofessional team to focus their interventions.

According to Rabow and colleagues,[1] physicians should focus on five areas when relating to family members caring for patients at the end of life:

1. Promoting excellent communication with the family
2. Encouraging appropriate advanced care planning and decision making, including discussing preferences, values, and contingencies for end-of-life care, as well as preparing advanced directives and identifying a proxy for decision making
3. Supporting the patient and family to manage home care
4. Demonstrating empathy and understanding for family emotions and relationships
5. Attending to family members' grief and bereavement

The remainder of this chapter focuses on specific strategies for establishing effective communication and a collaborative relationship with the family.

Strategies to Optimize Communication and Collaboration

As George Bernard Shaw once said, "The single biggest problem in communication is the illusion that it has taken place." In palliative care, discussion related to the patient and family's perceptions and information needs should occur regularly. Approaching interactions by engaging the family in discussion, not only providing information, is imperative. This approach may be new to the family, especially if for the first time members are taking on the roles of spokesperson or decision maker, and they may need support. The objective is to create a relationship that supports collaboration—working with the family toward a common goal.

ACKNOWLEDGING EMOTIONS

Clinicians must be prepared for intense emotional responses. Anger is a common emotion for patients and families to experience and express. It is often rooted in fear and worry about the unknown. When responding to anger, care providers must validate the patient's and family's feelings, explore the underlying source, and examine ways to help manage their specific concerns.[13]

In addition, clinicians must carefully consider the nature and quality of communication with families, particularly in cross-cultural situations. This can be key to establishing a collaborative relationship, minimizing the risk of conflict, and providing the needed support and information to help them optimally cope.[10]

HANDLING LANGUAGE DIFFERENCES

Whenever possible, the team should use trained interpreters, not family members, to bridge language gaps and to ensure accurate interpretation.[12,14] This is especially important when determining that informed consent has been obtained. Equally important, using an interpreter ensures that family members (especially children) are not put in the difficult position of being responsible for delivering difficult news.

USING FAMILY CONFERENCES

Family conferencing (also known as family meetings) can be a valuable way for members of the health care team to assess a family's needs and to address the presence of conflict. The family conference is an intervention that is consistent with the interprofessional focus of palliative care and acknowledges the unit of care as the patient and their family.[15]

A meeting serves a number of purposes. It is an opportunity to provide information and patient and family education, discuss and determine goals of care, and ensure optimal planning for care transitions[8,15–18] (Boxes 16-1 and 16-2).

Conferences are most often led by social workers, physicians, or the two together. Nurses are often present. Other professionals, such as case managers, psychologists, occupational or physical therapists, chaplains, nutritionists, and ethicists, may also attend. Based on issues that arise to suggest a need for the meeting, teams decide who should attend and chair the meeting. Several authors[8,15–18] have suggested that family conferences can be useful for the following purposes:

- Set the stage for partnership in care
- Provide specific medical information and advice to achieve goals of care
- Share other information with the patient and family (e.g., options for support, community resources)
- Gain a better understanding of family dynamics
- Identify and affirm individual relationships (e.g. those responsible for decision making, those providing direct care) and the response of individual members to the illness and its effects
- Identify areas of difficulty in family communication and relating
- Identify previously unspoken or unidentified concerns
- Normalize fears and concerns as appropriate
- Correct misinformation
- Model and encourage shared decision making
- Reach consensus on health care decisions and work out points of disagreement
- Demonstrate respect and support for the family's involvement

---

BOX 16-1. *Common Reasons for Family Conferences in Palliative Care*

- Establishing or reviewing the needs for change in goals of care
- Considering withholding or withdrawing medical interventions
- Complex planning for discharge from hospital (e.g., coordination of family caregivers and community supports)
- Transition in care settings (e.g., referral to hospice palliative care program)
- Admission to new care setting (e.g., inpatient hospice care)
- Resolving conflict

Adapted from references 1, 8, 15–18.

BOX 16-2. *Recommendations for Planning and Facilitating Family Conferences*

Family conferences can be conceptualized as having three phases, each with special points for consideration by the physician and participating team members: preparation, meeting, and follow-up.

PREPARATION: TASKS AND CONSIDERATIONS BEFORE THE CONFERENCE

- Identify the right participants, with patient confidentiality fully considered.
- Prepare the patient and family (empower them).
- Clarify the purpose of the meeting and the subjects that must be covered.
- Reach a consensus about recommendations and key messages among palliative care team members and other consultants who may be involved.
- Determine the logistics of the meeting (time, location, appropriate room for uninterrupted meeting).
- Establish who will lead the conference.

MEETING: TASKS AND CONSIDERATIONS DURING THE CONFERENCE

- Facilitate introductions and state the purpose and goals of the meeting.
- Determine what the patient and family understand.
- Review the relevant information and options.
- Ensure that the patient and family understand the information that has been presented.
- Make recommendations.
- Allow for reactions and questions while at the same time doing the following:
  - Keep the patient at the center of the discussion.
  - Demonstrate that the team values and appreciates what the family members have to say, acknowledge the family members' emotions, and ask questions that help the team to understand who the patient is as a person.
- Ask for clarification if responses are not clear.
- Summarize consensus, points of disagreement, and decisions reached—that is, restate the plan.
- State responsibilities for implementation of the plan and timeframe (if relevant).
- Indicate availability for further communication; plan a subsequent meeting if needed to facilitate further decision making.

FOLLOW-UP: TASKS AND CONSIDERATIONS AFTER THE CONFERENCE

- Provide needed support.
- Implement the conference decisions.
- Follow-up to ensure that the issues raised in the conference are dealt with.
- Create a summary document and ensure that it is available for those team members who were not present. Include a list of those present, the key points of discussion, the action plan, and any necessary follow-up. A standardized form might be helpful.

Adapted from references 1, 8, 15–18.

Potential Sources of Conflict

"Interactions between families and health care providers can bring tremendous satisfaction or may be a source of great frustration".[14] Relationships in health care are very dynamic, and conflict can arise between family and the health care team, often to the surprise of the care providers. Perceived breakdown in communication and differences in perception of the situation are perhaps the most common sources of conflict in the family-team interaction.

DISCORDANT COMMUNICATION STYLE

Establishing relationships with patients and families is an intensely interpersonal process.[14] Often these relationships need to be developed quickly, involving behaviors or interactions within minutes of meeting a care provider that might be considered inappropriate or very uncomfortable in any other social context. This includes directly asking personal questions about health behaviors and physical touch related to clinical examinations. Relationships are negotiated by how we communicate with one another. People in interactions negotiate the definition of their relationship through verbal and nonverbal cues, which can present challenges in cross-cultural situations or situations that are emotionally charged. Often care providers are not aware of this and their body language does not fit their verbal messages, creating a cognitive dissonance in the listener. This can be magnified by the reality that there is a differential in "power" in the health care provider–patient–family relationship. Patients and families, for example, may perceive that a provider is too busy to listen to their concerns or does not feel they are important because the provider stood rather that sat during the interaction. Similarly, family members may feel troubled by the interaction if the clinician didn't make eye contact, left the discussion to respond to a page, didn't acknowledge each person in the room, or didn't follow up with information promptly. Conflict may also be a direct result of differences in communication style (e.g., open vs. closed, direct vs. indirect) or cultural nuances influencing communication between the family and the care provider. Carefully considered verbal and nonverbal communication that is adjusted to the communication and decision-making style of the other can be experienced as validation and respect. Cultural sensitivity is of paramount importance.[11]

DIFFERENCE IN MEANING AND REASONING ABOUT WHAT IS HAPPENING AND WHAT TO DO ABOUT IT

Conflict may result from discord related to involved individuals' specific conclusions about the situation and (more often the case) what they believe the course of action should be. These conclusions are typically based in beliefs, past experiences, or observations. A patient, family, and health care professional may all begin with similar information—for example, the patient with metastatic cancer is experiencing more intense pain—but what they each conclude this means, and what they believe is best to do about it, may not be the same. Consider the range of possible beliefs about the role and nature of pain and its treatment that may conflict with health care professionals' approaches and views about optimal pain management.

1. "People living on the street are addicted to drugs like morphine. Taking pain medication will result in addiction. Therefore, my family member must refuse it."

2. "The pain is a sign that the treatments are now finally working. Taking pain medication might interfere with this progress. Therefore, my family member must avoid it."
3. "If my family member experiences any pain, he or she is not receiving good care."
4. "All that giving pain medications will do is hasten my family member's death."
5. "Pain medications make my family member too drowsy. We can't have meaningful interactions when he or she takes them."

Each of these beliefs requires a different approach by the care team in terms of patient and family education and ongoing engagement. It is important for the care team to help the family articulate their understanding and how they came to this conclusion, and avoid making assumptions.

PEARLS

- Families value the clinician's ability to communicate. Communication is the basis for trust in the health care provider–family relationship.
- It is important for the care team to help the family articulate their understanding.
- Family conferences can be a valuable intervention to achieve a number of goals, not just providing information and facilitating decision making.
- Trained interpreters should be used when there are language differences.

PITFALLS

- When engaging a patient's family members, it is imperative to determine who the patient wants to have involved and share information with and who will be involved in decision making. It should never be assumed. Establishing this early on will avoid challenging situations and ensure that patient privacy is not breached later.
- Making assumptions about a family's beliefs and understanding, especially related to ethnicity, can risk stereotyping and lead to conflict.
- The majority of patient and family complaints about health care providers relates to their experience of poor communication and lack of information given. This can be proactively addressed by focusing on communication strategies (Box 16-3).

Summary

Trust is a critically important ingredient in a successful relationships with families receiving care.[14] Communication is essential to ensure that expectations are defined and to establish trust. Trust evolves over time; this can be challenging because time is limited in palliative/hospice care. Expectations (both articulated and implied) greatly influence interactions. Excellent communication requires skills, time, consistency, and strong team work.

Approaching delivery of information should always be considered in the context of the following variables:

BOX 16-3. *Case for Reflection*

Mr. J., age 67, was admitted to the palliative care unit located at an academic hospital 2 weeks ago. It is the same hospital that houses the oncology clinic he has gone to for the past 18 months for treatment of lung cancer. He has brain metastases. Radiation treatment finished 3 weeks ago. He is moderately short of breath and presented on admission as confused. He fell twice at home, resulting in an admission through the emergency department when his wife could not get him back into bed. His condition has deteriorated and he is sleeping most of the day, completely bed bound and interacting minimally with visitors.

Mr. J is the father of two sons and has been married for 44 years. He was living at home with his wife. She has been his caregiver since his diagnosis and has taken a leave of absence from her job in the past month. She has expressed that if his symptoms are better controlled, she would like to take him home. When he was admitted, she told the unit's social worker that she was open to having a hospice care team come to their home, which she had previously declined.

Mr. J's younger son has not been to see his father since he was admitted to the unit.

Mr. J. oldest son arrived from Canada this week. He had not seen his father for 4 months. He has been asking the nurses for an explanation of "what the doctors are going to do" about his father's "situation." He wants to know what additional therapies can be tried. He has become angry when attempts have been made to explain palliative care and why his father is admitted to this unit, instead of the oncology inpatient unit where he has been cared for before.

Mrs. J is visibly upset when her son interacts this way with the nurses.

QUESTIONS

- In a situation such as this, how can the team promote trust and clarify expectations?
- How might earlier discussions about what to expect have been helpful in this situation?
- How can palliative care providers incorporate assessment of patient and family information needs into routine assessment?
- How would you use a family meeting? Who would you include? Which family members? Which health care team members?
- What might the team's key messages and recommendations be in this situation?
- What would your "opening remarks" be to the family?
- How would you help to prepare them for this meeting?

1. The family's cultural location (i.e., beliefs and values)
2. The learning style of the recipient of the information or education (i.e., auditory, visual, kinesthetic)
3. The recipient's educational background and comprehension level

Clinicians must remember, "Dying is not only what the patient experiences but also what the family remembers".[17]

References

1. Rabow M, Hauser J, Adams J: Supporting family caregivers at the end of life: "they don't know what they don't know," *JAMA* 291:483–491, 2004.
2. Grunfeld E, Coyle D, Whelan T, et al: Family caregiver burden: results of a longitudinal study of breast cancer patients and their principal caregivers, *CMAJ* 170(12):1795–1801, 2004.

3. Lynne J, Teno J, Phillips R, et al: Perceptions by family members of the dying experience of older and seriously ill patients, *Ann Intern Med* 126:97–106, 1997.
4. Bass DM, Bowman K, Noelker LSP: The influence of caregiving and bereavement support on adjusting to an older relative's death, *Gerontologist* 31:32–42, 1991.
5. Jeffrey D: What Do We Mean by Psychosocial Care in Palliative Care? In Lloyd-Williams M, editor: *Psychosocial issues in palliative care*, Oxford, UK, 2003, Oxford University Press, p 4.
6. King D, Quill T: Working with families in palliative care: one size does not fit all, *J Palliat Med* 9:3, 704–715, 2006.
7. Levine C, Zuckerman C: The trouble with families: toward an ethic of accommodation, *Ann Intern Med* 130:148–152, 1999. Available at www.annals.org/cgi/reprint/130/2/148.pdf.
8. Blacker S, Jordan A: Working with families facing life threatening illness in the medical setting. In Berzoff J, Silverman P, editors: *Living with dying: a handbook for end-of-life care practitioners*, New York, 2004, Columbia University Press, pp 548–570.
9. Loscalzo M, Zabora J: Care of the cancer patient: response of family and staff. In Bruera E, Portenoy R, editors: *Topics in palliative care*, vol. 2, New York, 1998, Oxford Press, pp 205–245.
10. Bowman KW: Communication, mediation and negotiation: dealing with conflict in end-of-life decisions, *J Palliat Care* 16:17–23, 2002.
11. Kagawa-Singer M, Blackhall LJ: Negotiating cross-cultural issues at the end of life: "you got to go where he lives," *JAMA* 286:2993–3001, 2001.
12. Houts P, Rusenas I, Simmonds MA, Hufford DL: Information needs of families of cancer patients: a literature review and recommendations, *J Cancer Ed* 6(4):255–261, 1991.
13. Jenkins C, Bruera E: Conflict between families and staff: an approach. In Bruera E, Portenoy R, editors: *Topics in palliative care*, vol. 2, New York, 1998, Oxford Press, pp 311–325.
14. Lynn-McHale D, Deatrick J: Trust between family and health care provider, *J Fam Nurs* 6(3):210–230, 2000.
15. Hudson P, Quinn K, O'Hanlon B, et al: Family meetings in palliative care: multidisciplinary clinical practice guidelines, *BMC Palliative Care* 7:1–12, 2008. Available at www.biomedcentral.com/1472-684x/7/12.
16. Curtis JR, Engelberg RA, Wenrich MD, et al: Missed opportunities during family conferences about end-of-life care in the intensive care unit, *Am J Respir Crit Care Med* 171:844–849, 2005.
17. Ambuel B, Weissman DE: Fast fact and concept #016: Conducting a family conference, *End-of-Life/Palliative Education Resource Center*, Milwaukee, WI, 2005. Available at www.eperc.mcw.edu/fastFact/ff_016.htm. 2005.
18. Curtis JR, Patrick DL, Shannon SE, et al: The family conference as a focus to improve communication about end-of-life care in the intensive care unit: opportunities for improvement, *Crit Care Med* 29(Suppl 2):N26–N33, 2001.

CHAPTER 17

Local Wound Care for Palliative and Malignant Wounds

KEVIN Y. WOO and R. GARY SIBBALD

Palliative Wounds	Patient-Centered Concerns with Malignant Wounds
Malignant Wounds	Local Wound Care Issues (HOPES)
Management of Malignant and Other Wounds	
HOPES	Diagnosis of Wound Infection
Treatment Approach	Treatment of Wound Infection
Prevention	
Antitumor Therapies	Summary

Chronic cutaneous wounds often are complex, recalcitrant to healing, and may not follow a predictable trajectory of repair despite standard interventions.[1] The exact mechanisms that contribute to poor wound healing remain elusive but likely involve an interplay of systemic and local factors. To establish realistic objectives, wounds are classified as healable, maintenance, and nonhealable based on prognostic estimation of the likelihood to achieve healing.[2] (See Table 17-1 for definitions.)

Palliative Wounds

As a result of the deterioration of the body and multiple system failures that are intrinsic to the dying process, patients at the end of life are vulnerable to skin breakdown that may not always be preventative. Underlying physiologic changes lower tissue perfusion, which compromises cutaneous oxygen tension, delivery of vital nutrients, and removal of metabolic wastes.[3] In fact, observable signs of skin changes and related ulceration have been documented in more than 50% of individuals in the 2 to 6 weeks before death.[4]

Wounds and associated skin changes that develop in palliative patients are generally considered nonhealable in light of poor health condition and the demands of treatment, which may outweigh the potential benefits. These patients often suffer from conditions that are incurable and life limiting, including malignancy, advanced diseases associated with major organ failure (renal, hepatic, pulmonary, or cardiac), and, in some cases, profound dementia.[5,6] Management of these cutaneous palliative wounds are challenging to patients and their health care providers. Although wound healing may not be realistic, it is imperative to maintain patients' dignity and quality of life by addressing psychosocial concerns (e.g., fear of dying or pain), empowering patients' independence, promoting the highest achievable quality of life, enhancing the ability to perform activities of daily living, and optimizing pain management.[7]

223

Table 17-1. Wound Prognosis and Realistic Outcomes

Wound Prognosis	Can the Cause Be Treated?	Effect of Coexisting Medical Condition/ Drugs on Prognosis	Goals/Objectives
Healable	*Yes, can be corrected or compensated with treatment* Examples: pressure redistribution; correction of incontinence; friction/shear and poor nutrition for pressure ulcers; compression for venous leg ulcers	Coexisting medical conditions and drugs do not prevent healing.	Promote wound healing. Example: Venous ulcers 30% smaller by week 4, to heal by week 12[3]
Maintenance	*No, cannot be treated because of poor treatment adherence or lack of appropriate resources* Examples: lack of financial resources to acquire appropriate footwear for foot ulcers	Coexisting medical conditions and drugs may stall healing, such as hyperglycemia.[4]	Prevent further skin deterioration or breakdown, trauma, and wound infection. Promote patient adherence. Advocate for patients to acquire appropriate resources. Optimize pain and manage other symptom.[5]
Nonhealable: Palliative or malignant	*No, the cause is not treatable.* Examples: widespread metastasis including the skin, advanced stages of cutaneous malignant conditions, chronic osteomyelitis	Coexisting medical conditions prevent normal healing,[6] such as: • Advanced terminal diseases • Malignant conditions • Poor perfusion • Malnutrition with low albumin (<20 mg/dL) or negative protein balance • Significant anemia (Hgb <80 g/dL) • High-dose immunosuppressive drugs	Prevent further skin deterioration or breakdown, trauma, and wound infection. Promote comfort. Optimize pain and manage other symptoms.[5]

Hgb, hemoglobin.
© KY Woo 2009

Malignant Wounds

A malignant wound can result from tumor necrosis, fungating tumor cells, an ulcerating cancerous wound, or a malignant cutaneous wound. Infiltration of malignant cells in these wounds is secondary to local invasion of a primary cutaneous lesion or metastatic spread. Clinicians should raise the index of suspicion of malignancy in the following scenarios:

1. *Wounds that are manifestation of primary skin cancer and certain types of malignancies.* These include basal cell carcinoma, squamous cell carcinoma, melanoma, Kaposi sarcoma, cutaneous lymphomas, and cutaneous infiltrates associated with leukemia.[8]

2. *Wounds in patients with history of cancer to rule out cutaneous metastasis.* Malignant wounds have been estimated to affect 5% to 19% of patients with metastatic disease.[9–10] Another study[11] reported that 5% of cancer patients develop malignant wounds. The chest and breasts, head and neck, and abdomen are the most common sites where metastatic malignant wounds develop.[12]

3. *Wounds that do not heal over a long time.* These types of wounds may undergo malignant transformation. A Marjolin ulcer or a squamous cell carcinoma may develop in an area of chronic inflammation.[13] These changes have been documented from a chronic osteomyelitis sinus, persistent trauma, and burn scar.[14]

4. *Chronic wounds in patients with chronic immunosuppression.* Patients at risk include those receiving azathioprine, methotrexate, and cyclosporin therapy and those with other immunodeficiency disorders, including human immunodeficiency virus infection.[9,14]

5. *Wounds secondary to treatment of malignancies.* This includes patients such as those undergoing late radiation therapy change with the development of a secondary malignancy.[15]

Extension of a tumor to the surface of the skin may initially present as localized, raised induration and evolve to a fungating or ulcerative skin lesion (Figure 17-1).

Figure 17-1. Fungating lesions related to metastatic cervical cancer.

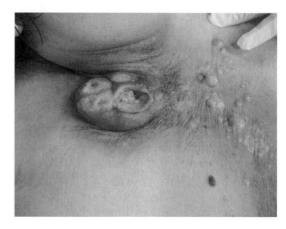

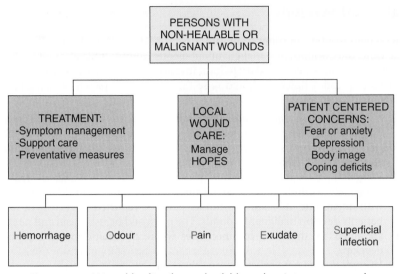

Figure 17-2. Wound healing for nonhealable and maintenance wounds.

Fungating lesions are fast growing and resemble a cauliflower or fungus, extending beyond the skin surface.[16] On the other hand, ulcerative lesions are characterized by deep craters with raised margins. As the tumor continues to grow, disrupting blood supply and outstripping local tissue perfusion, hypoxia is inevitable. This creates areas of necrosis. The presence of necrotic tissue establishes an ideal milieu for secondary bacterial proliferation. Vertical extension of the tumor, however, may reach the deeper structure, leading to sinus or fistula formation. Obstruction of normal vascular and lymphatic flow has been linked to copious exudate production and edema.[17]

Management of Malignant and Other Wounds

HOPES

A systematized and comprehensive approach is required to manage the complexity of malignant and palliative wounds and optimize patient outcomes. The plan of care begins with treating the wound cause, when possible, and addressing patient concerns before local wound care. Based on previous study results,[18,19] local wound care must be modified to address several key concerns: *h*emorrhage, *o*dor, *p*ain, *e*xudate, and *s*uperficial infection (HOPES). Wound management for malignant wounds is outlined in Figure 17-2 and described in the rest of the chapter.

Treatment Approach

PREVENTION

Although the care of palliative and advanced malignant wounds is centered on symptom management, other supportive strategies to prevent exacerbation of existing wounds and emergence of new ulcers are equally important.[20]

To prevent pressure ulcers, at-risk individuals benefit from therapeutic support surfaces and regular repositioning. (Frequency is determined by the patient's condition. Some clinicians recommend repositioning at least every 4 hours.)[21] Although best practice recommendations are targeted at pressure redistribution and shear elimination, the plan of care must be customized to promote comfort and meet the needs of patients, including their circle of care.[20] Suboptimal nutrition is common due to various combinations of cancer-related factors, including impaired absorption; increased metabolic demand; and decreased oral intake as a result of poor appetite, swallowing difficulties, nausea, vomiting, taste alteration, and mucositis.[22] Nutritional supplementation with enriched protein and other micronutrients (zinc, vitamins A, E, and C) should be considered.[23] Meticulous skin care after each incontinent episode, together with the use of a mild cleanser and skin protectant, may reduce irritation to skin.[24]

ANTITUMOR THERAPIES

Depending on disease trajectory, therapies including radiotherapy, surgery, laser therapy, chemotherapy, and hormonal blocking agents may be considered to reduce the tumor size and alleviate associated symptoms.[25] Topical application of anticancer agents such as miltefosine and imiquimod may delay tumor progression.[26, 27]

Patient-Centered Concerns with Malignant Wounds

It is unequivocal that malignant wounds constitute a significant source of emotional distress to patients and their families.[7] In a survey of patients living with malignant wounds,[10] pain, aesthetic distress, and mass effect were the three most commonly expressed symptoms. In several qualitative studies, recurring themes revolve around powerlessness, anxiety, embarrassment, and the bleak feeling of isolation due to wound related stigma; however, they also involve willpower to maintain a positive outlook.[28] To address patient-centered concerns, clinicians must engage, empathize, educate, and enlist their patients in the overall plan of care.[29] Individualized education and appropriate information should be provided to help patients understand the parameters of care.

LOCAL WOUND CARE ISSUES (HOPES)

H: Hemorrhage or Bleeding

The granulation tissue within a malignant wound bleeds easily due to local stimulation of vascular endothelial growth factor (VEG-F), resulting in excess formation of abundant but fragile blood vessels. Reduced fibroblast activity and ongoing thrombosis of larger vessels in infected and malignant wounds may compromise the strength of collagen matrix formation, rendering the granulation less resilient to trauma.[30] Even minor trauma from the removal of wound dressings that adhere to wound surface can provoke bleeding.[31] Other health conditions (e.g., abnormal platelet function, vitamin K deficiency) may also put patients with cancer and other terminal diseases at risk of bleeding. Frank hemorrhage can occur as the tumor erodes into a major blood vessel.

A variety of hemostatic agents can be applied topically to control hemorrhage (Table 17-2). In severe cases, suturing a proximal vessel, intravascular embolization,

Table 17-2. Topical Hemostatic Agents

Categories	Example	Comments
Natural hemostats	Calcium alginates	Used to control minor bleeding
	Collagen	Available as a dressing material
	Oxidized cellulose	Can absorb moderate to large amount of wound exudate
		Bioabsorbable
Coagulation agents	Gelatin sponge	Expensive
	Thrombin	Increases risk of embolization
Sclerosing agents	Silver nitrate	May cause stinging/burning
	Tricholacetic acid	Leaves coagulum that can stimulate inflammation
Fibrinolytic antagonists	Tranexamic acid	Oral agent; can produce gastrointestinal side effects (nausea/vomiting)
Astringents	Aluminum sucralfate	May leave residue on wound

Woo 2009 ©

laser treatment, cryotherapy, radiotherapy, or electrical cauterization may be necessary.[32]

O: Odor

Unpleasant odor and putrid discharge are associated with increased bacterial burden, particularly involving anaerobic and certain gram-negative (e.g., *Pseudomonas*) organisms.[30] Bacterial metabolic byproducts produce this odor. To eradicate wound odor, metronidazole, as an anti-inflammatory and anti-infective agent against anaerobes, has been demonstrated to be efficacious.[33] Topical metronidazole is readily available as a gel and cream. Alternatively, gauze can be soaked with intravenous metronidazole solution to use as a compress or tablets can be ground into powder and sprinkled onto the wound surface. Some patients derive the greatest benefit from oral metronidazole administration.

Activated charcoal dressing has been used to control odor with some success. To ensure optimal performance of charcoal dressing, edges should be sealed and the contact layer should be kept dry.[16] If topical treatment is not successful or practical, putting odor-absorbing agents such as cat litter or baking soda (not charcoal; it only works as a filter) beneath the bed may reduce odor.

P: Pain

Pain is consistently reported by patients as one of the worst aspects of living with chronic wounds, which profoundly affect their quality of life.[28] Wound-related pain is frequently experienced during dressing changes. Dressing materials adhere to the fragile wound surface due to the glue like nature of dehydrated or crusted exudate; each time the dressing is removed, potential local trauma may evoke pain. Granulation tissue and capillary loops that grow into the product matrix, especially gauze, can also render dressing removal traumatic.[31] According to a review of dressings and topical agents for secondary intention healing of postsurgical wounds, patients experienced significantly more pain with gauze than with other types of occlusive dressings.[34] Nonetheless, gauze continues to be a commonly used dressing materials, indicating a need to bridge research to practice.[18] Careful selection of dressings with atraumatic and nonadherent interfaces, such as silicone, has been documented to limit skin damage and trauma with dressing removal and minimize pain at dressing changes.

Avoidable pain may also result from damage to the periwound skin. Repeated application and removal of adhesive tapes and dressings pull the skin surface from the epithelial cells, which can precipitate skin damage by stripping away the stratum corneum.[35] In severe cases, contact irritant and allergic dermatitis results in local erythema, edema, and blistering on the wound margins. Enzyme-rich exudate may spill onto the periwound skin, causing maceration and tissue erosion with a subsequent increased risk of trauma and pain. To minimize trauma induced by adhesives, a number of sealants, barriers, and protectants are useful on the periwound skin (Table 17-3).[36]

Topical agents or dressings play a critical role in alleviating wound-related pain. Slow-release ibuprofen foam dressings have demonstrated reduction in persistent wound pain between dressing change and temporary pain on dressing removal.[37] The use of topical morphine and lidocaine/prilocaine (EMLA) may be considered for acute or procedure-related pain.[38] However, lack of pharmacokinetic data precludes the routine clinical use of these compounds at this time. There are many advantages to using local rather than systemic treatment. Any active agent is delivered directly

Table 17-3. Strategies to Protect Periwound Skin

Types	Description	Application	Comments
Silicone	Polymers that include silicone together with carbon, hydrogen, and oxygen	Apply to periwound skin.	Allergy is rare. Certain types of silicone products are tacky, facilitating dressing adherence to the skin without any adhesive.
Zinc oxide/ petrolatum	Inorganic compounds that are insoluble in water	Apply a generous quantity to skin.	May interfere with the activity of ionic silver.
Acrylates	Film-forming liquid skin preparation to form a protective interface on skin attachment sites	Spray or wipe on skin sparingly.	Allergy is uncommon. Facilitates visualization of periwound skin.
Hydrocolloid	Hydrocolloid wafer consists of backing with carboxymethylcellulose as filler, water-absorptive components such as gelatin and pectin (commercial gelatin desserts), and adhesive	Window frame the wound margin to prevent recurrent stripping of skin.	Allergies have been reported from some colophony-related adhesives (Pentylin H) associated with some hydrocolloid dressings.

Woo & Sibbald 2009 ©

to the affected area, bypassing the systemic circulation, and the dose needed for pain reduction is low with minimal risk of side effects.

For severe pain, it may be necessary to consider combining long-acting opioids with adjunctive agents for the neuropathic component.

Next to dressing removal, wound cleansing is also likely to evoke pain during the dressing change. Patients with chronic wounds rated cleansing as the most painful part of dressing change.[39] Avoid using abrasive materials such as gauze to scrub the wound surface. Techniques that involve compressing and irrigation may be less traumatic and painful. In the presence of unexpected pain or tenderness, clinicians should consider antimicrobial therapy for wound infection. A validated checklist of 12 clinical signs and symptoms to identify localized chronic wound infection can be used. Subjects with no indications of wound infection did not express increased levels of pain. Pain is a useful indicator of infection.

A systematized approach to wound-related pain is summarized in Figure 17-3 based on a previous published model for the management of wound-related pain.[40]

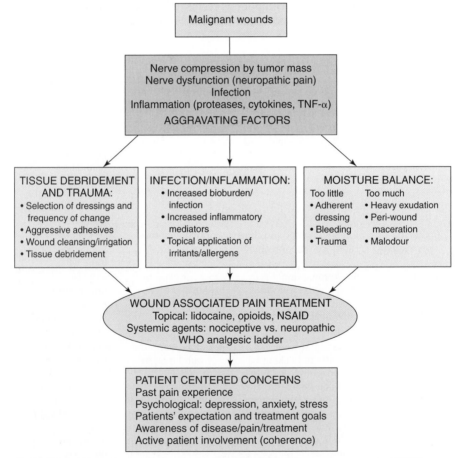

Figure 17-3. Wound management for nonhealable and maintenance wounds. NSAID, nonsteroidal anti-inflammatory drugs; TNF-α, tumor necrosis factor alpha; WHO, World Health Organization.

E: Exudate

Exudation is promoted by inflammation that may be associated with infection. Excessive moisture creates an ideal wound environment for bacteria to proliferate, especially when the host defense is compromised. Moisture is contraindicated in nonhealable wounds; hydrating gels and moisture-retentive dressings (hydrocolloids) should be avoided.[39] To contain and remove excess exudate from the wound, a plethora of absorbent dressings have been developed. Major categories of dressings include foams, alginates, and hydrofibers.[41]

- *Foams.* The micro-architecture of the foam dressings is arranged like a honeycomb with an air-filled center and polyurethane wall. Foams that have variable pore sizes are superior in fluid management because they lock in some moisture even under compression. Permeable backing of the dressing allows water molecules to pass through the dressing and evaporate into the ambient environment at a variable rate, depending on the water-vapor transmission rate (WVTR) of the backing material.
- *Alginates.* Calcium alginates are derived from kelp or brown seaweed. Calcium alginate is unique for its hemostatic property. This dressing is completely absorbable, and residual alginate fibers can be removed by adding water or saline, saving the patient a painful removal procedure.
- *Hydrofibers.* Hydrofibers are carboxymethylcellulose strands available in pads or packing materials. They have a water-hating component (hydrophobic methylcellulose) that gives this dressing its tensile strength, as well as a water-loving component (hydrophilic carboxyl) that sequesters fluid. As the dressing absorbs fluid, the hydrofiber consistency converts to a gel, weakening its tensile strength. Despite new stitching technology to reinforce the strength of the dressing, packing hydrofibers into deep sinuses and tunnels warrants careful monitoring to avoid material left in dead spaces.

For large volumes of exudate, incontinence products and fluid containment devices are effective in removing fluid and effluent from the skin surface; however, these products can be bulky. Creative use of ostomy pouches can be beneficial to patients with an active fistula.

When drainage volume exceeds the fluid handling capacity of dressings, enzyme-rich and caustic exudate may spill over to wound margins, causing maceration or tissue erosion and pain.[41] Irritant dermatitis is not uncommon from the damage of wound effluent; topical steroids continue to be the mainstay of therapy.

The moist and warm wound environment is also ideal for proliferation of fungi and yeast, including *Candida*. Individuals with coexisting conditions that affect the immune system (such as diabetes mellitus, kidney disease, and hepatitis C) or receiving immunosuppressive drugs (e.g., steroids) or chemotherapy are more susceptible to fungal infection. In addition, antibiotic use may disrupt the normal ecology of skin flora, permitting the overgrowth of fungi. Besides the typical raised red lesions with satellite lesions extending around the wound margin, the patient may complain of burning and itching. As a treatment option, *Candida* can be effectively treated with topical nystatin. For the treatment of infection related to fungi, terbinafine (Lamisil) has been shown to be the most effective. Clotrimazole cream is only effective against 70% to 80% of infections related to dermatophytes or yeasts, but it also possesses anti-inflammatory and minor antibacterial properties.[42]

S: Superficial Infection

All chronic wounds contain bacteria. Critical to wound management is whether bacterial balance is maintained (contamination or colonization) or bacterial damage (critical colonization or infection) has occurred.[30] In brief, *contamination* refers to bacteria on the surface of a wound. When bacteria attach to tissue and proliferate, colonization is established. Bacteria can cause local tissue damage in the superficial wound compartment. This is referred to as critical colonization, increased bacterial burden, covert infection, or localized infection. Some bacteria prefer the superficial and relatively hypoxic wound environment—not all species have the virulence to invade the deep compartment. When the bacteria invade and damage the surrounding and deeper structures, the classic signs and symptoms of deep tissue infection are revealed.[30]

Diagnosis of Wound Infection

The assessment of infection in a chronic wound is a bedside skill and the decision to prescribe antibiotics or apply topical antimicrobial agents should be based primarily on the clinical presentation. The clinical values of a culture should be limited to the identification of multiresistant bacteria such as methicillin-resistant *Staphylococcus aureus* (MRSA) and to determine the antimicrobial sensitivity of bacterial organisms associated with clinical infection.

Wound bacterial damage can be divided into superficial and deep component[43] (Figure 17-4, a color version of this figure can be found online at www.expertconsult.com). Signs of increased surface bacterial burden may include the signs represented by the letters in the mnemonic NERDS and of deep and surrounding-skin bacterial infection include the components of the mnemonic STONEES. The presence of three or more signs of NERDS or STONEES indicates probable superficial critical colonization or bacterial damage or deep infection, respectively. By focusing on salient clinical signs to separate superficial and deep compartment involvement, the clinician can consider therapeutic options that are most appropriate and cost-effective. Superficial bacterial burden can be reduced by topical antimicrobial agents, whereas deep and surrounding wound infection usually requires systemic antimicrobial therapies (69).[30]

Osteomyelitis should be suspected if ulcers probe to bone, especially in the neuropathic foot. Elevation of the erythrocyte sedimentation rate (ESR) and C-reactive protein (CRP), in the absence of other inflammatory conditions, are both valuable diagnostic indicators to validate the diagnosis of osteomyelitis[2] (see Table 17-2).

TREATMENT OF WOUND INFECTION

Debridement is a crucial step to remove devitalized tissue such as firm eschar or sloughy material, which serves as growth media for bacteria. Aggressive debridement is not recommended in malignant wounds in light of the potential risk of causing pain and bleeding and creating a larger and deeper portal for bacterial invasion.[44] Conservative debridement of nonhealable wounds may be appropriate by trimming loose fibrin to reduce necrotic mass and associated odor. The purpose of conservative debridement is to enhance quality of life and decrease the risk of bacterial proliferation and infection, not to facilitate healing.

Cleansing solutions, saline, and water are usually recommended to remove surface debris because of their low tissue toxicity. Topical antimicrobial products are available, but no one product is indicated or suitable for all patients.[2] Many active

		Definition/defining features	Comments
N	Non-healing wound 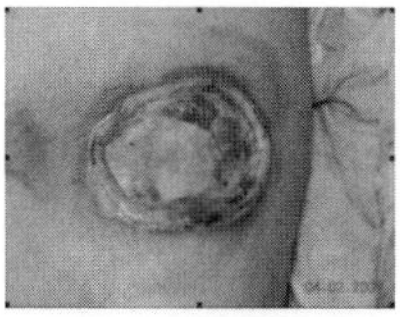	• Wounds that are not 20–40% smaller in 4 weeks according to patients' history or existing documentation	• Bacterial damage has caused an increased metabolic load in the chronic wound creating a pro-inflammatory wound environment that delays healing. • If the wound does not respond to topical antimicrobial therapy, consider a biopsy after 4 to 12 weeks to rule out an unsuspected diagnosis such as vasculitis, Pyoderma gangrenosum, or malignancy.
E	Exudative wound 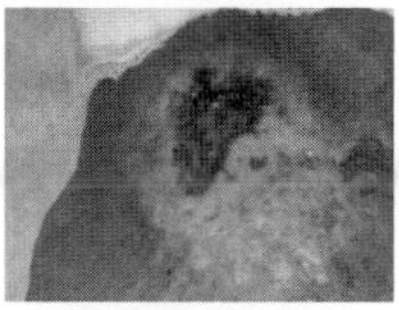	• An increase in wound exudate can be indicative of bacterial imbalance and leads to periwound maceration. • More than 50% of the dressing was tainted with exudate.	• Exudate is often clear before it becomes purulent or sanguineous. • Protect periwound area using the LOWE© memory jogger (Liquid film forming acrylate; Ointments; Windowed dressings; External collection devices) for Skin Barrier for Wound Margins.
R	Red & bleeding wound 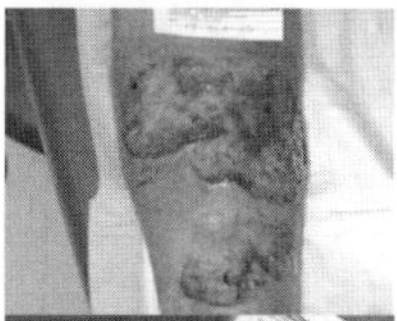 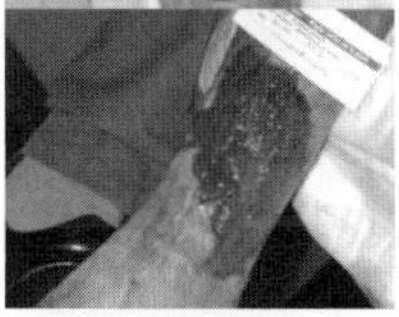	• The wound bed tissue is bright red with exuberant granulation tissues. • Tissue that is easy to bleed with gentle manipulation	• Granulation tissue should be pink and firm. The exuberant granulation tissue that is loose and bleeds easily reflects bacterial damage to the forming collagen matrix and an increased vasculature of the tissue.
D	Debris in wound 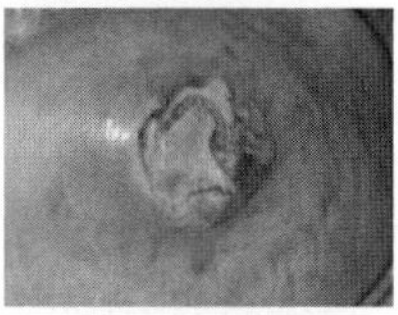	• Presence of discolouration of granulation tissue, sloughy, material and necrotic/non-viable tissue	• Necrotic tissue and debris in the wound is a food source for bacterial and can encourage a bacterial imbalance. • Necrotic tissue in the wound bed will require debridement.
S	Smell from the wound 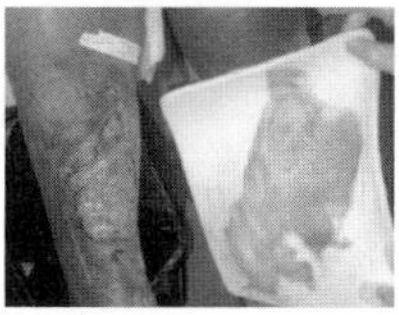	• Unpleasant or sweet sickening odour	• Smell from bacterial byproducts caused by tissue necrosis associated with the inflammatory response is indicative of bacterial damage. Metabolism of negative organisms and anaebrobe organisms can cause a putrid smell. Pseudomonas is associated with a sweet characteristic smell/green color.

Figure 17-4. NERDS and STONEES.
MRI, Magnetic resonance imaging.   *Continued*

		Definition/defining features	Comments
S	**Size is bigger**	• Wound size is increasing. • Size as measured by the longest length and the widest width at right angles to the longest length. Only very deep wounds need to have depth measured with a probe.	An increased size from bacterial damage is due to the bacteria spreading from the surface to the surrounding skin and the deeper compartment. This indicates that a combination of bacterial number and virulence has overwhelmed the host resistance.
T	**Temperature increased**	• Increased periwound margin temperature by more than 4 °F difference between two mirror image sites	Temperature differences can also be attributed to: • A difference in vascular supply (decreased circulation is colder) • Extensive deep tissue destruction (Acute Charot joint)
O	**Os (probes to or exposed bone)**	• Wounds that had exposed bone or that probed to bone	• High incidence of osteomyelitis if the wound is probed to the bone • X-rays, Bone Scans, and MRIs of underlying bone to confirm osteomyelitis
N	**New areas of breakdown**	• New areas of breakdown or satellite lesions	• Check for local damage and consider infection, increased exudate, or other sources of trauma.
E	**Erythema, Edema Exudate**	• Reddened skin in the peri-wound area • Presence of swelling in the periwound wound area • Increased amount of drainage	• With increased bacterial burden, exudate often increases in quantity and transforms from a clear or serous texture to frank purulence and may have a hemorrhagic component. The inflammation leads to vasodilatation (erythema) and the leakage of fluid into the tissue will result in edema. Match the absorbency of the dressing (none, low, moderate, heavy) to amount of exudate from the wound.
S	**Smell**	• Unpleasant or sweet sickening odour	• Systemic antimicrobial agents are indicated that will treat the causative organisms and devitalized tissue should be aggressively debrided in wounds with the ability to heal.

Figure 17-4, cont'd NERDS and STONEES.

MRI, Magnetic resonance imaging.

Table 17-4. Use of Silver Dressings

S	Signs of increased bacterial burden	Silver should be used when bacterial damage is a concern (differentiate superficial from deep wound infection using NERDS and STONEES signs).
I	Ionized silver	Only ionized silver exerts an antimicrobial effect. Requires an aqueous environment.
L	Log reduction over time	A quick kill time is desirable.
V	Vehicle for moisture balance	Select dressing materials to match moisture level.
E	Effects on viable cell	Watch for a toxic effect on viable cells.
R	Resistance	Resistance is rare. Three mutations are required to develop resistance to silver.

Woo & Sibbald 2007 ©[2]

ingredients in dressings are released into the wound surface compartment, but they require wound fluid or exudate to diffuse into the tissue. Despite the lack of randomized, controlled trials showing evidence of complete wound healing,[45] silver dressings are one of the most popular topical agents. For silver to exert an antimicrobial effect, it must be activated into ionic form in the presence of an aqueous wound environment, which is contraindicated for nonhealable wounds (Table 17-4).

Alternatively, bacteria can be entrapped and sequestered in the micro-architecture of a dressing, where they may be inactivated. In nonhealable wounds, when bacterial burden is of more concern than tissue toxicity, antiseptics such as povidone-iodine, chlorhexidine, and their derivatives are propitious treatment options[2] (Table 17-5). Unlike silver products, which require an aqueous environment to be released and activated, these antiseptics can exert their antimicrobial effect even in a relatively dry environment.

Other topical antimicrobial agents are summarized in Table 17-6. If the infection is promulgated systemically, systemic agents must be administered. Prophylactic use of antibiotics has not been demonstrated to facilitate wound healing.[46] All these agents except metronidazole and silver sulfadiazine creams have been associated with an increased incidence of allergic sensitization. Silver sulfadiazine (SSD) is not recommended to be used in patients with sulfa sensitivity. The documented rate of sensitization to silver sulfadiazine remains low, possibly because the sulfa molecule is bound in a large organic complex. Creams, ointments, and gels are antibacterial, but they do not have the autolytic debridement or moisture balance properties of moist interactive dressings. However, they are still excellent topical treatment options for some malignant and palliative nonhealable wounds.

Summary

Management of patients with malignant wounds is challenging. Key local wound care issues include hemorrhage, odor, pain, exudates, and superficial infection. A holistic approach is crucial to enhance the quality of life of patients suffering from malignant wounds.

Table 17-5. Antiseptic Agents

Class and Agent	Action	Effect on Healing	Effect on Bacteria	Comments
Alcohols Ethyl alcohol Isopropyl alcohol	Dehydrates proteins and dissolves lipids	Cytotoxic May cause dryness and irritation on intact skin	Bactericidal and viricidal	Used as a disinfectant on intact skin Not for use on open wounds (stings and burns)
Biguanides Chlorhexidine (≤2%) Polyhexamethylene biguanide (PHMB)	Acts by damaging cell membranes	Relatively safe Little effect on wound healing Toxicity: small effect on tissue	Highly bactericidal against gram-positive and gram-negative organisms	Highly effective as hand-washing agent and for surgical scrub Binds to stratum corneum and has prolonged residual effect
Halogen compounds Sodium hypochlorite (Hygeol, Eusol, Dakins)	Lyses cell walls	Acts as a chemical debrider and should be discontinued with healing tissue (high tissue toxicity)	Dakins solution and Eusol (buffered preparation) selective for gram-negative microorganisms	High pH causes irritation to skin
Organic iodine 10% povidone-iodine (Betadine)	Oxidizes cell constituents, especially sulfoxyl protein groups; iodinates and inactivates proteins	Povidone iodine Cytotoxicity depends on dilution Potential toxicity in vivo related to concentration and exposure	Prevents and controls bacterial growth in wounds No reports of resistance Broad-spectrum activity, but decreased in presence of pus/exudate	Toxicity concern with prolonged use or application over large areas Potential for thyroid toxicity (measure sTSH if used on large wounds for >3 months; relatively+ contraindicated in thyroid disease)
Organic acid Acetic acid (0.25%–1%) or diluted vinegar, (1 part vinegar, 5 parts water)	Lowers surface pH	Cytotoxic in vitro; concentration-dependent in vivo	Effective against *Pseudomonas* May be useful for other gram-negative rods and *S. aureus*	Often burns and stings on application; effect minimized with pain medication or neuropathy
Peroxides 3% Hydrogen peroxide	May induce cell death by oxidative damage	Can harm healthy granulation tissue May form air emboli if packed in deep sinuses	Very little to absent antimicrobial activity (only for seconds when fizzing)	Acts more like a chemical debriding agent by dissolving blood clots and softening slough Safety concerns with deep wounds (reports of air embolisms)

sTSH, sensitive thyroid-stimulating hormone.
Sibbald & Woo 2008 ©

Table 17-6. Topical Antimicrobial Agents

Agent	Vehicle	S. Aureus	Streptococcus	Pseudomonas	Anaerobe	Comments
Gentamicin sulphate cream, ointment	Alcohol cream base or petrolatum ointment	✓	✓	✓		Good broad-spectrum treatment for gram-negative organisms Discourage topical use due to increased resistance
Metronidazole cream/gel	Wax-glycerin cream and carbogel 940/propylene glycol gel				✓	Good anaerobe coverage and wound deodorizer
Mupirocin 2% cream, ointment	Polyethylene glycol (ointment)	✓	✓			Good for MRSA Excellent topical penetration Used predominantly via perirectal route, nasal colonization
Bacitracin zinc/polymyxin B sulfate (Polysporin)	White petrolatum ointment	✓	✓	✓		Broad spectrum Low cost Increased incidence of allergic sensitivity
Bacitracin zinc/neomycin/polymyxin B sulfate (Neosporin, Septa)	White petrolatum ointment	✓	✓	✓		Neomycin is potent sensitizer and may cross-react with other aminoglycosides in 40% of cases
Polymyxin B/gramicidin	Cream	✓	✓	✓		Broad-spectrum coverage
Silver sulfadiazine (SSD)	Water-miscible cream	✓	✓	✓		Short half life Neutropenia possible May leave pseudoeschar on wounds *Do not use in sulpha-sensitive individuals*

Sibbald & Woo 2007©

Resources

1. Cutting KF, White R: Defined and refined: criteria for identifying wound infection revisited, *Br J Community Nurs* 9(3):s6–s15, 2004.
2. Winter GD: Formation of the scab and the rate of epithelization of superficial wounds in the skin of the young domestic pig, *Nature* 193:293–294, 1962.
3. Hutchinson JJ, Lawrence JC: Wound infection under occlusive dressings, *J Hosp Infect* 17(2):83–94, 1991.
4. Sasseville D, Tennstedt D, Lachapelle JM: Allergic contact dermatitis from hydrocolloid dressings, *Am J Contact Derm* 8(4):236–238, 1997.
5. Vermeulen H, Ubbink D, Goossens A, et al: Dressings and topical agents for surgical wounds healing by secondary intention, *Cochrane Database Syst Rev* 2:CD003554, 2004.
6. Palfreyman SJ, Nelson EA, Lochiel R, et al: Dressings for healing venous leg ulcers, *Cochrane Database Syst Rev* 3:CD001103, 2006.
7. Briggs M, Torra I, Bou JE: Pain at wound dressing changes: a guide to management. In Pain at wound dressing changes, *EWMA Position Document*, 2002, 12–17. Available at www.ewma.org.

References

1. Woo K, Ayello EA, Sibbald RG: The edge effect: current therapeutic options to advance the wound edge, *Adv Skin Wound Care* 20(2):99–117, 2007.
2. Woo KY, Ayello EA, Sibbald RG: Silver versus other antimicrobial dressings: best practices, *Surg Technol Int* 17:50–71, 2008.
3. Langemo DK, Brown G: Skin fails too: acute, chronic, and end-stage skin failure, *Adv Skin Wound Care* 19(4):206–211, [Review.] 2006.
4. Sibbald RG, Woo KY, Ayello E: Wound bed preparation: DIM before DIME, *Wound Heal South Africa* 1(1):29–34, 2008.
5. O'Brien T, Welsh J, Dunn FG: ABC of palliative care. Non-malignant conditions, *Br Med J* 316(7127):286–289, 1998.
6. Liao S, Arnold RM: Wound care in advanced illness: application of palliative care principles, *J Palliat Med* 10(5):1159–1160, 2007.
7. Ferris FD, Al Khateib AA, Fromantin I, et al: Palliative wound care: managing chronic wounds across life's continuum: a consensus statement from the International Palliative Wound Care Initiative, *J Palliat Med* 10(1):37–39, 2007.
8. Naylor W: Malignant wounds: aetiology and principles of management, *Nurs Stand* 11–17;16(52):45–53, 2002.
9. Alexander S: Malignant fungating wounds: epidemiology, aetiology, presentation and assessment, *J Wound Care* 18(7):273–274, 276–278, 280, [Review.] 2009.
10. Maida V, Corbo M, Dolzhykov M, et al: Wounds in advanced illness: a prevalence and incidence study based on a prospective case series, *Int Wound J* 5(2):305–314, 2008.
11. Lookingbill DP, Spangler N, Sexton FM: Skin involvement as the presenting sign of internal carcinoma. A retrospective study of 7316 cancer patients, *J Am Acad Dermatol* 22(1):19–26, 1990.
12. Lookingbill DP, Spangler N, Helm KF: Cutaneous metastases in patients with metastatic carcinoma: a retrospective study of 4020 patients, *J Am Acad Dermatol* 29(2 Pt 1):228–236, 1993.
13. Esther RJ, Lamps L, Schwartz HS: Marjolin ulcers: secondary carcinomas in chronic wounds, *J South Orthop Assoc* 8(3):181–187, 1999.
14. Schiech L: Malignant cutaneous wounds, *Clin J Oncol Nurs* 6(5):305–309, 2002.
15. Walton A, Broadbent AL: Radiation-induced second malignancies, *J Palliat Med* 11(10):1345–1352, 2008.
16. Grocott P: Care of patients with fungating malignant wounds, *Nurs Stand* 21(24):57–58, 60, 62, 2007.
17. McDonald A, Lesage P: Palliative management of pressure ulcers and malignant wounds in patients with advanced illness, *J Palliat Med* 9(2):285–295, [Review.] 2006.
18. Probst S, Arber A, Faithfull S: Malignant fungating wounds: a survey of nurses' clinical practice in Switzerland, *Eur J Oncol Nurs* 13(4):295–298, 2009.
19. Schulz V, Triska OH, Tonkin K: Malignant wounds: caregiver-determined clinical problems, *J Pain Symptom Manage* 24(6):572–577, 2002.
20. Langemo DK, Black J, National Pressure Ulcer Advisory Panel: pressure ulcers in individuals receiving palliative care: a National Pressure Ulcer Advisory Panel white paper, *Adv Skin Wound Care* 23(2):59–72, 2010.
21. Krapfl LA, Gray M: Does regular repositioning prevent pressure ulcers? *J Wound Ostomy Continence Nurs* 35(6):571–577, [Review.] 2008.

22. Chasen MR, Bhargava R: A descriptive review of the factors contributing to nutritional compromise in patients with head and neck cancer, *Support Care Cancer* 17(11):1345–1351, [Review.] 2009.

23. Dorner B, Posthauer ME, Thomas D, National Pressure Ulcer Advisory Panel: The role of nutrition in pressure ulcer prevention and treatment: National Pressure Ulcer Advisory Panel white paper, *Adv Skin Wound Care* 22(5):212–221, [Review.] 2009.

24. Woo KY, Sibbald RG: The ABCs of skin care for wound care clinicians: dermatitis and eczema, *Adv Skin Wound Care* 22(5):230–236; quiz 237–238, 2009.

25. Stephen Haynes J: An overview of caring for those with palliative wounds, *Br J Community Nurs* 13(12):S24, S26, S28 passim, [Review.] 2008.

26. Adderley U, Smith R: Topical agents and dressings for fungating wounds, *Cochrane Database Syst Rev* 18(2):CD003948, [Review.] 2007.

27. Spaner DE, Miller RL, Mena J, et al: Regression of lymphomatous skin deposits in a chronic lymphocytic leukemia patient treated with the Toll-like receptor-7/8 agonist, imiquimod, *Leuk Lymphoma* 46(6):935–939, 2005.

28. Lo SF, Hu WY, Hayter M, et al: Experiences of living with a malignant fungating wound: a qualitative study, *J Clin Nurs* 17(20):2699–2708, 2008.

29. Keller VF, Carroll JG: A new model for physician-patient communication, *Patient Educ Couns* 23:131-140, 1994.

30. Sibbald RG, Woo K, Ayello EA: Increased bacterial burden and infection: the story of NERDS and STONES, *Advance Wound Care* 19(8):447–461, 2006.

31. Woo KY, Harding K, Price P, Sibbald G: Minimising wound-related pain at dressing change: evidence-informed practice, *Int Wound J* 5(2):144–157, 2008.

32. Harris DG, Noble SI. Management of terminal hemorrhage in patients with advanced cancer: a systematic literature review, *J Pain Symptom Manage* 38(6):913–927, 2009.

33. Paul JC, Pieper BA: Topical metronidazole for the treatment of wound odor: a review of the literature, *Ostomy Wound Manage* 54(3):18–27, quiz 28–29, [Review.] 2008.

34. Ubbink DT, Vermeulen H, Goossens A, et al: Occlusive vs gauze dressings for local wound care in surgical patients: a randomized clinical trial, *Arch Surg* 143(10):950–995, 2008.

35. Woo K, Sibbald G, Fogh K, et al: Assessment and management of persistent (chronic) and total wound pain, *Int Wound J* 5(2):205–221, 2008.

36. Woo KY, Sibbald RG, Ayello EA, et al: Peristomal skin complications and management, *Adv Skin Wound Care* 22(11):522–532; 2009.

37. Gottrup F, Jørgensen B, Karlsmark T, et al: Reducing wound pain in venous leg ulcers with Biatain Ibu: a randomized, controlled double-blind clinical investigation on the performance and safety, *Wound Repair Regen* 16(5):615–625, 2008.

38. Evans E, Gray M: Do topical analgesics reduce pain associated with wound dressing changes or debridement of chronic wounds? *J Wound Ostomy Continence Nurs* 32(5):287–290, 2005.

39. Woo KY: Meeting the challenges of wound-associated pain: anticipatory pain, anxiety, stress, and wound healing, *Ostomy Wound Manage* 54(9):10–12, 2008.

40. Woo KY, Sibbald RG: Chronic wound pain: a conceptual model, *Adv Skin Wound Care* 21(4):175–188; quiz 189–190, 2008.

41. Okan D, Woo K, Ayello EA, Sibbald G: The role of moisture balance in wound healing, *Adv Skin Wound Care* 20(1):39–53, 2007.

42. Alavi A, Woo K, Sibbald RG: Common nail disorders and fungal infections, *Adv Skin Wound Care* 20(6):358–359, 2007.

43. Woo KY, Sibbald RG: A cross-sectional validation study of using NERDS and STONEES to assess bacterial burden, *Ostomy Wound Manage* 55(8):40–48, 2009.

44. Kirshen C, Woo K, Ayello EA, Sibbald RG: Debridement: a vital component of wound bed preparation, *Adv Skin Wound Care* 19(9):506–517, 2006.

45. Vermeulen H, van Hattem JM, Storm-Versloot MN, Ubbink DT: Topical silver for treating infected wounds, *Cochrane Database Syst Rev* 24(1):CD005486, [Review.] 2007.

46. O'Meara SM, Cullum NA, Majid M, Sheldon TA: Systematic review of antimicrobial agents used for chronic wounds, *Br J Surg* 88(1):4–21, [Review.] 2001.

PART C

Personal Contexts

CHAPTER 18

Loss, Bereavement, and Adaptation

SARA J. KNIGHT and LINDA L. EMANUEL

Approaches to grief for bereaved family members are an important focus of theoretical, empirical, and clinical work in palliative care. However, it is essential also to focus on the experiences of the dying person as losses occur in health, physical and mental function, and social roles and responsibilities. A conceptual framework for how a person adapts to losses can provide a road map for how to intervene effectively in palliative care. We therefore describe a reintegration model that includes comprehension, creative adaptation, and reintegration processes for adapting to losses at the end of life. We describe adjustment processes from both the perspectives of the dying person and the bereaved survivor. For each, we consider the implications of adjustment processes for the palliative care team and for families and others with significant relationships. We provide examples of how caregivers can use knowledge of adjustment processes to provide focused interventions aimed at improving decision making and the quality of care at the end of life (Table 18-1).

Brief Overview of Adaptive Processes

News about a terminal prognosis, the experience of functional decline, and an acute health crisis are among the losses commonly experienced by persons approaching the end of life. Significant others may experience the same news and events as losses, and they also experience the death, the funeral, and other rituals and face continuing in life without the deceased. For both it is often a time of multiple accumulating

Table 18-1. Reintegration Model: Process, Experience, and Activities of Palliative Care

Process	Patient Experience	Key Activities of Palliative Care Team
Comprehension		
Realize the loss	Shock, numbness, sadness, anxiety	Empathic listening
	Awareness of the loss	Verbal and nonverbal support
		Discussion of the practical consequences of the loss
	Uncertain goals and values	Avoidance of premature decision making
Creative adaptation		
Explore ways of living without what was lost	Ambivalence, mixed emotions	Discussion of alternatives for living
	Exploration and experimentation through action and imagination with new or alternate ways of living without what was lost	Support for efforts to try adaptive behaviors
	Changing values, goals, preferences	Tolerance for changing emotions and ambivalence
		Support for distress
	Life review and legacy building	Values clarification, if decisions need to be made
		Education for family members and significant others
Reintegration		
Consolidate revised self-concept and view of life without what was lost	Emotional equilibrium	Encouragement and support for revised self-concept and new ways of living
	Consolidation of revised self-concept and new ways of living	
	Stable values, goals, preferences	Reevaluation of decisions for care made during comprehension and creative adaptation

losses interspersed with periods of recovery and gains in strength and stability, followed by further loss.

Losses that occur close to the end of life can precipitate great distress. Yet these losses have the potential to stimulate psychological growth. For both the person who is close to the end of life and the survivor, these experiences can provide opportunities to resolve conflict in relationships, heighten spiritual awareness, and offer new perspectives on living. In the following section we describe adjustment processes, comprehension, creative adaptation, and reintegration from the perspectives of the dying person and the bereaved survivor. We present a conceptual framework, termed the *reintegration model,* to understand the adjustment processes of the dying person, and we consider relevant conceptual and empirical research on bereavement.[1] For each, we discuss implications for palliative care.

Losses for the Dying Person

The trajectory to death differs according to the type of illness or injury. For some patients, the path involves a rapid decline to death; others experience a series of acute crises followed by periods of relatively stable health; still others see a slow deterioration in function and well-being.[2] Adjustment to the losses that occur along any of these trajectories begins when the dying person becomes aware of limitations in function, well-being, and life. Awareness of end-of-life loss can occur when a person observes an acute, noticeable deterioration in function or compares a gradual decline with a previous higher level of health. This awareness can also occur when a person receives news of a terminal prognosis from clinicians or a referral to hospice care. A significant characteristic of many end-of-life losses is that they are irreversible; the person will not recover the previous level of function or well-being. A related characteristic is that many losses close to the end of life are associated with awareness of impending death.

When a person becomes aware of an end-of-life loss, adjustment occurs across several domains. A person may adjust physically, as when a walker is used to compensate for weakness in the legs or unsteady gait. Other adjustments may be psychological, social, or spiritual. For example, a person who is unable to work because of advanced pulmonary disease may focus greater attention on those close relationships with family and friends. With the loss of work, self-concept may shift from an emphasis on oneself as a worker to views of oneself in other roles such as friend, partner, or parent. Purpose in life may be realized through one's relationships with family, humanity, nature, or a higher power rather than through contributions at work. With greater awareness of impending death, meaning may be found through leaving one's legacy to loved ones, through considering beliefs about what happens after death, and through awareness of spiritual connections. These physical, psychological, social, and existential or spiritual domains are consistent with those that Cicely Saunders identified some three decades ago at the outset of the hospice movement, and they have been incorporated into contemporary conceptual models of palliative care.[3,4] We describe three processes—comprehension, creative adaptation, and reintegration—that occur across these four domains as people adjust to losses at the end of life, and we discuss how palliative care professionals can use understanding of these processes to improve end-of-life care.

COMPREHENSION

Theories of coping with stress postulate that an appraisal process occurs after the onset of stress.[5] Appraisal serves to evaluate the characteristics of the stressful situation and to assess the resources one has to cope with it. Similarly, when a person observes deterioration in health and function or receives "bad news" in terms of prognosis, we suggest that he or she engage in a process of *comprehension* that identifies the experience as an irreversible loss. To adapt to functional decline, a person has to interpret diminishing abilities as an irreversible loss. Some losses may be so gradual that they are not interpreted as such. Other losses may appear temporary. For example, a fall and a fractured hip may be interpreted as a short-term setback in life. Conversely, if this injury signifies a sequence of losses leading to death, the comprehension process for irreversible loss may be initiated.

The emotional experience associated with comprehension includes shock, numbness, sadness, and anxiety. However, it is possible for a person to experience a range of positive responses as well as negative affect. For example, a person may feel relieved when the loss eliminates responsibility that is no longer manageable. Anger, sadness, relief, and regret may represent the range of emotion for a frail elderly man who has been struggling for several years to maintain independent living when a fall and broken hip result in a transition to long-term care. Regardless of the emotion, during comprehension, the loss itself is highly salient cognitively and behaviors are directed toward determining that a loss has occurred (e.g., asking questions about prognosis, requesting information about what to expect in the future). Recognition of what will be missed and evaluation of the importance of what is lost to the person's identity, in turn, disrupt equilibrium across the core domains. For example, a loss in the physical domain, such as in congestive heart failure, initiates activity in the psychological domain about what this means in terms of ability to work or care for oneself, the ability to think of oneself as an independent person, the need for assistance from others, the relevance of the health prognoses of family members, and the meaning of heart disease in terms of one's religious or spiritual beliefs. These psychological activities contribute to further disruption in the social and existential domains. Especially when a loss is realized suddenly and is central to a person's self-concept, comprehension may be associated with acute stress responses in the physical domain. In addition, because of the effort needed to process the loss, a person may appear to be self-focused, having little energy for other people and low capacity for making decisions about care and living situations.

For seriously ill people, comprehending loss may be made more difficult by cognitive impairment related to medications or disease. Similarly, comprehension cannot be expected to occur if caregivers withhold prognostic news. In addition, the type of loss is an important factor that influences the comprehension process. Losses associated with shame or stigma may be particularly difficult to process emotionally. For example, in many Western cultures where people take pride in independence, shame associated with becoming more dependent on others (e.g., needing assistance with dressing, bathing, and toileting) may make it difficult for a person to experience fully his or her feelings about the loss of independence, and therefore to engage in comprehension processes.

Palliative care clinicians can support the person by allowing the time and space for comprehension processes to occur. Clinicians can expect that the person who has experienced the loss may have many and repeated questions about what has happened and what it means for life and living. Clinicians can provide opportunities for the person to think about the loss, to discuss his or her perception of the news, to ask questions about what the loss means in practical terms, and to confer with significant others. The onset of a loss often becomes a time when health care decisions need to be made about a new treatment approach or the start of hospice care. The person who is in the process of understanding the loss and what it means may not have the cognitive capacity to evaluate alternatives and to make informed choices at this time. It may be useful for the clinician to allow comprehension to occur before engaging the person in clinical decision making. If a decision about care or living arrangements cannot be delayed, then it may be important to provide additional support to the person by involving significant others, focusing attention on most likely alternatives, and allowing the person to reevaluate the decision once he or she fully comprehends the loss and its implications.

CREATIVE ADAPTATION

Once a loss is comprehended as something that cannot be restored completely, a person begins a transition to living without what has been lost. We term this process *creative adaptation*. The person may experiment, through action and imagination, with new ways of thinking about oneself and living without what has been lost. New relationships may be formed, or new ways of interacting and being in existing relationships may occur. For example, a person who has fatigue and functional decline that affects mobility may develop alternate means of maintaining important social relationships. The case study in Box 18-1 illustrates the processes of adaptation.

Although several researchers have proposed that awareness of impending death is an important, if not necessary, stage of adjustment to dying, more recent work suggests that most people fluctuate in their awareness of death, and some never reach a state of complete awareness or avowal of impending death. It is not clear that awareness or acknowledgement of imminent death is necessary for good psychological adjustment during dying.[6,7] However, when a loss is interpreted as leading to death, the transition that occurs with creative adaptation incorporates the idea of dying and death. Some people may imagine what it is like to die, and many have fears as they envision this process. The process of dying and what happens at and after death may be considered with new awareness and immediacy.

An important aspect of the creative adaptation process is that it involves experimenting with novel thoughts and behaviors, as well as drawing on existing skills and abilities. This type of coping has been described previously in the literature on aging and in reports on studies of disability.[8,9] When losses occur close to the end of life, previous avenues of coping are no longer available, and ultimately when a person is close to death, few options for new behaviors or ways of relating to others may appear to be open. The only possibility for adaptation at these times may be to find new psychological or spiritual perspectives. This approach may involve leaving a legacy to loved ones; reviewing one's life, experiences, and accomplishments; or considering beliefs about what happens after death with an immediacy and urgency that was not possible before facing death so closely.

During the creative adaptation process, new self-perspectives emerge that transcend previous self-concepts.[10] A person who focused earlier in life on work and the meaning in life that is derived from work contributions may have a renewed appreciation of family relationships and close friendships. The perspective of earlier roles and self-concepts becomes one of the past rather than the present (e.g., "I once was an engineer, and now I am…"). Although new perspectives develop during creative adaptation, this process is one of shifting affect, behavior, and self-concepts. A person's values, goals, and preferences are likely to be in flux at this time. During the time that new behaviors and perspectives are being tested, it may be difficult for the person to express stable preferences for activities or care.

Caregivers, including palliative care clinicians, can support a person during creative adaptation by accepting the person's ambivalence through acknowledgement of changing emotions, by supporting the person's exploration of alternatives for living through empathic listening and focused discussion, and by allowing for changes in plans of action as the person's needs evolve. Creative adaptation can be distressing for the person as well as for significant others, and family members may

BOX 18-1. CASE STUDY

B. G. was a 58-year-old man who lived alone and started therapy for metastatic malignant melanoma, but he found that he did not have the energy, attention, or concentration to work full time in his job as a vice president of a publishing company. He scaled back his responsibilities and, with some difficulty, continued in his position. Although his part-time work schedule allowed him greater time to rest, he was no longer included in the decision making of the inner management of the firm. B. G. found this highly discouraging and told his doctors that he was considering ending therapy early, before he had received the recommended dose. His doctor listened to him express his frustration and his desire to discontinue treatment. They discussed options and described what they thought were the advantages and disadvantages of each. After serious consideration of the alternatives, B. G. decided to continue on his current course. He felt that his physician understood his situation and supported him in considering the possible options fully.

When his disease progressed following his initial treatment, B. G. started an alternate treatment course and left his position at the publishing company. At this time, B. G. was aware that his prognosis was poor and that he was not expected to live beyond the year. Most of his social relationships were with coworkers at his firm, and his few family members lived at some distance away. He felt lonely and dispirited on days at home, and as he thought about dying, he ruminated about what he had not been able to accomplish in his life. Initially, he attended a support group at his hospital, and although this offered connections to others, he missed the sense of importance that he had always found in his work. After a call from an old friend with whom he had lost touch, he started writing letters that reestablished closeness with friends he had not seen in more than a decade. The friends who knew B. G. before his success as a publisher reminded him of the many ways in which his life had mattered to them. Through the letters, he became engaged in telling his story, and he often illustrated his letters with line drawings and watercolors, activities that he had always enjoyed and that he could do even with reduced concentration. The renewed means of self-expression and his reaching out to others became a way that B. G. reestablished self-worth and identity apart from work roles and contributions. As B. G. reflected on his life, he was able to think of himself as someone who had made a difference to his friends and family. He came to think of his letters as part of his legacy.

B. G.'s experience illustrates the creative adaptation process, which for him started with losses in his ability to work, and depicts the exploration of alternative ways of living and finding meaning that are characteristic of this process. As shown in this example, creative adaptation may involve struggles to maintain earlier roles and activities and unsuccessful attempts to find new ways of coping. At times, the struggle to find ways of coping with loss may result in conflict with others. In this example, the clinician caring for B. G. was able to avoid conflict by supporting B. G. in an exploration of what it could mean to discontinue treatment. For B. G., the creative adaptation process ultimately contributed to revisions in his self-concept that incorporated a past-tense view of himself in a specific job and reaffirmed a broader image of himself as a writer and friend.

have difficulty understanding the person's shifting preferences and plans. It may be important for clinicians to provide emotional support and education during creative adaptation to reduce distress and to minimize potential sources of conflict. As avenues for new behaviors become severely curtailed close to the end of life, life review and legacy building activities may be important sources of finding new ways of living through transcendence of earlier self-concepts. Especially as the person develops greater awareness of dying, it becomes important to answer questions about the dying process and to provide opportunities to talk about what happens at death and after death. When decisions need to be made, values clarification may be important because core beliefs may be reevaluated during creative adaptation as the person adjusts to the loss.

REINTEGRATION

Finally, a process of *reintegration* occurs that consolidates the new perspectives, adjustments in social relationships, and new behaviors. Whereas the comprehension and creative adaptation processes are characterized by realization of a loss, transition, and experimentation, reintegration rebuilds the stability of the revised self-concept, expectancies about the future, and goals. In contrast to the flux in preferences that occurs during creative adaptation as the person experiments with alternatives for living, there is continuity in values and goals during reintegration.

Reintegration allows for greater psychological and social stability, and a person in this process may feel more "settled." We see this as a process rather than as an outcome at the end of life for several reasons. First, in contrast to a stable state, the consolidation that occurs during reintegration is an ongoing activity that involves the enactment and validation of the revised self-concept, worldview, and new course of living. Second, in many situations of deteriorating health, it is likely that new losses will occur, resulting in reiterative cycles of comprehension, creative adaptation, and reintegration.

The palliative care team can support the person during reintegration by providing affirmation of the revised self-concept and new ways of living and by offering practical support that helps the person to stabilize function and well-being. Because values and preferences change during creative adaptation and stabilize during reintegration, it may be important for palliative care clinicians to work with the person to reevaluate important decisions about care. Choices made during comprehension and creative adaptation may no longer be consistent with the revised self-concept and goals that emerge during reintegration.

Journey through the Processes

The successful adaptive processes can be thought of as generally progressive, in which the primary direction of movement is from comprehension to creative adaptation and from creative adaptation to reintegration. However, like other psychological and behavioral adaptations, this is often a recursive process that includes iterations. Similar recursive processes have been described in the literature on bereavement and in previous work on adaptation at the end of life.[11,12] Thus, during a process that is overall one of creative adaptation, a person may return to the comprehension process (i.e., realization that the loss has occurred). Similarly, during reintegration, a person may return to the creative adaptation processes (i.e., experimentation with new possibilities for the future without what was lost). Return to an earlier aspect rather than unidirectional progression may occur when a person has not reached equilibrium or when that person's resources are not sufficient to handle the demands of processing the loss. It may also be possible to enter the creative adaptive process or even reintegration and then confront the comprehension process, perhaps little by little, later on. A dying person may not possess the psychological, social, existential, or physical resources needed to progress completely or linearly toward reintegration when multiple significant losses are experienced in rapid succession. Alternatively, that person's sense of depletion may enhance his or her ability to let go and progress to departure-oriented adaptations. If the losses are compiled to such an extent that adaptation is overwhelmed and then blocked, complex or maladaptive responses may arise. These possibilities will require further investigations in the future.

The features of the comprehension, creative adaptation, and reintegration processes that are characteristic of dying may be characterized by the specific challenges, roles, tasks, and opportunities of the final life stage. For instance, people can attain a state of giving, and all the reciprocity that results from it, that may be dependent on knowing that there is no use gathering things or relationships or roles for themselves that can no longer be; or they may attain a spiritual state that is heightened by the imminent end of life; or they may discover relationships of dependence as a result of their physical state that give them unexpected difficulty or gratification.

The final dying process has some unique features in that the adaptation process involves a nonrecursive handing over to family, friends, and others. This process has been described as "leaving a legacy".[10,13] However, we see this as part of a broader process sometimes described as *self-transcendence,* a diminishing emphasis on independent functioning as an individual as one loses physical capabilities, functional abilities, and social relationships, contrasted with an emerging emphasis on the creative use of dependence and spiritual connections. In the end-of-life experience the patient may reach a point, through comprehension processes, in which he or she acknowledges death as imminent, and the patient may let go. Family members and friends may even be involved in giving permission, by telling the dying person that it is all right to die. Hospice and palliative care workers often describe a kind of withdrawal when the dying person may talk to dead relatives or friends and may seem less engaged in the living world.[14] The creative adaptation and reintegration processes of the real-time world are left to the living as they transition into bereavement and carry forward the dying person's legacy as part of the final reintegration pathway.

Growth and Development Near the End of Life

Some commentators describe the phenomenon of growth and development among elders and those near the end of life and among their loved ones.[10,15,16] Age, illness, and the adjustment processes may trigger the growth, and it is often highly valued. The ability to engage in life review and to make a connection to those expected to live on, whether with a legacy document made in a process called dignity therapy or in some other way, is highly fulfilling to both patients and loved ones.[16,17] It can be helpful for the clinician to think of the patient and loved ones having roles to fulfill, because these roles carry tasks and relationships that can guide the parties through this difficult life stage. For instance, the person in the dying role has jobs to do that include passing on his or her life story, gleanings, and wisdoms (these could be small gestures of love such as passing on cooking recipes); preparing the loved ones for living without him or her; passing on roles such as leading the family business or being care provider to a minor; making practical plans for care decisions if unable to communicate; and making practical after-death arrangements. Often the least tangible are the most important: settling fraught relationships, saying "I love you," or giving a blessing (of whatever nature) to relevant people. People who have started to withdraw but then realized they have these tasks to do often rally, gain gratification, and even continue to live well for some time; that is, foreseeable death is not necessary for entering these roles. Those who are close to the dying person usually appreciate these activities as gifts of great value and often find that these communications ease the transition to life without their loved one. It also may be that the states of mind that these types of activities both engender and foster help with prudent care decisions. Some have termed these types of settled states of mind equanimity and existential maturity.[18,19] The task of the clinician is to know the importance of these activities and to facilitate the circumstances that allow them— whether by arranging for home care, through family visits, by offering prompting reading materials, or by engaging in relevant prompting conversations.

Factors that Influence Adjustment

Various factors influence the course of adjustment to and quality of end-of-life losses. These range from the type of illness or injury to psychological and social factors, including developmental stage, previous experience with loss, personality, social support network, and spiritual beliefs and practices. For example, a person whose illness is characterized by a gradual decline in function may slowly become aware of significant losses over time and may have little need to make major adjustments in quick succession. For this person, comprehension of losses may be gradual and associated with little distress. Creative adaptation may involve little exploration of new avenues for functioning, and reintegration may involve little change in self-concept. In contrast, a person who has rapidly progressing metastatic breast cancer may suddenly lose the ability to walk because of fractures and may experience a rapid cascade of other losses, including work and social activities. The loss of mobility, for this person, may require major shifts in her roles, responsibilities, and relationships. The ramifications of a sudden and significant loss may be difficult to comprehend and may be accompanied by greater distress. Creative adaptation may involve a larger struggle to find new ways of functioning and meaning in life, and reintegration may require more time for consolidation of a revised self-concept once alternate ways of living are established.

Depression, anxiety, and other psychiatric disorders can limit a person's ability to engage in the adjustment processes. For example, a person with a severe major depression may not have the energy or cognitive flexibility to envision alternative ways of functioning as a part of creative adaptation. For seriously ill people, adjustment may be impeded by cognitive impairment, related medications, or disease. Moreover, failure to comprehend a loss is often discussed in the context of denial, a coping process that is thought to protect a person from information associated with intense, painful affect.[20] In this sense, adaptation to a loss may vary according to a person's ability to be aware of and to process painful information.

Losses for the Bereaved Survivor

Theoretical perspectives have offered frameworks for understanding why we grieve. Bowlby suggested that grief occurs when an attachment necessary to one's safety and security is disrupted.[21] Others have conceived grief as a part of the healing process, reestablishing equilibrium in a person's life after the loss of a loved one. Most theories conceptualize grief as multidimensional, encompassing emotional (e.g., sadness, anxiety, anger), physical (e.g., loss of appetite, fatigue), cognitive (e.g., preoccupation, confusion), and behavioral (e.g., restlessness, searching) sensations and experiences. The type of loss and closeness of the relationship are significant factors in the intensity and duration of grief. For some losses, grief continues for 6 months to several years. Grief may continue longer in some situations, such as the death of a child. Other factors that determine the duration of grief include the mode of death (e.g., natural or traumatic), historical antecedents (e.g., depression, stress), personality variables (e.g., coping and resilience), and social and cultural context (e.g., traditions, rituals, social network).

Clinicians have long observed that thoughts, emotions, and behaviors evolve during the grief process. Kubler-Ross proposed that grief occurs in stages: denial, anger, bargaining, depression, and acceptance.[22] Although this theory has been important in its recognition of grief as a multifaceted and developmental process, it has been criticized for its limitations. It does not appear that grief involves all these stages or that people progress linearly through the stages. However, a similar conceptual framework often cited as being clinically useful is that of Worden,[23] who suggested four tasks of grief:

1. Accepting the reality of the loss
2. Experiencing the pain of grief
3. Adjusting to an environment in which the deceased is missing
4. Withdrawing emotional energy from the deceased and reinvesting in other relationships

According to Worden's framework, immediately after the death of a loved one, it is critical for the bereaved to accept that the loss has occurred and that it is irreversible. The second task involves the bereaved's experiencing the pain of grief, such as sadness, anxiety, and anger. Although more recent work on bereavement suggests that the range of emotional response to the death of a loved one is wide, this model indicates that both cognitive processing and affective processing of a significant loss are important. The third task involves adjusting to an environment without the deceased. This task involves both practical accommodations and psychological adjustments. For example, the bereaved may need to find ways of meeting the responsibilities that had been previously handled by the deceased. The fourth and final task of grief involves disengaging from the relationship with the deceased and becoming involved in other relationships or endeavors.

Worden and others defined benchmarks from which to judge the resolution of the grief process.[23,24] One indication is when the bereaved is able to talk about the deceased without intense, fresh feelings of loss. Another is when the survivor is able to invest energy in new relationships, roles, and responsibilities without the disabling guilt and feelings of disloyalty toward the deceased. Previous theories described processes, called masked grief and delayed grief, characterized by the lack of experience or lack of expression of emotions in response to significant loss. These views raised concern that suppression or displacement of emotions associated with a loss would lead to subsequent depression. However, Bonanno and Kaltman found that psychological resilience is more common during bereavement than previously thought.[25] This work suggested multiple trajectories for the grief process, including those that involve little intense, negative emotional experience throughout the course and those that involve psychological growth.

Interventions for the Bereaved

Clinicians can support a grieving person in several ways. Before the loss, clinicians can encourage significant others to spend time with their loved one who is dying and can acknowledge the importance of these relationships. Clinicians can show appreciation for the contributions of the significant others to caregiving and to the well-being of the dying person. Immediately after a loss, it is important to provide a time and place for the bereaved to express feelings. Clinicians can extend sympathy, support cultural rituals, encourage reminiscing, and listen to the bereaved talk about the deceased.

During the weeks and months before and after the death, clinicians can provide education and communicate that painful feelings about a loss, such as sadness and anxiety, are understandable. It may be valuable to confirm that ambivalent feelings (e.g., sorrow and anger, anxiety and relief) in grief are common because most relationships have difficult times as well as wonderful ones. It can alleviate guilt if the clinician clarifies that anticipatory grief (i.e., occurring in expectation of the loss) is a normal response. As the bereaved adjusts to life without the deceased, clinicians can provide support in problem solving. This may involve discussing the survivor's new roles, helping the survivor to reorganize overwhelming tasks into small steps, and identifying sources of social support. Ultimately, when the bereaved is ready, clinicians can encourage investment in new relationships. Although many individuals do not need professional counseling for grief, they may benefit from opportunities to receive education about the grief process, to express emotions with others who have similar feelings, and to receive guidance with problem solving during adjustment to life without the deceased.

Grief and Clinical Depression

Grief can occur without clinical depression. However, depression can develop during the grieving process, and preexisting depression can complicate grief. Because both grief and depression are associated with intense, low mood, difficulty with the experience of pleasure, sleep disturbance, and appetite loss, it may be difficult to distinguish between them. Although a full depressive reaction may accompany a normal grief response, grief typically does not include the loss of self-esteem, worthlessness, or overall sense of guilt that characterizes depression. The depressed person has consistently low mood or an absence of emotion, has little enthusiasm for previously enjoyable activities, and has little interest in others. In contrast, the grieving person has variable emotions and is likely to shift from being able to enjoy some activities to refusing activities and from wanting to be with others to preferring to be alone.

PEARLS

- Introduce the idea of loss and creative adaptation early in the course of illness to assist people near the end of life and their loved ones with coping resources during each transition.

- During comprehension processes, allow time for the patient and family members to realize that a loss has occurred before they make final decisions about care.

- Acknowledge that a range of emotions (e.g., numbness, sadness, anger, anxiety, relief), some quite intense and variable, may follow awareness of loss for both the dying person and loved ones.

- Recognize that during creative adaptation processes, a patient's preferences for care may fluctuate as various adaptive strategies are considered.

- Revisit decisions about care during reintegration processes when adaptive strategies, self-concept, and preferences are relatively stable.

- Identify psychological, social, and spiritual distress.

- Involve a mental health professional early in the course of persistent depression, anxiety, and other distress symptoms.

PITFALLS

- Health care policies and other health system pressures may influence clinicians to ask for final decisions about care before dying persons and their loved ones have fully comprehended a loss.

- Because negative emotions can be difficult to tolerate and positive emotions may be missed close to the end of life, clinicians may fail to affirm the full range of affect experienced by dying persons and their loved ones.

- During the creative adaptation process, clinicians and families may find that it is difficult to accept and to work with the fluctuating adaptive strategies and values of dying persons.

- During the reintegration process, it is possible to miss the opportunity to confirm previous decisions about care.

- Because the mental health needs of dying persons and their loved ones may be less clearly expressed than other needs for support, clinicians may have difficulty recognizing opportunities to address persistent psychological, social, and spiritual distress that emerges close to the end of life.

Summary

The losses of function, health, and well-being that occur at the end of life are among the most stressful of human experiences, and palliative care clinicians have little theoretical or empirical literature on which to base interventions. In this chapter, we describe adjustment to end-of-life losses from the perspective of the dying person. Awareness of a significant, irreversible loss, particularly one that signals a decline toward dying and death, can initiate adjustment processes that include comprehension, creative adaptation, and reintegration aspects. Clinicians can intervene more effectively in the care of the dying if their communications are guided by awareness of the adjustment process in which a person is engaged at a particular time. Worden's tasks of grief provide a similar framework for considering how best to provide support to the bereaved survivor.

Resources

Casarett D, Kutner JS, Abrahm J: Life after death: a practical approach to grief and bereavement, *Ann Intern Med* 134:2008–2015, 2001.

Endlink Resource for End of Life Care Education www.endoflife.northwestern.edu

Rando TA: *Clinical dimensions of anticipatory mourning: theory and practice in working with the dying, their loved ones, and their caregivers,* Champaign, IL, 2000, Research Press.

Worden WJ: *Grief counseling and grief therapy: a handbook for the mental health practitioner,* ed 3, New York, 2002, Springer Publishing.

References

1. Knight S, Emanuel L: Processes of adjustment to end-of-life losses: a reintegration model, *J Palliat Med* 10:1190–1198, 2007.
2. Covinsky KE, Eng C, Lui LY, et al: The last 2 years of life: functional trajectories of frail older people, *J Am Geriatr Soc* 51:492–498, 2003.
3. Saunders C: The evolution of palliative care, *Patient Educ Couns* 41:7–13, 2000.
4. Steinhauser KE, Clipp EC, McNeilly M, et al: In search of a good death: observations of patients, families, and providers, *Ann Intern Med* 132:825–832, 2000.
5. Folkman S, Lazarus RS, Gruen RJ, et al: Appraisal, coping, health status, and psychological symptoms, *J Pers Soc Psychol* 50:571–579, 1986.
6. Chochinov HM, Tataryn DJ, Wilson KG, et al: Prognostic awareness and the terminally ill, *Psychosomatics* 41:500–504, 2000.
7. Seale C, Addington-Hall J, McCarthy M: Awareness of dying: prevalence, causes and consequences, *Soc Sci Med* 45:477–484, 1997.
8. Baltes PB, Staudinger UM, Lindenberger U: Lifespan psychology: theory and application to intellectual functioning, *Annu Rev Psychol* 50:471–507, 1999.
9. Brennan M, Cardinali G: The use of preexisting and novel coping strategies in adapting to age-related vision loss, *Gerontologist* 40:327–334, 2000.
10. Block SD: Perspectives on care at the close of life. Psychological considerations, growth, and transcendence at the end of life: the art of the possible, *JAMA* 285:2898–2905, 2001.
11. Stroebe M, Schut H: The dual process model of coping with bereavement: rationale and description, *Death Stud* 23:197–224, 1999.
12. Weisman AD: *On dying and denying: a psychiatric study of terminality,* New York, 1972, Behavioral Publications.
13. Breitbart W, Gibson C, Poppito SR, et al: Psychotherapeutic interventions at the end of life: a focus on meaning and spirituality, *Can J Psychiatry* 49:366–372, 2004.
14. Rando TA: *Grief, dying, and death: clinical interventions for caregivers,* Champaign, IL, 1984, Research Press.
15. Byock I: *Dying Well: The prospect for growth at the end of life,* New York, 1997, Riverhead Books.
16. Butler RN: The life review, *J Geriatr Psychiatry* 35:7–10, 2002.
17. Chochinov HM: Dignity-conserving care—a new model for palliative care: helping the patient feel valued, *JAMA* 287:2253–2260, 2002.
18. Mack JW, Nilsson M, Balboni T, et al: Peace, Equanimity, and Acceptance in the Cancer Experience (PEACE), *Cancer* 112:2509–2517, 2008.
19. Emanuel LL: Decisions at the end of life: have we come of age? *BioMed Central* 2010 [in press].
20. Zimmermann CL: Denial of impending death: a discourse analysis of the palliative care literature, *Soc Sci Med* 59:1769–1780, 2004.
21. Bowlby J: Attachment, vol. 1. In *Attachment and loss,* ed 2, New York, 1982, Basic Books.
22. Kubler-Ross E: *On death and dying, 40th anniversary ed,* New York, 2009, Macmillan.
23. Worden WJ: *Grief counseling and grief therapy: a handbook for the mental health practitioner,* ed 4, New York, 2009, Springer Publishing.
24. Casarett D, Kutner JS, Abrahm J: Life after death: a practical approach to grief and bereavement, *Ann Intern Med* 134:208–215, 2001.
25. Bonanno GA, Kaltman S: The varieties of grief experience, *Clin Psychol Rev* 21:705–734, 2001.

CHAPTER 19

Understanding and Respecting Cultural Differences

KERRY W. BOWMAN

Background and Significance

Although death is universal, dying is very much a culturally specific experience. *Culture* refers to learned patterns of behaviors, beliefs, and values shared by individuals in a particular social group. It provides humans with a sense of identity and belonging, and it gives us a framework for understanding experience. When referring to culture in its broadest sense, the term usually implies a group of people with similar ethnic background, language, religion, familial beliefs, and worldview. Culture is a strong determinant of people's views of the very nature and meaning of illness and death. Culture also influences whether health-related or end-of-life–related decisions can or should be controlled, how bad news should be communicated, and how decisions (including end-of-life decisions) should be made.

As a result of profound demographic changes that affect many Western nations, physicians increasingly care for patients from diverse cultural backgrounds. Differences in beliefs, values, and traditional health care practices are of profound relevance at the end of life. Culture shapes the expression and experience of dying and death as families prepare to lose a loved one. There is growing awareness that the care of the dying is deficient despite many advances in the field of medicine and multiple initiatives to improve this care. The burgeoning field of end-of-life care is receiving increased attention, and experts in the field are attempting to improve the care of

255

the dying by clarifying priorities and establishing humane and respectful palliative care standards and practices. Simultaneously, Western nations are being transformed by rapidly changing demographics related to the growing numbers of immigrants from diverse backgrounds. Because culture provides the primary framework for understanding experience, it is critical to consider culture in relation to end-of-life care.

The heart of the problem is that health care providers, patients, and family members may have dissimilar beliefs about the meaning of illness or death, and they may not agree on which strategies are the most appropriate to alleviate pain and suffering or in planning for the end of life. Good palliative care may be compromised by disagreements between physicians and patients, by miscommunication, or by decisions or beliefs that are not understood or valued.[1] Values that are ingrained in a physician may be alien to patients from different backgrounds. Because of the significant potential for misunderstanding, it is imperative that health care workers be cognizant of potential cultural differences and develop the skills necessary to identify such differences.

A way in which we often go wrong in medicine, and especially in palliative care, is that we see "cultural differences" as something rooted solely in the patient's perspectives. As health care workers, we also represent a "culture" in which perspectives on end of life have a social and cultural history. It is imperative, therefore, to recognize that working with patients new to our society represents the interface of two cultures: theirs and ours. It is naive and unrealistic to believe that differences in patient perspectives can be taken into account without first understanding the genesis of our own perspectives. To this end, we must explore the historic and contemporary perspectives on end-of-life care. The terms *Western* and *non-Western* are used in this chapter. This distinction is not geographic, but rather it is philosophical and anthropologic. In the context of medicine, this distinction is grounded primarily in different beliefs about the primacy of the individual as well as the adherence to the biological views of health and illness.

Sociocultural Development of Palliative Care

An empirical and philosophical analysis of cultural differences in end-of-life care[2,3] has started to identify significant differences in perspectives that are rooted in culture.[4,5] However, this limited analysis has not yet had a significant influence on the fundamental assumptions of end-of-life care. When considering culture and end-of-life care, it is important to note that, despite the broadening of perspectives in the field of end-of-life care, moral agency and individual autonomy remain at the heart of contemporary attitudes and may cause cultural conflicts. Many health care workers who deal with people at the end of life recognize the importance of culture, but they argue that despite significant cultural differences, fundamental, inherent, universal ethical principles can and should to be applied across cultures, nations, and all forms of human boundaries as death approaches. The argument is founded in the belief that essential elements are embedded within the world's apparently diverse moral systems, such as *humanness* (defined as compassion for the pain and suffering of others) and recognition of the equal worth and basic autonomy of every human being.

These concepts of equal worth and autonomy stem from the European Enlightenment of the 18th century. Moral agency and individual autonomy were strongly expressed by Immanuel Kant, were later refined into the political philosophy of liberalism expressed by John Stuart Mill, and, in turn, were developed and refined by many subsequent philosophers. These concepts are fundamentally Western and may be truly foreign to many patients.

If these concepts are applied as universal and are seen as our guiding light in the face of death, what then, for example, of Asian philosophical traditions grounded in Taoism, Confucianism, or Buddhism, in which moral perspective and direction are illuminated by *interdependence* rather than independence? Such cultures are perplexing to most Westerners because they do not contain references to autonomy or self. We often believe that having an "open mind" and "taking our cues from patients" will ameliorate cross-culture misunderstanding. We must first acknowledge, however, that our deepest beliefs related to death and dying are also shaped by culture.

Table 19-1 is developed from three paradigms from the social sciences: *cultural context*, as first described Edward Hall[6]; *health locus of control*, described by Rotter[7]; and the *explanatory model of illness*, described by Kleinman.[8] This table represents trends in dealing with individual patients and families at the end of life.

The following common clinical situation illustrates some of these conceptual differences in perspective.

> A patient who is in a cognitively incompetent state is brought into an intensive care unit (ICU). When the ICU team meets with the patient's family, they focus first on biomedical explanations of illness and the potential for brain death. They then ask whether the patient expressed any personal wishes about treatment before becoming incompetent and thus encourage an open and direct conversation about the severity of the situation and the potential for death. By exploring the patient's perspectives and values with the family, the team hopes to formulate the best plan for the medical care of the patient.

> However, the focus on individual rights and choices, the direct and blunt verbal communication about such a personal and difficult situation, the introduction of the element of choice, and the focus on a purely biomedical explanation of illness and death may be so confusing for this family of non-Western origin that the result is a complete breakdown in communication.

Inherent in this relatively standard approach is a belief in the Western definition of illness and death, a belief that the timing and circumstances of dying can and should be controlled. At the heart of each of these paradigms is the fundamental belief in the inherent value of respect for autonomy, even if the patient and the family are unaware of that concept.

Elements That Can Limit Cultural Understanding

MARGINALIZING ETHNOGRAPHIC AND PSYCHOSOCIAL INFORMATION

Many medical approaches and bioethical models rely on comparative cases and examination of competing principles. Although these methods may be useful in defining some ethical issue, to understand end-of-life dilemmas fully, we must examine the social and cultural context within which the situation is embedded. Medical perspectives or comparative cases alone tend to marginalize many relevant factors such as culture or the personal and social meaning of a situation. Thus, the common effort to render end-of-life analyses as objective, rational, and unbiased by defining "value-neutral" concepts such as futility risks making end-of-life decisions socially and culturally neutral. Concepts such as *futility* and the lived experience of

Table 19-1. Trends in Dealing with Patients and Families at the End of Life

	Contemporary Medical Perspectives	Non-Western Perspectives	Clinical Approach
Beliefs about causation of death and dying	Death is biologically determined. Dying occurs when medicine can no longer stave off, treat, or reverse illness. Death most often occurs in hospitals, and the declaration of death is ultimately in the hands of medical personnel.	Death may be seen in a broader and seemingly less tangible manner. It may be viewed as being linked to religious, social, spiritual, and environmental determinants. Some cultural groups may perceive illness and death as separate entities. Declaration of death is also socially and culturally determined.	Anticipate nonmedical perspectives on death. Allow cultural rituals. Allow flexibility with time spent with the dying or deceased. Explore perceptions about the causes of the critical illness, its treatment, and death.
Social structures	Equality and independence are valued. Strong acceptance and value are given to autonomy.	Hierarchy is respected. Moral value is given to interdependence and family decision making.	Allow patients and families to make collective decisions (in the absence of coercion).
Communication about dying with patients and others	Information should be explicitly communicated. Clinicians have a moral obligation to truth telling because the patient has a right to know and must make autonomous decisions. Information is best communicated overtly.	People have a moral duty to protect loved ones from negativity. Cues are taken from social context. Frank communication about death is often unacceptable. Truth telling is highly problematic.	Ask the patient how much medical information he or she wishes. Ask how that information should be communicated.
Perception of a religiously/ culturally meaningful death	Individual choice is valued. There is no direct association to medicine. These attitudes can be an impediment to the acceptance of the futility of further treatment.	Religion/culture norms may be the most critical aspect of death. These values greatly shape the bereavement process.	Allow rituals and flexibility with the number and timing of visitors. Accept nonmedical perspectives.

Table 19-1. Trends in Dealing with Patients and Families at the End of Life (Continued)

	Contemporary Medical Perspectives	Non-Western Perspectives	Clinical Approach
Perception of negotiating death (levels of negotiating treatment)	Patients are largely responsible for defining the "kind of death" they wish.	Suffering and death are largely a matter of fate and may hold profound spiritual meaning.	A trial of therapy allows patient outcomes to be determined more by "fate."
Timing of death	The timing and circumstances of death can and ought to be controlled as much as possible to respect a patient's autonomous choices.	The timing and circumstances of death and dying are preordained and a matter of fate.	Allow as natural a process as possible. If the patient is on life support, withdraw it gradually.
Nonverbal communication	Direct communication, even about difficult matters, is the most ethical approach.	Consider body language, and respect silences and rituals.	Listen more than speak. Consider body language. Allow and respect silences; consider their meaning.

patients and families are separated by a substantial distance. Health care workers and medical literature often describe social and cultural factors as external "constraints" and frequently use the term *cultural barrier,* usually with the intent to analyze and clarify. However, the word *barrier* implies that culture blocks access to the resolution of the ethical issue, thus implying something universal on the other side of this barrier. Is there?

SECULAR FOCUS

Despite the significant Judeo-Christian contributions to end-of-life care and although many health care workers are aware of the profoundly religious and spiritual beliefs and contributions to end-of-life perspectives, health care in general continues to adhere to a largely secular perspective. This is understandable because a secular approach in medicine is a practical, political, and moral response that seeks to apply a unitary approach to the demands of complex and diverse cultures. Many would also endorse the idea that palliative care philosophy is emerging as a secular alternative to religious perspectives and is better able to serve a pluralistic, morally diverse society. However, by doing this we often isolate cultural issues from their spiritual and social context to achieve an institutionally sanctioned method of avoiding potential conflict. Unfortunately, our efforts to examine issues from a nonspiritual or nonreligious perspective make our approach limited, incomplete, and sometimes devoid of meaning and difficult to understand for many patients and families who are new to Western health care.

FOCUS ON INDIVIDUAL AUTONOMY

Although challenges to the principle of autonomy are becoming increasingly apparent in medicine in general and in end-of-life care in particular,[9] this awareness has not deeply affected standard medical practice. For example, much of the contemporary discourse in medical ethics equates autonomy with personhood, as though autonomy exists universally for all people independently of cultural perspectives. The extreme opposite of autonomy would be experienced by people who live in remote tribal societies where the concept of the individual is virtually nonexistent and holds little social relevance. Although we do not have people from remote tribal societies living in Western industrialized nations, this difference in perceptions of the self in relation to others illustrates the power and influence of culture. Despite this, the concept of autonomy remains the intellectual and moral foundation of Western medicine,[10] and it is a direct manifestation of the Western concept of individualism: a belief in the importance, uniqueness, dignity, and sovereignty of each person and the sanctity of each individual life. According to this belief, every person is entitled to individual rights such as autonomy of self, self-determination, and privacy. For most cultures, this focus on individuality neglects the vital role of personal interconnectedness and the social and moral meaning of these interrelationships.

TRUTH TELLING, NEGATIVE FOCUS

Generally, Western medicine (and, in turn, end-of-life care) has responded to the cultural trends of placing a high value on truth telling. Yet in the presence of serious illness, many cultures believe that giving negative information may induce negative outcomes.[11,12] This belief reflects the considerable cultural differences concerning the interaction between mind and body. Some cultures are strongly protective of the critically ill and believe that ill loved ones require the same supervision and protection as well-loved children. Western medicine derives the physician's obligation to communicate the truth to patients from the rarely questioned belief in the patient's "right to know," which, when considered as unconditional, requires that patients must deal with the truth overtly and rationally. The belief is that patients will ultimately be better off, and this perspective is particularly powerful in oncology. Sometimes we meet the patient's refusal to accept the truth with impatience and believe they are in denial, a state that is understandable but generally considered unacceptable. From a Western perspective, we usually agree quickly about what the truth is as we anticipate outcomes based solely on medical perspectives, yet this view may mystify people of other cultural perspectives.

Attitudes toward truth telling are largely determined by culture. A qualitative study showed that Chinese seniors did not see truth telling as a moral absolute but instead believed that in many cases truth telling could produce more harm than good and should be dealt with in a cautious way that involved the family more than the patient.[13] Another study that examined the attitudes of 200 seniors from four ethnic groups (African American, Korean American, Mexican American, and European American) found that Korean Americans and Mexican Americans were significantly less likely than European Americans and African Americans to believe that patients should be told about a diagnosis of metastatic cancer. A study of American Navajo perspectives concluded that the Navajo culture views medical information as harmful.[14] In Taiwan, neither Western-oriented nor traditional Chinese doctors give information related to diagnosis and prognosis to patients who are facing life-threatening illness; instead, this information is given to family members, who, in turn, are expected to inform and support the patient. These findings have been supported by further studies involving Asian populations.[15] Neither patients nor physicians view truth telling as an ethical issue. In the West, however, this practice would be considered a direct violation of the principle of autonomy.

DIFFERENT DEFINITIONS OF DEATH

Although many of us accept the standard medical determinations of death, there can be profound cultural variation in this area. The following example illustrates this variation.

In Western health care, organ donation from brain-dead patients may be seen as something positive and without a great deal of moral ambiguity. This is not the case from some non-Western perspectives. Japanese views of brain death and organ transplantation clearly illustrate such differences. One study, for example, suggested that in Japanese society, Shinto and Buddhism have strongly supported "natural" processes and approaches to dying.[16] According to Buddhist belief, aging, illness, and death are inevitable once a person has entered the cycle of life. From a traditional Japanese perspective, a human being is the integration of body, mind, and spirit. After death, a person remains an integrated whole. The metaphorical center of the body, *kokoro*, has traditionally been located in the chest. Therefore, removal of an organ from a brain-dead human, especially from the chest, may be perceived as disturbing this integrated unit. The Japanese find a fragment of the deceased's mind and spirit in every part of a deceased person's body. It follows that the Japanese believe a dead person goes to the next world as a soul. Similar to a living person, this soul has its own body, senses, and feelings. The dead body must remain whole because if some parts are missing, the soul becomes unhappy in the next world. Such latent yet formative cultural views are not specific to the Japanese. For example, although not homogeneous in their views, many North American aboriginal people are profoundly uncomfortable with organ donation.[17] In many non-Western cultures, death is viewed as a social event rather than a scientific phenomenon.

What are the cultural, historical, philosophical, and religious influences that have made certain ideas about death acceptable in the West? Perhaps it is because in the West, human beings have often been perceived as the blending of body and soul. Christianity has shaped the West just as Buddhism, Shinto, and Confucianism have shaped Japan. In Christianity, people are expected to respect the body after death because it was an essential part of the person during life; however, a body without a soul is no longer considered a person. With regard to organ procurement, many Christians perceive the donation of one's organs as an act of love and generosity.[18] The spiritual value of nonreciprocal giving is central to Christian belief. This, in part, may have contributed to the widespread social acceptance of organ donation. In general terms, Western medicine and, in turn, end-of-life care, have accepted brain death as death and have embraced transplantation. Clearly, there are profound cultural differences in perceptions of validity of brain death and the moral value of organ transplantation; this cultural difference cannot be addressed by the often-stated need for better education of new immigrants.

Communication and Context

It is imperative to understand the influence of culture on communication. All cultures have verbal and nonverbal approaches to giving and receiving messages. Although we as health care providers working the realm of end-of-life care can easily acknowledge the medical and ethical complexities of end-of-life decisions, we have barely begun to acknowledge the psychological and sociocultural complexities. For many people new to scientifically advanced Western nations, several factors—including the absence of life-sustaining technology, a far shorter life expectancy, a higher child mortality rate, and a closer geographic proximity for many families—made death a more frequent, home-based experience that had little to do with choice. In Western nations, however, end-of-life decisions abound, and the stakes are high. These decisions involve life or death, views about the quality and meaning of life, high costs, moral principles, and legal rights. Not surprisingly, such decisions can generate intense emotions, particularly for those with no familiarity with the concepts involved, and can increase the potential for conflict.

Moreover, substantial differences in culture, combined with social class and education, often exist between physicians and families. What is known or valued by health care workers may be elusive or irrelevant to families. When differences exist, so too will perspectives on choices, and this disparity creates a greater opportunity for conflict. Conflicting perspectives become increasingly obvious when major decisions must be made. Large health care teams with shifting and inconsistent members, each trained in specific professions with separate working cultures, often fracture communication and make for an environment that is not conducive to balanced discussion and negotiation. Furthermore, all these factors occur in the climate of continuing change that defines the contemporary health care system. For families, end-of-life decisions are not abstract philosophical questions or matters of clear-cut clinical judgment; rather, they are painful emotional experiences, greatly shaped by cultural and religious beliefs that can generate profound revelations about mortality and family relationships. As previously stated, rather than viewing culture as an integral part of a patient's identity and life, much of the health care literature depicts culture in terms of a barrier. Families, central to the end-of-life experience in most cultures, are frequently described by health care workers as being a help or a hindrance, as supportive or difficult.[19] Furthermore, the cultural meaning of illness in the context of the family is often not identified and is poorly understood by health care workers. This patient-centered perspective in health care may be rooted in the strong focus on patient autonomy and the sanctity of the physician–patient relationship.

Hispanic Perspectives

BACKGROUND

Although cultural generalizations as a means of anticipating behavior are not useful and run the great risks of stereotyping and producing further conflict, exploring the general cultural trends outlined in Table 19-1 can be a useful means of examining *existing* behavior (as opposed to prediction). The first point that must be considered when referring to Hispanics is that the term is a label of convenience for a cultural group with a common cultural heritage stemming from Spain's colonization of the Americas. Hispanics can be of any racial group (e.g., indigenous American, black,

Asian, white, or of multiple racial ancestry). Hispanic immigration to most Western nations has been rising steadily and is particularly extensive in the United States, where the Hispanic population of 31 million will soon surpass African Americans as the largest minority group in the country. Although significant differences exist among Hispanic subgroups, virtually all share a common language, religion, and traditional family structure and have many common values. In addition to differences in subgroups, they differ in terms of their level of acculturation or assimilation into mainstream culture. Language use is one very good example of these differences. For instance, although many Hispanics are bilingual, the degree to which they speak either Spanish or English varies considerably.

CULTURAL FEATURES

Religion

One value shared by most Hispanics, as evident in the Carillero family in Box 19-1, is religion. Although the degree of practice and church participation varies, most Hispanics are Christian, predominantly Roman Catholic. However, many Hispanics practice other religious beliefs that they have incorporated into their Christianity, such as forms of ancestor worship with rituals dating back to pre-Columbian times among Central American Indians. For example, many Caribbean Hispanics practice *Santería,* a fusion of Catholicism and the Yoruba religion that was brought to Cuba by African slaves. Such rituals are described as *Espiritismo,* a belief in good and evil spirits that can affect health and well-being and that includes views on dying and death. The rituals performed by the Carillero family that others found loud and disruptive and the attending Roman Catholic nurse felt were not Catholic in nature were likely rooted in this cultural trend. As evident with the Carillero family, it is common to hold a continued vigil over an older family member with a terminal illness. These and other practices honor the loved one and form part of the bereavement ritual.

BOX 19-1. CASE STUDY: THE CARILLERO FAMILY

Mrs. Carillero is a 70-year-old Hispanic woman who was admitted to the ICU with metastatic bone disease from a primary site of breast cancer that has now spread to her lungs and possibly her brain. Mrs. Carillero has a large extended family that essentially never leaves her side. Earlier in the illness, the Carillero family had been asked to consider a palliative care facility in the future because of the possibility that Mrs. Carillero's care could become complex and demanding. The family steadfastly refused and asked that the topic not be brought up again. These family members have consistently advocated for full and aggressive treatment. The ICU rule of two visitors at a time is rarely being followed, and the ICU staff is becoming frustrated and upset. When visitors are asked whether they are immediate family, they fall silent.

Although the ICU staff assured the Carillero family that prayer was welcomed, the family repeatedly engages in fairly loud ritualized prayer sessions. The ICU staff members now feel that these sessions have become disruptive to the unit and disturbing to the other patients and their families.

In addition, the Carillero family had identified themselves as Catholics. A Roman Catholic nurse has stated that at first she had joined them in prayer, but many elaborate rituals have been introduced, and many of the prayers are unfamiliar to her. She has openly questioned whether they are truly Roman Catholic and respectful of Catholic traditions.

Through negotiation, Mrs. Carillero's son Everett was chosen as spokesperson. When the physician told Everett about his mother's poor prognosis and the "futility" of further treatment, Everett appeared to not acknowledge the severity of the situation and insisted that his mother be fully treated. He told the doctor that he had the skill to do miracles. The health care team repeatedly asked Everett and other family members whether Mrs. Carillero had previously expressed wishes about what she would want if she were in her current circumstances. The family did not respond to this question. The team also asked: "If she could speak to us now, what would she tell us she wanted?" The Carillero family was again consistently silent on this question.

Everett says that he wishes to deal with things one day at a time and states that his mother's fate should be in God's hands, not determined by decisions made by either the doctors or the family. The family's unresponsiveness to these questions and their insistence on continued treatment have been interpreted by some as a means of focusing on their "agenda" rather than on Mrs. Carillero's wishes and best interests.

The Carilleros told a patient relations officer that they are very upset by the constant staff changes. They said that they feel like they have no one really to talk to and they are feeling pressured to end Mrs. Carillero's life.

Everett has also demanded that should his mother regain consciousness even briefly, she not be told about her condition or asked questions about her wishes, because it would "kill her spirit." The physician explained to Everett that he had a legal and ethical obligation to inform his mother of her medical situation and to clarify her wishes should she become conscious and capable. Family members are now refusing to leave even when procedures are being done and state that they are afraid that medical staff will give up on their mother. Tension is growing, and the ICU team has deemed this case a serious ethical dilemma.

Lack of Focus on Individual Patient Perspectives and Large Number of Visitors

The large extended Carillero family network can be understood in a context of the strong role of family for many Hispanics, highlighted by powerful ties within an extended network of uncles, aunts, cousins, grandparents, and family friends. Included in this is the important role of the family in the concept of *familismo*, an emphasis on the welfare of the family over that of the individual, perhaps illustrated by the family's silence and reluctance to identify Mrs. Carillero's *independent* wishes.

Discomfort with Constant Staff Changes

The Carillero family informed a patient relations representative that they found the constant staff changes very disturbing at such a difficult time. This could possibly be attributed to the Hispanic concept of *personalismo,* a term that refers to trust building over time and is based on the display of mutual respect.

Reluctance to Partner with Physicians for Planning and Unrealistic Expectations

Everett's reluctance to discuss family issues and values with the physician as well as his potentially unrealistic expectations of physicians could be related to *jerarquismo,* a term that refers to respect for hierarchy.

Focusing on the Present and Avoiding Long-Term Plans

Everett's persistent wish to take things day by day may be tied to the concept of *presentismo,* defined as maintaining important focus on the present instead of on the past or the future.

Avoiding End-of-Life Decisions

The family's fervent wish to avoid human influence in the timing of Mrs. Carillero's death may be seen as *fatalismo,* the belief that fate determines life outcomes, including health, and that fate is basically unbeatable.

TRUTH TELLING AND ADVANCED MEDICAL PLANNING

In a study that compared beliefs of Mexican Americans, Korean Americans, African Americans, and European Americans on several issues related to patient autonomy, researchers found that Mexican Americans and Korean Americans were less likely to believe that a patient should be told about a terminal diagnosis or make decisions about using life support. The researchers also found that Mexican American and Korean American elders were more likely than African American and European American elders to want family members to make these decisions.[20]

LIFE-PROLONGING TREATMENTS

When it came to the issue of life-prolonging treatments at the end of life, Hispanic Americans and African Americans were more likely than non-Hispanic whites to report wanting their doctors to keep them alive regardless of how ill they were (42% and 37% vs. 14%, respectively). Furthermore, only 59% of Hispanics and 63% of African Americans agreed to stop life-prolonging treatment, compared with 89% of non-Hispanic whites.[21] It is possible that this trend reflects a mistrust of the system or religious beliefs related to not killing and the sanctity of life.

Palliative Care Perspectives

As seen in the Carillero family, some studies have suggested a significantly low use of palliative care services in Hispanic populations. Reasons may include unfamiliarity with palliative care, language barriers, and unpleasant experiences with or distrust of the health care system. Cultural factors may well be at play, however, and further research is required in this area.

HOW COULD THE CARILLERO FAMILY BE BETTER RESPECTED?

Because Hispanics have a significant demographic representation in our culture, it is wise to increase our knowledge about Hispanic culture by becoming familiar with the history of the subgroups we dealing with, as well as the family, social, and religious values associated with Hispanic culture. This will help providers to display respect and to build trust. The provider should include family members in discussions with the patient regarding treatment planning and palliative care. There may be situations in which the patient does not want to have the family included, and this wish, of course, should be respected.

Finally, it is important to have open and clear communication with the patient and family, because deference to and respect for the provider as a result of *jerarquismo* may lead the Hispanic patient to withhold information or to hesitate to communicate honestly. The provider must ascertain whether the patient understands the treatment being offered and whether he or she fully agrees with the treatment plan. This is particularly important when it comes to end-of-life decision making and advance directives, because several cultural factors discourage discussions of these topics. *Jerarquismo* may lead the patient and family to have unrealistic expectations about what conventional treatment can offer. The family may be expecting a miracle cure for the terminally ill patient and thus may refuse to consider palliative care treatment options. Appropriate religious representation is imperative to avoid perceived conflicts between the patient's religion and the withdrawal or withholding of treatment.

Cross-Cultural Awareness in Practice

Keep in mind the following questions when working cross-culturally with patients:

- Does this patient value individuality and personal choice, or does he or she focus more on family and collective choices?
- Does he or she value open communication, or does the patient tend to draw cues from the context of the situation?
- Does he or she believe a person can and should influence his or her health or death?
- Does he or she believe in a Western explanation of illness, or does the patient hold an alternative culturally based view, and is this view blended with Western perspectives on illness?

PEARLS

- Cultural differences vary extensively. Do not assume; always ask.
- When working cross-culturally, there is a good chance that your patient and his or her family may not value individuality over interdependence. Ask your patient how he or she would like decisions to be made.
- Not everyone believes in Western medicine. To understand your patient's perspective better, ask: "What do you think is causing your illness, and how should it best be treated?"
- Truth telling is often not valued when working cross-culturally. Accommodate for this possibility by asking how and to whom information should be given and how and with whom decisions should be made.

PITFALLS

- Be careful when assessing emotional reactions cross-culturally.
- Do not assume to know another's cultural views. Always ask.
- Do not assume that patients are aware or accepting of a Western biomedical view of illness. Inquire, give your perspectives, and negotiate a treatment plan.

Summary

Cultures are maps of meaning through which people understand the world and interpret the things around them. When patients and health care workers have different cultural backgrounds, they frequently follow different "maps," and this can hinder effective communication.

As a result of profound immigration and the resultant demographic changes, health care workers increasingly care for patients from cultural backgrounds other than their own. Culturally constructed differences in beliefs, values, and traditional health care practices are of profound relevance at the end of life. Culture greatly determines the expression and experience of death and dying as patients and families prepare to lose a loved one. As much as contemporary end-of-life care critiques and acknowledges cultural differences, it remains questionable whether we have truly explored the profound significance of the cultural differences of the values given to independence and interdependence, present or future orientation, intervention with the timing and circumstances of death, and the way in which families and patients understand the nature and meaning of death. Nor have we compensated for how greatly these factors lead to substantial differences in cognitive processes, perception, social structures, values, and beliefs in both patients and health care workers.

Those who work in the domain of end-of-life care must undertake a deeper exploration of those social and cultural realities that shape end-of-life experiences. Although end-of-life care increasingly identifies and values interrelationships with others, autonomy and, in turn, the individual, remain at the heart of end-of-life analysis. Our organizational and legal structures assume that the person experiencing the illness is the best person to make health care decisions. This raises profound questions about the adaptability of end-of-life care in a culturally pluralistic society. Because many cultures vest the family or community with the right to receive and disclose information, and to organize and make decisions about patient care, we must be constantly cognizant that the cross-cultural application of the concept of autonomy will mean accepting each person's terms of reference for their definition of self. Specifically, we should respect the autonomy of patients and families by incorporating their cultural values and beliefs into the decision-making process. Although this may sound straightforward, it is easy to lose sight of this principle in our busy practices.

Ultimately, the most effective way to address cultural differences in end-of-life decision making is through open and balanced communication. When health care workers are uncertain about how a patient or family perceives a situation, it is best simply to ask. Differences can frequently be negotiated easily. Many people now living in Western cultures already hold blended views of culture, illness, and death. The mere acknowledgment of such differences will usually lead to improved communication. In health care, we often assume that respect and acceptance of cultural diversity are givens, yet it is important for us to remember that despite our openness to other cultures, our attitudes toward end-of-life care are as much an effect of *our* cultural beliefs as they are of the many diverse cultures we see in practice. We must make a significant effort to raise our awareness and to alter our practices in this crucial area.

Resources

AT&T LanguageLine. The AT&T language bank does translation. These interpreters are not trained in medical interpretation. Further, because they are on the telephone, they do not have access to the visual information in the setting.
1–800–752–0093, extension 196
www.languageline.com

Ekblad S, Marttila A, Emilsson M: Cultural challenges in end-of-life care: Reflections from focus groups' interviews with hospice staff in Stockholm, *J Adv Nurs* 31:623–630, 2000.

Hallenbeck J: High context illness and dying in a low context medical world, *Am J Hosp Palliat Care* 23:113–118, 2006.

Sarhill N, LeGrand S, Islambouli R, et al: The terminally ill Muslim: Death and dying from the Muslim perspective, *Am J Hosp Palliat Care* 18:251–255, 2001.

Xculture. This web site has a short and long glossary of medical terms in several languages.
www.xculture.org

References

1. Jecker NS, Carrese JA, Pearlman RA: Caring for patients in cross cultural settings, *Hastings Cent Rep* 25:6, 1995.
2. Kunstadter P: Medical ethics in cross-cultural and multi-cultural perspectives, *Soc Sci Med* 14:289, 1980.
3. Games AD, Robert AH: Physicians of western medicine: five cultural studies, *Cult Med Psychiatry* 6:215, 1982.
4. Carrese JA, Rhodes LA: Western bioethics on the Navajo reservation, *JAMA* 247:10, 1995.
5. Blackhall LJ, Murphy ST, Frank G, et al: Ethnicity and attitudes toward patient autonomy, *JAMA* 274:820, 1995.
6. Hall ET: How cultures collide, *Psychol Today* 10:66, 1976.
7. Rotter JC: *Locus of control: current trends in theory and research*, ed 2, New York, 1966, Wiley.
8. Kleinman A: *Patient and healers in the context of culture: an exploration of the borderland between anthropology, medicine, and psychiatry*, Berkeley, CA, 1980, University of California Press.
9. Fagan A: Challenging the bioethical application of the autonomy principle within multicultural societies, *J Appl Philos* 21:15, 2004.
10. Barker JC: Cultural diversity-changing the context of medical practice. In Cross-Cultural Medicine: A Decade Later [special issue], *West J Med* 157:248, 1992.
11. Caralis PV, Davis B, Wright K, Marcial E: The influence of ethnicity and race on attitudes toward advance directives, life-prolonging treatments, and euthanasia, *J Clin Ethics* 4:155, 1993.
12. Blackhall LJ, Murphy ST, Frank G, et al: Ethnicity and attitudes toward patient autonomy, *JAMA* 274:820, 1995.
13. Bowman KW, Singer PA: Chinese seniors' perspectives on end of life care, *Soc Sci Med* 53:455–464, 2001. Available at http://econpapers.repec.org/article/eeesocmed/.
14. Carrese JA, Rhodes LA: Western bioethics on the Navajo reservation, *JAMA* 247:10, 1995.
15. Hui E, Ho SC, Tsang J, et al: Attitudes toward life-sustaining treatment of older persons in Hong Kong, *J Am Geriatr Soc* 45:1232, 1997.
16. Tanida N: Japanese religious organizations view on terminal care, *J Asian Int Bioethics* 10:34, 2000.
17. Emory M: Native America Calling. Available at www.nativeamericacalling.com.
18. Scorsone S: Christianity and the significance of the human body, *Transplant Proc* 22:943, 1990.
19. Levine C, Zuckerman C: The trouble with families: toward an ethic of accommodation, *Ann Intern Med* 130:148, 1999.
20. Blackhall LJ, Murphy DT, Frank G, et al: Ethnicity and attitudes toward patient autonomy, *JAMA* 274:820, 1995.
21. Caralis PV, Davis B, Wright K, Marcial E: The influence of ethnicity and race on attitudes toward advance directives, life-prolonging treatments, and euthanasia, *J Clin Ethics* 4:155, 1993.

PART D

Specific Situations and Skill Sets

CHAPTER 20

Advance Care Planning

HELENE STARKS, ELIZABETH K. VIG, and ROBERT ALLAN PEARLMAN

Overview

Advance care planning is a process that aims to align medical decisions with patient values and preferences in the event that the patient cannot communicate. In the context of palliative care, advance care planning discussions offer a framework for exploring a patient's current values and goals, as well as how these could change as the illness evolves. To facilitate the implementation of advance care planning in palliative care, this chapter explores the following questions:

1. Which patients should engage in advance care planning?
2. Can patients with cognitive impairments also have these conversations?
3. How is the ability to communicate preferences assessed?
4. When should conversations occur?
5. Who should initiate the conversation?
6. What communication strategies are most helpful?
7. How should the conversation be introduced?
8. What topics should be addressed?
9. What strategies can be used when patients and families are reluctant to discuss these issues?

Ideally, advance care planning should begin early in the clinical relationship and should be revisited periodically, especially when changes in health status or goals of care occur. When possible, family members, especially designated substitute decision

270

makers, should be included in these conversations because it is important for them to be aware of any changes in the patient's values and preferences. Exploring the reasons behind any changes can be very helpful in bringing discordant views into alignment.

Advance care planning is a process that aims to inform and facilitate medical decision making that reflects patients' values and preferences in the event that patients cannot communicate. This process is achieved in many ways, including conversations with patients and families, the use of written advance directives that document a patient's wishes, and the participation of substitute decision makers who can represent a patient's interests, values, and preferences. In this chapter, we first define the terms *advance care planning* and *advance directives* and provide a review of the evolution of these terms and mechanisms in practice. We then explore how to practice advance care planning in the context of palliative care and include a set of questions that can be used to guide advance care planning discussions with patients and family members.

Definitions

The Institute of Medicine defines advance care planning as "not only the preparation of legal documents but also discussions with family members and physicians about what the future may hold for people with serious illnesses, how patients and families want their beliefs and preferences to guide decisions (including decisions should sudden and unexpected critical medical problems arise), and what steps could alleviate concerns related to finances, family matters, spiritual questions, and other issues that trouble seriously ill or dying patients and their families".[1] As such, advance care planning is a process—not a single event—with the goal of learning about both what patients *want* and what they *do not want* for themselves in the future. A recent literature review outlined a framework of six goals that commonly arise in advance care planning discussions. These goals include being cured, living longer, improving or maintaining function or quality of life, being comfortable, achieving life goals, and providing support for family caregivers.[2] Some of these goals may coexist, and they may also shift over time. The focus for advance care planning is to elicit what values, goals, and outcomes are important to patients and their families so that care decisions can meet the goals.

Advance care planning includes two basic components: thinking about preferences and goals of care, and communicating these preferences to loved ones, substitute (or proxy) decision makers, and health care providers.[3] For the first component, a patient needs to consider the many factors that influence care preferences, including beliefs about the sanctity of life, estimated life expectancy, current and future quality of life, suffering, the probability of achieving a desirable outcome if treatment is pursued, withholding and withdrawing treatments, and the cost of treatment or nontreatment to the patient and family (in both monetary and nonmonetary terms). Ideally, the person who engages in this deliberation process will be able to identify a personal threshold of acceptability for the benefits and burdens of future treatment and how treatments help them realize their goals of care. For the second component of advance care planning, the patient must communicate preferences to those persons who will be involved in making decisions on his or her behalf. These individuals include legally appointed powers of attorney or proxy decision makers, family members, and intimate others. Values and preferences can be communicated through formal conversations about the person's wishes as well as through informal discussions about the serious illness or death of family members or friends or about current events in the news that represent good and bad dying experiences. Communication also includes documenting the person's wishes through advance directives or other means, such as letters or video recordings.

Advance directives can be informal verbal agreements; health care providers' written summaries of patient values and preferences in the medical record; or formal, legal, written documents. The formal documents have the potential advantage of providing the "clear and convincing" evidentiary standard that is required in some states in the United States (e.g., New York and Missouri) as proof of the person's wishes in the event of a legal dispute. These documents have two forms: a *durable power of attorney for health care,* in which the person identifies a designated proxy or substitute decision maker (or decision makers), and an *instructional directive* (commonly known as a living will), which is a written statement of instructions to guide medical decision making. Living wills often specify treatment preferences under conditions of terminal illness or a persistent vegetative state.

History and Critique

Laws that allow advance directives to guide the use or nonuse of life-sustaining treatments were first drafted in United States in the mid-1970s, about the same time as the sentinel court case involving Karen Ann Quinlan. This young woman was in a persistent vegetative state. When her physicians declined to remove her breathing tube, her parents petitioned the court to remove it. The Quinlans eventually won the case, thus setting a legal precedent for the right to refuse unwanted medical treatments. State laws to the same effect began to appear throughout the United States, and a similar case regarding Nancy Cruzan was settled in favor of the same right in the United States Supreme Court. The legal effort continued in the United States with passage of the Patient Self-Determination Act in 1990, which required that all health care facilities receiving Medicare or Medicaid funding offer patients information about advance directives and inform them of their right to refuse unwanted medical treatments.[4]

The durable power of attorney for health care and instructional directives are recognized as legal mechanisms everywhere in the United States. In Canada, advance directives legislation was passed starting in the late 1980s. Currently, 11 of the 13 provinces have advance directives legislation; the exceptions are New Brunswick and Nunavut. Of the 11 provinces with advance directive laws, all include specific language about appointing substitute decision maker(s). Instructional directives are explicitly included in the legislation in five provinces and recognized as part of health consent legislation in four others; Nova Scotia and Quebec are the two exceptions with no specific language covering instructional directives.

Since the 1970s a great deal of work has been devoted to increasing the access, availability, usability, and completion of advance directives. This was complemented by research and interventions designed to increase the use of advance directives in health care systems and to simplify the language and process of documenting preferences. Additional community-based initiatives were developed to educate the public and to increase completion rates. Elements that contribute to success include a combination of educational materials directed toward patients and their family members and proxy decision makers coupled with systematic efforts to encourage patient–provider discussions over multiple visits.[5] Even with these multimodal interventions, most of these efforts have had modest effects on the rate of directive completion. Currently, approximately 30% of U.S. residents complete written advance directives, although the number of those who have discussed the issue may be larger. Yet even among those who have advance directives, some steps in the advance care planning process may not be complete. Providers may not know that a directive exists, the directive may not be located or brought in when a patient is admitted to the hospital, or it may be ignored or overruled during the hospital stay.[6] There are multiple aspects of written instructional directives that make the application of these documents problematic in practice:

1. People must obtain and complete the forms.
2. They must predict their future assessments of quality of life and preferences for life-sustaining treatments.
3. They must state these preferences in writing.
4. The documents must be available for use when necessary.
5. The substitute decision makers, family members, and health care providers who interpret these documents must be able to understand them in the context of the current situation.
6. The substitute decision makers must then follow the written instructions as originally intended.[7]

Critics argue that these conditions are virtually impossible to meet and that society should abandon this approach to extending autonomy at the end of life. They advocate continued use of substitute decision makers and also endorse the general shift in focus away from the legalistic documents toward the iterative process of advance care planning, which emphasizes eliciting the patients' values and goals of care rather than specific treatment preferences.

In spite of the critique of living wills, documentation of advance care planning discussions is still necessary to facilitate the transfer of information between institutions, to provide evidence of the patient's wishes in the event of a dispute, and to guide and support substitute decision makers. Several authors have developed worksheets and workbooks to facilitate this documentation. These documents take different forms. (See the Resources section for links to these different types of documents.) Some emphasize patient values (e.g., the Values History Form), and others offer a range of situations and treatment choices and allow for the identification of personal thresholds for medical intervention (e.g., Your Life, Your Choices and the Medical Directive). Another effort that has had positive effects on the outcomes and processes of care is the Physician Orders for Life-Sustaining Treatment (POLST) form. Technically, the POLST is not an advance directive because it is completed by a physician rather than by the person whose wishes it conveys. It was developed to provide standing physicians' orders for emergency medical personnel (who cannot legally follow advance directives in emergency situations) and to serve as a transportable document to guide health care decisions between and across health care institutions. However, use of the POLST improves both identification of and compliance with patients' wishes in multiple settings.[8,9]

Advance Care Planning in Palliative Care

In the context of palliative care, advance care planning discussions also offer a framework for exploring a patient's current values, goals, and treatment choices, as well as how these may change over the trajectory of illness. For example, early in the course of cancer, palliative care may primarily serve as a symptom management approach, with the goal being to alleviate symptoms associated with the cancer and disease-modifying treatments. As the cancer progresses, palliative care can become the primary goal of care. Goals of care may shift toward staying at home, maximizing comfort regardless of how that affects participation in daily activities, or finding a balance between controlling pain and still maintaining cognitive function. To the extent that the patient is capable of participating in these discussions, these goals will be established and updated in real time, but these discussions also serve as advance care planning to guide care when the patient can no longer express his or her wishes.

Putting advance care planning into practice requires the consideration of several issues. These include determining which patients are appropriate, deciding when and how to introduce the discussion, selecting members of the health care team who are best suited to initiate these discussions, and establishing the specific areas to be covered.

WHICH PATIENTS?

All older adults and all patients with chronic or serious illness could benefit from advance care planning discussions, especially those who are likely to experience exacerbations of the illness that could cause loss of decisional capacity and require emergency therapy. Advance care planning offers the opportunity to identify goals of care, to explore contingency plans, and to prepare patients with serious illness for the probable trajectory of the illness. All patients in transition to a terminal phase of illness are ideal candidates.

CAN COGNITIVELY IMPAIRED PATIENTS PARTICIPATE?

Patients with dementia, delirium, and psychiatric illness present unique challenges for advance care planning, but they may still be capable of participating. Patients with dementia, especially those in the early stages, may be able to express preferences for aspects of care, such as their preferred substitute decision maker. Keys to success include initiating the discussion when patients are doing their best and framing questions in simple terms. It is far better to try to elicit preferences and to assess how much is understood than to assume that persons with dementia cannot participate at all. Patients with psychiatric illness also may be able to participate in advance care planning. During periods of remission or when their illness is well controlled, they can express preferences for future situations of decisional incapacity. They may complete two kinds of directives: a living will to guide end-of-life care and a mental health advance directive to guide care during acute exacerbations of mental illness (see the Resources section for links to examples of both types of directives).

HOW IS DECISIONAL CAPACITY ASSESSED?

For their stated preferences to be legally and ethically valid, patients need to have intact decision-making capacity. However, it is not appropriate to use a diagnosis of dementia, delirium, or other psychiatric illness to connote decisional incapacity because patients with cognitive impairments or psychiatric diagnoses may be able to assess the risks and benefits of some decisions but not others.[10]

Decisional capacity to choose a medical treatment is also not the same as capacity to complete an advance directive. Voicing preferences in a directive is more complicated than choosing to receive or forego a recommended treatment in a contemporaneous situation. Formulating preferences for a directive requires a patient to consider a future time and hypothetical circumstances involving interactions between treatments and health states. Decisional capacity to execute an advance directive presupposes meaningful, comprehensive communication between the health care provider and the patient. Health care providers should try to ensure that the patient understands and appreciates that the choices articulated in a directive will be used in the future when the patient is no longer capable of participating in the decision-making process. Moreover, the health care provider should ensure that the patient understands that choices can involve medical treatments and the designation of a substitute decision maker, as well as the relative strengths and weaknesses of alternative approaches to advance directives. The patient should be able to understand that choices can change over time, and if they do, that he or she can and should change the directive.

When a patient's decision-making capacity is in doubt, clinicians should assess the elements of decisional capacity. For patients to make decisions about preferred future treatments, they need to have the capacity to do the following:

1. Understand broadly that they are thinking about future situations in which treatment may be needed and what that treatment could entail
2. Appreciate that these choices would be applicable in future situations in which they develop an illness requiring treatment
3. Use their reasoning to reach an opinion about whether the benefits and burdens of having treatment would be acceptable to them
4. Choose and voice a goal of care or treatment preference. Difficult cases can be referred for psychiatric or ethics consultation.

WHEN SHOULD CONVERSATIONS OCCUR?

The best time for advance care planning discussions is before the patient becomes acutely ill. Many patients are willing to have these conversations but prefer that clinicians raise the topic. Ideally, these conversations should happen in an outpatient setting, before a crisis occurs that could impede the patient's ability to think through values and preferences carefully. Other opportune times are those that could be viewed as "teachable moments," for example, after a recent hospitalization or health crisis, when patients raise specific concerns about their care, or when they share stories about the death or serious illness of a close friend or family member. Such moments offer the opportunity to explore a patient's hopes and fears and the values that shape these feelings.

Many palliative care clinicians meet the patient for the first time in a hospital setting. The challenge then is first to determine whether or in what ways the patient is able to participate in discussions. Even when the patient is seriously ill, clinicians should attempt to include him or her in advance care planning discussions to the extent that he or she is able to participate. However, some situations will require that clinicians identify the substitute decision maker who will be able to assist with determining appropriate goals of care and decision making. For example, this is common in intensive care units, where more than 90% of patients are unable to communicate at the time decisions need to be made about withholding or withdrawing life-sustaining treatments.

WHO SHOULD INITIATE THE CONVERSATION?

Any of the clinicians who establish a relationship with the patient and family can initiate advance care planning conversations. Physicians, nurses, social workers, and other team members each bring different expertise and points of entry. Because advance care planning is an iterative process, it can be enhanced when more members of the health care team participate. However, in order for clinicians to initiate advance care planning conversations routinely, this activity needs to be made part of the culture of health care delivery. Health care leaders need to make explicit their expectation that advance care planning is an important component of high-quality care and reinforce its value in patient-centered care. Moreover, leaders need to institute mechanisms that make advance care planning easy to accomplish. Thus, there is the need for more than mere policies. In outpatient settings, clinic schedules need to allow for sufficient time to discuss advance care plans. In inpatient settings, attending physicians need to be champions and role models for trainees by demonstrating how to engage patients in these discussions and elicit patient preferences regarding future decisions.

Physicians bring the perspective of medical facts and available treatment options to advance care planning conversations. Their knowledge of the patient's condition and probable trajectories of illness can help patients and families to understand the range of possible outcomes of future decisions. Regardless of who initiates the conversation, it is important to ensure physician involvement at some point in the process because physicians have the ultimate responsibility for implementing medical decisions and they can probe for inconsistencies in the patient's preferences. For example, some treatment preferences may not match with one another or with stated goals of care, such as, "I want CPR but do not want to be hospitalized."

Nurses bring their expertise in patient education and may be better suited to exploring the psychosocial aspects of the patient's life. In hospital settings, nurses frequently elicit patient and family values with respect to treatment goals. They often serve as information brokers, before and after advance care planning discussions, by answering additional questions, clarifying misunderstandings, explaining details of medical treatments, and revisiting topics addressed in earlier advance care planning discussions.

Social workers can initiate advance care planning conversations by introducing the topic of advance directives and by helping patients and families complete legal documents. In their exploration of social support and service needs, social workers may uncover important values and beliefs that shape patient and family preferences. In addition, their understanding of family dynamics is very helpful when the need arises to negotiate differences of opinion or achieve family consensus about changing goals of care.

Other team members, such as chaplains, may have a significant trust relationship with the patient and family and can also be helpful in advance care planning.

WHAT COMMUNICATION STRATEGIES ARE MOST HELPFUL?

Research has identified that good communication skills are vital to the success of advance care planning discussions. Skills that are particularly valued include being able to listen without interrupting, being open to questions, being sensitive to when patients choose to engage or not engage in these discussions, using plain and honest language, ensuring that patients and families understand what is being said, and appearing comfortable when talking about death and dying.[11] Effective communication strategies that invite an open dialogue include using empathy to respond to the patient or family's emotion and using techniques such as "ask-tell-ask" and "tell me more" to ensure understanding and to elaborate on important values.[12] In "ask-tell-ask," the clinician asks the patient and family to explain their understanding of the current situation, then tells them the objective for the conversation (e.g., to deliver bad news about prognosis or the need to revisit goals of care given the patient's change in condition), and then asks again for the patient and family to restate their understanding. "Tell me more" is a strategy that allows clinicians to determine whether patients and families need more information to understand the situation or the decisions that need to be made, how they are responding emotionally to the conversation, and what the conversation means to them. All of this is useful in deciding how to pace the conversation and what topics should be addressed.

HOW SHOULD THE TOPIC BE INTRODUCED?

There are many ways to introduce the topic of advance care planning, and the choice depends on the clinician–patient relationship and the setting where the conversation takes place. Normalizing the topic and being comfortable discussing it help to put patients and families at ease. In outpatient settings, it is important to explain why the topic is being raised during this particular appointment. Box 20-1 offers some possible scripts that could be used under different circumstances.

Box 20-1. *Scripts for Introducing Advance Care Planning*

ROUTINE VISIT WITH NO RECENT CHANGES IN HEALTH STATUS
"It looks like you are doing well right now, and I expect it to continue that way in the near future. I like to talk with all my patients about their preferences for care in case they get very sick and to determine who they would want to make decisions for them if they were too sick to make their own decisions. I think it's best to talk about these things when patients are feeling well and long before we have to react to a crisis. That gives both of us plenty of time to talk about what matters to you so that I can give you the kinds of care that match your goals. Would it be okay for us to talk about this today?"

EPISODE OF ACUTE ILLNESS OR HOSPITALIZATION
"To make sure that we are working together while you are so sick, it is important that we talk about your goals for care at this time. I know it can be hard to think about these things when you are ill, but would it be okay for us to spend a little time talking about this right now?"

FOLLOW-UP VISIT AFTER ILLNESS EXACERBATION
"You were pretty sick last time I saw you. Are you feeling better now? It's times like this that I like to talk about goals of care to make sure that I'm up to date with what you would want in case you have another episode like that and others might have to make decisions for you. Would it be okay for us to talk about this now?"

WHAT TOPICS SHOULD BE ADDRESSED?

A range of topics can be addressed, depending on how willing the patient is to engage in the process. At a minimum, patients should be asked to identify the person or persons who should speak on their behalf if that becomes necessary. It is important to inform patients about relevant laws on the legal hierarchy of substitute decision makers, especially in the absence of a legally appointed proxy health care agent. Typically, the hierarchy is as follows (although this should be verified against state or provincial laws):

1. Court-appointed guardian
2. Proxy health care agent
3. Spouse
4. Adult children
5. Parents
6. Adult siblings

Hierarchy laws may cause problems for some patients, particularly those with large families or nontraditional family relationships, such as common-law or same-sex partners. For example, many patients do not know that some laws require consensus among multiple persons in a category (e.g., all adult children must agree) or that estranged spouses still have legal authority over others to make decisions for the patient. Patients who believe there may be debate and disagreement among family members or who have family relationships that may not be recognized by law should be encouraged to complete a durable power of attorney for health care or similar document to give their substitute decision maker more legal standing as the preferred and legal decision maker.

Most patients are willing to identify a substitute decision maker. Although cognitively impaired individuals may not be able to make decisions about treatment, they may still be capable of identifying which person they would prefer to make decisions on their behalf. Box 20-2 provides a set of criteria for evaluating who would be the best candidates to act as a substitute decision maker. After a substitute decision maker has been identified, it may be best to end the first advance care planning conversation by encouraging the patient to have the substitute decision maker attend the next visit to discuss preferences and goals of care.

Box 20-2. *Recommendations for Choosing a Durable Power of Attorney for Health Care*

Consider the following qualifications and traits when choosing which person is best suited to act as the durable power of attorney for health care:
- Meets the legal criteria for appointing a proxy/health care agent
- Willing to speak on behalf of the patient
- Able to act on the patient's wishes and separate his or her own feelings
- Lives close by or could travel if needed
- Knows the patient well and understands what is important to him or her
- Could handle the responsibility, physically and emotionally
- Will talk with the patient now about sensitive issues
- Available in the future if needed
- Able to handle conflicting opinions among family members, friends, or medical personnel

> **Box 20-3.** *Specific Questions to Elicit Preferences and Goals of Care*
>
> "Who should speak for you if you're too sick to speak for yourself?"
> "What is your understanding of your current illness?"
> "What are you hoping for?"
> "We're always hoping for the best, but we also know that sometimes we need to plan for the worst. What are your fears about your illness and how it's going to affect you in the future? If what you fear were to happen, what would you hope for then?"
> "What are your past experiences caring for someone who is or was seriously ill? What did you learn from those experiences about how you want to be cared for?"
> "Who do you count on for support? Is there anyone specifically you would want to be involved in your care [including family, friends, and religious or spiritual advisers]?"

When the substitute decision maker is present, it is helpful to restate the goal of the advance care planning discussion and the role of the substitute decision maker, including a reminder that the substitute's authority as a decision maker takes effect only when the patient becomes decisionally incapacitated. The clinician can then review what is known about the patient's wishes and can give the patient an opportunity to expand on preferences and goals of care. Box 20-3 lists questions that clinicians can use to discuss a patient's preferences and goals of care.

Topics to explore include gaining an understanding of patient and family values and beliefs with respect to their hopes and fears about their illness. For some, this topic may involve a discussion of religious beliefs and cultural values. For others, this topic may lead to a discussion of undesirable outcomes or situations in which the patient would choose to die rather than rely on medical technologies that support life. If they mention these situations, it is important to explore the features of the circumstances that makes them so extremely unacceptable, especially because patients frequently end up in situations that do not exactly match their conceptualizations.

Another point to consider is what people mean when they use certain terms. For example, some people might mention that having dementia would be unacceptable without understanding the full range of abilities and time course of the illness. Thus, when people use such terms, it is important to probe what it is about dementia (or other health conditions) that is of concern. Similarly, some patients have strong feelings about "*never* being on machines." Again, it is important to explore the source of these feelings because often they are based on misunderstandings of what the treatment entails or because they do not know about the option of therapeutic trials that can be stopped after a short time. Discussions about specific treatments should always be framed around goals of care and how those treatments will be used to reach the desired outcome, not the treatments in and of themselves.

The patient and the substitute decision maker should discuss the degree of interpretive leeway that can be exercised in adhering to the patient's previously expressed preferences. Research has documented that many patients are comfortable with allowing substitute decision makers some leeway in decision making.[13] Additionally, although autonomy is the major principle that guides advance care planning, some patients who still retain decision-making capacity prefer to defer to the judgment of their substitute decision makers and acknowledge that the best outcome may be one that does not always maximize their personal autonomy. One reason that patients defer decision making and allow substitute decision makers leeway in interpreting their preferences is because they recognize that family members should be able to consider the big picture, including their own needs and interests.

It is important to determine whether the substitute decision maker is comfortable with the plan and to discuss any anticipated difficulties (e.g., discomfort making the decision to withdraw life support) or fundamental differences in values (e.g., sanctity of life vs. quality of life). Substitute decision makers often need support with coming to terms with their loved one's illness and impending death. Sometimes differences in values reflect substitute decision makers' difficulty with letting go and may signal the need for help with anticipatory grief or with feeling overwhelmed by the responsibility for making life-and-death decisions. It can be helpful to reassure substitute decision makers that the clinical team will be responsible for making treatment recommendations and making treatment decisions about life support. The substitute decision maker's role will be to represent the patient's values and preferences with respect to the goals of care. This can help to relieve the substitute decision maker's feelings of responsibility for causing the patient's death when, for example, decisions about withholding or withdrawing life-sustaining treatments are made.

For patients with chronic illness or those whose trajectory of decline is somewhat predictable, it is very useful to discuss contingency plans for how the patient and family may respond to acute exacerbations or other sudden changes in health status. Patients and families report that being prepared for the next steps on their illness journey is highly valued.[11] Knowing who to call and where to go in an emergency helps patients and families to manage the uncertainties of illness and dying.

Some people advocate discussing prognosis with patients as part of advance care planning, especially if the patient may die in the next 12 months. The benefits of discussing prognosis with those patients who are willing to do so is that it can help them and their families prioritize how they would like to spend their remaining time. In addition, a patient's preferences for life-sustaining treatment may be shaped by his or her understandings of the prognosis. For example, patients who are optimistic about their survival are more likely to choose more aggressive therapies, even those therapies that health care providers consider futile. In contrast, patients who acknowledge a shorter life expectancy are more likely to accept palliative care referrals and the shift in goals to palliative care.[14]

WHAT IF PATIENTS AND FAMILIES ARE RELUCTANT TO DISCUSS THESE ISSUES?

Patients and family members have legitimate reasons to resist engaging in advance care planning discussions. These include perceiving that the topic is irrelevant, trusting family members to make good decisions, cultural traditions that discourage discussing bad news to keep it from manifesting, a desire to avoid thinking about death and dying as a coping mechanism, and an unwillingness to focus on future events either because it distracts from the present or because there is no point in speculating about events that cannot be controlled.[15-18] For all these reasons, it is a good idea to ask permission to discuss the topic before fully launching into the agenda. If the patient appears hesitant, the discussion should focus on appointing a substitute decision maker. One way for the clinician to frame further exploration of preferences is to explain that this is a means of helping the patient hope for the best while preparing for the worst. The "ask-tell-ask" and "tell me more" strategies can be useful ways to explore the patient's hopes and fears. Responding to emotions allows for exploration of possible barriers to engaging in advance care planning discussions. If the patient is reluctant to talk about death and dying, exploring that reluctance may allow the health care provider to discover a way to approach the topic that feels more comfortable to the patient and family. Although they may be uncomfortable imagining themselves with a life-threatening illness, some patients are willing to discuss the illnesses and deaths of people in their lives or in the media. Probing a patient's opinions about the situations of these other individuals can be an indirect way to obtain information about their preferences. If patients choose not to engage in the specifics of advance care planning discussions, it is reasonable to describe how future decisions likely will be made and by whom, so the patient is aware of the consequences of his or her choice.

PEARLS

- Initiate advance care planning discussions as a component of early goal planning conversations because patients are often waiting for clinicians to raise this topic.

- Include substitute decision makers in these discussions whenever possible to ensure shared understanding of goals of care among all stakeholders (patients, substitute decision makers and other family members, and health care providers). If substitute decision makers cannot participate, encourage patients to discuss their goals, values, and preferences with their substitute decision makers and family members.

- Use the patient's (and family's) values and goals of care (rather than specific treatment preferences) to focus advance care planning discussions.

- Check in early and regularly throughout a patient's illness while he or she still is capable and when clinical changes occur, to ascertain whether the patient's goals of care have changed.

- Use communication strategies that include lay language and invite open-ended dialogue to ensure that patients and family members understand what is being said and to provide opportunities for patients to express their values and preferences.

PITFALLS

- Do not wait until the patient is near death to engage in advance care planning conversations.

- Do not confuse the collaborative, ongoing process of advance care planning with completion of advance directives or a POLST form.

- It is a mistake to assume that patients with dementia cannot express their wishes. Especially in the early stages, these patients are often capable of expressing their preferences for their proxy decision maker.

- Failure to check with substitute decision makers to see what help they may need in implementing the patient's care plan can result in an inability to meet the patient's stated goals of care.

- Forcing patients and families to engage in specific conversations when they are not ready or willing to discuss details about death and dying can derail advance care planning.

Summary

Advance care planning is an integral part of palliative care and is one way to monitor changing goals of care as the illness progresses. Because people continue to accommodate to new challenges presented by their illnesses, it is important to check periodically to ensure that earlier values and preferences continue to be relevant and applicable. Patients may be more or less willing to discuss details about their prospective preferences for future treatments. For this reason, we recommend that advance care planning focus on establishing goals of care, given the likely trajectory of the patient's illness, and the appointment of one or more designated substitute decision makers. When possible, these proxies should be present for any discussions about shifting goals of care because it is important for them to be aware of any changes in the patient's values and preferences. Exploring the reasons behind any preferences, including the reasons behind any changes in preferences, can be helpful in bringing discordant views into alignment. This process can also identify areas in which family members may need support to help them manage anticipatory grief or closure with their loved one.

Resources

National Hospice and Palliative Care Organization Caring Connections. Advance directive forms by state (United States) and province (Canada).
   www.caringinfo.org/stateaddownload
Dalhousie University's Health Law End of Life Project.
   http://as01.ucis.dal.ca/dhli/cmp_advdirectives/default.cfm
Medical Directive: Aids for personalized instructions.
   www.medicaldirective.org/current/index.asp.
Your Life, Your Choices: Planning for Future Medical Decisions.
   www.rihlp.org/pubs/Your_life_your_choices.pdf
   (Updates forthcoming on www.myhealth.va.gov)
Values History Form
   http://hsc.unm.edu/ethics/advdir/vhform_eng.shtml
Five Wishes
   www.fivewishes.org
National Resource Center on Psychiatric Advance Directives. A source for psychiatric advance directives.
   www.nrc-pad.org
Balaban RB: A physician's guide to talking about end-of-life care, *J Gen Intern Med* 15:195–200, 2000.
Physicians Orders for Life Sustaining Treatment (POLST): From the Center for Ethics in Health Care, Oregon Health Sciences University.
   www.ohsu.edu/polst

References

1. Field MJ, Cassel CK, editors: *Approaching death: improving care at the end of life*, National Washington, DC, 1997, Academy Press.
2. Kaldjian LC, Curtis AE, Shinkunas LA, et al: Goals of care toward the end of life: a structured literature review, *Am J Hosp Palliat Care* 25:501–511, 2009.
3. Pearlman RA, Cole WG, Patrick DL, et al: Advance care planning: eliciting patient preferences for life-sustaining treatment, *Patient Educ Couns* 26:353–361, 1995.
4. Luce JM: End-of-life care: What do the American courts say? *Crit Care Med* 29(Suppl):N40–N45, 2001.
5. Ramsaroop SD: Completing an advance directive in the primary care setting: what do we need for success? *J Am Geriatr Soc* 55:277–283, 2007.
6. Morrison RS: The inaccessibility of advance directives on transfer from ambulatory to acute care settings, *JAMA* 274:478–482, 1995.
7. Fagerlin A: Enough: the failure of the living will, *Hastings Cent Rep* 32:30–42, 2004.
8. Tolle SW, Tilden VP, Nelson CA, et al: A prospective study of the efficacy of the physician order form for life-sustaining treatment, *J Am Geriatr Soc* 46:1097–1102, 1998.

9. Meier DE: POLST offers next stage in honoring patient preferences, *J Palliat Med* 12:291–295, 2009.
10. Kim SYH: *Evaluation of capacity to consent to treatment and research*, New York, 2010, Oxford University Press.
11. Steinhauser KE, Christakis NA, Clipp EC, et al: Factors considered important at the end of life by patients, family, physicians, and other care providers, *JAMA* 284:2476–2482, 2000.
12. Back AL, Arnold RM, Baile WF, et al: Approaching difficult communication tasks in oncology, *CA Cancer J Clin* 55:164–177, 2005.
13. Hawkins NA, Ditto PH, Danks JH, et al: Micromanaging death: process preferences, values, and goals in end-of-life medical decision making, *Gerontologist* 45:107–117, 2005.
14. Weeks JC, Cook EF, O'Day SJ, et al: Relationship between cancer patients' predictions of prognosis and their treatment preferences, *JAMA* 279:1709–1714, 1998.
15. Perkins HS, Geppert CM, Gonzales A, et al: Cross-cultural similarities and differences in attitudes about advance care planning, *J Gen Intern Med* 17(1):48–57, 2002.
16. Carrese JA, Mullaney JL, Faden RR, et al: Planning for death but not serious future illness: qualitative study of housebound elderly patients, *BMJ* 325:125–129, 2002.
17. Kwak J: Current research findings on end-of-life decision making among racially or ethnically diverse groups, *Gerontologist* 45(5):634–641, 2005.
18. Schickedanz AD, Schillinger D, Landefeld CS, et al: A clinical framework for improving the advance care planning process: start with patients' self-identified barriers, *J Am Geriatr Soc* 57(1):31–39, 2009.

CHAPTER 21

Responding to Requests for Euthanasia and Physician-Assisted Suicide

NUALA P. KENNY

The palliative care movement developed in response to concerns that care at the end of life had been badly done in the midst of the acute care and technologic advances of 20th-century medicine. The need for special attention to end-of-life issues emerged not because of modern medicine's failures, but from its successes. Phenomenal advances in medical science and technology during the 20th century increased fears of dying and loss of control to a sterile and terrifying technology at the end of life. We had become not just a death-denying but a death-defying society, with an almost limitless possibility of medical benefit where something *more* could always be done. Those same technologies that can save life can also prolong dying.

Palliative care, with its goals of providing better medical care for pain and symptom control and attending more appropriately to the personal, emotional, and spiritual issues at the end of life, has become an important component of health care in most developed nations. Despite significant challenges to the recognition of the limits of medicine to cure and to the acknowledgment of dying, serious issues of access to high-quality palliative care, and the need for research in the difficult symptoms at the end of life, palliative care has made significant improvements in the care of the dying.[1] Despite these advances, a renewed interest in the "right to die" through legalizing assisted death (AD)—euthanasia and physician-assisted suicide

284

(PAS)—has emerged. In order to understand this interest and to respond appropriately, palliative care practitioners and supporters need to reflect on the context of death and dying today as well as the evolution of medical decision making.

Changes in where and how we die in developed nations have been profound. Historically, death was common, normal, and quick. The elderly died of pneumonia, "the old man's friend," and death occurred at home. Today, death increasingly comes in hospitals for individuals who are still undergoing aggressive treatment directed at cure. Our institutions are structured for the old way of dying, where the doctor is central, the priest and family peripheral. It has been suggested that we need a new art of dying because whereas in earlier times many worried about death coming too early, many of us now worry that death will come too late.[2] Today, because of the almost endless possibilities of modern technology, we need to reflect carefully on how we would want to use technology at our end. We even have to think of these things in advance of our dying in case we cannot express our wishes. Dying, previously seen as a natural matter of fate or personal faith, is seen now as a matter of personal choice. Requests for assisted death can be seen as an extension of modern bioethics with its centrality of respect for patient autonomy in medical decision making. This includes the competent patient's right to refuse care and the development of advance directives as a mechanism of promoting the patient's autonomy when the patient is incompetent. From an ethical perspective, a major shift occurs with movement from the right to refuse treatments considered nonbeneficial or burdensome by the patient to the right to assistance in death.

There has been a long-standing prohibition in society and in Western medicine against the intentional ending of life. Legal changes in the last decades in some jurisdictions have fueled the debate. In Europe, after a long series of judicial decisions, the Netherlands formally legalized both euthanasia and PAS in 2002. Belgium has legalized PAS; Switzerland has legalized AD and so allows people other than physicians to end life; Luxembourg legalized both euthanasia and PAS in 2008. Northern Australia adopted AD legislation in the late 1990s, but it was rescinded; Southern Australia rejected narrowly AD legislation in late 2009. In North America, the state of Oregon legalized PAS by lethal prescription in 1997; Washington state approved the same in 2009, and Montana legalized AD by judicial fiat. State initiatives are constantly proposing various bills. Many other jurisdictions, including the United Kingdom and Canada, are actively debating PAS. Clearly there has been a major shift in the traditional prohibition in many jurisdictions.

Although this shifting context presents fundamental ethical and moral issues for societies and medicine, it poses some urgent and very particular questions to the palliative care communities. Changes in legal and social policy surrounding assisted death will have profound effects on the practice of palliative care and on individual palliative care practitioners. It is crucial for palliative care providers to understand the issues and to reflect on their position with regard to PAS and euthanasia. With the renewed interest in the legalization of PAS, those committed to palliative care at the end of life face some crucially important questions:

1. Is the renewed interest in euthanasia and PAS a consequence of the failure of palliative care to improve end-of-life care?
2. Is physician-assisted death by euthanasia or assisted suicide an essential tool of last resort in palliative care?
3. Or is physician-assisted death inherently contradictory to the philosophy and goals of palliative care?

Any approach to these questions requires reflection on the goals of palliative care, an understanding of the philosophical arguments supporting and rejecting assisted death, and knowledge of the actual reasons for requests for assisted death and the experience of palliative care practitioners where such practices have been legalized. These questions will require individual responses from clinicians when requests for assistance in dying are made and communal responses from palliative care communities after careful reflection on the implications of PAS and euthanasia on their commitments to the dying. Fortunately, we now have some empirical information from palliative care experience to assist in deliberation on these crucially important questions.

Philosophy and Goals of Palliative Care

Palliative care emerged in the United Kingdom, the United States, and Canada during the 1960s. With the enormous scientific and technologic advances of the 1960s and early 1970s, critics began to warn of the medicalization of dying (e.g., use of the portable ventilator, renal dialysis, and cardiopulmonary resuscitation) and feared these interventions could lead to a loss of the capacity to accept death and dying as normal, a rejection of the importance of personal and family care at the end of life, a disregard for traditional religious and cultural rituals surrounding death and dying, and medical control of the dying person conceptualized as *a patient* until the end.

A concern for fostering the dignity of dying persons and a commitment to restoring care of the dying as a proper goal of medicine was the inspiration for the founders of the palliative care movement. The vision of Dame Cecily Saunders was actualized with the founding of St. Christopher's Hospice in the United Kingdom in 1967. The term *palliative care* describes the parallel development of medical expertise in end-of-life care. These movements demonstrated renewed commitment to the care of the dying and to improving pain and symptom control as soon as possible in the course of any chronic, ultimately fatal illness.

These approaches stress the multifaceted, multidimensional nature of the experience of living with an acknowledged time-limiting illness and the priority of working as a team to achieve the relief of suffering and the enhancement of the last days of life. Supporting the patient, family, and loved ones as a unit became a hallmark of palliative care. The sense of medical abandonment of the dying, seen as a failure of medicine, was replaced by a return to the traditional medical goal of care for the dying. The idea of a *good death* has been central to palliative care. A *good death* has been described as one that is pain free, where dying is acknowledged and preferably occurs at home in the presence of family and friends, with the patient aware and alert as long as possible so the unresolved business of life can be accomplished.

The underlying norms and values of palliative care have been articulated by the World Health Organization (WHO) and the European Association for Palliative Care (EAPC) among others. WHO's definition states that palliative care "affirms life and regards dying as a normal process.... Intends neither to hasten nor postpone death".[3] EAPC affirms the WHO definition and has concluded that "the provision of euthanasia and physician-assisted suicide should not be part of the responsibility of palliative care".[4] Generally then, the palliative care community has been opposed to practices of AD[4-6]; however, a small minority appear open to such legislation and see good palliative care as the standard, with access to physician-assisted death as a "last resort".[7] For palliative care this is not just another debate about differences of opinion in pluralistic societies. It represents a profoundly important set of questions regarding the philosophy, goals, and practices of palliative care.

Language, Rhetoric, and Definitions

Many different terms and concepts are used in the general societal debates about euthanasia and PAS. Much of the confusion surrounding these issues has arisen because of a lack of clarity regarding the issues and concepts. This is not surprising because each term is related to a profoundly value-laden set of concepts and practices. Public opinion polls show varying degrees of support for the right to assistance in death in the face of unrelieved pain and suffering. All these polls demonstrate confusion regarding the right to refuse interventions, the role of palliative care, and the current state of pain and symptom control.

Palliative care practitioners need to be clear in their understanding of the various important terms and concepts involved in the practice of palliative care. There is considerable confusion regarding palliative care itself. First and foremost for palliative care is the confusing use of "assistance in dying" language in the debates. Palliative care at end of life is committed to assistance in the process of dying. Euthanasia and AS are actions aimed at assistance in achieving death.

The right of a competent patient to refuse medical interventions, based on his or her judgment of the benefits and burdens, is central to modern practice. Termination of life-sustaining treatments generally refers to the withholding or withdrawing of life-sustaining treatment at the request of a competent patient or that patient's representative, a proxy or surrogate. The broad consensus is that physicians are not only allowed to honor these requests, they are also legally and ethically bound to do so.

The two practices that are the focus of legislation are PAS and euthanasia. PAS involves the physician's providing the means for a patient to end life, usually by prescribing a lethal dose of a medication or furnishing information to enable the patient to perform the life-ending act. It requires a suicide—that is, the patient performs the act that causes death. In contrast to the agreement regarding the termination of treatment, there is no consensus on PAS. Most health care professional organizations oppose PAS on ethical grounds, and most jurisdictions have clear legal prohibitions. The ongoing debates question whether these prohibitions should be lifted.

In contrast to PAS, euthanasia involves the physician's performing an intervention, usually a lethal injection, which ends the patient's life. Euthanasia is categorized as voluntary, involuntary, and nonvoluntary. *Voluntary euthanasia* is requested by the patient; *involuntary euthanasia* is performed despite the objections of the patient; and *nonvoluntary euthanasia* occurs when the patient's decision has not been sought or, as in the case of infants and young children, there is a lack of decisional capacity.

Palliative care practitioners have developed intermediate practices such as aggressive pain management and terminal sedation that, for some, challenge the traditional distinction between forgoing treatment and actively assisting death.

Most observers would be able to distinguish classic cases of forgoing treatment (say, by withdrawing artificial ventilation) from assisting suicide (say, by providing a lethal prescription). The claim, however, is that it would be harder to distinguish two practices from assisted suicide or euthanasia: first, pain relief that may suppress respiration and hasten death, and second, sedation combined with withdrawal of artificial nutrition.[8]

There have been concerns that *aggressive pain relief with opioids* may hasten death. Even if this were accurate, the use of aggressive pain relief has been considered ethically acceptable when there is no less dangerous way to provide pain relief, the competent patient is informed of the risks and benefits and gives consent, and the physician's intent is therapeutic, not to hasten death. The empirical data are increasingly clear about effects. Competent palliative care practice utilizing opioids for pain control does not hasten death.[9-13]

Terminal sedation raises other issues. Definitions differ, but the term usually means sedating a patient to unconsciousness while withholding artificial nutrition. If sedation to loss of consciousness is necessary to provide good pain or symptom relief and the patient agrees to it and to the withdrawal of artificial nutrition, this is considered acceptable practice. The primary goal of terminal sedation is effective relief of refractory symptoms. However, terminal sedation is used judiciously because it results in the loss of capacity for interaction, the other crucial goal of end-of-life care.[14,15]

These two standard practices of palliative care have been justified by the ethical *principle of double effect,* meaning the following: The act must be good or morally neutral; only the good effect is intended, whereas the bad effect is merely foreseen; the bad effect must not be the means to the good effect; and the good effect must outweigh the bad. The principle is not a simple mathematical formula but rather requires judgment regarding which effects are good or bad. Here, the intention of the doctor (to relieve pain and suffering, not to end the life of the patient) is crucially important.

Arguments for and against Euthanasia and Physician-Assisted Suicide

It is important for palliative care physicians to understand, at least in a general way, the reasons put forward in support of PAS and euthanasia and the long-standing arguments against allowing physicians to end life intentionally. This is an area of deep and highly contested issues and values.

FOR

Arguments in favor of PAS include the principle of respect for the autonomy of competent persons, the duty of physicians to care for patients who are in pain and suffering, and rejection of the distinctions considered morally and ethically relevant in the current practice of palliative care, such as that between killing and letting someone die. Proponents believe that the practices can be regulated, and regulation is dealt with in the next section.

The central argument for PAS is based on patients' rights and on respect for autonomy in modern society and health care in particular. This would extend the right to make decisions to include the right to determine the course of one's own dying. Under this argument, no competent person should have to endure what they judge to be unbearable pain, suffering, loss of dignity, or loss of quality of life. The right is based on principles of dignity, respect, and autonomous choice. It is seen as a control on the unrestrained use of technology at the end of life. This reasoning rests on a conception of autonomy as "negative liberty"—that is, the right to act in accordance with one's beliefs and choices without interference as long that behavior does not harm others. Proponents of PAS argue that this right should include an individual's control over the timing and circumstances of death, up to and including assistance in dying. In this understanding, PAS is a personal decision, an application of the right to self-determination that should be free from paternalistic interference from any source. It is seen as a type of rational suicide.

Some arguments for PAS are based on the claim that physicians have a duty to provide assistance in dying if the patient's suffering cannot be relieved by standard care. This argument is based on understanding PAS as a compassionate response to medical failure. Others go farther and argue that a physician's refusal of requests for AD by competent, terminally ill patients constitutes a kind of abandonment. These proponents argue that the traditional prohibitions of the Hippocratic Oath—against abortion and surgery, for example—have been lifted in response to changing social situations. In this understanding, the Hippocratic tradition requires a physician to alleviate suffering, and this can include PAS if that is the only solution. Moreover, PAS is distinct from euthanasia in that it does not involve the ending of life by a physician; the person takes his or her own life, a suicide.

Some argue that no principled difference exists between acceptable practices such as terminating life-sustaining treatment and aggressive pain control (omission) and euthanasia and PAS (commission) and also no meaningful distinction between letting die and killing.

AGAINST

The main arguments against PAS and euthanasia understand these life-ending procedures as contradictory to the physician's role so rejection of such procedures is crucial to the integrity of medicine; these procedures do not promote patient autonomy but further medicalize both human suffering (in contrast to pain and other physical symptoms) and dying; the practice is not necessary for efficient and compassionate care at the end of life and allowing the procedures will lead to error and abuse that cannot be regulated.

Although there were early debates about the practice, the Hippocratic prohibition against a physician's intentional ending of life is long standing. Today, with notable exceptions, most professional organizations (e.g., the American Medical Association and the Canadian Medical Association) hold that euthanasia and PAS are incompatible with the physician's role as healer. Trust is central in the patient–doctor relationship, and it requires a clear commitment to restore and promote life. Violations of this trust are possible when death is a legitimate option. Some believe that the "false promise of beneficent killing"[16] unalterably changes the patient–doctor relationship.

A physician must respect a competent patient's right to refuse potentially lifesaving treatment. However, this does not translate into an obligation to end life, even at the patient's request. In addition, a physician who is caring for a patient at the end of life should provide adequate and effective pain and symptom control. Opponents argue that PAS and euthanasia do not promote patient autonomy but give more power and authority to the physician and medicalize suicide.

Assisted death has also been described as "self-determination run amok".[17] Respect for autonomy is important, but other interests and values are at stake. Even if voluntary euthanasia and PAS were accepted as instruments of personal autonomy, limits should be set for the sake of other goods. A paradox emerges here. PAS is seen as a radically individual manifestation of autonomy, but it requires the agreement and participation of physicians and society. As long as PAS requires the assistance of others, it cannot be conceived of as solely an extension of individual autonomy. PAS is an impediment to an individual's autonomy rather than an extension of it. It medicalizes an act, a practice, and the social ethos of death and suicide. Ideally, the patient is not abandoned, so the physician must be present. PAS becomes a medical act.

Opponents argue that euthanasia and PAS are not needed to provide good end-of-life care. Much of the public support for these practices is based on a belief that they are necessary in some circumstances of intractable pain, but advances in palliative care have made such circumstances extremely rare.[1] Moreover, as long as doctors can provide aggressive pain relief, including terminal sedation if necessary, intractable pain is not a necessary or usual experience at the end of life.

Finally, opponents have grave concerns about error and abuse of PAS and euthanasia. Recognizing the prevalence of depression in the chronically and terminally ill and the tendency for doctors to underestimate depression, substantive concerns exist regarding the patient's competence to request PAS and euthanasia. Depression and hopelessness are important because treatment, if provided, could alter the request for PAS or euthanasia.[18,19] Opponents have significant concerns for vulnerable populations, such as the disabled and chronically ill, who already experience subtle pressures to accept limits. There are special concerns for discrimination against women and children, who can be perceived as burdensome. Because health care costs are a concern for many, especially those with no insurance coverage, these concerns about pressures and limits are real. Although proponents of PAS and euthanasia base their arguments on the free choice of competent adults to make decisions regarding their dying, there is grave concern for the "slippery slope" extension to practices involving others who have not made or who cannot make such choices.

Regulation and the "Slippery Slope"

Debate is vigorous over the effectiveness of regulating practices such as PAS and euthanasia. These debates turn on the notion of the slippery slope. The slippery slope connotes a concern that some practices, once allowed for specific reasons, gradually slide from an acceptable to an unacceptable state. Therefore, the argument for these practices of AD is made for the right of competent persons to determine the circumstances of their own death. However, once AD is allowed for these persons, the practice slides to include others who have not requested assistance in dying and those who have no capacity to make such a request. If intentionally ending death is a good thing for rational persons, then it ought to be provided to others; this is how the slippery slope occurs. Philosophers and others argue that there is a logical and an empirical slippery slope and that reasons for allowing a practice at the top of the slope can be logically distinguished from reasons for allowing practice at the bottom of the slope. Regulation of these practices is based on the importance of such logical distinctions. The empirical slippery slope is complex because it relates to societal acceptance of practices that were never intended at the outset, but with which society becomes comfortable over time. The empirical evidence of a practice should assist us in judging whether the slide has actually occurred.

Some propose that it is better to regulate covert practice and believe that safeguards regarding the slippery slope are possible through legislation and professional regulation. Guidelines have been suggested to ensure that the request is voluntary, the procedure is a last resort, and there is public accountability. Empirical data from the two jurisdictions with experience (Oregon and the Netherlands) have given rise to competing assessments of the effectiveness of regulations.

The Oregon Death with Dignity Act provides that a capable adult suffering from a terminal disease and who voluntarily expresses a wish to die may make a request for medication for the purpose of ending his or her life. Reports are dependent on physician reporting. Subsequent studies and their conclusions have been criticized on methodologic grounds. Since the Oregon assisted suicide law was enacted, 297 Oregonians have used PAS to die between 1998 and 2006. The ratio of PAS deaths to total deaths in Oregon has increased from 5 per 10,000 to 19.4 per 10,000 in 2008. Thus, the Oregon experience seems to demonstrate that although an increase in PAS deaths has occurred, a tidal wave of PAS and euthanasia has not. Without accurate reporting, however, valid judgments on the practice are impossible. A recent review continues the questioning of adequate reporting and monitoring in Oregon:

> "In the absence of adequate monitoring, the focus shifts away from relieving the distress of dying patients considering a hastened death to meeting the statutory requirements for assisted suicide."[20]

This is an example of a shift in social concern subsequent to legalization of AD.

Interpretations of the Dutch experience regarding a slippery slope are conflicting as well.[21] The Netherlands implemented euthanasia and PAS before palliative care services were developed. Since 1973, courts in the Netherlands have dealt with cases of both PAS and euthanasia, but prosecutors mostly dismissed physicians from prosecution if they adhered to a set of minimum requirements. In 2001, the Dutch Parliament legalized both practices. An official reporting procedure was established in 1993. In 2005, 1.7% of all deaths were euthanasia as compared with 2.6% in 1990. Assisted suicide was less common in each year reported. Reporting has been a difficulty here as well as in Oregon. The reporting rate for euthanasia has increased from 18% in 1990 to 80.2% in 2005, but significant numbers of Dutch physicians do not comply with reporting requirements, and this issue raises serious questions regarding oversight.

Some conclude that there is a cautious use of PAS and euthanasia in a well-regulated practice in the Netherlands. However, in the past 2 decades, the Netherlands has moved to legalize PAS and euthanasia for those who are chronically ill or in psychological distress. Moreover, the Dutch experience of nonvoluntary euthanasia involving children and incompetent adults legitimizes the concern that euthanasia can be abused more readily than PAS. This finding reinforces concerns regarding the slippery slope.

Understanding Requests for Assisted Death: From Argument to Experience

Most palliative care practitioners have received requests for euthanasia or PAS. Understanding the issues underlying both desires for hastened death and reasons for actual requests for assisted death are crucially important. Even while acknowledging methodologic flaws and the ethical complexities in research around end of life, research is helping to clarify a number of issues about the reasons for the requests and responses of health care professionals within and without palliative care. Some representative samples of the growing body of empirical evidence, both quantitative and qualitative, are included here.

The first published study assessing the attitudes and experiences regarding PAS and euthanasia found that "the key determinants of interest in euthanasia relate not to physical symptoms but to psychological distress and care needs".[22] A U.S. study of how experienced physicians respond to not infrequent requests for assisted death, even where illegal, identified a code of silence among physicians about discussing these requests and their effects on physicians. These investigators identified three categories of issues and physician responses[23]:

Physical symptoms: Responded to by increased pain and symptom management
Psychological issues: Responded to by attending to issues of depression and anxiety
Existential suffering: Most frequently responded to by assistance in death

Here, physicians were surprised requests came from persons who were "alert and functional" and not in pain.[23]

In a systematic review on understanding and appropriately responding to desire-to-die statements from patients with advanced disease, Hudson and colleagues categorized (1) feelings and current reactions to circumstances (fears regarding death and loss of control); (2) communication of distress and suffering or a communication exploring ways to relieve distress; (3) asking for information regarding euthanasia and physician-assisted suicide because of feelings described in categories 1 and 2; and (4) specifically seeking assistance with hastening death or acknowledging the intent to commit suicide.[24] Zylicz identifies five main profiles[25]:

1. Patients whose request is based on fear of the future (anxiety)
2. Patients who are exhausted by their disease course (burnout)
3. Patients who desire to control a disease process they experience as out of control
4. Patients with depression
5. Patients whose main motive is based on a belief that it is their right to determine the circumstances of their death

Other studies have now explored directly the reasons patients and their family members give for their requests. One such study of patients who were seriously considering PAS and their family members, recruited through advocacy organizations that counseled hastened death, identified seven issues in three major categories[26]:

1. Illness-related experiences, including feeling weak, tired, and uncomfortable; pain and or unacceptable side effects of pain medications; and loss of function
2. Sense of self and the desire not to lose control
3. Fears about the future, focusing on fears for future quality of life and dying and negative past experiences of dying

This same study noted "that pain is often not the most salient motivating factor".[26] Another study of family members of 83 Oregon decedents who had made explicit requests for legalized physician-assisted death, including 52 who received prescriptions and 32 who died of physician-assisted death, were asked for the reasons for the request.

"According to family members, the most important reasons for PAD were: wanting to control the circumstances of death and die at home, and worries about loss of dignity and future losses of independence, quality of life and self-care ability. No physical symptoms at the time of the request were rated higher than a median of 2 (of 5) in importance. Worries about symptoms and experiences in the future were."[27]

Most of the reported requests for physician-hastened death come from patients with terminal cancer. A Norwegian study of patients with advanced cancer at a palliative medicine unit focused on understanding wishes for and attitudes about euthanasia. The study's authors found that wishes were generally "fluctuating and ambivalent" and that "*fear* of future pain, rather than actual, perceived pain, was the predominant motivation for a possible future wish for euthanasia".[28] A Canadian study surveyed patients receiving palliative care for cancer to determine attitudes toward the legalization of euthanasia and physician-assisted death and personal interest in a hastened death. Approximately 62% of these patients endorsed the legalization of euthanasia and physician-assisted suicide. They endorsed it as a future possibility. Only 5.8% said that if it were legal they would have used it. This study highlighted again the importance of physical and psychological findings. More than 50% had a sense of self-perceived burden to others; 40% of those with a desire for euthanasia or physician-assisted suicide met diagnostic criteria for major depression.[29]

The issue of depression has been the subject of a growing and increasingly robust body of research. Chochinov and colleagues found a strong relationship between the desire for hastened death and clinical depression.[18] Breitbart and colleagues found that the "diagnosis of depression was significantly associated with desire for hastened death".[19] These investigators also pursued the notion of "hopelessness" as a cognitive functioning style, not as a prognostic factor, and found that "the presence of both depression and hopelessness increased desire for hastened death considerably".[19] This body of research for a treatable condition has important consequences for medicine's and palliative care's response.

Effect on Physicians and Other Health Care Practitioners

The effects of AD on the practicing physicians have also been the object of some research. Recognizing that many doctors have difficulty with death and dying, an Australian study explored the role of doctors' attitudes and experiences, particularly experiences of terminally ill patients, and the doctor–patient relationship in patients' wishes to hasten death (WTHD). It concluded that "dissatisfaction with the level of care the patient had received for emotional symptoms was a salient theme among the doctors with patients in the high WTHD group".[30] Early after legalization of PAS in Oregon, investigators studied how these requests for assisted death affect physicians who receive and respond to the requests. The report suggested that the experience is emotionally intense and highly time-invested and provoked feelings of discomfort.[31] As with the Kohlwes findings,[23] doctors did not discuss these requests or their experience of them with colleagues. The Dobscha study[31] did find that doctors felt there was more open discussion with patients regarding end of life after the legalization of PAS. In the Dutch experience, participating physicians believed that they had done the right thing but also believed that "ending a person's life was inherently an unnatural act and felt unacceptable". [32]

The dilemmas encountered by palliative care workers when patients wish to hasten death have been identified[33]:

- Increased responsibility to adequately manage symptoms
- Challenges to beliefs regarding patient autonomy

- Concerns that physician-assisted death is antithetical to the philosophy of palliative care
- Missed opportunities for spiritual transformation
- Conflicts over when and how to help patients redefine quality of life
- Confusion regarding their advocacy role when patients and their families are in conflict over PAS

Considerations of hastening death among palliative care patients and their families have also been studied through the experience of social workers in the southeastern United States. These considerations were not rare in palliative care. The most common reasons given for the request were poor quality of life and concerns for suffering. Investigators concluded that "subjects in this study overwhelmingly perceived that unmet needs contributed to the consideration of hastening death".[34]

Very relevant to palliative care providers' response to AD is the recent Swiss experience at the Centre Hospitalier Universitaire Vaudois, the first hospital in Switzerland to allow AS (remember Switzerland allows AS, not only PAS) within the hospital. Careful analysis of the palliative care team's response concluded:

> Clearly, the decision to allow access to AS within the hospital has had a significant impact on the palliative care consult service which does not endorse the practice of AS or euthanasia. It has created tensions between the philosophy and beliefs of the palliative care team and the institution's directive on AS…. It has prompted significant discussion within the team and a deeper understanding of the implications of principles such as non-abandonment, patient autonomy and caregiver values and positions, and larger impact on society as a whole.[35]

A set of important themes emerge strongly from the growing empirical literature. As exemplified in the Oregon experience, most patients who request PAS or euthanasia do not experience intractable pain or other physical symptoms.[22,36] There is no significant association between desire for hastened death and either the presence of pain or pain intensity.[19,26] Fear of future pain, rather than actual, perceived pain, is a strong motivation for a possible future wish for euthanasia.[27,28] Rather, persons indicating desires for hastened death are concerned about loss of control, autonomy, being a burden, and loss of dignity.[34,37] Moreover, depression and hopelessness are significant contributors to wishes and requests for assisted suicide or euthanasia.[18,19,22] On the other hand, doctors have "difficulty addressing patients' existential suffering",[23] yet feel an obligation to "do something."

We also know now that AD takes a toll on physicians, even when they believe it was the right thing to do in a particular case. Finally, the experience of AD within palliative care has brought confusion and distress. AD is being provided most often for issues that extend far beyond the care of those who are at the end of life and those with terminal illness. They go beyond the medical issues of pain and other physical symptoms to an array of social and emotional circumstances that cause human suffering.

Is There a Role for Euthanasia or Physician-Assisted Suicide in Palliative Care?

The debate over legalizing AD is complex and requires attention to ethical, legal, and professional arguments. As empirical data emerge, it also requires careful scrutiny of what we know of the reasons for actual requests and the practice of AD. This debate has particular significance for those who provide palliative care. In the spirit of honest disclosure about attitudes and beliefs regarding end-of-life care, I acknowledge that I oppose the legalization of PAS and euthanasia. My opposition is based on my personal religious belief that life is sacred. As a physician, my opposition is based on a belief that these practices irrevocably compromise both the role of the physician as a moral agent and principles of justice (especially protection of the vulnerable). I believe that a social slippery slope has been well demonstrated thus far in studies on the actual reasons for and responses to requests for AD. More specifically, for palliative care, AD is a contradiction of the fundamental philosophy of neither prolonging nor hastening death. It is, as the empirical literature now makes abundantly clear, primarily about issues of control and the medicalization of suffering.

So we can now return to the fundamental questions raised in the beginning of this chapter.

1. Is the renewed interest in euthanasia and PAS a consequence of the failure of palliative care to improve end-of-life care?
2. Is physician-assisted death by euthanasia or assisted suicide an essential tool of last resort in palliative care?
3. Or is physician-assisted death inherently contradictory to the philosophy and goals of palliative care?

It is crucial for the palliative care community to note that the majority of requests for euthanasia and PAS are not related to inadequate pain and symptom control. The requests emphasize the need for education about excellent palliative care for patients, families, and health care professionals. They present a compelling case for ensuring that high-quality palliative care is accessible for all. These requests strengthen the need for research into the full range of difficult symptoms at the end of life, but they are not evidence of failure of palliative care.

There are two levels at which physicians involved in palliative care need to reflect on the appropriate response to the role of PAS and euthanasia. The first is at the bedside, when the clinician receives such a request. The second level is within the palliative care community.

INDIVIDUAL RESPONSE

Even when not legalized, physicians and members of palliative care teams receive requests for AD. As stated earlier, reports suggest that the experience of a request for a hastened death is often emotionally intense, highly time-invested, and provokes feelings of discomfort. There is an obligation to respond competently and compassionately but a lack of evidence-based strategies.[24]

We do know that a request for PAS or euthanasia may be a sign of unrelieved pain or existential suffering or fear of future suffering, and physicians need to treat these requests seriously. Palliative care teams should explore the issues that underlie the request and should use scientific and other available resources to relieve those underlying causes. We have seen that requests for PAS often come from those who suffer some existential distress rather than refractory pain or other symptoms. Social work and pastoral care colleagues have much to offer here. Because they are so common, identifying and treating depression and hopelessness are crucial.

Despite the best efforts of the palliative care team, some patients will request PAS or euthanasia not for intractable pain or other symptoms, but for issues of control or spiritual and emotional distress—that is, suffering. How ought a palliative care physician respond? This is an incredibly challenging situation, one that requires the support and advice of colleagues. Requests for assisted death have personal, ethical, and legal ramifications. Most requests are resolved by attending to the pain and suffering. In almost all jurisdictions, PAS is illegal. In declining a request for PAS, however, the commitment to the care of the patient remains unchanged.

PALLIATIVE CARE'S RESPONSE

What does the palliative care movement make of the role of PAS? There is not a single unified response across palliative care, though there appears to be a dominant view. For some, these requests are expressions of patient autonomy and a means to liberate patients from pain and suffering. However, it does medicalize dying at both the professional and societal level. How would these practices affect the philosophy and ethics of palliative care? If legalized, PAS would become the prerogative of physicians. If AD is a medical option, does a new medical specialty develop? Is it a sub-specialty of end-of-life palliative care? Must the person be terminally ill? If loss of meaning and emotional and spiritual suffering are reasons for requests, are we expanding the scope of medicine here to consider euthanasia and PAS for reasons unrelated to health status?

A thoughtful assessment of the reasons that AS and euthanasia should not be practiced in palliative care units has been provided for us[6]:

Intentionally hastening death is contrary to palliative care philosophy.

It sends mixed messages to a public that is already poorly informed about palliative care.

It is a source of distress for some patients and families in palliative care.

It is a source of tension and conflict among palliative care staff.

It is a source of personal distress for some staff.

It places palliative care teams in the position of gatekeepers.

Dynamics of care are altered once the decision is made to proceed with assisted suicide or euthanasia.

Palliative care may become a "dumping site" for assisted suicide (or euthanasia).

For many working in palliative care, dignity is a core concept that conveys a particular respect for patients as they prepare for death. Loss of dignity is one of the most common reasons for requesting assistance in ending life. In a landmark study, Chochinov and colleagues explored the meaning of dignity from the perspective of terminally ill patients. They identified critically important factors for the maintenance of a sense of dignity in terminal illness, including "illness-related concerns, a dignity conserving repertoire and a social dignity inventory".[37] This research has profound implications for palliative care because the loss of a sense of dignity is a crucial factor that underlies requests for assistance in dying. Attention to patients' identified illness-related concerns regarding independence and symptom distress, sensitivity to the policies and practices that either conserve or erode dignity, and the development of an inventory of the social concerns and relationship dynamics that enhance or erode a sense of dignity must now be part of palliative care philosophy and practice. As the authors concluded:

> Further empirical work is necessary to develop and evaluate interventions that promote dignity and the quality of life of dying patients. Whether lost dignity leads to a wish for hastened death, or merely explains the patient's compromised quality of life, understanding dignity offers an opportunity to respond more sensitively and purposefully to those nearing death.[37]

Regardless of the legal and social situation, the decision regarding inclusion of AD in palliative care is crucial to its founding philosophy—neither hastening nor prolonging dying—its goals of restoring dying to the normal, spiritual, and familial; and to an understanding of death with dignity that is radically different from that of AD.

PEARLS AND PITFALLS

- It is important to understand that patients may request a hastened death for many reasons, including unrelieved pain or other symptoms, fear of being a burden, loss of dignity, depression, and fear of loss of autonomy and control.

- Identifying and treating the underlying reasons for the request are crucial because most of these issues can be managed.

- Aggressive management of pain and other symptoms, including terminal sedation, with the intent of relieving suffering is ethically acceptable and is almost always effective in relieving intractable symptoms.

- PAS involves a physician's providing the means for a patient to end life, usually by prescribing a lethal dose of medication.

- Euthanasia involves the physician's performing an intervention, usually an injection, to end the patient's life.

- Most enduring requests for PAS and euthanasia arise not from inadequate pain and symptom control but from a patient's beliefs about dignity, autonomy, and control over the circumstances of one's death.

Summary

There is a clear imperative to improve care at the end of life. Palliative care research needs to be enhanced, access to palliative care expertise needs to be improved, and information on the effectiveness of palliative care needs to be disseminated more effectively. These initiatives can reduce the perceived need for euthanasia and PAS, although to what extent is unclear. The ethical, legal, and professional debates about PAS and euthanasia require ongoing empirical work, serious reflection on the philosophy of palliative care, and continual improvements in the care of the dying. Those committed to a philosophy of "neither hastening death nor prolonging dying" must make a renewed commitment to understanding and facilitating dignity at the end of life.

Resources

American Medical Association Council on Ethical and Judicial Affairs: Physician assisted suicide. In *Reports on End of Life Care*, Chicago, 1998, American Medical Association.

Beauchamp TL, editor: *Intending death: the ethics of assisted suicide and euthanasia*, Toronto, 1996, Prentice-Hall.

Foley KM, Hendin H, editors: *The case against assisted suicide for the right to end-of-life care*, Baltimore, 2002, Johns Hopkins University Press.

Keown J, editor: *Euthanasia examined: ethical, clinical and legal perspectives*, New York, 1995, Cambridge University Press.

Quill TE, Battin MP, editors: *Physician-assisted dying: the case for palliative care and patient choice*, Baltimore, 2004, Johns Hopkins University Press.

References

1. Lorenz KA, Lynn J, Dy SM, et al: Evidence for improving palliative care at the end of life: a systematic review, *Ann Intern Med* 148:147, 2008.
2. Hardwig J: Going to meet death: the art of dying in the early part of the twenty-first century, *Hastings Center Rep* 39:37–45, 2009.
3. Sepúlveda C, Marlin A, Yoshida T, et al: Palliative care: the world health organization's global perspective, *J Pain Symptom Manage* 24:91–96, 2002.
4. Materstvedt LJ, Clark D, Ellershaw J, et al: Euthanasia and physician-assisted suicide: a view from an EAPC ethics task force, *Palliat Med* 17:97–101, 2003.
5. Finlay IG, Wheatley VJ, Izdebski C: The House of Lords Select Committee on the Assisted Dying for the Terminally Ill Bill: implications for specialist palliative care, *Palliat Med* 19:444–453, 2005.
6. Pereira J, Anwar D, Pralong G, et al: Assisted suicide and euthanasia should not be practiced in palliative care units, *J Palliat Med* 11:1074–1076, 2008.
7. Quill TE, Battin MP: Conclusion—Excellent palliative care as the standard, and physician-assisted dying as a last resort. In Quill TE, Battin MP, editors: *Physician-assisted dying: the case for palliative care and patient choice,* Baltimore, 2004, Johns Hopkins University Press, pp 323–334.
8. Wolf SM: Physician-assisted suicide, *Clin Ger Med* 21:179–192, 2005.
9. Bercovitch M, Adunsky A: Patterns of high-dose morphine use in a home-care hospice service. Should we be afraid of it? *Cancer* 101:1473–1477, 2004.
10. Clemens KE, Quednau I, Klaschik E: Is there a higher risk of respiratory depression in opioid-naïve palliative care patients during symptomatic therapy of dyspnea with strong opioids? *J Palliat Med* 11:204–216, 2008.
11. Clemens KE, Klaschik E: Effect of hydromorphone on ventilation in palliative care patients with dyspnea, *Support Care Cancer* 16:93–99, 2008.
12. Sykes NP: Morphine kills the pain, not the patient, *Lancet* 369:1325–1326, 2007.
13. Portenoy RK, Thomas J, Moehl Boatwright ML, et al: Subcutaneous methylnaltrexone for the treatment of opioid-induced constipation in patients with advanced illness: a double-blind, randomized, parallel group, dose-ranging study, *J Pain Symptom Manage* 35:458–468, 2008.
14. Hasselaar JG, Verhagen SC, Vissers KC: When cancer symptoms cannot be controlled: the role of palliative sedation. [Miscellaneous Article,] *Curr Opin Support Palliat Care* 3:14–23, 2009.
15. Cherny NI: Sedation for the care of patients with advanced cancer, *Nat Clin Pract Oncol* 3:492–500, 2006.
16. Pellegrino E: The false promise of beneficent killing. In Emanuel LL, editor: *Regulating how we die: the ethical, medical, and legal issues surrounding physician-assisted suicide,* Cambridge, MA, 1998, Harvard University Press, pp 71–91.
17. Callahan D: When self-determination runs amok, *Hastings Center Rep* 22:52–55, 1992.
18. Chochinov HM, Wilson KG, Enns M, et al: Desire for death in the terminally ill, *Am J Psychiatr* 152:1185–1191, 1995.
19. Breitbart W, Rosenfeld B, Pessin H, et al: Depression, hopelessness, and desire for hastened death in terminally ill patients with cancer, *JAMA* 284:2907–2911, 2000.
20. Hendin H, Foley K: Physician-assisted suicide in Oregon: a medical perspective, *Mich Law Rev* 106:1613–1639, 2008.
21. van der Heide A, Onwuteaka-Philipsen BD, Rurup ML, et al: End-of-life practices in the Netherlands under The Euthanasia Act, *N Engl J Med* 356:1957–1965, 2007.
22. Emanuel EJ, Fairclough DL, Emanuel LL: Attitudes and desires related to euthanasia and physician-assisted suicide among terminally ill patients and their caregivers, *JAMA* 284:2460–2468, 2000.
23. Kohlwes RJ, Koepsell TD, Rhodes LA, et al: Physicians' responses to patients' requests for physician-assisted suicide, *Arch Intern Med* 161:657–663, 2001.
24. Hudson PL, Kristjanson LJ, Ashby M, et al: Desire for hastened death in patients with advanced disease and the evidence base of clinical guidelines: a systematic review, *Palliat Med* 20:693–701, 2006.
25. Zylicz Z: Palliative care and euthanasia in the Netherlands: observations of a Dutch physician. In Foley KM, Hendin H, editors: *The case against assisted suicide for the right to end-of-life care,* Baltimore, 2002, Johns Hopkins University Press, pp 122–143.
26. Pearlman RA, Hsu C, Starks H, et al: Motivations for physician-assisted suicide: patient and family voices, *J Gen Intern Med* 20:234–239, 2005.
27. Ganzini L, Goy ER, Dobscha SK: Why Oregon patients request assisted death: family members' views, *J Gen Intern Med* 23:154–157, 2008.
28. Johansen S, Holen JC, Kaasa S, et al: Attitudes towards, and wishes for, euthanasia in advanced cancer patients at a palliative medicine unit, *Palliat Med* 19:454–460, 2005.

29. Wilson KG, Chochinov HM, McPherson CJ, et al: Desire for euthanasia or physician-assisted suicide in palliative cancer care, *Health Psychol* 26:314–323, 2007.
30. Kelly B, Burnett P, Badger S, et al: Doctors and their patients: a context for understanding the wish to hasten death, *Psychooncology* 12:375–384, 2003.
31. Dobscha SK, Heintz RT, Press N, et al: Oregon physicians' responses to requests for assisted suicide: a qualitative study, *Psychosomatics* 45:168–169, 2004.
32. Obstein KL, Kimsmay G, Chambers T: Practicing euthanasia: the perspective of physicians, *J Clin Ethics* 15:223–231, 2004.
33. Harvath T, Miller L, Ganzini L, et al: Dilemmas encountered by hospice workers when patients wish to hasten death, *Gerontologist* 45:4, 2005.
34. Arnold EM, Artin KA, Person JL, et al: Consideration of hastening death among hospice patients and their families, *J Pain Symptom Manage* 27:523–532, 2004.
35. Pereira J, Laurent P, Cantin B, et al: The response of a Swiss university hospital's palliative care consult team to assisted suicide within the institution, *Palliat Med* 22:659–667, 2008.
36. Sullivan AD, Hedberg K, Fleming DW: *Oregon's Death With Dignity Act: The Second Year's Experience*, Portland, OR, 2000, Oregon Health Division.
37. Chochinov HM: Dignity-conserving care—a new model for palliative care: helping the patient feel valued, *JAMA* 287:2253–2260, 2002.

CHAPTER 22

Withholding and Withdrawing Life-Sustaining Therapies

ROHTESH S. MEHTA, WENDY G. ANDERSON, SUSAN HUNT, ELIZABETH K. CHAITIN, and ROBERT M. ARNOLD

One of the advances of modern medical technology has been the creation of therapies to sustain life. These therapies, such as artificial nutrition and hydration, mechanical ventilation, dialysis, and cardiopulmonary resuscitation, allow patients to be supported through episodes of reversible illness while the cause of their illness is treated. The use of life-sustaining therapies in patients with curable illness is rarely questioned, but it is not always clear how such therapies should be used in patients with progressive, late stage, incurable disease. In patients with incurable illness, the potential benefits of life-sustaining therapy are not always great enough to justify the burdens the treatment imposes. This may be because the patient feels that his or her current quality of life is low, the expected quality of life after treatment is too low, or the burden of treatment is too great. In these cases, treatments should be withheld or withdrawn. Because withholding or withdrawing life-sustaining therapies is at times the right decision for the patient, it is important that providers understand the ethical and legal consensus involved in making these decisions and can discuss withholding or withdrawing therapies with patients and their families in an accurate and sensitive manner. Moreover, clinicians must be skilled in the palliation of symptoms that may arise when these therapies are withheld or withdrawn.

Epidemiology of Withholding and Withdrawing Life-Sustaining Therapy

Both adult and pediatric patients often die in technologically intensive situations, and it is common for life-sustaining therapies to be withdrawn or withheld before death. One in five adults in the United States receives care in intensive care units (ICUs) before death, and 80% of deaths in ICUs in North America are preceded by limitation of therapy.[1-3] In U.S. nursing homes, cardiopulmonary resuscitation (CPR) is withheld in more than 60% of all adult patients, a rate that has been steadily increasing; withholding of CPR is more common among whites, women, and patients with dementia.[4] The mortality rate of children admitted to ICU varies from 18% to 43%.[3] More than half of children who die in ICUs in the United States die after life-sustaining therapy is withdrawn or withheld.[5] There is considerable regional variation in withholding and withdrawing of life-sustaining therapies. In the United States, fewer ICU deaths are preceded by forgoing life-sustaining therapy in New York and Missouri than in the Middle Atlantic and Midwest regions.[1]

Forgoing life-sustaining treatment is not an all-or-nothing phenomenon. CPR is commonly withheld while other therapies are provided.[1] One study of adult patients receiving prolonged mechanical ventilation reported that 35% had orders to withhold CPR.[6] In a study of children who died in the ICU, 40% had a life-sustaining treatment withdrawn before death, but another 20% to 25% had a do not resuscitate (DNR) order before death.[7] Although DNR orders are common in nursing homes, fewer than 5% of patients have orders to forgo hospitalization and about 10% have orders to restrict artificial feeding.[4] A study of adults indicates that when multiple therapies are withdrawn in the ICU, they are withdrawn in a specific order: blood products first, followed by hemodialysis, vasopressors, mechanical ventilation, and finally antibiotics, nutrition, and hydration.[2]

In the ICU setting, discussions about limiting therapy are usually initiated by physicians, and decisions to withhold or withdraw therapy are almost always made by a surrogate or substitute decision maker (SDM) because the patient is too ill to participate. SDMs agree with recommendations to withhold or withdraw therapy most of the time, although in some cases multiple meetings are held before a decision to withdraw therapy is made. Withdrawal is usually initiated within hours after the decision is made, and most patients die within a few hours, although a few survive to hospital discharge. Despite an SDMs agreement with physician recommendations, conflict frequently occurs between families and medical staff. Families may feel they are not given enough information about the patient's condition, or they may disagree with the manner in which providers discuss withholding or withdrawing therapies.

Ethical Consensus Regarding Withholding and Withdrawing Therapies

An ethical consensus regarding withholding and withdrawing of medical treatments emerged as the use of life-sustaining therapies became more common in the latter half of the 20th century. The current consensus was crystallized in the 1983 report on forgoing life-sustaining treatment that was issued by the President's Commission, a group mandated by United States Congress to study ethical problems in medicine and research. The Commission examined who should decide whether to withhold or withdraw life-sustaining therapies and the criteria by which the decisions should be made. The Commission found that, ethically, the withholding or withdrawal of life-sustaining therapies is no different than the withholding or withdrawal of other medical therapies. Thus, the withholding or withdrawal of life-sustaining therapies does not require a unique decision-making process. Further, the same criteria should be used regardless of whether a treatment was withdrawn or not started in the first place. Similar support for the ethics and legality of withdrawing and withholding these treatments exists in Canada.

The primary factor driving the decision-making process should be patient self-determination, or autonomy. When patients lack the capacity to make decisions, a surrogate should be used with the goal of preserving the patient's autonomy by replicating the decisions the patient would have made. When the patient's wishes are not clear, a surrogate who knows the patient and his or her values and interests should make decisions. Surrogates should base their decision making either on what the patient had said they would want (best interest) or on what, given their knowledge of the patient, they feel the patient would have wanted (best interest). Patients or their surrogates and clinicians should engage in the process of shared decision making to promote patient autonomy. What constitutes quality of life is defined from the patient's perspective, and the physician's role is to recommend treatment consistent with the patient's goals and to explain the benefits and burdens of therapy. The patient or surrogate has the authority to accept or reject the treatment plan. Patients and surrogates do not have the right to specify which therapies they receive, and physicians are not obligated to offer treatment they believe would be ineffective or inconsistent with professional treatment standards.

The President's Commission also examined four moral distinctions that traditionally had been used to determine whether life-sustaining therapies should be forgone:

1. Whether death occurs as a result of an *action* on the part of the clinician as opposed to an *omission*
2. Whether a treatment is *withheld* as opposed to *withdrawn*
3. Whether a consequence of a treatment is *intended* or *unintended*
4. Whether treatment is *ordinary* (usual care) as opposed to *extraordinary* (heroic measures)

The Commission found that these four distinctions oversimplify both the clinical reality and the physician's moral responsibility and therefore are not ultimately useful in guiding decision making.

Decisions about life-sustaining therapies in children are unique in several ways. First, because children are not yet felt to have decision-making capacity, surrogates usually make all decisions about their medical care. (In certain situations, children can make decisions themselves, such as when they are emancipated minors. The definition of emancipated minors varies among jurisdictions but generally includes factors such as whether the child is self-supporting, married, pregnant, or a parent; in the military; or declared by a court to be emancipated.) Second, because many children have not yet had developed values and preferences, it may not be possible to base decisions on what they would have wanted. Therefore, the child's best interest is often used as a standard. This is challenging because different family members and providers may disagree about what is in the child's best interest.

When a surrogate gives consent for treatments for a child, the concept of assent can be used to incorporate older children's perspective into decision making. Assent involves similar elements to informed consent, including information giving, assessment of understanding, and assessment of agreement to commence on a plan of care, with modifications for the developmental stage of the child; however, it lacks the formal elements of consent. Though children may not be able to weigh all the risks and benefits of a therapy, and thus fulfill the requirements of informed consent, they can talk about their opinions and feelings about their medical treatment and its impact on their life. The child's perspective is taken into consideration in decision making.

Legal Consensus Regarding Withholding and Withdrawing Therapies

LEGAL CONSENSUS IN THE UNITED STATES

In the United States, a legal consensus has developed over the past 30 years regarding withholding and withdrawing medical therapies (see Meisel and Cerminara). This consensus can be described as follows:

1. Patients have a right to refuse any medical treatment, even if the refusal results in their death.
2. There is no legal distinction between withholding and withdrawing therapies.
3. Decisions to withhold or withdraw medical interventions are usually made in the clinical setting, and courts rarely need to be involved.
4. When patients die after they request that life-sustaining therapies be withheld or withdrawn, their death is considered neither homicide nor suicide, and their providers are not held liable.

The right of patients to refuse life-sustaining therapy has been repeatedly and consistently upheld. The sources of the right to refuse medical treatment lie in the common law doctrine of battery and in the constitutional right to liberty. *Battery* is defined as the unwanted invasion of one's bodily integrity, and this includes undesired medical therapy. The law of battery provides legal recourse for persons whose bodily integrity has been violated against their will. A person found guilty of battery is subject to punishment by fines or imprisonment and, in the case of health care providers, by suspension or revocation of licensure. The U.S. Supreme Court and other courts have suggested a constitutional basis for the right to be free from unwanted interference with bodily integrity, based on the protection of liberty contained in the 14th Amendment.

In patients who are unable to consider their own medical situation and voice their wishes, autonomy is preserved for them through the use of advance directives and surrogate decision makers (see also Chapter 20). While competent, patients may voice their wishes through oral or written directives (also called living wills). These directives are helpful in that they document the patient's wishes. However, they may not address all clinical situations, because it is difficult to anticipate all possible scenarios when writing the directive. Further, it is often difficult to apply them in clinical situations. For instance, the phrase "if there is no hope of recovery...," without a description of what level of recovery would be acceptable to a patient, does not elucidate a patient's desires sufficiently. Thus, even when an advance directive is present, a surrogate is still used.

Most legal cases regarding withholding and withdrawing therapies involve incompetent or incapable patients. *Competence* is a legal term that defines the decision-making capacity of an individual who is able to comprehend the treatment in question and its risks, benefits, and consequences, as well as the alternatives. Every adult is legally presumed to be competent unless proved otherwise. In medical terminology, the term *capacity* is often used. Though incapable patients have the same right to forgo life-sustaining therapy as competent patients, controversies have arisen related to who should make decisions for incapable patients and what type and level of proof of the patient's wishes is required.

Who Should Make Decisions about Life-Sustaining Therapies for Incapable Patients?

A patient may appoint a surrogate (durable power of attorney) before becoming incapable. If an incapable patient has not designated a surrogate, the choice is guided by either state law or by the clinician's judgment regarding who best knew the patient. Some states have legally specified a hierarchy of surrogates. For married couples, spouse is generally the first decision maker, followed by eldest adult child, parents, siblings, and then other relatives and people who know the patient. When no one is identified who knows the patient, a court-appointed guardian or physicians may make decisions. This order of designation does not always accomplish the goal of surrogate decision making, which is to represent the patient's perspective by involving the person who knew him or her best in decision making. When families disagree on surrogacy, disputes can arise about who should make decisions for the patient, as the Terri Schiavo case illustrated.

The Evidence Surrogates Should Use to Guide their Decision Making

Two standards are used to establish the patient's wishes: *subjective judgment* and *substituted judgment.* The subjective judgment standard requires the patient to have stated verbally or in writing what he or she would want done in the specific situation in question. The substituted judgment standard does not require that the patient's actual wishes be established, but rather that the designated surrogate be familiar enough with the patient's values and beliefs to infer what he or she would have decided. A third standard is the *best interest standard,* in which the surrogate and/or physician make decisions about withholding or withdrawing therapies guided by what they feel to be the patient's best interest. States are allowed to set the type and level of proof of an incapable patient's wishes that life-sustaining therapy be withheld or withdrawn. The subjective standard is preferred by states because it is believed to reflect the patient's wishes most closely. Because a patient's actual wishes are often not known, however, most states allow a substituted judgment standard. In some states, if the evidence of the patient's values and beliefs is insufficient to permit the use of a substituted judgment standard, a best-interest standard may be used. If the type and level of proof designated by the state are not met, life-sustaining therapies cannot be withdrawn. The Cruzan case emphasizes these points (see Meisel and Cerminara).

Nancy Cruzan, a woman from Missouri in her 30s, entered a persistent vegetative state after a car accident in 1983. Four years later, her parents and husband requested that her feeding tube be withdrawn. After opposition from the director of the hospital, the probate judge, and the Missouri Supreme Court (all of which denied their request for removal of the feeding tube), her case was eventually brought before the U.S. Supreme Court, which upheld her right to refuse unwanted medical treatment but also ruled that states have a right to protect the interests of incapable persons. States are thus permitted, although not required, to specify the type and level of evidence required to document an incapable person's wishes.

LAWS ON WITHHOLDING AND WITHDRAWING THERAPIES IN OTHER COUNTRIES

The comparative legal literature about withholding and withdrawing of therapies is limited. Mendelson and Jost studied Australia, Canada, France, Germany, Japan, the Netherlands, Poland, and the United Kingdom and found that, in all these countries, competent patients have the right to refuse any medical therapy, even if doing so may result in their death.[8] However, the laws differ in the legality of withholding and withdrawing therapies from incapable patients. A subjective or substitute judgment standard is employed in some countries, whereas others use a best-interest standard. In some countries, the patient's physician may act as the surrogate and may withhold or withdraw therapies on the basis of his or her evaluation of what is in the patient's best interest. Some courts have also found that life-support measures need not be continued for incapable patients. A seminal case involving Anthony Bland, a young man in a persistent vegetative state who was sustained with a feeding tube, was decided in the United Kingdom in 1993. The House of Lords ruled that incapable patients should be treated according to their best interests when their wishes are not known. Life-support measures, including artificial nutrition and hydration, are not in the best interest of a patient who cannot be returned to his previous state; thus, such treatments can be stopped.

Discussing Withholding and Withdrawing Therapies with Patients and Families

Many of the key points involved in discussing withholding and withdrawing therapies are common to general communication (see Chapter 3). A six-step protocol for discussing withholding and withdrawing of therapies, adapted from recommendations for communicating serious information, is presented in the following subsections and in Table 22-1. Depending on the patient's or surrogate's understanding and acceptance of the current situation and the clarity of overall goals of care, the following steps may be covered in one conversation or may require several discussions.

STEP 1: ESTABLISH THE SETTING FOR THE DISCUSSION

Before the discussion, the clinician should review the pertinent parts of the patient's case, including the prognosis, the evidence for that prognosis, and the likely effects of the treatment in question. Although many patients want to hear detailed information about their diagnosis and prognosis, some do not. Patients should be asked how much information they would like and what level of detail they prefer. Some patients may prefer to designate family members to receive information or make decisions. Clinicians should use shared decision making, and it is important to ensure that all people relevant to the decision are present: the patient's loved ones, nurses, social

Table 22-1. Communicating about Withholding or Withdrawing Therapies

1. Establish the Setting

Review relevant information.	Patient's prognosis Outcome of therapy in question in this patient
Make sure the right people are there.	Patient's or surrogate's loved ones Staff
Find a comfortable, quiet location.	Places for everyone to sit Seclusion from others Ability of everyone to see and hear each other
Introduce everyone at the beginning.	"Could we start by introducing everyone?" "How are you related to Ms. Jones?"
Introduce the topic for discussion.	"I was hoping we could talk about the next steps in your care."

2. Review the Patient's Situation

Elicit the patient's or surrogate's understanding.	"Can you tell me your understanding of what is going on with your medical situation?" "What have the other doctors told you about your dad's medical situation?"
Educate as needed.	"That's right, the cancer has spread. What that means is that although there are treatments to control the symptoms, we can't cure the cancer."

3. Review Overall Goals of Care

Elicit goals from the patient or surrogate.	"Did you talk with Dr. Smith about what the goal of your treatments should be?"
Summarize to confirm.	"So it sounds like the most important thing is to make sure your father is comfortable."

4. Relate Your Recommendation for Withholding or Withdrawing Treatment

Introduce the specific treatment to be discussed.	"Today I wanted to talk about what we should do if your breathing gets worse, including whether we should use a breathing machine."
Ask about previous experience with the intervention in question.	"Has anyone ever asked you about being on a breathing machine?"
Describe the intervention in question and its benefits and burdens for this patient.	"Based on what we've talked about—the fact that this cancer isn't curable—the chance of being able to come off the breathing machine would be very low."
State your recommendation.	"I recommend that if your breathing gets worse we don't put you on a breathing machine."
Describe how you feel your plans are consistent with the patient's overall goals.	"The reason I think we shouldn't is that you said you wouldn't want your life to be prolonged if there wasn't a good chance of recovering to where you are now."
Describe what treatments will be provided.	"We will use medicines to improve your breathing and comfort."

Table 22-1. Communicating about Withholding or Withdrawing
Therapies (Continued)

5. Respond to Patient or Surrogate Reaction	
Acknowledge emotions.	"It's hard getting to this point, isn't it?"
Is the recommendation consistent with patient's values and goals?	"How does that plan sound to you?"
Answer questions.	"I'll be around if you think of things you want to ask me later, but are there questions can I answer now?"
6. Summarize and Establish Follow-Up	
Summarize.	"Good. So we'll keep the antibiotics going and give you medicines if the breathing gets worse, but we won't put you on a breathing machine."
Explain the next steps in treatment.	"We'll plan on keeping you here in the hospital for the next few days and see how things go."
Arrange for the next meeting.	"I'll see you tomorrow on rounds. Please have your nurse page me if you need anything before then."

workers, and spiritual advisor, as appropriate and if acceptable to the patient. It may be beneficial to involve other physicians to help the family members and patient better understand the patient's condition and prognosis. For instance, an oncologist may be more proficient in answering questions about a patient's cancer. The patient may also have a particular relationship with certain providers and prioritize information from them.

The discussion should take place in a location where everyone is able to sit comfortably and hear and see one another. After introducing everyone and explaining each person's relationship to the patient or the role in the patient's care, the clinician should begin the discussion with a general statement about the purpose of the meeting. The specific treatment in question can be introduced later, but the fact that the meeting is being held to discuss the next steps in the patient's care should be stated to focus the discussion.

STEP 2: REVIEW THE PATIENT'S CURRENT SITUATION

Before withholding or withdrawing therapies can be discussed, the patient or surrogate should understand the patient's medical situation. The patient should be asked and be given opportunity to describe his or her understanding, with the clinician then providing additional information and education as necessary. The patient's prognosis is a key element of the current situation (see Chapter 5). Although not all patients desire prognostic information, many appreciate it and use it to make treatment decisions. Although the majority of patients want the information, patients are less likely to request life-prolonging therapies if they know that their overall prognosis is poor.[9]

STEP 3: REVIEW OVERALL GOALS OF CARE

Decisions to withhold or withdraw life-sustaining therapies should be based on the benefits and burdens to the patient and the potential effectiveness of the treatment.

Effectiveness can be evaluated only with respect to a specific goal, so the overall goals of therapy should be agreed on before specific therapies are discussed. Therapies may be aimed at curing disease (curative), slowing the progression of disease (life-prolonging), or alleviating symptoms (palliative) (see Chapter 4). The goals of therapy are influenced by the patient's disease state, the available treatments, and the patient's values. To provide care consistent with the values of terminally ill patients, the clinician must determine how the patient defines prolonging life and palliating symptoms. Whether life should be prolonged depends on the patient's definition of quality of life, the kinds of burdens the patient feels are worth tolerating, and the chance of success that would make a treatment worthwhile. Once the clinician has an understanding of the patient's values and preferences for medical care, this information can be used in combination with knowledge of the patient's prognosis and the effectiveness of specific therapies to formulate a treatment plan, including recommendations regarding whether to initiate or continue a specific therapy.

STEP 4: DISCUSS RECOMMENDATIONS FOR WITHHOLDING OR WITHDRAWING THERAPY

Next, the specific treatment in question should be introduced. Asking about previous discussions of or experiences with the therapy can be a useful way to start. If the patient or surrogate has discussed the therapy, asking about her or his previous preference can expedite the conversation. In addition, previous experiences may have created biases that the physician needs to explore and consider when providing education. The treatment, its likely benefits and burdens for the patient, and the physician's recommendation should be stated clearly and concisely, avoiding medical language. Enough detail should be given so the patient can make an informed decision in agreeing or disagreeing with the recommendation. Because patients use the likelihood of success of a given therapy to make decisions,[9] information about the effectiveness of the therapy in question should be included. It is useful to ask patients how much detail they want to hear about the treatment, because preferences differ. The physician should describe the reasons for the recommendation, specifically how it is consistent with the physician's understanding of the overall goals of care. It is also important to describe the withholding or withdrawing of treatment in the overall picture of the patient's care, by specifically describing what treatments *will* be given. The withholding or withdrawing of therapies is not an absence of treatment, but rather a tailoring of treatment to meet the patient's unique needs and goals.

STEP 5: RESPOND TO PATIENT OR SURROGATE REACTION

Conversations about limiting therapy are, by their nature, upsetting because they make those involved aware of the nearness of death. Patients should give permission for these discussions, and clinicians should be aware of patients' emotional reactions throughout the discussion. Emotional reactions are common and are to be expected. They should be acknowledged and responded to before attempting to proceed, because continuing a conversation in an emotionally wrought situation is unproductive and can be interpreted as insensitive. In addition, responding to the emotion shows that the clinician cares about the patient or surrogate. This can be as simple as acknowledging that the conversation is difficult ("It's hard to talk about this, isn't it?") and allowing time for the emotion to lessen. Emotions that do not subside after simple steps are taken may require more attention and exploration (see Chapter 3).

Finally, the patient's or surrogate's opinion of the plan should be elicited and any questions answered. Lack of immediate agreement is not a failure on the part of the clinician, the patient, or the surrogate; it is a signal that further discussion is required. Conflict between providers and families is not uncommon when withholding or withdrawal of therapies is considered, so it is important to learn how to respond constructively. Most conflict relates to communication issues, and multiple meetings are often required before a decision is reached, so focusing on communication and allowing time are usually all that is needed. If time is truly of the essence and a plan has not been agreed on, treatment should be given, with the understanding that it can be withdrawn when the patient's wishes are clarified.

STEP 6: SUMMARIZE AND ESTABLISH FOLLOW-UP

Finally, to provide a sense of closure and because information retention is usually poor in highly emotional conversations, the physician should summarize the results of the discussion and should establish what will happen next, both with the medical therapy and in the next meeting.

Considerations for Withholding and Withdrawing Specific Therapies

ARTIFICIAL NUTRITION AND HYDRATION

Patients who are unable to eat and drink because of illness can receive support through artificial nutrition and hydration (ANH). Nutritional therapy can sustain patients with reversible illness until they are able to eat and drink on their own again. Deciding whether to provide such therapy to patients with nonreversible illness requires consideration of ethical, legal, emotional, religious, and clinical issues. The ethical and legal consensus in the United States and Canada is that artificial nutrition and hydration are medical therapies and should be treated as such when making treatment decisions. Ethicists and courts have both affirmed that in dying patients, it is the terminal illness that causes the patient's disinterest or inability to eat and drink, and not the act of withholding or withdrawing artificial nutrition and hydration, that results in death.

Food and water have social and symbolic significance. They are part of celebrations with family and friends, and sustenance is seen as a source of strength. Some patients and families feel, on the basis of their religious beliefs, that it is wrong to withhold or withdraw food or water.[10] Others, even those who logically understand that patients are unable to eat and drink as a result of their underlying illness, may feel, on an emotional level, that it is wrong to deprive them of food and water as this is "basic care."

Artificial Nutrition

Artificial nutrition can be provided parenterally as total parenteral nutrition or enterally as tube feedings via nasogastric, gastrostomy, and jejunostomy tubes. More than 160,000 percutaneous endoscopic gastrostomy (PEG) tubes are placed annually in the U.S. Medicare patient population alone, and more than one third of nursing home residents with advance cognitive impairment receive artificial nutrition support via tube feeds.[11] The question whether to provide long-term artificial nutrition frequently arises in patients who are unable to take oral nutrition or who have anorexia or weight loss. Inability to take food orally is commonly the result of advanced cata-strophic neurologic injury (e.g., stroke, ischemic encephalopathy, traumatic brain injury) or advanced dementia. Decreased appetite and weight loss are also associated with cancer and other chronic diseases.

Over the past decade, a clinical consensus has developed that artificial nutrition should not be routinely provided to patients with advanced dementia because it does not provide clinical benefit. An evidence-based review of tube feeding in patients with advanced dementia did not find any survival benefit with a feeding tube. Rather, operative and perioperative mortality associated with feeding tube placement was substantial and ranged up to 25%.[12] Median survival after percutaneous endoscopic gastrostomy tube placement is less than 1 year, and mortality is 60% at 1 year and 80% at 3 years. Moreover, tube feeding does not decrease aspiration pneumonia, skin breakdown, or infections or increase functional status; rather, it can add to morbidity by increasing the risk of local and systemic infections.[12] It is not possible to know with certainty whether patients with advance dementia experience hunger, but their global decline in mental status suggests that they do not. The tube itself may be a source of discomfort.

Most patients with metastatic cancer and other terminal illnesses, in whom weight loss and decline in functional status are caused by the underlying disease, also do not benefit from artificial nutrition. On the other hand, enteral nutrition can prolong life in patients with malignancies such as head and neck cancers and abdominal tumors that block the proximal gastrointestinal tract; in those with neurologic illnesses such as persistent vegetative state or amyotrophic lateral sclerosis; and in patients with extreme short-bowel syndrome. In these cases, the decision to withhold or withdraw therapy should be based on the patient's definition of quality of life.

Artificial Hydration

Artificial hydration can be provided intravenously, subcutaneously, or enterally. Although the potential benefits and burdens of artificial hydration at the end of life have been debated extensively, clinical outcome data to guide decision making are only beginning to emerge,[13] and there is no clear clinical consensus about when artificial hydration should be provided. Families are most often concerned about their loved one not experiencing thirst. The reported incidence and severity of thirst in terminal patients vary among studies. It is not clear whether thirst is related to systemic dehydration, nor is it clear that parenteral fluids relieve it, although mouth swabs effectively do so, and mouth care should be an important part of care for dying patients. One randomized controlled trial (RCT) in terminally ill cancer patients concluded that hydration improved myoclonus and sedation in more than 80% of the patients, without any significant effect on hallucinations or fatigue.[13] However, another multicenter prospective trial found no differences in the prevalence of hyper-active delirium, agitation score, communication score, myoclonus, bedsores, or bron-chial secretions and no statistically significant differences in the blood urea and serum creatinine levels in terminally ill cancer patients receiving hydration therapy compared with those who did not.[14] Furthermore, those in the hydration group had worsening of ascites, pleural effusion, and peripheral edema.[14] However, these results should be interpreted with caution because these studies were of short duration and included cancer patients exclusively; thus, they are not representative of the wider palliative care population.[15] The potential burdens of parenteral fluids at the end of life include increased respiratory secretions and resulting "death rattle," as well as volume overload with resulting pulmonary and peripheral edema. Evidence is insufficient to establish the frequency and severity of these burdens, although administration of large fluid volumes would seem likely to produce them.

MECHANICAL VENTILATION

Mechanical ventilation can be provided either by invasive means (such as endotracheal intubation) or noninvasively though methods such as noninvasive positive pressure ventilation (NIPPV). Although the withholding and withdrawing of interventions are considered equivalent from an ethical and legal perspective, the two may be very different emotionally, especially in the case of withdrawal of mechanical ventilation. Because patients who are withdrawn from mechanical ventilators often die shortly after withdrawal, removing the ventilator can be seen as actively causing the patient's death. Critical care physicians report that withdrawing mechanical ventilation is more likely to cause patient distress than is withdrawal of other life-sustaining treatments. Because of this, in patients who are receiving multiple life-sustaining treatments, therapies such as renal replacement therapy, artificial hydration and nutrition, and vasopressors should be withdrawn before ventilation is withdrawn. In one study, this stepwise and gradual withdrawal process, as well as a longer duration of the withdrawal process, was associated with higher satisfaction in family members of ICU patients.[16]

Methods of Ventilator Withdrawal

When the burdens of mechanical ventilation outweigh its benefits in a given patient, it should be withdrawn. Mechanical ventilation must be withdrawn while maintaining patient and family comfort. The two methods of ventilator withdrawal are *terminal weaning* and *terminal extubation*.[17] In terminal weaning, the artificial airway is maintained while ventilator support is gradually reduced. In terminal extubation, ventilator support is more rapidly reduced and the artificial airway is removed. The decision to extubate, either before or after reduction in ventilator support, should be made on the basis of the anticipated amount of airway secretions and the availability of staff to manage them[17] and whether the patient is awake, can express a preference, and whether there is an expectation that he or she may be able to talk even briefly with family after extubation. A recent systematic review of literature suggested no definite evidence to support one method over the other.[17] Both these methods carry their own pros and cons. Terminal weaning facilitates minimizing the "death rattle" because it helps reduce the accumulation of upper respiratory secretions, but it may protract the dying process. Terminal extubation has an advantage of removing the endotracheal tube, which itself is an immense source of discomfort to the patient, but it may cause sudden respiratory distress and "death rattle." However, these symptoms can be treated with increasing doses of opioids, sedatives, and antimuscarinic agents. In addition, "death rattle" is mostly distressing to the family members and medical staff and probably not to that extent to the patient. In a survey of ICU physicians, only 13% preferred terminal extubation, roughly one third favored terminal weaning, and the rest practiced both. Those who preferred weaning were mostly surgeons and anesthesiologists, while extubation was favored mostly by internists and pediatricians.[18] In one study, terminal extubation before death was associated with higher family satisfaction.[16] Irrespective of the method of ventilator withdrawal, the comfort of the patient and prompt treatment of any distressing symptoms is paramount. Experienced clinicians should remain at the bedside until the withdrawal

Box 22-1. *Protocol for Terminal Ventilator Weaning*

PREPARATION

Write do-not-resuscitate (DNR) order in chart.
Document the discussion with surrogate and rationale for withdrawing ventilator.
Discuss the procedure of withdrawal with loved ones and answer questions.
Discontinue monitoring, therapies, and devices not necessary for patient comfort.
Have support for loved ones available (pastoral care, social work, as appropriate).

SEDATION AND ANALGESIA

Continue infusions at current rates, or initiate with:
Opiate
• Fentanyl 100 µg/hr; *or* morphine 10 mg/hr; *or* dilaudid 1 mg/hr
Benzodiazepine
• Midazolam 10 mg/hr; *or* lorazepam 5 mg/hr
For signs of discomfort, appearance of pain, dyspnea, or respiratory rate >20, every 10
  minutes as needed :
• Bolus of opiate and benzodiazepine equivalent to hourly rate
• Increase infusion rates by 25%

VENTILATOR

Reduce ventilator alarms to minimum settings.
Reduce fractional inspired oxygen to room air and positive end-expiratory pressure to
  0 (over approximately 5 minutes).
Wean intermediate ventilation or pressure support incrementally.
Monitor for signs of discomfort, give boluses, and adjust opiate and benzodiazepine
  infusion rates.
Do not decrease support until the patient is comfortable at current settings (weaning
  is usually accomplished in approximately 15 minutes).
When intermediate ventilation is 4/min or pressure support 5 mm Hg, depending on
  anticipated airway secretions and ability to control:
• Extubate with suction immediately available
or
• Disconnect ventilator, connecting artificial airway to T-piece with air.

AFTER WITHDRAWAL

Allow time for the family to remain with the patient; be available for support.
If the patient has not died, continue comfort measures and arrange a comfortable space for
  the patient and family.

Adapted from Treece PD, Engelberg RA, Crowley L, et al: Evaluation of a standardized order form for the
  withdrawal of life support in the intensive care unit, *Crit Care Med* 32:1141, 2004.

has been completed. Protocols detailing the sequence of events during ventilator
withdrawal (Box 22-1) are useful to ICU staff.

Noninvasive Positive Pressure Ventilation

Noninvasive positive pressure ventilation is a newer technology that may be used as
(1) a "life-prolonging measure" in a full code patient, (2) as a life support in a patient
who has decided not to be intubated, or (3) as a palliative measure to relieve dyspnea
in a patient who has decided for "comfort measures only".[19] Several randomized trials

have demonstrated the beneficial role of NIPPV in management of the first category of patients with acute exacerbation of chronic obstructive pulmonary disease, hypoxic respiratory failure in immunocompromised subjects, and acute respiratory failure with cardiogenic pulmonary edema. In the second category, NIPPV reverses acute respiratory failure and prevents hospital mortality in patients with chronic obstructive pulmonary disease and those with cardiogenic pulmonary edema, especially those with strong cough and who are awake, but not in those with pneumonia, end-stage cancer, or other primary diagnoses such as hypoxemic respiratory failure, postextubation failure, and so forth. For patients in the third category, on the other hand, there is a paucity of data either for or against the use of NIPPV.[19] Pulmonologists often perceive NIPPV as a palliative intervention to relieve dyspnea in terminally ill patients. The question of how to balance this against other treatments for dyspnea and the discomfort that NIPPV may cause is unanswered. NIPPV may offer the patient time to resolve personal objectives and allow sufficient time for geographically distant family members to visit the dying relative.

Palliation of Dyspnea and Respiratory Distress

Dyspnea and respiratory distress should be differentiated from one another. The former is a subjective feeling of breathing discomfort and can be perceived only by the person feeling it. Respiratory distress can be observed and measured objectively. Terminally ill patients for whom withdrawal of ventilation is being considered are often neurologically and cognitively impaired and therefore are not able to describe dyspnea.[17] Opioid therapy is the primary treatment for dyspnea and respiratory distress associated with the withholding or withdrawing of mechanical ventilation. Other therapies include supplemental oxygen (if the patient is hypoxic); benzodiazepines, which are considered second-line agents[17]; and treatment of the underlying cause of respiratory failure. Most experienced clinicians administer bolus doses of opioids before ventilator withdrawal, use intermittent doses of opiates and benzodiazepines to target a respiratory rate less than 20 to 25 or to achieve patient comfort, and increase the doses at any indication of discomfort such as agitation, anxiety, grunting, uncomfortable facial expressions, use of accessory muscles, or nasal flaring. Frequently, mechanically ventilated patients are receiving neuromuscular blocking drugs, and these must be stopped several hours before withdrawal is initiated because neuromuscular blockade will mask signs of distress.

Depending on the severity of respiratory failure, patients may require doses of opiates and benzodiazepines that produce sedation. Medications should be given until the patient is no longer in distress. Ethically and legally, when medication is given with the intention of relieving suffering, any secondary effect the medication has that hastens death is seen as that, and the physician is not considered morally or legally culpable. Studies have shown no correlation between survival time after ventilator withdrawal and doses of opiates and benzodiazepines given during withdrawal.[17]

Family Education and Support

Because most patients are unconscious when the withholding or withdrawal of mechanical ventilation is considered, the decision to withhold or withdraw this treatment is usually made by surrogates. Families are comforted by being told how medications will be used to prevent and treat respiratory distress. Families should be offered opportunity to be present at the bedside during withdrawal, although they should not be made to feel obligated. Before the ventilator is withdrawn, the process should be explained and any questions should be answered. The possible outcomes should also be reviewed. When ventilator support is withdrawn in anticipation of death, most patients die within minutes of withdrawal. However, some patients live for hours or even days, and a few survive to be discharged from the hospital. An experienced clinician should be present at the bedside during the withdrawal. As with any patient near death, support should be provided by staff, and social workers or pastoral care providers should be present as needed. Monitors can be distracting, and removing them as appropriate can restore a sense of humanness and closeness. After a patient's death, the family should be offered ample time to remain at the bedside, and religious traditions should be accommodated.

CARDIOPULMONARY RESUSCITATION

Cardiopulmonary resuscitation (CPR), initially consisting of closed chest compressions and artificial respiration, was developed in 1960 as a means of sustaining circulatory and respiratory function in patients who suffered from anesthetic-induced cardiac arrest in the operating theater. The technique was subsequently included in hospital policies recommending use of CPR for all cardiac arrests. Although generally healthy patients with reversible causes of cardiac arrest benefited from CPR, it soon became apparent that CPR could simply prolong the dying process in patients with terminal illness and thus cause suffering. In the mid-1970s, hospitals began to use do not resuscitate orders to designate patients for whom CPR was inappropriate. By 1988, the United States Joint Commission on Accreditation of Healthcare Organizations required hospitals to have DNR policies to be accredited. A similar situation exists in Canada.

Most recent estimates indicate that the frequency of CPR is 1 to 5 per 1000 hospital admissions. Though the frequency of CPR overall has been stable over the past decade, the number of deaths preceded by CPR seems to be increasing. Survival rates after CPR depend on the site of resuscitation; the cause of cardiac arrest; the time to resuscitation; and the patient's age, functional status, and comorbidities. In general, about 40% to 44% of the patients undergoing CPR achieve spontaneous resumption of circulation and about 13% to 17% survive to discharge.[20] In the past, resuscitation in patients with cancer was felt to be uniformly fatal. However, recent data suggest that outcomes in these patients now approach those of resuscitation in populations without malignancy: Survival to discharge is less than 10% in patients with localized disease and about 6% in those with metastatic disease.[21] Sepsis, metastatic cancer, dementia, coronary artery disease, and elevated serum creatinine are some of the adverse prognostic factors associated with a poor outcome after CPR.[20]

Because the provision of CPR is prescribed by hospital and emergency medical response policies, CPR is unique from an ethical and legal perspective. A physician must take a positive action (e.g., write a DNR order) for CPR to be withheld. This procedure is appropriate, given that CPR candidates are clinically dead when CPR is initiated and any delay in initiation to consult with family members will lower survival rates. However, it leaves unresolved the issue of whether patient or surrogate consent is required for CPR to be withheld. From a legal perspective, the right of physicians unilaterally to write DNR orders has not been established. The position of professional associations, including the American Medical Association and the American Heart Association, is that physicians are not obligated to provide CPR if they believe that it would be ineffective, but the recommendation should be based on an understanding of the patient's goals and code status discussions with the patient in anticipation of the possible need for CPR.

The objective of a discussion regarding resuscitation preferences is to increase patient autonomy by matching a patient's care to his or her goals. Studies have raised concern about the effectiveness of code status discussions. CPR is discussed at hospital admission in about 10% to 25% of patients.[22] Code status discussions are more frequent in patients with previous DNR orders and those who are seriously ill, but still take place only for about half of seriously ill patients who are admitted to the hospital.[22] Even when these discussions occur, only a small number of patients actually comprehend the components of CPR or its success rates, and there is frequent discrepancy between what the patient or the surrogate thinks and what the physician thinks was discussed, which can result in placement of orders that are not in accord with patient preferences.[22]

DIALYSIS

Since the invention of dialysis and the end-stage renal disease amendment to the Social Security Act in 1972, use of this treatment has become more prevalent. In 2000, about 300,000 patients in the United States were undergoing maintenance dialysis and 95,000 were starting dialysis.[23] More than 36,600 Canadians were living with end-stage renal disease, otherwise known as kidney failure, at the end of 2008—an increase of 57% since 1999. According to a new report from the Canadian Institute for Health Information (CIHI), about three out of five of these patients[20] were on dialysis and two out of five[14] were living with a functioning kidney transplant. Patients with end-stage renal disease have a high rate of comorbid disease and a mortality rate comparable to that of patients with cancer.[23] Average 5-year survival rates for dialysis patients are 39%, and their life span is one third to one sixth that of patients who are not receiving dialysis.[24] One of every five patients undergoing dialysis in the United States discontinues it before death.[23]

In 2003, the Renal Physicians Association and the American Society of Nephrology convened a working group and published the *Clinical Practice Guideline on Shared Decision making in the Appropriate Initiation of and Withdrawing from Dialysis.*[23] The guideline emphasizes shared decision making, considering the patient's overall prognosis and quality of life when recommending dialysis, and respecting the patient's right to refuse therapy. Surveys have assessed nephrologists' attitudes toward withholding or withdrawing dialysis and other life-sustaining interventions. Trends in these surveys indicate that nephrologists are becoming more likely to respect patients' wishes for DNR status and are more likely to be willing to withdraw dialysis from severely demented or permanently unconscious patients.[25]

More studies have focused on patients who withdraw from dialysis than on those who choose not to initiate it. Those who discontinue dialysis are demographically similar to the general dialysis-treated population; that is, most of them are elderly and have a high rate of comorbid disease. Most discontinue dialysis after only a few years. Death occurs within days to weeks after dialysis withdrawal. The most common reasons for withdrawal of dialysis are deterioration because of a chronic condition, acute deterioration as a result of a new diagnosis, medical complications, or generalized failure to thrive.

The quality of death in patients who withdraw from dialysis is usually good in that it is free from suffering, brief, and peaceful. Symptoms in those dying of renal failure are caused by uremia, volume overload, general debilitation, and comorbid disease. In one study, pain, agitation, and dyspnea were most prevalent during the last 24 hours of life and symptoms were not severe. Opiates should be used to treat pain and dyspnea, with selection of agents based on renal function. Because nausea is secondary to the effect of urea on the chemoreceptor trigger zone, centrally acting antiemetics such as phenothiazines (chlorpromazine) and butyrophenones (haloperidol) should be used. Antipsychotic agents are useful in treating delirium. Finally, although they should be used cautiously, benzodiazepines can reduce dyspnea and agitation (see also Chapter 15).

PEARLS

- Ethical and legal guidelines support the right of a patient to have any medical therapy withdrawn or withheld, including therapies that are sustaining life.
- If a patient cannot participate in medical decision making, medical therapies may be withdrawn or withheld by a surrogate.
- The clinician's role in decision making about withholding and withdrawing of therapies is to use shared decision making and make recommendations for treatment based on the patient's values and beliefs, prognosis, and overall treatment goals.
- The role of the clinician is to clarify goals, not to impose his or her own judgment or values.
- Any recommendation to withhold or withdraw therapy should be preceded by a discussion of the overarching goals of care for the patient.
- Surrogate-physician conflict surrounding withholding and withdrawing of therapies most commonly relates to communication.
- Patients and their surrogates are less likely to prefer life-sustaining therapies if they understand the prognosis and the likelihood of success of the treatment being considered.
- Providers should be aware of and should respond to patient and surrogate emotions.

PITFALLS

- Physicians should be aware of the ethical and legal consensus regarding withholding and withdrawing of therapies.
- Avoid asking patients to decide about treatments without educating them about treatments and the accompanying risks and benefits.
- Do not assume that we know how a patient should define quality of life.
- Never underestimate the significance of listening to the patient and family.
- Do not expect that decisions to withhold or withdraw therapies will be made after a single meeting.
- Be acquainted with withholding or withdrawing therapies while maintaining patient comfort.

Summary

Life-sustaining therapies are frequently withheld or withdrawn. Ethically and legally, the decision to withhold or withdraw therapies is guided by the principle of autonomy; patients or their surrogates have the right to refuse any therapy, even if it results in death. Decisions to withhold or withdraw therapies should be made jointly between clinicians and patients or their surrogates, based on the patients' values and preferences for medical care. Each decision should be based on the patient's overall prognosis, the effectiveness of the therapy in question, its benefits and burdens to the patient, and the overall goals of care. Good communication is essential to increasing patient autonomy. Artificial nutrition and hydration, mechanical ventilation, CPR, and dialysis are commonly withheld and withdrawn. It is appropriate clinically, ethically, and legally to withhold or withdraw therapies when the burden to the patient outweighs the benefit. Distress of patients and their families can be minimized by symptom palliation and by ongoing communication about the patient's condition, prognosis, and treatment alternatives.

Resources

President's Commission for the Study of Ethical Problems in Medicine and Biomedical and Behavioral Research: Deciding to Forgo Life-Sustaining Treatment. Washington, DC, 1983, United States Government Printing Office.

Post SG, editor: *Encyclopedia of Bioethics*, 3rd ed, New York, 2004, Macmillan Reference USA.

Meisel A, Cerminara KL: *The Right To Die: The Law of End-of-Life Decisionmaking*, 3rd ed, 2005 supplement. New York, 2005, Aspen Publishers.

Back A, Arnold R, Tulsky J: *Mastering Communication with Seriously Ill Patients*, Cambridge, UK, 2009, Cambridge University Press.

American Academy of Hospice and Palliative Medicine: Fast Facts. Available at www.aahpm.org/cgi-bin/wkcgi/search?fastfact=1&search=1.

References

1. Prendergast TJ, Claessens MT, Luce JM: A national survey of end-of-life care for critically ill patients, *Am J Respir Crit Care Med* 158:1163–1167, 1998.
2. Asch DA, Faber-Langendoen K, Shea JA, et al: The sequence of withdrawing life-sustaining treatment from patients, *Am J Med* 107:153–156, 1999.
3. Angus DC, Barnato AE, Linde-Zwirble WT, et al: Use of intensive care at the end of life in the United States: an epidemiologic study, *Crit Care Med* 32(3):638–643, 2004.
4. Resnick HE, Schuur JD, Heineman J, et al: Advance directives in nursing home residents aged > or = 65 years: United States 2004, *Am J Hosp Palliat Care* 25(6):476–482, 2008.
5. Vernon DD, Dean JM, Timmons OD, et al: Modes of death in the pediatric intensive care unit: withdrawal and limitation of supportive care, *Crit Care Med* 21(11):1798–1802, 1993.
6. Camhi SL, Mercado AF, Morrison RS, et al: Deciding in the dark: advance directives and continuation of treatment in chronic critical illness, *Crit Care Med* 37(3):919–925, 2009.
7. Zawistowski CA, DeVita MA: A descriptive study of children dying in the pediatric intensive care unit after withdrawal of life-sustaining treatment, *Pediatr Crit Care Med* 5(3):216–223, 2004.
8. Mendelson D, Jost TS: A comparative study of the law of palliative care and end-of-life treatment, *J Law Med Ethics* 31:130–143, 2003.
9. Murphy DJ, Burrows D, Santilli S, et al: The influence of the probability of survival on patients' preferences regarding cardiopulmonary resuscitation, *N Engl J Med* 330:545–549, 1994.
10. Clarfield AM, Gordon M, Markwell H, et al: Ethical issues in end-of-life geriatric care: the approach of three monotheistic religions—Judaism, Catholicism, and Islam, *J Am Geriatr Soc* 51:1149–1154, 2003.
11. Mitchell SL, Teno JM, Roy J, et al: Clinical and organizational factors associated with feeding tube use among nursing home residents with advance cognitive impairment, *JAMA* 290(1):73–80, 2003.
12. Finucane TE, Christmas C, Travis K: Tube feeding in patients with advance dementia: a review of the evidence, *JAMA* 282:1365–1370, 1999.
13. Bruera E, Sala R, Rico MA, et al: Effects of parenteral hydration in terminally ill cancer patients: a preliminary study, *J Clin Oncol* 23:2366–2371, 2005.
14. Morita T, Hyodo I, Yoshimi T, et al: Association between hydration volume and symptoms in terminally ill cancer patients with abdominal malignancies, *Ann Oncol* 16(4):640–647, 2005.

15. Good P, Cavenagh J, Mather M, Ravenscroft P: Medically assisted hydration for palliative care patients, *Cochrane Database Syst Rev* (2):CD006273, 2008.
16. Gerstel E, Engelberg RA, Koepsell T, et al: Duration of withdrawal of life support in the intensive care unit and association with family satisfaction, *Am J Respir Crit Care Med* 178(8):798–804, 2008.
17. Campbell ML: How to withdraw mechanical ventilation: a systematic review of the literature, *AACN Adv Crit Care* 18(4):397–403, 2007.
18. Faber-Langendoen K: The clinical management of dying patients receiving mechanical ventilation. A survey of physician practice, *Chest* 106(3):880–888, 1994.
19. Curtis JR, Cook DJ, Sinuff T, et al: Noninvasive positive pressure ventilation in critical and palliative care settings: understanding the goals of therapy, *Crit Care Med* 35(3):932–939, 2007.
20. Ebell MH, Becker LA, Barry HC, et al: Survival after in-hospital cardiopulmonary resuscitation. A meta-analysis, *J Gen Intern Med* 13(12):805–816, 1998.
21. Reisfield GM, Wallace SK, Munsell MF, et al: Survival in cancer patients undergoing in-hospital cardiopulmonary resuscitation: a meta-analysis, *Resuscitation* 71(2):152–160, 2006.
22. Heyland DK, Frank C, Groll D, et al: Understanding cardiopulmonary resuscitation decision making: Perspectives of seriously ill hospitalized patients and family members, *Chest* 130(2):419–428, 2006.
23. Cohen LM, Germain MJ, Poppel DM: Practical considerations in dialysis withdrawing: "To have that option is a blessing," *JAMA* 289:2113–2139, 2003.
24. Cohen LM, Moss AH, Weisbord SD, et al: Renal palliative care, *J Palliat Med* 9(4):977–992, 2006.
25. Holley JL, Davison SN, Moss AH: Nephrologists' changing practices in reported end-of-life decision-making, *Clin J Am Soc Nephrol* 2(1):107–111, 2007.

CHAPTER 23

Last Hours of Living

FRANK D. FERRIS, MARIA DANILYCHEV, and ARTHUR SIEGEL

The death of someone close is never easy. No one can escape the experience of dying or death. Everyone at the dying person's bedside will be watching the potential for his or her own future end-of-life experience and death. If symptoms are not well managed, there may be unnecessary suffering. If the dying process is prolonged unnecessarily, those who watch may be left with memories that the death was not good or fears that their own death will be similar.[1]

Because much of end-of-life care and dying takes place in hospitals and long-term care facilities, most people have never witnessed death. Most people have never seen a dead body except in a funeral home. They have only seen media dramatizations on television or in the cinema. Based on their own experiences, many observers imagine what the patient must be feeling and suffering. They do not realize that the patient's experience may be very different.

For the patient, along with the end of life come losses of functional capabilities, body image, sense of future, independence, control, and dignity. There are major transitions in roles, responsibilities, and family dynamics. Under stress, social support systems change. Some people remain loyal to the patient and family. Others abandon them out of fear or any number of other reasons.

As the patient's physical capabilities diminish, he or she has an increased need for care, particularly as goals of care and treatment priorities start to shift frequently. Although individual family members may be willing to care for their loved one, they

319

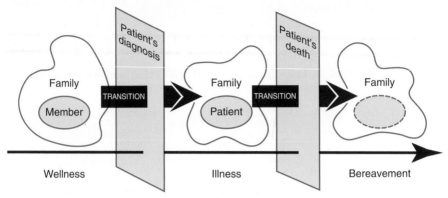

Figure 23-1. Family transitions.

will benefit from considerable training and support from their physicians and other health care professionals.

Ultimately, when the patient dies, the original family group adjourns. Those who survive will form a new family group without the patient, except in their memory. Most families benefit from ongoing help from their physicians and other health care professionals to help them storm and norm all over again before can begin to perform effectively and establish equilibrium once again[2,3] (Figure 23-1).

Prepare the Patient and Family

Care during the last hours of life is a core competency of every physician and health care worker.[4-6] People who know what to expect have a very different experience of dying and death than those who are ignorant of the process. Time spent preparing patients, family members, and caregivers for the end of life will reduce their anxiety and fear. Preparing family members and caregivers increases their competence and confidence to provide care; increases their sense of value and gifting during the process; creates good memories of the experience; prepares them for impending losses; shifts their roles, responsibilities, and support systems; and reduces their dependence on health care professionals (i.e., the frequency of visits and urgent phone calls).

CONDUCT A FAMILY MEETING

To help people prepare, conduct one or more family meetings. These meetings can help to convey information, facilitate the development of an effective care team, facilitate life closure, help arrange for rites and rituals, and encourage planning for funeral or memorial services. When communicating with family, however, be sensitive to personal and cultural differences related to information sharing and decision making.

The process for conducting a family meeting is an application of the six steps of effective communication.[7]

1. Set the stage carefully. Ensure that everyone who wants to be present is present.
2. Ask "What is known about the patient's illness and prognosis?"

3. Ask "How you would like to receive information?"
4. Once the family are clear that they would like to know, discuss the facts about the patient's illness and prognosis—that is, that he or she is dying—and then stop talking.
5. Wait for emotional responses, and provide support.
6. Once emotions have settled, check for understanding, questions, and preparedness for more information. If emotions have been intense and participants don't settle, it may be better to schedule a follow-up meeting.

If participants are prepared for further discussions, provide an overview of changes and events that are likely during the dying process (Table 23-1). Inquire who the caregivers might be and ask about their caregiving skills and experience. Facilitate decision making regarding goals of care and treatment priorities. Develop a plan of care that includes personal activities that the patient may wish to complete before dying. Clarify who the surrogate decision maker will be once the patient loses capacity to make decisions. Review advance directives. Discuss the appropriateness and comfort of the family with the current setting of care, such as home, as the place for the patient's end-of-life care and death. If family are not prepared for the patient to die at home, plan for a change in setting of care far enough in advance of the patient's death to ensure that it is safe for the patient, family, and all caregivers. Try to minimize the risk of sudden changes in the setting of care simply because the patient is dying. Transfers from a nursing home to hospital or vice versa can be very disruptive and distressing to everyone.

DEVELOP AN EFFECTIVE CARE TEAM

Most family members are not skilled at caring for someone who is dying. Frequently, those who volunteer to provide care need considerable training and support from the health care team.

As a care team forms, find out who would like to provide personal care versus help with other activities, such as cleaning, shopping, and scheduling of visitors. Give everyone permission to be family first and bedside caregivers only if they are prepared for the role. To help minimize guilt, offer everyone an appropriate task so they feel helpful. Establish who will coordinate the care team—that is, which clinician will lead the health care team and who will coordinate family, friends, and caregivers.

Once the care team has been selected, educate family and caregivers about changes to the patient's condition that may occur during the dying process (see Table 23-1), including the unexpected; how to communicate during the dying process; signs that death has occurred (Box 23-1); what to do when death occurs (Box 23-2); and specific caregiving skills, such as changing a bed with a patient in it, turning, massage, passive movement of joints, management of urine and stool, mouth, nose, lip, and eye care, and how to deliver medications when the patient is unable to swallow. Ensure that everyone present knows how to practice universal body fluid precautions.

Because having many visitors can be fatiguing for the patient and the family, have a care team member take on the task of scheduling visits so that everyone gets an appropriate length of time with the patient.

Use a logbook to facilitate communication between caregivers and minimize repetitive questioning of patients and families about the following ongoing issues:

Table 23-1. Changes During the Dying Process

Change During the Dying Process	Manifested by/Signs
General Changes	
Fatigue, weakness	Decreased function, hygiene Inability to move around bed Inability to lift head off pillow Loss of muscle tone
Cutaneous ischemia	Erythema over boney prominences, cyanosis Skin breakdown Wounds
Pain	Facial grimacing Tension in forehead, between eyebrows
Decreased food intake, wasting	Anorexia Poor intake Weight loss of muscle and fat, notable in temples
Loss of ability to close eyes	Eyelids not closed Whites of eyes showing (with or without pupils visible)
Altered handling of fluids	Decreased fluid intake Peripheral edema caused by hypoalbuminemia Dehydration, dry mucous membranes/conjunctiva
Cardiac dysfunction	Tachycardia and bradycardia Hypertension and hypotension Peripheral cooling Peripheral and central cyanosis (bluing of extremities) Mottling of the skin (livedo reticularis) Venous pooling along dependent skin surfaces
Renal failure	Dark, concentrated urine Oliguria, anuria
Neurologic Dysfunction	
Decreasing level of consciousness	Increased drowsiness Decreased awareness of surroundings Difficulty awakening Nonresponsive to verbal or tactile stimuli
Decreasing ability to communicate	Decreased concentration, decreased attention Difficulty finding words Monosyllabic, short sentences Delayed or inappropriate responses Verbally nonresponsive
Terminal hyperactive delirium	Early signs of cognitive failure (e.g., confusion, day-night reversal) Agitation, restlessness, hallucinations Purposeless, repetitious movements Moaning, groaning
Respiratory dysfunction	Dyspnea Change in ventilatory rate—increasing first, then slowing Decreased tidal volume Abnormal breathing patterns—apnea, Cheyne-Stokes respirations, agonal breaths

Table 23-1. Changes During the Dying Process (Continued)

Change During the Dying Process	Manifested by/Signs
Loss of ability to swallow	Dysphagia Coughing, choking Loss of gag reflex Buildup of oral and tracheal secretions Gurgling, noisy breathing
Loss of sphincter control, urinary retention	Incontinence of urine or bowels Maceration of skin Perineal infections (e.g., candidiasis)
Other	
Fever	
Sweating	
Seizures	
Defibrillator shocks	
Bursts of energy just before death occurs (e.g., the "golden glow")	
Aspiration, asphyxiation	
Hemorrhage, hemoptysis, bleeding out	

1. Goals of care
2. Active treatments
3. Patient preferences, such as food, conversation, and turning
4. Summaries of conversations, care provided, and fluid and nutritional intake
5. Contact information for all professional and informal caregivers
6. What to do in an emergency
7. What to do and who to call when death occurs

DISCUSS COMMUNICATING WITH THE DYING PATIENT

During the last hours of life, families frequently want "just a little more time" to communicate with their loved one and become very distressed when they are not

---

Box 23-1. *Signs That Death Has Occurred*

Ensure that the family, caregivers, and other health care providers are familiar with the signs of death and potential events that may occur as the patient dies:
- Heart stops beating
- Breathing stops
- Pupils become fixed and dilated
- Body becomes pale and waxen as blood settles
- Body temperature drops
- Muscles and sphincters relax (muscles stiffen 4–6 hours after death as rigor mortis sets in)
- Urine and stool may be released
- Eyes generally remain open
- Jaw can fall open
- Observers may hear trickling of fluids internally, even after death

---

Box 23-2. *What to Do When Death Occurs*

Always be sensitive to and respectful of personal, cultural, and religious values, beliefs, and practices.

Ensure that family, caregivers, and health care providers know what to do when death occurs:

- There are no rules or regulations governing what happens after the patient dies.
- There is no need to call 911.
- There is no need to rush to call a physician or other health care provider. Invite the family and caregivers to call whenever they want support.

Encourage everyone to take time as needed after the death:

- Loved ones and caregivers should spend the time they need to witness and realize what has happened and say their goodbyes.
- They may touch, hold, and even kiss the person's body, as they feel most comfortable.
- They may complete the desired rites and rituals at the appropriate time.

Sufficient time spent at the bedside beginning to "realize" that their loved one has died will benefit everyone as they start to adapt to the changes in their lives.

When family members are ready for or need support, make sure they know who to call (i.e., the physician, the hospice, etc.).

---

able to. The degree of distress seems inversely related to the extent to which advance planning and preparation occurred.

Although we do not know what unconscious patients can hear, experience suggests that their awareness may be greater than their ability to respond. *Presume that the unconscious patient hears everything.* Advise families and caregivers to talk to the patient as if he or she is conscious. Surround the patient with the people, pets, things, music, and sounds that he or she would like. Encourage family to say the things they need to say. Share "bad" news away from the bedside, in another room, behind closed doors. Encourage family to give the patient permission to "let go and die" using words that are comfortable to them. Suggest phrases such as, "I know that you are dying, please do so when you are ready" and "I love you. I will miss you. I will never forget you. Please do what you need to do when you are ready."

Encourage everyone to show affection in ways they are used to, including touching and lying beside the patient. Encourage as much intimacy as family feel comfortable with. Maintain the privacy of the family as they are with the patient.

FACILITATE LIFE CLOSURE

If they have the opportunity, many patients approaching the end of their lives want to finish their business, organize their financial and legal affairs, and reconcile both close and estranged relationships. Help them engage in activities to create memories, including reminiscence and life review through stories and photos, family reunions and celebrations, letter writing, and the creation of audiotapes or videotapes. Patients can engage in gift giving of thoughts, personal treasures, family heirlooms, or money. They can also discuss the possibility of organ donation such as corneas, or say a last "hurrah" and goodbye. Some patients even want to have a celebration before their death to give gifts and say goodbye to close family and friends.

RITES AND RITUALS, FUNERALS, AND MEMORIAL SERVICES

Ensure that everyone is aware of personal, cultural, and religious traditions, rites, and rituals that may dictate how prayers are to be conducted, how a person's body is to be handled after death, whether health care professionals can touch it, and when and how the body can be moved.

Help the patient and family plan funeral or memorial services, burial, or cremation.

PROVIDE ONGOING SUPPORT

Throughout the last hours of life of the patient, the family will benefit from repeated contact with their physicians and health care team. Review the status of the patient with family and caregivers regularly. Repeat and clarify the goals of care, the futility of life-prolonging therapies (especially artificial hydration and nutrition), and the irreversibility of unfolding events. Modify the plan of care as needed to address the changing situation and goals of care. Assess the potential for an intense, acute grief reaction and who is at high risk for a complicated grief reaction.

Because delays in communication only heighten anxiety, ensure that knowledgeable clinicians, including a physician, are available by telephone 24 hours per day, 7 days per week. Families and caregivers will have the best outcome if their questions and concerns are addressed promptly, so they don't feel compelled to call 911 or visit the emergency room.

DYING IN INSTITUTIONS

Because many patients die in hospitals, nursing homes, and prisons and jails, a few remarks are warranted regarding the particular challenges of ensuring a comfortable death in institutions where the culture is not focused on end-of-life care. Tradeoffs previously acceptable because the patient would get better, such as the loss of privacy and no opportunity for intimacy, are no longer acceptable because this is the last chance for the patient and family to be together.

Provide privacy so that confidential conversations are possible and family can be present continuously (or move other patients out of a multibed room). Encourage the family to surround the patient with a few of his or her favorite personal belongings and photos.

Because this is the last chance for family members to be close, encourage intimacy. Teach them how to pillow side rails and curl up safely in a hospital bed beside their loved one. Provide privacy signs to hang on closed doors that staff will respect.

Ensure that the staff is knowledge and skilled in last-hours-of-life care and collaborates to provide a single plan of care across nursing shifts and changes in house staff. If the provision of environments conducive to end-of-life care proves to be difficult on the general medical/surgical units, establish or move the patient to a specialized palliative care unit where patients and families can be assured of the environment and the skilled care they need.[8]

Manage the Dying Process

The many common, irreversible signs and symptoms that develop during the last hours of life can be alarming if not understood (see Box 23-1). Reassess the need for every therapeutic intervention. Stop all therapies that are inconsistent with the patient's goals of care. Continue only medications needed to manage symptoms such

Table 23-2. Medications Used During the Last Hours of Life

Drug	Dosing	Notes
Lorazepam	1–2 mg buccal mucosal/ PR/SL/SC/IV, q1h to titrate, then q4–6h to maintain	If paradoxical agitation observed, choose a nonbenzodiazepine for sedation.
Haloperidol	2–5 mg PR/SC/IV q1h to titrate then q6h to maintain	Relatively nonsedating at low doses. May require 10–30 mg daily to sedate.
Chlorpromazine	10–25 mg PR/SC/IV q4–6h	Parenteral route may require special exemptions from standard nursing policy in some settings.
Scopolamine (hyoscine hydrobromide)	10–100 µg/hr SC/IV continuous infusion; or 0.1–0.4 mg SC q6h; or 1–10 patches q72h	Transdermal preparation only: delivers approximately 10 µg/hr and takes 12–24 hours to reach therapeutic levels.
Glycopyrrolate	0.2–0.4 mg SC q2–4h and titrate	Does not cross blood–brain barrier.

as pain, breathlessness, and terminal hyperactive delirium or to reduce secretions and prevent seizures (Table 23-2).

Base pharmacologic and nonpharmacologic management on the etiology and underlying pathophysiology of each symptom. Always use the least invasive route of administration, usually the oral or buccal mucosa routes; occasionally the subcutaneous or intravenous routes; never the intramuscular route.

WEAKNESS AND FATIGUE

As patients approach death, fatigue and weakness usually increase. Eventually, most will not be able to move around the bed or raise their head.[9] Discontinue therapy to alleviate fatigue. Because joint position fatigue and significant achiness can develop if a patient remains in the same position without moving for prolonged periods, move joints passively every 1 to 2 hours to minimize any sense of achiness.

SKIN CARE

During the last hours of life, skin care focuses on hygiene, moisture, protection, pressure reduction, and massage. Bathe the patient routinely to maintain body hygiene, remove dead skin, clean up body fluids like urine and stool, and minimize body odor. Use warm water and a gentle skin-cleansing agent. Dry thoroughly to minimize the risk of maceration. Avoid soaps that are drying or abrasive and perfumes that may be irritating.

Moisturize the skin routinely to minimize the risk of dry, flaking skin and pruritus, maintain elasticity, and minimize the risk of tears. Avoid rubbing areas that are erythematous or have broken down.

Protect thin, fragile skin to minimize the risk of skin tears. This is particularly important in cachectic patients who have lost skin elasticity and resilience. Thin, transparent membranes reduce shearing forces. Hydrocolloid dressings add a cushioning effect.

Continuous pressure, particularly over bony prominences, increases the risk of ischemia, skin breakdown, and pain. To minimize sacral pressure, keep the head of the bed to elevations less than 30 degrees. Raise it only for short periods of social interaction. Avoid resting one limb on another. Use a pillow or another cushioning support to keep legs apart. Protect bony prominences with hydrocolloid dressings.

Turning helps to maintain comfort, reduce pressure, and minimize the risk of ischemia, skin breakdown, and joint position fatigue. When patients are unable to move themselves, turn the patient from side to side every 1 to 1.5 hours. Use a careful "log-roll" technique with a draw sheet to distribute forces evenly across the patient's body and minimize pain on movement and to reduce shearing forces that could lead to skin tears. If turning is painful, turn the patient less frequently or place the patient on a pressure-reducing surface, such as an air mattress or air bed. As patients approach death, the need for turning lessens as the risk of skin breakdown becomes less important.

Massage intermittently to stimulate circulation, shift edema, spread out moisturizing lotions, and provide comfort. This is particularly helpful in dependent areas subject to increased pressure, before and after turning. Avoid massaging skin that is erythematous or has broken down.

WOUND CARE

During the last hours of life, wound care focuses exclusively on comfort, not healing. Minimize the frequency of dressing changes. Use nonstick pain-reducing dressings, such as hydrogels, alginates, and soft silicones. Control infections with topical antibacterials such as iodine, metronidazole, or silver sulfadiazine, and antifungals such as ketoconazole. Contain exudate flow with foam dressings. Absorb odors with kitty litter or activated charcoal placed in a pan under the bed or a candle burning in the room. Consider masking odors with alternate smells like vanilla or vinegar. Avoid scented deodorizers or perfumes.

DECREASED NUTRITIONAL INTAKE AND WASTING

Most patients lose their appetite and reduce food intake long before they reach the last hours of life. Families and professional caregivers may often interpret cessation of eating as "giving in" and worry that the patient will starve to death. In fact, most dying patients are not hungry; food is not appealing and may even be nauseating. Parenteral or enteral feeding at the end of life does not improve symptom control and it does not lengthen life.[10-12]

Clinicians can help reframe families' understanding of anorexia from "starving to death" to "metabolic abnormalities due to cancer that may be protective." Intellectual function remains intact for longer. Ketosis can also increase the patient's general sense of well-being.[13]

Clinicians can help families and caregivers realize that food pushed on an unwilling patient or one who is incapable of eating inadvertently may cause nausea, aspiration, or asphyxiation and increase tensions and bad feelings. Clenched teeth may be the only way for the patient to exert control and should be respected. As an alternative, help family members and caregivers find different ways to provide appropriate physical care and emotional support to the patient.

Loss of Ability to Close Eyes

During the last hours of life, patients frequently leave their "eyes open," though their irises and pupils are not visible. This is *not* a sign of neurologic dysfunction. Advanced wasting leads to loss of the retro-orbital fat pad. Muscles pull the orbit back into its socket. The patient's eyelids are not long enough to extend the additional distance backward and fully cover the conjunctiva. As a result, the eyelids no longer appose and some conjunctiva remains exposed, even when the patient is sleeping. Educate the family and caregivers about the cause so they will understand what is happening and not find it distressing. When conjunctiva is exposed, maintain moisture using ophthalmic lubricants, artificial tears, or physiologic saline (see Oral, Nasal, and Conjunctival Care section).

Decreased Fluid Intake and Dehydration

Most patients reduce their fluid intake or stop drinking before they die.[13] This frequently causes distress to family and caregivers, who worry that the patient will become dehydrated, thirsty, and suffer. Clinicians can help families and caregivers understand that this is an expected event and suggest alternate ways for them to give care.

When Fluid Intake Is Reduced. If the patient is still taking some fluid but not eating, salt-containing fluids, such as soups, soda water, sport drinks, and red vegetable juices, can facilitate rehydration, maintain electrolyte balance, and minimize the risk of nausea from hyponatremia. Fluids such as water, fruit juices, sodas, and soft drinks that are effectively "free water" and do not contain sodium bicarbonate are not rehydrating. Fluids that contain caffeine, like coffee, tea, and colas, are diuretics and worsen dehydration, as can alcohol. Discontinue all diuretics and antihypertensives.

As patients develop cachexia and hypoalbuminemia, their oncotic pressure and intravascular volume decrease, and mild peripheral edema is expected. The absence of mild peripheral edema signals severe dehydration. Increased fluid intake increases the risk of peripheral and pulmonary edema. It does not replenish the intravascular volume.

An albumin infusion can restore temporarily intravascular oncotic pressure, produce a transitory diuresis, and reduce edema for a short period (hours to 1 or 2 days). Especially when combined with a loop diuretic, this may allow the patient to participate in a specific activity, such as a family reunion. Routine albumin infusions are not recommended in cachectic patients. The albumin is catabolized within hours as a nutritional source for the patient (or tumor), and it does not reverse the underlying protein deficit. It is also an expensive procedure.

When the Patient Stops Taking Fluids. When a patient stops taking oral fluids, explain to the family that patients with peripheral edema or ascites have excess body water and salt and are not dehydrated. They will not get lightheaded or dizzy if they are not elevated in bed. Low blood pressure and a weak pulse are part of the dying process, not just an indication of dehydration. Most experts believe that dehydration in the last hours of life does not cause distress. It may stimulate endorphin release and add to the patient's sense of well-being.[14–16]

The most frequent symptoms that dehydrated patients complain of are thirst, dry mouth, and fatigue. At the end of life these symptoms are most likely to be caused by disease progression, mouth breathing, analgesics, anxiolytics, and anticholinergics used to control secretions.[17,18] Several studies have shown that parenteral fluids do not affect the sensation of thirst and dry mouth that patients experience at the end of life. The best treatment for these symptoms is frequent and good oral care, ice chips, swabs with water, and nystatin if thrush is present. Parenteral fluids may help to reduce sedation and myoclonus, either from hydration or increased elimination of active opioid metabolites. However, parenteral fluids have not been shown to lengthen life, and may even shorten life. They can worsen peripheral edema and ascites and increase gastrointestinal and respiratory secretions, which may result in breathlessness, pain, nausea and vomiting, and increased urination that requires catheter placement.

Oral, Nasal, and Conjunctival Care

During the last hours of life, meticulous oral, nasal, and conjunctival hygiene are essential to maintain comfort.

To minimize bad odors and tastes and the sense of thirst and reduce the risk of painful cracking and bleeding, moisten and clean oral mucosa every 15 to 30 minutes with either a baking soda mouthwash (5 mL salt plus 5 mL baking soda mixed in 1 L tepid water) or an artificial saliva preparation. If oral candidiasis is present and the patient is still able to swallow, treat with systemic fluconazole. Otherwise, dab white plaques with topical nystatin. Avoid swabs containing lemon and glycerin because glycerin is desiccating and lemon irritating, particularly on open sores.

To reduce evaporation, drying, and painful cracking of lips and nares, coat lips and anterior nasal mucosa with a thin layer of petroleum or other nonaqueous jelly every 4 hours. Be careful not to occlude nasal cannulae. Although not flammable, petroleum jelly could soften some plastics if exposure is prolonged. Avoid perfumed lip balms because these can be irritating.

To minimize the risk of painful dry eyes, particularly when eyes remain open, moisten conjunctiva with an ophthalmic lubricating gel every 3 to 4 hours or artificial tears or physiologic saline solution every 15 to 30 minutes (though these drain through tear ducts and evaporate quickly).

CARDIAC DYSFUNCTION AND RENAL FAILURE

Cardiac output, intravascular volume, and urinary output normally decrease toward the end of life. As oliguria develops, the remaining urine typically becomes very dark and "tea" colored. Ultimately, most dying patients become anuric. Rehydration with parenteral fluids is unlikely to reverse this circulatory shutdown or renal failure, particularly when the patient is hypoalbuminemic.[38]

NEUROLOGIC DYSFUNCTION: THE TWO ROADS TO DEATH

Neurologic changes typically manifest as one of two patterns that have been described as the two roads to death (Figure 23-2).[19] Approximately 70% to 90% of patients follow the "usual road" and die quietly, likely a hypoactive delirium. Another 10% to 30% or more of patients follow the "difficult road" and experience a terminal hyperactive delirium.

The Usual Road

Patients following the "usual road" to death typically experience increasing drowsiness, decreasing ability to communicate, changes in their perception of pain,

2 ROADS TO DEATH

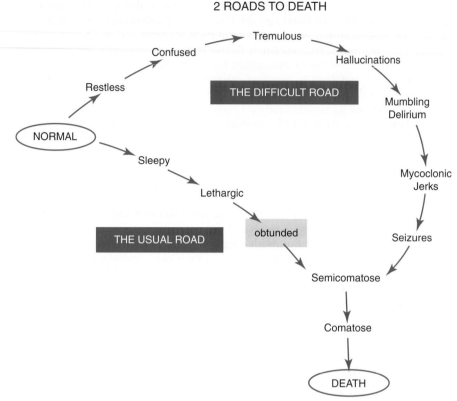

Figure 23-2. The two roads to death. (Modified from Ferris FD, Flannery JS, McNeal HB, et al editors: *Palliative Care*, vol. 4. In A Comprehensive Guide for the Care of Persons with HIV Disease. Toronto, Mount Sinai Hospital and Casey House Hospice, 1995, pp. 118–120.)

respiratory dysfunction, loss of ability to swallow, loss of sphincter control, coma, and finally a quiet death.

Eyelash Reflex. The eyelash reflex is a useful indicator to estimate the patient's level of consciousness during the dying process. Previously used by anesthetists to guide the induction of anesthesia, its disappearance suggests a profound level of coma equivalent to full anesthesia and lack of any awareness of what is happening.

Pain. Many people fear that pain will suddenly increase during the last hours of life. In fact, the experience of pain during the dying process may lessen as a result of decreasing neurologic activity, decreasing awareness and perception, and buildup of endorphins and other endogenous metabolites that have analgesic properties, such as ketones.

Though difficult to assess in the semiconscious or obtunded patient, continuous pain may be associated with grimacing and continuous facial tension, particularly across the forehead and between the eyebrows. Physiologic signs, such as transitory tachycardia, may also signal acute changes.[20]

Clinicians must be careful not to diagnose pain when fleeting forehead tension comes and goes with movement, passage of gas, mental activity, dreams, or hallucinations. They must also be careful not to confuse pain with the restlessness, agitation, moaning, or groaning that accompany a terminal hyperactive delirium. If the diagnosis is unclear, a time-limited therapeutic trial of opioids administered as needed may help to establish whether pain is driving the observed behaviors.

Knowledge of opioid pharmacology is critical to managing pain during the last hours of life. Codeine is metabolized into morphine. Morphine, oxycodone, and hydromorphone are conjugated into glucuronides by the liver and then 90% to 95% of the metabolites are renally excreted. Some of these metabolites are potent analgesics like morphine 6-glucuronide; others may cause central nervous system (CNS) excitation but no analgesia, like morphine 3-glucuronide (M3G); the effects of others, such as metabolites of hydromorphone and oxycodone, are less certain.

As renal clearance decreases during the dying process (manifested by oliguria and anuria), decrease the routine administration of morphine (including continuous infusions) by 50% if urine output is less than 500 mL/24 hours and stop routine dosing once urine output is less than 200 mL/24 hours in order to avoid the accumulation of potentially toxic metabolites and minimize the risk of terminal hyperactive delirium. Maintain analgesia by administering breakthrough doses of morphine to manage expressions suggestive of pain. Alternately, consider the use of opioids like fentanyl or hydromorphone, which have inactive or less active metabolites.

Respiratory Dysfunction. Before the last hours of life, correct reversible causes of respiratory dysfunction when appropriate. Treat pneumonia, perform a therapeutic thoracentesis or paracentesis, and use dexamethasone to reduce inflammation or diurese edema caused by heart failure.

During the last hours of life, altered breathing patterns may indicate significant neurologic compromise.[21] As the patient fatigues, breaths may become shallow and frequent with a diminishing tidal volume. As the respiratory control center malfunctions, periods of apnea or Cheyne-Stokes pattern respirations frequently develop. Accessory respiratory muscle use may become prominent. A few last reflex breaths may signal death. These "agonal breaths" can persist for minutes to hours, with significant gaps between each breath, and can be "agonizing" for everyone who watches.

Families and caregivers frequently find changes in breathing patterns to be one of the most distressing signs of impending death. Many fear that the comatose patient is suffocating. They are frequently comforted to know that the unresponsive patient may not be experiencing any sense of breathlessness or "suffocating" and that oxygen will not be of benefit, and may actually prolong the dying process.

Because dyspnea is subjective, clinicians have to rely on patient self-report rather than objective measures such as respiratory rate or oxygen saturation.[22] Administer low doses of opioids using standard dosing guidelines to manage any perception of breathlessness without risk of shortening the patient's life. Bronchodilators can be helpful for some patients.

Oxygen is generally helpful regardless of the degree of hypoxia or cause of dyspnea, and it can be delivered via nasal cannula or an Oxymizer. Patients tend to tolerate these devices better that facial masks, which can be uncomfortable but not necessarily more helpful. Air flow may be as helpful as oxygen in treating breathlessness.[23] A stream of air from a fan can also be very useful in managing dyspneic patients.

Chlorpromazine (12.5–25 mg PO/PR/SC every 4 hours as needed) may provide a beneficial effect and reduce dyspnea.[24] Benzodiazepines, such as lorazepam (1–2 mg PO/SC/IV/buccal mucosa [elixir or tablet predissolved in 0.5–1 mL water, or injectable] every hour as needed) may also help alleviate any associated anxiety. Their use will not shorten the patient's life.[25]

Difficulty Swallowing. In the last hours of life, as the patient dies, weakness and decreased neurologic function present as difficulty swallowing and coughing and loss of the gag reflex. Fluids build up in the tracheobronchial tree. Crackling or gurgling noises are caused by the movement of air through or over these pooled secretions. When these noises occur in the presence of other signs of the dying process, they are a strong predictor that death will occur within 96 hours.[26] These noisy respirations, also known as the "death rattle," occur in 23% to 92% of patients.[27] They are most common in patients with lung and brain tumors, either primary or secondary.[27]

Family members are frequently disconcerted when their loved ones develop the "death rattle" because they are afraid the patient is suffocating or drowning when they hear the noise. Other causes of noisy respirations in a dying patient are respiratory infections or pulmonary edema.

When a patient is unable to swallow, stop *all* oral intake. Warn families and caregivers of the risks of aspiration and asphyxiation. Before using medications, it is useful to try simpler nursing interventions, such as repositioning the patient, postural drainage, educating the family, and suctioning:

- Reposition the patient on the side or semi-prone. This may shift enough of the secretions that air flows over the fluid without making a sound.
- Secretions can also be cleared by postural drainage using Trendelenburg position. In this position, gravity may draw fluids into the oropharynx, where they can be removed with a sponge, gauze on a stick, or oropharyngeal suction. However, because of the risk of reflux and aspiration of gastric contents, do not maintain Trendelenburg position for more than a few minutes.
- Educate families that the patient is not suffocating. This can reassure to families and take away some of their angst.
- When secretions have reached the pharynx but are not clearing by repositioning, try oral suctioning. Suctioning is less effective when secretions remain beneath the pharynx and are difficult to get to with typical suctioning maneuvers. Avoid deep suctioning whenever possible. It can be highly stimulating and painful to an otherwise peaceful patient and may cause distress to family members who are watching.

Medications. Oropharyngeal and tracheobronchial secretions come from the production of saliva by the salivary glands and secretions from the bronchial mucosa. Because these glandular tissues contain muscarinic receptors, antimuscarinic medications such as atropine, scopolamine hydrobromide, scopolamine butylbromide, and glycopyrrolate are effective treatments for the death rattle. Although similar in action, there are significant differences between these medications. Scopolamine hydrobromide has a more rapid onset of action, but a lower response rate, than scopolamine butylbromide or glycopyrrolate.[27] Scopolamine butylbromide has a significantly more powerful action compared with atropine. Although atropine may be equally effective in similar doses, it has an increased risk of producing undesired cardiac or central nervous system excitation.[28] Glycopyrrolate and scopolamine butylbromide have the potential added benefit that they do not cross the blood–brain barrier. As a result, there is much less risk of short-term memory deficits and increased confusion.[29]

To minimize the accumulation of secretions, particularly in an unconscious patient, start one of these medications early and administer them routinely.

All these medications have the potential to worsen open angle glaucoma. To prevent worsening of acute eye pain, continue glaucoma medications until death.

Atropine is administered as 0.4 to 0.6 mg SC every 4 hours or 1 drop of atropine solution (containing 0.5 mg atropine in 1% wt/vol solution) SL every 4 hours.

Glycopyrrolate is given as 0.2 to 0.4 mg or more SC every 4 to 6 hours or 0.4 to 1.2 mg or more every 24 hours by intravenous or subcutaneous infusion (64,65).

Scopolamine is given as 0.2 to 0.4 mg or more SC every 4 hours, 1 to 3 transdermal scopolamine patches every 72 hours, or 0.1 to 1 mg/hour by continuous intravenous or subcutaneous infusion.

Loss of Sphincter Control. In the last hours of life, fatigue and loss of sphincter control may lead to incontinence of urine or stool. Both can be very distressing to patients, family members, and caregivers, particularly if they are not warned in advance that this may happen. If incontinence occurs, clean the patient promptly and provide appropriate skin care. If urine flow is minimal, try to manage recurrent incontinence with absorbent pads placed under the patient. If urinary incontinence persists, a condom or indwelling urinary catheter may reduce the need for frequent changing and cleaning prevent skin breakdown. Although convenient for caregivers, an indwelling urinary catheter may be uncomfortable for the patient, particularly males. Always instill lidocaine 2% gel into the urethra 10 to 15 minutes before catheterizing males. If diarrhea is considerable and relentless, a rectal tube may help to contain the liquid stool, minimize skin maceration, and maintain patient dignity.

The "Difficult Road"

Terminal Hyperactive Delirium. Terminal hyperactive delirium is an irreversible acute confusional state in the last hours or days of life that is associated with other signs of the dying process (see Box 23-1). It occurs in up to 88% of dying patients. It may be the first change to herald the "difficult road to death." Failure to recognize terminal hyperactive delirium may result in worsening of the patient's agitation. If left unmanaged, myoclonus and seizures can ensue, particularly when cerebral metastases are present.

Before the onset of terminal hyperactive delirium, many patients have an altered sleep–wake cycle. Day–night reversal is common. Attention and ability to focus decrease. Patients lose touch with the environment surrounding them and appear to be "in their own world."

In its initial stages, terminal hyperactive delirium may be difficult to distinguish from reversible delirium. If signs of the dying process are not present, and if it is consistent with the goals of care, look for potentially reversible causes of delirium, including hypoxia, metabolic disturbances (e.g., electrolyte imbalance, acidosis), infections, toxin accumulation as a result of liver and renal failure, adverse effects of medications, disease-related factors, and reduced cerebral perfusion. Always assess for urinary retention and fecal impaction because they are common and easily correctable causes of reversible delirium. Review medications for recent changes, potential adverse effects, and medication interactions.

As with reversible delirium that occurs at other times in life, terminal hyperactive delirium can be associated with significant patient distress as it evolves, including intermittent restlessness, agitation, and hallucinations. Symptoms typically wax and wane, interspersed with periods of calm and even moments of lucidity. Whether slowly or abruptly, it frequently evolves into a highly agitated state. Repetitious and purpose-less movement, such as pulling blankets on and off, sitting up and lying down, or tossing and turning in bed, are very common. Unintelligible speech may be present.

Terminal hyperactive delirium is often associated with moaning and groaning. When this occurs, it is frequently mistaken for pain. Escalating "pain" near the end of life in the setting of rapidly titrated opiates may be a manifestation of terminal agita-tion. To differentiate the moaning and groaning of terminal hyperactive delirium from pain, look for tension across the forehead, furrowing of eyebrows, or facial grimacing. When these are absent, the vocalization is more likely related to delirium than pain. Although a time-limited trial of opioids may be diagnostic, when renal clearance is compromised, such as when perfusion decreases as a patient is dying, extra opioid doses can lead to metabolite accumulation and increase the hyperactive delirium.

Terminal hyperactive delirium may also be difficult to differentiate from a psy-chological or spiritual crisis at the end of life, although these crises do not typically occur in the patient who has been previously calm and prepared for the end of his or her life.

There is a significant difference between the management of irreversible terminal hyperactive delirium in dying patients and the management of potentially reversible delirium in patients who are not dying. In reversible delirium, neuroleptics are the mainstay of pharmacologic treatment. Benzodiazepines are not appropriate because of their potential to worsen the symptoms of delirium and short-term memory defi-cits, particularly in the elderly.

If the possibility of terminal hyperactive delirium is discussed in advance, most patients will not want to experience or have any memory of it. They, and their fami-lies, will want the process to be quiet, and to die peacefully. In contrast to the man-agement of reversible delirium, the management of irreversible terminal hyperactive delirium focuses on settling the patient and the family and ensuring that the patient does not experience bad dreams, hallucinations, myoclonus, or seizures.

Utilize any nonpharmacologic interventions that may be comforting. Reduce agitation and improve day–night cycle reversal. Avoid restraints and provide a quiet, relaxed atmosphere (minimize external stimulation), preferably in a familiar envi-ronment. Use appropriate lighting (light during the day, dark at night).

If routine opioids are believed to be the cause and the patient is dehydrated, a trial of intravenous or subcutaneous fluids could help reduce the patient's symptoms.

In contrast to their contraindication in the management of reversible delirium, benzodiazepines are ideal for the management of terminal hyperactive delirium for four reasons:

1. As anxiolytic/sedatives, they will settle the patient and minimize his or her awareness.
2. As muscle relaxants, they will relax both skeletal muscles and contracted vocal cords (which lead to moaning and groaning).
3. As amnestics, they will ensure no short-term memory of the experience.
4. As antiepileptics, they will act prophylactically against possible seizures.

Typically benzodiazepines settle the patient quickly and, in turn, everyone who is watching.

Lorazepam is a moderately long-acting benzodiazepine that is ideal for managing terminal hyperactive delirium. Place lorazepam 1 to 2 mg elixir or tablet predissolved in 0.5 to 1 mL of water against the buccal mucosa every 1 hour as needed and titrate until the patient is settled.[30] Once the patient is settled, administer the dose used over 4 hours to settle the patient, every 4 hours to maintain the desired state. Typically 2 to 10 mg of lorazepam every 4 hours will settle most patients. A few extremely agitated patients may require 20 to 50 mg lorazepam or more in 24 hours.

As an alternative, midazolam is a fast-acting benzodiazepine that has been used in several studies.[31,32] Start with 0.5 to 2 mg IV or SC every 15 minutes and titrate to effect. Once the patient is settled, use midazolam 1 to 5 mg SC or IV every 1 hour to maintain sedation.

Although intravenous administration produces a quicker effect, if intravenous access is not available, benzodiazepines may be easily administered subcutaneously (as individual injections or an infusion), via buccal mucosa, or rectally.

If benzodiazepines are not available, chlorpromazine (10–25 mg or more PO/PR/IV q4h) is preferred over haloperidol for the management of terminal hyperactive delirium because it is more sedating.[33] Use caution with neuroleptics because there is a small risk that they will lower a patient's seizure threshold and increase the risk of seizures.

Occasionally, a combination of a neuroleptic and a benzodiazepine is necessary for symptom control.[34] If ineffective, barbiturates or propofol have been suggested as alternatives.[35–37]

Seizures. If seizures occur during the dying process, manage them with high doses of benzodiazepines, such as subcutaneous or intravenous lorazepam or midazolam. Rectal diazepam gel administered in doses of 0.05 mg/kg PR q4–12h can be very effective. If seizures are resistant, other medications may be needed to establish control, such as parenteral or intravenous phenytoin, subcutaneous fosphenytoin, or phenobarbital. Phenobarbital can be started with initial dose of 100 to 200 mg PR/IV/SC/IM, followed by additional doses up to a maximum of 600 to 1000 mg at maximum rate of 100 mg/minute. Phenobarbital is usually effective in doses of 200 mg/24 hours.

Other Symptoms and End-of-Life Issues

Hemorrhage. Bleeding may be present during the last hours of life.[38] If extensive, it can be a frightening experience for everyone involved, from patient to family, caregivers, and staff. Bleeding generally is due to superficial tumor friability, tumor eroding into a blood vessel, coagulopathy, low platelet count, or platelet dysfunction. It may also be secondary to a combination of these factors. Hemorrhage may be precipitated by minor trauma or pressure, but it may also happen spontaneously without warning.

If there is a possibility of bleeding, especially of an extensive hemorrhage, advance planning is very helpful. Attempt to correct the coagulopathy or other potential causes if this is consistent with the patient's goals of care. Provide interdisciplinary support. Keep dark towels easily accessible in the room in case there is acute bleeding. They will minimize the visibility of blood and help reduce patient and family distress. At the time of acute bleeding, midazolam 2 to 10 mg IV or SC can be given to minimize the anxiety and produce amnesia. If the hemorrhage is severe, the patient may die within a few minutes and it may not be possible to provide sedating medication quickly enough.

For superficial bleeding, apply pressure to the area. Topical hemostatic agents can be helpful unless the bleeding is extensive (Table 23-3). In case of bleeding wounds, good wound care is essential. Procedures such as radiotherapy, embolization, and

Table 23-3. Treatment Options for Bleeding

Type of Treatment	Examples	Notes
Temporary Reversal of a Bleeding Disorder	Platelet transfusions Fresh frozen plasma Vitamin K Clotting factor replacement	If used, should be done before the last hours
Local Therapy	Radiotherapy Embolization Cryotherapy Variceal banding	If used, should be done before the last hours
Systemic Therapy	Tranexamic acid 1 g PO q8h Aminocaproic acid 1 g PO q6h Octreotide, vasopressin	
Topical Therapy	Epinephrine 1:1000 Thrombin 1000–2000 units/mL Calcium alginate Silver nitrate (sticks or liquid)	

endoscopic hemostasis may be helpful in the last weeks or months of life but are not appropriate during the last hours, because the burden will outweigh the benefit. In case of variceal bleeding, medical management with octreotide or vasopressin may be helpful.

Fever. Fevers during the last hours of life are frequently multifactorial. They can be the result of infections, cancer, or medications or can be central in origin. Most often their cause remains uncertain.

For the symptomatic management of fever, acetaminophen or other antipyretics may be effective. Nonsteroidal anti-inflammatory drugs (NSAIDs) are particularly helpful if the fever is tumor related.[39] Often these medications will need to be given parenterally once the patient stops swallowing. Topical cooling methods such as bathing with tepid water, alcohol sponging, or the use of cooling blankets can also be synergistic.[40]

For most patients, antibiotics will not provide any significant symptom relief. Discontinue them once the patient stops swallowing, if not beforehand.

If a neuroleptic malignant syndrome is present (a rare side effect of neuroleptics), discontinue all neuroleptics and use dopaminergic and anticholinergic drugs in conjunction with benzodiazepines to provide relief.

Turning Off Defibrillators. As the prevalence of cardiovascular disease in our aging society increases, automatic implantable cardioverter-defibrillators (AICDs) are becoming more common. AICDs can detect rapid life-threatening heart rhythms and perform a cardioversion—delivery of an electrical shock to the heart that is intended to restore a normal heartbeat. If a dying patient with an AICD has a rapid life-threatening rhythm, the device will attempt to deliver a shock as long as a "shockable" rhythm is present.

Although when life-threatening arrhythmias are present the patient is frequently unconscious, it is not always the case. Sequential shocks could be uncomfortable to the patient and distressing to family members observing them, especially if it is clear that the patient is dying.

Unfortunately, because an AICD is introduced as life-saving device, when its implantation is recommended some of the details of the potential end-of-life issues are frequently overlooked. When discussing goals of care with patients who have AICDs, inquire whether having an active defibrillator is consistent with the patient's overall goals. Obtain information about the manufacturer and the type of defibrillator. If the decision is made to keep the device active, offer pain relief and a sedative in case the device starts delivering a shock in the last days or hours of life, because most patients report significant discomfort at the time of cardioversion. For those patients who choose to deactivate the AICD, ask the manufacturer or a cardiologist to turn off the device using special equipment (no invasive procedures necessary). For patients who have a combination pacer and defibrillator, pacemaking function can be maintained even after the cardioverter-defibrillator function is switched off. If a cardiologist or a company representative is not available, a deactivating magnet can be held over the device to prevent continuous shocks in a dying patient.

When Death Occurs

When expected death occurs (see Box 23-1), the focus of care shifts from the patient to the family and caregivers (see Box 23-2). Everyone will have a different experience and a very personal sense of loss. Even though the death has been anticipated for some time, no one will know what the loss feels like until it actually occurs. Encourage family and caregivers to spend the time they need with the body to help them address their acute grief. It may take hours to days to weeks or even months for each person to realize the full impact of the changes.[41-43]

It is rarely obligatory for physicians or health care professionals to attend quickly to witness what has happened, unless the patient has requested organ donation or made an anatomic gift to a medical school. However, the presence of a professional may be helpful if family members are distressed and need immediate support with their acute grief reactions or if they have questions.

Members of the health care team who have not been present for the death can assess how family members are handling their loss by listening to a recounting of how things went leading up to the death and afterward. Listen for signs of acute grief reactions that are beyond cultural norms. They may suggest a significant risk of complicated grief reactions. Watch for individuals who are showing little or no emotional reactions to the death, or who may be catatonic. They will need significant acute support and interventions to push them to realize what has just happened. They are almost certainly at high risk for complicated grief reactions. Spiritual advisors or other interdisciplinary team members may be instrumental in orchestrating events to facilitate the transition that those present are experiencing.

RITES AND RITUALS

After death occurs, ensure that all cultural and religious values, beliefs and practices, prayers, and rites and rituals are observed.

PRONOUNCING AND CERTIFYING DEATH

In teaching hospitals, medical students and residents are typically called to "pronounce" death. In nonteaching settings, the attending physician or nursing staff may be the ones to do it. When a patient dies at home with hospice care, it is usually a nurse who confirms the absence of vital signs. Although local regulations differ, if an expected death occurs at home without hospice care and the patient has a physician willing to sign a death certificate, then transport of the body to a hospital for a physician to confirm death may not be needed.

First, confirm that it is culturally acceptable for the physician to touch the patient to confirm that death has occurred. Then, verify the patient's identify. Ask those present for the patient's full name; verify it with the hospital identification tag if available. Observe the patient for several minutes. Note the general appearance of the body, particularly its color, and the presence of mottling (livedo reticularis) or venous pooling along dependent skin surfaces. Look and listen for the absence of spontaneous respirations. Listen for the absence of heart sounds. Feel for the absence of carotid pulse. Observe the size of the pupils. Test for the absence of pupillary light reflex. Test for response to verbal or tactile stimuli. Overtly painful stimuli, such as nipple or testicle twisting, or deep nailbed or sternal pressure are neither appropriate nor necessary.

If you have known the patient, *stop*—spend a few moments taking in what has happened. This may your only personal opportunity to say goodbye. Once the pronouncement is complete, document all activities in the medical record.

All funeral directors require a completed death certificate to proceed with any body preparation and registration of the death. Some will insist on having one before they pick up the body. Ensure that the physician has the information he or she will need to complete the death certificate and ample warning of the time by which one will be required.[44]

NOTIFYING THE CORONER

The medical coroner exists to review cases where the circumstances surrounding a death are unknown or there is suspicion of wrongdoing. In most jurisdictions, regulations also exist to trigger mandatory scrutiny of deaths that occur under specific circumstances, such as deaths that occur in acute care facilities within 48 or 72 hours of transfer of the patient from a long-term care facility. Because regulations vary, health care professionals must know the regulations in effect within the local jurisdiction. If there are any doubts about the circumstances surrounding a death, call the coroner's office, review the case, and ask for advice. If you are calling the coroner's office, don't move the patient, leave all lines and tubes in place, don't touch medications, and move nothing in the room until the coroner has "reviewed and released" the case. Make sure family and friends also know not to touch or move anything. If the coroner investigates a case, he or she will typically complete the death certificate before closing the case.

NOTIFYING FAMILY

Once the patient has been pronounced dead, let the family know what has happened, even if the coroner has not completed his or her investigation. Try to avoid breaking unexpected news by telephone, because communicating in person provides much greater opportunity for assessment and support.

PREPARING THE BODY FOR VIEWING

Once the pronouncement is complete (and the coroner, if called, has released the body), you may wish to create a visually peaceful and accessible environment to make viewing of the body easier. Some cultures permit only designated people to touch the body after death. Before starting to prepare the body, ensure that your proposed preparation will be acceptable to the family.

Once you have permission to proceed, spend a few moments alone in the room to position the body, disconnect any lines and machinery, remove catheters, and clean up any mess.[45] If eyes remain open, hold the eyelids closed for a few minutes (they will usually remain closed once they dry). If they still remain open, a small amount of surgical tape or a short adhesive surgical strip will hold them closed without risk of pulling out eyelashes when the tape is removed. If the jaw falls open as muscles relax, place a rolled-up towel under the chin and elevate the head. This will usually hold the jaw closed until muscles stiffen. Remember that muscles will stiffen as rigor mortis sets in 4 to 6 hours after the death. To make transfers and funeral arrangements easier, make sure the patient's body is straight and flat and arms are placed across the chest before this occurs.

INVITING OTHERS TO BEDSIDE

When the body is ready for viewing, first invite family, then anyone who has been close to the patient, including friends, caregivers, and health care professionals, to come to the bedside to witness what has happened. Before taking visitors into the room, spend a few minutes to remind them of the changes in body color, temperature, and the scene they will see. This can reduce the surprise and make the transition easier for everyone. Make sure everyone knows that there is no need to rush, that each person can take the time he or she needs to witness what has happened and say goodbye.

Moving the Body

Once family and caregivers have had the time they need at the bedside to deal with their acute grief reactions and observe their customs and traditions, preparations can begin for the funeral or memorial service. Families who have not discussed funeral arrangements in advance may have many questions about embalming, burial, cremation, and/or different types of services. If the funeral director is not available, spend a little time answering questions. This will ease their anxiety about what happens next.

Invite family members or caregivers to help prepare the body for transfer to the funeral home or the hospital morgue. Some people will find the touching, bathing, and preparation to be very therapeutic. It will help them realize that the patient has in fact died. For many, such rituals will be one of their final acts of direct caring.

Occasionally, a family will want to keep the body at home (or in their room at the acute or long-term care facility) for 2 to 4 days until the funeral service, burial, or cremation. Although this is possible in most jurisdictions, some additional preparation of the body and good ventilation are essential. Ask the funeral home to help prepare the body before rigor mortis sets in by positioning the body appropriately and packing the throat and rectum so fluids and odors don't escape unexpectedly.

Once the family is ready for the body to be moved, they should call the chosen funeral service provider and arrange for removal of the person's body.

For many, the arrival of the funeral directors to remove the body is the next major confrontation with reality, particularly when the death has occurred at home. Some family members will wish to witness the removal. Others will find it very difficult. They may prefer to retire to another place and allow professional caregivers to handle things discreetly. For some, the thought that the person's body will be enclosed in a body bag is intolerable. Health care professionals and funeral directors should have the sensitivity to recognize when this is an issue and negotiate a suitable alternative like not closing the bag until it has been removed from the vicinity of the home. Institutional staff should be aware that there may be similar reactions by family members when they prepare the body for transfer to the morgue.

After the Body Has Been Moved

Once the body has been removed and family members are settled, offer to assist with some of the immediate next steps. Notify other health care professionals that the death has occurred, including attending and consulting physicians, all involved health care service agencies, and all caregivers on the patient's care team.

Health care professionals will need to be clear about local regulations governing ownership of medications after a death and waste disposal. Discuss how family members can properly dispose of medications, particularly opioids. Document the type and quantity of medications disposed of. Have the witness cosign the medical record.

Discuss how family members can dispose of biological wastes (typically double bagged and placed in trash) and sharps containers.

When family members are ready, they can be left to have some privacy together.

Before departing, let them know who to call and how, if they have questions or need help or support, and establish when the first follow-up calls from the team should be.

FOLLOW-UP

Most families expect the physician and other health care professionals who have known the patient to provide initial follow-up bereavement support. A phone call followed by a bereavement card, with or without attendance at the patient's funeral, may be an appropriate way to provide initial follow-up. A phone call to key family members within 2 to 5 days of the death can be used to offer condolences, find out how everyone is doing, and plan further follow-up. A condolence note sent within 2 weeks of the death is an opportunity to offer tribute to the deceased as someone who was important. Use standard stationery and write it by hand. Mourners appreciate that time taken to sit and compose a personal message to them or share a memory of the deceased.

Attendance at Funerals and Memorial Services

Health care professionals may choose to attend some funeral or memorial services. In addition to supporting the family, many find that it helps them personally to close long-standing relationships they have had with their patients and families. Let families know in advance so they will not be surprised, particularly if they are only planning for an intimate family gathering. Although most families don't expect health care providers to attend, many will be delighted at the prospect.

PEARLS

- If managed well, the last hours can lead to significant personal and family growth.
- Advance preparation and education of professionals, family, and volunteer caregivers are crucial.
- Use only essential medications. Stop routine dosing and continue to offer opioids as needed. Accumulating serum concentrations of active drug and metabolites may lead to toxicity and terminal delirium.
- Know the signs of the dying process and understand the causes, underlying pathophysiology, and appropriate pharmacology to use in management.
- Attend to acute grief reactions.

PITFALLS

- If managed poorly, life closure may be incomplete, unnecessary suffering may occur, family distress may continue long after the patient's death, and those who watch may worry that their own death will be similar.

- Maintaining parenteral fluids may have adverse effects that are not commonly considered.

- Oropharyngeal suctioning is not likely to be effective at clearing secretions, yet it is very effective at stimulating a gag, cough, or vomiting.

- Moaning, groaning, and grimacing that accompany agitation and restlessness are frequently misinterpreted as pain. Terminal delirium may be occurring.

- Removal of the body insensitively or too soon can be more distressing for families than the moment of death.

Summary

The last hours of living are some of the most important in the life of the patient and his or her family. Although the focus is on relieving the patient's suffering and ensuring a safe and comfortable death, the health care team is also caring for everyone at the bedside. Through an effective intervention by the physician and other health care professionals, everyone will have a very different experience of end-of-life care and bereavement, and survivors will rebuild their lives sooner and more effectively.

References

1. Hallenbeck J: Palliative care in the final days of life: "They were expecting it at any time," *JAMA* 293(18):2265–2271, 2005.
2. Tuckman B, Jensen M: Stages of small group development, *Group Org Stud* 2:419–427, 1977.
3. Ferris FD, Balfour HM, Bowen K, et al: *A model to guide hospice palliative care*, Ottawa, Calif, 2002, Canadian Hospice Palliative Care Association, pp 13. Available at www.chpca.net.
4. Field MJ, Cassel CK, editors: *Approaching death: improving care at the end of life*, Washington, DC, 1997, National Academy Press, pp 28–30.
5. Emanuel LL, von Gunten CF, Ferris FD: *The Education for Physicians on End-of-Life Care (EPEC) Curriculum*, Chicago, 1999, American Medical Association.
6. Ellersahw J, Ward C: Care of the dying patient: the last hours or days of life, *Br Med J* 326:30–34, 2003.
7. Emanuel LL, von Gunten CF, Ferris FD: Communicating bad news. In *The Education for Physicians on End-of-Life Care (EPEC) Curriculum*, Chicago, 1999, American Medical Association.
8. Keller N, Martinez J, Finis N, et al: Characterization of an acute inpatient hospice palliative care unit in a US teaching hospital, *J Nursing Admin* 26:16–20, 1996.
9. Twycross R, Lichter I: The terminal phase. In Doyle D, Hanks GWC, MacDonald N, editors: *Oxford textbook of palliative medicine*, ed 2, New York, 1998, Oxford University Press, pp 977–992.
10. Bruera E, Fainsinger R: Clinical management of cachexia and anorexia. In Doyle D, Hanks GWC, MacDonald N, editors: *Oxford textbook of palliative medicine*, ed 2, New York, 1998, Oxford University Press, pp 548–557.
11. Ahronheim JC, Gasner MR: The sloganism of starvation, *Lancet* 335:278–279, 1990.
12. McCann RM, Hall WJ, Groth-Juncker A: Comfort care for terminally ill patients. The appropriate use of nutrition and hydration, *JAMA* 272:1263–1266, 1994.
13. Billings JA: Comfort measures for the terminally ill. Is dehydration painful? *J Am Geriatr Soc* 33:808–810, 1985.
14. Ellershaw JE, Sutcliffe JM, Saunders CM: Dehydration and the dying patient, *J Pain Symptom Manage* 10:192–197, 1995.

15. Musgrave CF: Terminal dehydration. To give or not to give intravenous fluids? *Cancer Nurs* 13:62–66, 1990.
16. Musgrave CF, Bartal N, Opstad J: The sensation of thirst in dying patients receiving IV hydration, *J Palliat Care* 11:17–21, 1995.
17. Morita T, Tei Y, Tsunoda J, et al: Determinants of the sensation of thirst in terminally ill cancer patients, *Support Care Cancer* 9:177–186, 2001.
18. Bruera E, Sala R, Rico MA, et al: Effects of parenteral hydration in terminally ill cancer patients: a preliminary study, *J Clin Oncol* 23:2366–2371, 2005.
19. Freemon FR: Delirium and organic psychosis. In *Organic mental disease*, Jamaica, NY, 1981, SP Medical and Scientific Books, pp 81–94.
20. Warden V, Hurley AC, Volicer L: Development and psychometric evaluation of the Pain Assessment in Advanced Dementia (PAINAD) scale, *J Am Med Dir Assoc* 4(1):9–15, 2003.
21. Twycross R, Lichter I: The terminal phase. In Doyle D, Hanks GWC, MacDonald N, editors: *Oxford textbook of palliative medicine*, ed 2. Oxford, UK, 1998, Oxford University Press, pp 985–986.
22. Thomas JR, von Gunten CF: Management of dyspnea, *J Support Oncol* 1(1):23–32, 2003. Discussion 32–34.
23. Booth S, Kelly MJ, Cox NP, et al: Does oxygen help dyspnea in patients with cancer? *Am J Respir Crit Care Med* 153(5):1515–1518, 1996.
24. Walsh D: Dyspnoea in advanced cancer, *Lancet* 342:450–451, 1993.
25. Sykes N, Thorns A: The use of opioids and sedative at the end of life, *Lancet Oncol* 4:312–318, 2003.
26. Wildiers H, Menten J: Death rattle: prevalence, prevention and treatment, *J Pain Symptom Manage* 23:310–317, 2002.
27. Bennett M, Lucas V, Brennan M, et al: Using anti-muscarinic drugs in the management of death rattle: evidence-based guidelines for palliative care, *Palliat Med* 16:369–374, 2002.
28. Twycross RB, Lack SA: *Therapeutics in terminal cancer*, ed 2, Philadelphia, 1990, Churchill Livingstone, pp 134–136.
29. Bennett M, Lucas V, Brennan M, et al: Using anti-muscarinic drugs in the management of death rattle: evidence-based guidelines for palliative care, *Palliat Med* 16:369–374, 2002.
30. Twycross R, Lichter I: The terminal phase. In Doyle D, Hanks GWC, MacDonald N, editors: *Oxford textbook of palliative medicine*, ed 2, Oxford, UK, 1998, Oxford University Press, pp 987–988.
31. Bottomley DM, Hanks GW: Subcutaneous midazolam infusion in palliative care, *J Pain Symptom Manage* 5(4):259–261, 1990.
32. Ramani S, Karnad AB: Long-term subcutaneous infusion of midazolam for refractory delirium in terminal breast cancer, *South Med J* 89(11):1101–1103, 1996.
33. McIver B, Walsh D, Nelson K: The use of chlorpromazine for symptom control in dying cancer patients, *J Pain Symptom Manage* 9:341–345, 1994.
34. Kehl KA: Treatment of terminal restlessness: a review of the evidence, *J Pain Palliat Care Pharmacother* 18(1):5–30, 2004.
35. Truog RD, Berde CB, Mitchell C, et al: Barbiturates in the care of the terminally ill, *N Engl J Med* 337:1678–1681, 1992.
36. Moyle J: The use of propofol in palliative medicine, *J Pain Symptom Manage* 10:643–646, 1995.
37. Stirling LC, Kurowska A, Tookman A: The use of phenobarbitone in the management of agitation and seizures at the end of life, *J Pain Symptom Manage* 17(5):363–368, 1999.
38. Pereira J, Phan T: Management of bleeding in patients with advanced cancer, *Oncologist* 9(5):561–570, 2004.
39. Tsavaris N, Zinelis A, Karabellis A, et al: A randomised trial of the effect of three non-steroid anti-inflammatory agents in ameliorating cancer-induced fever, *J Int Med* 228:451–455, 1990.
40. Axelrod P: External cooling in the management of fever, *Clin Infect Dis* 31(Suppl 5):S224–S229, 2000.
41. Sheldon F: Communication. In Saunders C, Sykes N, editors: *The management of terminal malignant disease*, Boston, 1993, Edward Arnold, pp 29–31.
42. The Hospice Institute of the Florida Suncoast: *Care at the time of death. Hospice training program*, Largo, Fla, 1996, The Hospice Institute of the Florida Suncoast.
43. Doyle D: Domiciliary palliative care. In Doyle D, Hanks GWC, MacDonald N, editors: *Oxford textbook of palliative medicine*, ed 2, Oxford, UK, 1998, Oxford University Press, pp 957–973.
44. Physician's Handbook on Medical Certification of Death. Hyattsville, Md, Department of Health and Human Services, 2003.
45. Weber M, Ochsmann R, Huber C: Laying out and viewing the body at home: a forgotten tradition? *J Pall Care* 14:34–37, 1998.

CHAPTER 24

Legal and Ethical Issues in the United States

ARTHUR R. DERSE

As the field of palliative care has grown and evolved, so also has an evolution occurred in the ethical and legal issues that are associated with care at the end of life. A consensus has developed concerning the ability of patients to refuse life-sustaining medical treatment, the importance of patient informed consent, and autonomous choice. Although other ethical and legal issues such as physician-assisted suicide and futility have a preponderance of opinion in professional guidelines, there is no such clear consensus. This chapter discusses current ethical and legal issues for palliative care in the United States and highlights some pearls and pitfalls.

Ethics, Law, and End-of-life Care

Palliative medicine in the United States, with its emphasis on end-of-life care, has long been inextricably intertwined with difficult ethical issues and consequent legal concerns.[1] As technologic advances have extended the ability to prolong life (and to prolong the dying process), ethical and legal questions have arisen about the appropriate implementation or discontinuation of those technological interventions. Some U.S. legal cases that deal with ethical issues at the end of life have had a major impact on the law of medical practice, although the legal precedents generally follow medical ethical principles.

Major ethical and legal issues for end-of-life care include the issues of informed consent and refusal; limitation of treatment, including withholding and withdrawing life-sustaining medical treatment; the determination of a patient's decision-making capacity; and the way in which decisions should be made if the patient does not have decision-making capacity. Other ethical and legal issues include the use of advance directives, the proper use of opioids in end-of-life care, a patient's voluntary refusal of orally ingested nutrition and hydration, physician-assisted suicide, and palliative sedation.

Informed Consent

A basic tenet of Anglo-American law is the principle of *informed consent*. This doctrine is based on patient self-determination as well as the right of the patient to receive information that is material to making a decision to consent to a medical treatment or procedure. The principle of informed consent is based on a physician's duty to tell the truth about the patient's current medical condition and prognosis. In the past century, it was common to not tell patients who were diagnosed with a terminal condition about their diagnosis, but a sea change occurred when many inside and outside the profession recognized that it was essential for the physician to disclose the diagnosis and prognosis to the patient.

The patient needed to be told the truth not only about the diagnosis and prognosis but also about the proposed procedure or treatment, the risks associated with that treatment, the benefits of the treatment, and the alternatives to that treatment, including the alternative of no treatment (Salgo, Cal.App. 1957). Additionally, if patients refused treatment, they were also entitled to information about the consequences of that refusal (known as *informed refusal*) (Truman, Cal. 1980).

Often in end-of-life care, information that would normally be disclosed was forgone based on the assumption that it was lifesaving treatment, and, therefore, patients need not consent to that treatment. However, even life-sustaining medical treatment requires informed consent (Anderson, Ohio 1996), unless it is an emergency and the patient is no longer decisional and no legally authorized decision maker is available.[2] Informed consent for end-of-life care should include not only the benefits of treatment but also the burdens or risks of treatment that the patient will have to bear, as well as the prognosis of the disease (if known) both with and without treatment.

Before life-sustaining medical treatment is begun, the patient and family should understand that the burdens of treatment may become so great that they may outweigh the prospective benefits of treatment. Additionally, the patient should be told that physicians may limit or stop treatment if it is no longer effective. A timely discussion with the patient and family that leads to an understanding of treatment possibilities and limitations may preclude later, painful discussions of "futile" treatment. If treatment is not successful, then further discussion about stopping treatment may not surprise the patient or family. It also gives the patient and family an opportunity to discuss with physicians, long before a crisis occurs, the fact that there may come a time when treatment may no longer be of benefit to the patient and thus will not be indicated.

When palliative and end-of-life care are among reasonable alternative treatments for a patient's condition, informed consent may require that the patient be informed of these options. For instance, California statutory law requires that when a health care provider makes a diagnosis that a patient has a terminal illness, the health care provider shall, upon the patient's request, provide the patient with comprehensive information and counseling regarding legal end-of-life care options pursuant to this section (Cal. 2008).

Limitation of Treatment

In the United States, a legal and ethical consensus for limitation of treatment developed[3] between the time the first state court considered the issue of withdrawing life-sustaining medical treatment (Quinlan, N.J. 1976) and the time of the U.S. Supreme Court's determination of the same issue 14 years later (Cruzan, U.S. 1990).[4]

The consensus holds that patients have the right to refuse any intervention, including life-sustaining medical interventions. A series of state Supreme Court decisions determined that patients have the right to refuse medical treatments that include ventilators (Bartling, Cal.App. 1984), administered nutrition and hydration (Bouvia, Cal.App. 1986), and blood transfusions (Wons, Fla.App. 1987). Another tenet of this consensus is that all patients—even incapacitated patients—have the right to refuse any medical intervention.

The U.S. Supreme Court confirmed this principle in the Cruzan case (U.S. 1990), holding that patients have a liberty interest under the Constitution's 14th Amendment due process guarantee to refuse life-sustaining medical treatment, although states may require clear and convincing evidence of the patient's wishes if the patient is incapacitated. Another important principle of the ethical and legal consensus is that withholding and withdrawal of life-sustaining medical treatment are essentially equivalent and are not homicide or suicide (Barber, Cal.App. 1983) and that orders to do so are valid (Dinnerstein, Mass.App. 1978). An additional important principle of this consensus is that courts need not be routinely involved in end-of-life care decisions.

Decision Making for the Incapacitated

Because many patients for whom life-sustaining medical treatment decisions must be made have lost decision-making capacity, ethically and legally there is a consensus as to decision making for those who are incapacitated and unable to make their own decisions. If the incapacitated patient left directions in advance regarding his or her wishes (through either a living will or a power of attorney for health care document), those wishes should be followed. If no written directives were made but the patient's wishes are known, a guardian, health care agent, or designated surrogate may make decisions on the basis of what the patient would have wanted, a process called *substituted judgment*. If the patient's wishes are unknown, the decision maker must use the *best interest standard*—that is, consider what is best for the patient.

In the Terri Schiavo case (Schiavo, Fla.Ct.App. 2001, Fla. 2004), the spouse and parents of an incapacitated patient in a persistent vegetative state battled over whether life-sustaining medical treatment in the form of artificial nutrition and hydration could be withdrawn. This case encompassed many ethical and legal issues. As contentious as this case was, however, certain principles were reinforced: Patients have the right to refuse life-sustaining medical treatment, even if incapacitated; and if a patient has expressed those wishes clearly, then a guardian may act according to those wishes. The Schiavo case also reinforced the principle that artificial nutrition and hydration are considered medical treatments and may be legally and ethically withdrawn under appropriate circumstances. Nonetheless, it is important to recognize that some disagreement exists among religious communities as to whether it is ethical to remove artificial nutrition and hydration from an incapacitated patient in a persistent vegetative state. The Schiavo case also demonstrated that family members may disagree about who should serve as guardian or surrogate for the patient.

Determination of Decision-Making Capacity

Patients who have decision-making capacity have the right to refuse life-sustaining medical treatment. Thus, when a patient refuses such treatment, the determination of decision-making capacity is crucial.[5] *Decision-making capacity* has been defined as the ability to make decisions about medical care, and it can be contrasted with competence. The term *competence* is commonly used to indicate the ability to do something, but in the medical milieu it is more commonly used synonymously with *legal competence*—that is, the determination by a court as to the ability to make decisions about one's person or property. Not all patients who have lost the ability to make medical decisions will have been declared legally incompetent, nor will patients who have been declared legally incompetent necessarily be unable to make any decisions with respect to medical care.

Decision-making capacity is constituted by the ability to understand information, reason and deliberate about a choice, make a choice consistent with values and goals, communicate the choice, and maintain stability of that choice over time.[3] Although it has been noted wryly that questions of patient decision-making capacity typically arise only when the patient chooses a course other than the one the health care professional finds most reasonable,[4] this is, in fact, not so ironic. Health care professionals generally make a treatment recommendation that is in the best interest of patients, and when patients agree with this course of action, there is generally less concern about the patient's decision-making capacity. Thus, questions of decision-making ability arise when the patient chooses to refuse beneficial medical treatment.

Decision-making capacity is dependent on the individual abilities of the patient, the requirements of the task at hand, and the consequences of the decision. When the consequences of the decision are substantial, there is a greater need for certainty of the patient's decision-making capacity. Decision-making capacity is not necessarily established by simply expressing a preference, having the content of the patient's decision fit an "objectively correct" standard, or acting in accord with the physician's recommendation.[6] Some patients (e.g., the comatose) are clearly incapacitated, whereas decision-making capacity may be more difficult to determine in others (e.g., those in the early stages of dementia).[7]

Advance Directives

Advance directives are written expressions of medical decisions that are made by the patient while he or she is still capable of making those decisions. A *living will* is a directive to a physician when the patient is nondecisional and has a terminal condition (including, in some jurisdictions, persistent vegetative state) in which the patient refuses life-sustaining medical treatment. A *power of attorney for health care* is the appointment of an agent to represent the patient when the patient is no longer decisional. It applies during any incapacity and is often written with directions to the agent about the patient's treatment preferences, including preferences about nutrition and hydration.

Advance directives are appropriate planning tools for end-of-life decision making. However, only a minority of patients actually complete an advance directive, although the proportion is higher for patients facing the end of life. Additionally, studies show that proxy decision makers are often poor predictors of the patient's wishes.[8] There is also a current controversy about whether completion of advance directives significantly guides the course of patient care.[9] Nonetheless, failure to engage in advanced care planning is worse, and advance directives may be more effective when they are part of a larger advanced care planning regimen in which the patient expresses wishes about end-of-life care to family members.[10]

Advance directives are even more important in light of recent legal developments. In determining whether the guardian or surrogate may withdraw or withhold life-sustaining medical treatment of a patient who is no longer decisional, some state courts have required clear and convincing evidence of the incapacitated patient's wishes. This requirement results, in part, from legislative concerns about withdrawal of life-sustaining medical treatment without the patient's explicit consent, as well as the courts' concern that the consequences of decisions to withdraw life-sustaining medical treatment are, for the most part, ultimately irreversible.

Advance directives may satisfy legal requirements for clear and convincing evidence of the patient's wishes for withdrawal of life-sustaining treatment. The use of advance directives will allay legal concerns and may ensure that the patient's wishes are implemented.

Guardianship and Surrogates

Patients who are not able to make decisions about their medical treatment may already have a guardianship in place. *Guardianship* (known in some jurisdictions as *conservatorship*) is a legal mechanism that allows the appointment of a person who will make decisions for the patient as they relate to the patient and his or her property. Although guardians have power to make decisions, including health care decisions, they generally do not have the information about patients' preferences that a person who has been specifically appointed power of attorney for health care would have. Guardians are charged with acting in the best interest of the patient or, when possible, acting in the adult patient's substituted judgment when the patient's wishes are known. Additionally, parents are generally guardians of their child's best interest until the child reaches the age of majority or maturity. When the incapacitated patient does not have an advance directive, some states have an automatic hierarchy of surrogates or decision makers for incapacitated patients, including spouses, adult children, parents, and other relationships of significance (e.g., Ill. 1991).

Refusal of Orally Ingested Nutrition and Hydration

Patients have the right to refuse life-sustaining medical treatment; at the end of life, that ability to refuse treatment encompasses the patient's refusal of orally ingested nutrition and hydration. In the dying process, ketonemia causes the patient to have a lack of appetite. Oral discomfort (e.g., dryness of the mouth) can be alleviated with ice chips. To decline orally ingested nutrition and hydration, patients must have the decision-making capacity to make this choice and should also complete an advance directive that indicates their continued wish to refuse artificial nutrition and hydration so their wishes will still be honored after their decision-making capacity is lost.[11]

Opioids in End-of-Life Care

In the past, physicians reported that although they used opioids appropriately in end-of-life care by their own evaluation, nonetheless, medical examining boards could reprimand them for repeatedly prescribing narcotics to an individual patient, even if that patient was facing the end of life. There have, however, been significant changes in medical examining board policies. The Federation of State Medical Boards' model guidelines on the appropriate use of narcotics at the end of life[12] recognize that neither the amount nor the chronicity of opioid prescription for patients at end of life should automatically serve as an indication of inappropriate use of narcotics. In general, physicians have enjoyed a wide berth from medical examining boards that realize that patients at the end of life need appropriate opioid treatment.[13]

The current trend involves cases in which physicians who did not provide appropriate pain medication were found to be in violation of medical examining board regulations[14] or were found liable for malpractice (Bergman, Cal.Sup.Ct. 2001). The Federal Drug Enforcement Administration stated, "It is crucial that physicians who are engaged in legitimate pain treatment not be discouraged from providing proper medication to patients as medically justified. ... The longstanding requirement ... that physicians may prescribe controlled substances only for legitimate medical purposes in the usual course of professional practice should in no way ... cause any physician to be reluctant to provide legitimate pain relief".[12] Most cases dealing with inappropriate narcotic prescriptions have involved treatment of patients with chronic pain rather than treatment of patients who were facing the end of life. Despite physicians' fears about the possibility of criminal liability for appropriate end-of-life treatment, millions of patients are treated at the end of life each year, but in only a very few cases have physicians been charged and prosecuted for intentional homicide during treatment at the end of life, and in those cases almost uniformly the prosecution is dropped, physicians are acquitted, or a conviction is reversed. In one extremely rare case, a physician was convicted, and that conviction was upheld on appeal. Those rare cases often involve troubling aspects of care in which the claimed appropriate medical treatment was difficult to defend.[15] The U.S. Supreme Court recognized the principle of double effect: If the physician does not intend the patient's death but the patient's death comes as an unintended side effect of appropriate treatment, the physician should not be liable for intentionally causing the death of the patient.[16] Thus, physicians should continue to treat patients at the end of life with appropriate amounts of medications despite the possibility of an unintended side effect of hastened death.

Physician-Assisted Suicide

Although there was a movement to recognize legally that patients facing a terminal condition should be able to end their lives of their own voluntary accord, the U.S. Supreme Court found no constitutional right to physician-assisted suicide in the United States under either the due process or the equal protection provision of the 14th Amendment (Glucksberg, U.S. 1997; Vacco, U.S. 1997). However, the Court did recognize that the states were free to develop laws on physician-assisted suicide, and Oregon is the prime example of the few states in the United States that allow physician-assisted suicide under certain conditions.

The Oregon statute that was passed by referendum in 1994 and reaffirmed in 1997 allows a patient who is facing a terminal illness to ask a physician to write a prescription for a lethal dose of medication if that patient is both decisional and a resident of Oregon. The patient needs to make two separate requests 15 days apart, and the prescription may not be filled until 48 hours after being presented to a pharmacist (Ore. 1995). Legal challenges to the Oregon law have failed (Gonzalez, U.S. 2006). The Oregon experience shows that small numbers of end-of-life patients avail themselves of this option each year. The patients who choose this option tend to be those who are concerned about self-determination, self-control, and being a burden on others. Only a few of these patients are primarily concerned with unrelieved pain.[17] Washington state voters in 2008 passed a referendum similar to the Oregon statute legalizing physician-assisted suicide, and the Washington statute went into effect in March 2009.[18] In 2009, Montana's Supreme Court found no statutory or public policy basis for prohibition of physician-assisted suicide, effectively permitting the procedure (Baxter, Mont. 2009). In all other states in the United States, physician-assisted suicide is prohibited by either statute or common law.

Futility

One of the more contentious issues in medical ethics at the end of life is whether and under what circumstances physicians may determine that, despite the demand from patients and families that physicians "do everything," further treatment would lack benefit and would prolong the dying process. The American Medical Association's Code of Ethics states that providers are under no obligation to provide futile treatment.[19] Some hospitals and health systems have established policies to define and resolve these situations. Methods to resolve these difficult problems include identifying the goals of treatment and determining whether there is an objective benefit to the patient if medical treatment continues, obtaining a second opinion, considering ethics consultation, and offering transfer of care to another provider. Ultimately, if no willing provider is found, there is no obligation to provide nonbeneficial treatment.

Some hospitals have policies that address the issue of futility that may be applied when physicians determine that continued treatment would no longer be beneficial.[20] Texas has codified its approach to resolution of this vexing issue through a process that includes determination by an ethics committee, review by a court, and an opportunity for a patient and family to find other willing practitioners (Tex. 2002). The Texas experience has shown that physicians may appropriately determine futility within a legal and ethical framework.[21] The case law concerning the issues of futility varies depending on the facts of case and jurisdiction. Unilateral determinations of futility by physicians should be rare.

Palliative Sedation

A trial of palliative sedation is an option for end-of-life patients who have intractable pain or suffering if all other methods to relieve the suffering have been unsuccessful. In palliative sedation, the patient is sedated to the point of unconsciousness for palliative relief. An intermediate step is a trial of palliative sedation in which the patient is sedated to unconsciousness and, after a certain period, is reawakened to determine whether the pain or suffering has been alleviated. If not, the patient is sedated again.

Because the patient is not eating or drinking during this period, death would be caused by either the underlying disease or a known but unintended side effect of the treatment regimen.[22] Critics of the practice are concerned that the use of palliative sedation for so-called existential suffering would allow this practice to move toward euthanasia. Some health care systems have developed guidelines to ensure that palliative sedation is used for intractable and measurable pain.[23] An appellate level court in the United States has not yet made a full legal consideration of the issues of palliative sedation. Many ethical and legal commentators find this practice an acceptable alternative to physician-assisted suicide and argue that without this treatment there would be more pressure to allow physician-assisted suicide.

PEARLS AND PITFALLS

- All patients should be informed of the benefits and risks (burdens) of life-sustaining medical treatment. They should also be informed that treatment will be discontinued if it is no longer effective.
- Patients have the right to refuse life-sustaining medical treatment. The patient's right to refuse life-sustaining medical treatment may be asserted by a guardian, an agent of a power of attorney for health care, or a surrogate.
- Advance directives, used in a context of advanced care planning, are legally valid documents in which patient preferences concerning end-of-life care may be described.
- Opioids should be administered appropriately to patients at the end of life.
- Physician-assisted suicide is prohibited in almost all U.S. states; exceptions are Oregon, Washington, and Montana.
- Issues of futility may be resolved through a due process approach.
- The ethical and legal issues of palliative sedation should be carefully considered.

Summary

Patients who are facing the end of life should have informed consent regarding life-sustaining medical treatments. Patients may refuse all medical treatments, including artificial nutrition and hydration. Because many patients are unable to speak for themselves at the time that end-of-life choices must be made, advance directives (legal documentation of directions in advance of incapacity) have been created. For those patients without advance directives, physicians and surrogates should make choices on the basis of the patient's substituted judgment or best interest. Opioids should be administered appropriately to relieve suffering at the end of life. Other difficult ethical and legal issues include situations in which medical treatments are not indicated despite patient or surrogate demand and the practices of physician-assisted suicide and palliative sedation. These situations can, nonetheless, be guided by professional standards and legal precedent.

References

1. Derse AR: Legal issues in end-of-life care. In Emanuel LL, von Gunten CF, Ferris FD, Hauser JM, editors: *The Education in Palliative and End-of-life Care (EPEC) Curriculum: The EPEC Project*, Evanston, Ill, 2003, Northwestern University Feinberg School of Medicine.
2. Defenses to intentional interference with person or property. In Keeton WP, Dobbs DB, Keeton RE, Owen DG, editors: *Prosser and Keeton Oo Torts*, ed 5, St. Paul, Minn, 1984, West Publishing Company, pp 117–118.
3. Junkerman C, Derse A, Schiedermayer D: Competence and decision making capacity. In *Practical ethics for students, interns, and residents: a short reference manual*, ed 3, Frederick, Md, 2008, University Publishing Group, pp 20–23.
4. Roth LH, Meisel A, Lidz CW: Tests of competency to consent to treatment, *Am J Psychiatry* 134: 279–284, 1977.
5. Derse AR: Decision-making capacity. In Berger AM, Portenoy RK, Weissman DE, editors: *Principles and practice of palliative medicine*, ed 2, Philadelphia, 2002, Lippincott Williams & Wilkins.
6. President's Commission for the Study of Ethical Problems in Medicine and Biomedical and Behavioral Research: *Making Health Care Decisions*, vol. 1. Washington, DC, 1992, U.S. Government Printing Office, pp 55–68.
7. Derse AR: Making decisions about life-sustaining medical treatment in patients with dementia: the problem of decision making capacity, *Theoret Med* 20:55–67, 1999.
8. Sulmasy DP, Terry PB, Weisman CS, et al: The accuracy of substituted judgments in patients with terminal diagnoses, *Ann Intern Med* 128:621–629, 1998.
9. Teno JM, Lynn J, Wegner N, et al: Advance directives for seriously ill hospitalized patients: effectiveness with the Patient Self-Determination Act and the SUPPORT intervention, *J Am Geriatr Soc* 45:500–507, 1997.
10. Hammes BJ, Rooney BL: Death and end-of-life planning in one Midwestern community, *Arch Intern Med* 158:383–390, 1998.
11. Quill TE, Lo B, Brock DW: Palliative options of last resort: a comparison of voluntarily stopping eating and drinking, terminal sedation, physician assisted suicide, and voluntary active euthanasia, *JAMA* 278:2099–2104, 1997.
12. Dispensing of controlled substances for the treatment of pain, *Fed Reg* 69:67170–67171, 2004. Policy statement: dispensing of controlled substances for the treatment of pain, *Fed Reg* 71:52715–52723, 2006.
13. Ziegler SJ, Lovrich NP: Pain relief, prescription drugs, and prosecution: a four-state survey of chief prosecutors, *J Law Med Ethics* 31:75–100, 2003.
14. Charatan F: Doctor disciplined for "grossly undertreating" pain, *Br Med J* 319:728, 1999.
15. Alpers A: Criminal act or palliative care? Prosecutions involving the care of the dying, *J Law Med Ethics* 26:308–331, 1998.
16. Sulmasy DP, Pellegrino ED: The rule of double effect: clearing up the double talk, *Arch Intern Med* 159:545–550, 1999.
17. Oregon Department of Human Services: *Characteristics and end-of-life care of 401 DWDA patients who died after ingesting a lethal dose of medication, by year, Oregon*, Portland, Ore, 2006, Oregon Department of Human Services. pp 1998–2008. Available at http://egov.oregon.gov/DHS/ph/pas/ar-index.shtml. Accessed December 4, 2009.
18. Steinbrook R: Physician-assisted death. From Oregon to Washington state, *N Eng J Med* 359:2513–2515, 2008.
19. Council on Ethical and Judicial Affairs 2006–2007: *Medical Futility in End-of-Life Care. Opinion 2.037. Code of Medical Ethics: Current Opinions with Annotations*, Chicago, 2006, American Medical Association.
20. Furrow BR, Greaney TL, Johnson SH, et al: *Health law: cases, materials and problems*, ed 6, St. Paul, MN, 2008, Thomson West Publishing, pp 1518.
21. Fine RL, Mayo TW: Resolution of futility by due process: early experience with the Texas Advance Directives Act, *Ann Intern Med* 138:743–746, 2003.
22. Lo B, Rubenfeld G: Palliative sedation: "We turn to it when everything else hasn't worked," *JAMA* 294:1810–1816, 2005.
23. Quill TE, Lo B, Brock DW, Meisel A: Last-resort options for palliative sedation, *Ann Intern Med* 151:421–424, 2009.

Cases and Statutes

Anderson 1996: Anderson v. St. Francis–St. George Hospital, Inc (1996), 77 Ohio St. 3d 82w

Barber 1983: Barber v. Superior Court 147 Cal.App.3d 1006, 195 Cal.Rptr. 484 (Cal.Ct.App., 2nd Dist 1983)

Bartling 1984: Bartling v. Superior Court, 163 Cal.App.3d 186, 209 Cal.Rptr. 220 (1984)

Baxter 2009: Baxter v. State, 2009 MT 449 (Mont. 2009).

Bergman 2001: Bergman v. Chin, No. H205732–1, Superior Court of Cal., County of Alameda, Southern Div. (Complaint filed Feb. 16, 1999; jury verdict rendered June 13, 2001)

Bouvia 1986: Bouvia v. Superior Court, 179 Cal.App3d 1127, 225 Cal.Rptr. 297 (1986)

Cal. 2008: Cal. HSC Code §442.5(2008)

Cruzan 1990: Cruzan v. Director of Missouri Department of Health, 109 S.Ct 3240 (1990)

Dinnerstein 1978: In re Dinnerstein, 6 Mass.App.Ct. 466, 380 N.E.2d 134 (1978)

Gonzalez 2006: Gonzalez v. Oregon, 126 S.Ct. 94 (2006)

Illinois Health Care Surrogate 1991: Illinois Health Care Surrogate Act (Illinois Pub. Act 87–749, HB 2334, 87th Gen. Assembly, 91st Sess., 1991)

Ore. Rev. Stat. 1995: Ore. Rev. Stat. §127.800–127.995 (1995)

Quinlan 1976: In re Quinlan, 70 N.J. 10, 355 A.2d 647, cert. denied 429 U.S. 922, 97 S.Ct. 319, 50 L.Ed.2d 289 (1976)

Salgo 1957: Salgo v. Leland Stanford, Jr. University Board of Trustees, 152 Cal.App.2d 560, 317 P.2d 170 (1957)

Schiavo 2001: Guardianship of Schiavo, 780 So.2d 176 (Fla.Ct.App. 2nd Dist. 2001)

Schiavo 2004: Bush v. Schiavo, Case No. SC04–925 (Fla. 2004)

Tex. Health 2002: Tex. Health and Safety Code §166.046(a) (Vernon Supp. 2002)

Truman 1980: Truman v. Thomas, 27 Cal.3d 285, 611 P.2d 902, 165 Cal.Rptr. 308 (1980)

Vacco 1997: Vacco v. Quill, 521 U.S. 793, 117 S.Ct. 2293, 138 L.Ed.2d 834 (1997)

Washington v. Glucksberg 1997: Washington v. Glucksberg, 521 U.S. 702, 117 S.Ct. 2258, 138 L.Ed.2d 772 (1997)

Wons 1987: Wons v. Public Health Trust of Dade County, 500 So.2d 679 (Fla.App. 3 Dist. 1987)

Specific Types of Illness and Sites of Care

CHAPTER 25

Hematology/Oncology

TOBY C. CAMPBELL and JAMIE H. VON ROENN

Cancer survivors and their families face myriad challenges related to their disease and its treatment. This life-changing journey begins the moment they hear "cancer." Palliative care of the oncology patient involves the assessment and treatment of the multidimensional experience of cancer: the physical, emotional, and spiritual. Although each of these elements is important in the total care of patients, this chapter focuses on the physical manifestations of advanced disease and specific approaches to supportive care of the oncology patient. We present a practical approach to the presentation, evaluation, and supportive management of several common oncologic problems: brain, liver, and bone metastases; bowel obstruction; and malignant effusions.

Approach to Brain Metastases

INCIDENCE

Brain metastasis, a common complication of systemic cancer, is present in 98,000 to 170,000 new patients each year, approximately 30% of all patients with malignancy.[1] The frequency may be rising because of the use of more sensitive detection techniques and the prolonged survival of patients with metastatic disease from common malignant tumors. Most recently reported in a large population study, the incidence percentage for patients with primary lung (19.9%), melanoma (6.9%), renal (6.5%), breast (5.1%), and colorectal (1.8%) cancers account for the majority of individuals with brain metastases.[2] The prognosis is dependent on several factors: brain as the only site of metastasis, performance status, age, primary lesion (controlled versus uncontrolled), and number of lesions (single vs. multiple).[3]

PRESENTATION

Brain metastases may manifest with the rapid onset of symptoms or with subacute but progressive neurologic dysfunction. Common presenting symptoms include headache (49%), a focal neurologic deficit (30%), cognitive disturbance (32%), ataxia (21%) seizures (18%), dysarthria (12%), visual disturbances (6%), sensory disturbance (6%), and limb ataxia (6%).[1]

EVALUATION

Imaging studies are recommended for any patient with a history of cancer and new neurologic symptoms. Both contrast-enhanced computed tomography (CT) and magnetic resonance imaging (MRI) are appropriate evaluation tools, although gadolinium-enhanced magnetic resonance imaging is more sensitive and specific for the detection of central nervous system metastases. Of patients with enhancing metastatic lesions, approximately one third present with solitary lesions and two thirds present with multiple lesions. Metastatic lesions to the brain are commonly well circumscribed and associated with vasogenic edema. A biopsy is generally not necessary in patients with multiple metastatic lesions and known malignant disease, particularly if the primary tumor commonly metastasizes to the brain. If there is clinical uncertainty about the origin of brain lesions, a stereotactic biopsy can differentiate metastatic disease from a primary brain tumor or a nonmalignant cause, such as infection. A solitary brain metastasis in the setting of a patient with good performance status and otherwise well-controlled disease should be considered for resection. A biopsy should be considered in patients with acquired immunodeficiency syndrome, even when patients have multiple lesions, if *Toxoplasma* titers are negative, to differentiate cancer, particularly lymphoma, from infectious causes.

MANAGEMENT

Medical

The goal of medical therapy for patients with newly diagnosed symptomatic brain metastases is to control edema and to minimize symptoms while evaluating for more definitive therapeutic options. Treatment options include surgical resection, radiosurgery, whole-brain radiation therapy (WBRT), and medical therapy. Untreated, patients with multiple brain metastases have a median survival of approximately 1 month.[4] Corticosteroids reduce vasoedema and double the median survival to 2 months.[1] These agents are an important first step in the management of patients with brain metastases because nearly 70% of patients will experience significant relief of symptoms in the first 48 hours with corticosteroids.[5] Patients who do not improve in the first 2 days generally have a very limited life expectancy of days to weeks and face significant progressive neurologic disability. Although there is no evidence-based consensus on the optimal corticosteroid dose, dexamethasone at 16 to 24 mg/day in divided doses every 4 to 12 hours is a reasonable recommendation. Dexamethasone is the preferred corticosteroid because of its reduced mineralocorticoid effects and relatively long half-life. In patients with symptomatic brain lesions who are near the end of life, corticosteroids may be continued for the remainder of the patient's life or until he or she can no longer swallow.

Patients receiving high doses of corticosteroids experience several predictable acute side effects, including hyperglycemia, oral candidiasis, leukocytosis, and increased energy; subacute and chronic toxicity includes gastritis, central adiposity, and proximal myopathy. When steroid therapy is initiated, patients should simultaneously start prophylactic antifungal therapy, antacids, and regular blood glucose monitoring.

Interventional

Surgical resection of metastatic brain lesions is indicated for patients with a good performance status, a single lesion in a surgically accessible field, good neurologic function, and well-controlled systemic cancer.[6] Surgery should be followed by WBRT to reduce the risk of central nervous system recurrence. In a recent meta-analysis comparing surgery with surgery plus WBRT, survival was equivalent, but patients treated with combined-modality therapy tended to have greater improvement in function and a reduction in death from neurologic causes.[7]

For patients who are not surgical candidates or for those who present with multiple brain metastases, palliative WBRT is the standard of care. WBRT improves median survival over dexamethasone alone to 3 to 7 months. The best candidates for WBRT are younger than 65 years, with good performance status (KPS ≥70) and absent or controlled extra-cranial disease and have a median survival of 7.1 months.[3] WBRT may be administered as 10 to 15 fractions and is generally well tolerated. The most common side effects include fatigue, alopecia, and cognitive deficits, particularly problems with short-term memory.

Radiosurgery uses either γ-radiation or a linear accelerator to deliver a high dose of radiation to a defined target. It is a noninvasive alternative to surgery that can be administered quickly and can access regions of the brain not amenable to surgical resection. The median survival after radiosurgery appears to be equivalent to that after surgery, ranging from 7.4 to 12.9 months. Selection criteria for radiosurgery are similar to those for surgery: limited systemic disease, good performance status (Karnofsky Performance Scale [KPS] >70), and the presence of fewer than three metastatic lesions. Lesions amenable to radiosurgery should be well circumscribed, less than 4 cm, and without invasion deep into the brain tissue. Although single-institution studies are subject to significant selection bias, researchers have reported local control rates of 88% for patients treated with radiosurgery. Compared with WBRT alone, radiosurgery in combination with WBRT offers a survival advantage for patients with a single brain metastasis. In addition, patients with solitary metastasis treated with combined therapy were more likely to achieve a stable or improved KPS score than patients receiving WBRT alone.[8]

Approach to Liver Metastases

PRESENTATION

Patients with liver metastases may be asymptomatic or present with a range of abdominal or constitutional symptoms depending on the volume and location of disease in the liver. For many patients, liver metastases manifest with vague abdominal symptoms followed by increasing gastrointestinal and constitutional symptoms if left untreated. Liver metastases are routinely uncovered with routine surveillance imaging in patients with a history of cancer even before symptoms develop (e.g., lung cancer). Patients with extensive liver metastases may present with signs (ascites, jaundice, coagulopathy, encephalopathy) or symptoms (pain, fever, night sweats, early satiety, anorexia) of advanced liver disease. Liver metastases historically confer a poor prognosis, often less than a year. However, there is significant variability based on tumor type (e.g., colon vs. lung), treatment options, and comorbid disease.

EVALUATION

After a careful history and physical examination, evaluation includes imaging studies, typically a contrast-enhanced abdominal CT scan, to assess for the presence and extent of liver disease, biliary or hepatic obstruction, portal vein thrombosis, ascites, and peritoneal disease. Abdominal ultrasound is helpful in patients who cannot tolerate enhanced CT scan. Ultrasound can identify and characterize liver lesions and diagnose biliary obstruction but does not provide the same degree of diagnostic information as CT. Laboratory studies should include liver function tests, albumin, coagulation studies, chemistry profile, and complete blood cell count. If ascites is present, diagnostic paracentesis may be indicated to confirm the diagnosis or evaluate for infection with ascitic fluid analysis for cell count, culture, differential, albumen, and cytology.

MANAGEMENT

Medical

After a clear discussion of the goals of care, treatment may be directed at the tumor in concert with symptom management, or it may be focused on symptoms alone. Early satiety, pain, fever, sweats, anorexia, weight loss, pruritus, nausea, abdominal fullness, and confusion are all common symptoms attributable to bulky liver metastases.

Right upper quadrant pain or discomfort secondary to liver capsular stretch, distention, or bulky disease is common. Opioids are the mainstay of management for malignant pain. Even in patients with liver failure and impaired metabolism, opioids can be used safely and effectively when titrated to effect (see Chapter 7). Capsular distention is thought to produce pain, in part from a local inflammatory reaction, and corticosteroids are commonly used as adjuvant pain relievers. In addition, for patients with very advanced disease and multiple symptoms, corticosteroids may transiently ameliorate fatigue and nausea, stimulate appetite, reduce fever and sweats, and improve a patient's general sense of well-being. Evidence-based dosing recommendations are not available, although clinical experience suggests that modest doses of dexamethasone (6–10 mg/day) given orally or intravenously in the morning are often effective.

Fever and sweats associated with malignant liver disease are difficult to control. The treatment of choice is control of the cancer if possible. Palliative treatment options include antipyretics (nonsteroidal anti-inflammatory drugs, corticosteroids, and acetaminophen), sponging with cool water or an isopropyl alcohol solution, and hypothermic agents (chlorpromazine) that act by directly lower the core body temperature. Therapies for malignancy-associated sweats are not well studied, and reports of successful agents are largely anecdotal: low-dose thioridazine (10–30 mg), the H_2 receptor blocker cimetidine, and thalidomide (100 mg at bedtime) have been reported to improve sweats in patients with advanced cancer.[9,10]

Pruritus is a disruptive and troublesome symptom for patients. Pruritus secondary to liver disease is most often observed in the setting of obstructive jaundice; the severity of the pruritus, however, does not directly correlate with the degree of bilirubin elevation. Decompression or even partial decompression of the biliary tree, either through percutaneous or endoscopic approach, can provide significant and often permanent relief of the itching.

Interventional

Liver-directed treatment strategies now provide additional options for the treatment of liver metastases. Currently available liver-directed approaches include surgical resection, radiofrequency ablation (RFA), chemoembolization, cryotherapy, and brachytherapy with radiation-impregnated glass beads. The risks, benefits, and patient characteristics leading to a recommendation for one technique or another are highlighted in Table 25-1. In particular, patients with colorectal cancer and hepatic metastases, without evidence of other metastatic disease, have dramatically improved survival if their lesions are surgically resected (55%–80% survival at 1 year and 25%–50% at 5 years) compared with best supportive care (survival < 1 year).[11] Liver-directed therapies minimize systemic toxicity and spare most normal liver tissue. Patients with a good performance status (KPS > 70), fewer than four metastatic liver lesions, lesions 5 cm or smaller, and minimal systemic metastases are potential candidates for liver-directed therapy.

Approach to Bone Metastases

PRESENTATION

Patients with bone metastases commonly present with pain, usually localized to the site of the metastasis. The growth of malignant tumors creates pressure inside the bone and stimulates nociceptors sensitive to pressure. Locally active substances, such as prostaglandin E_2 and osteoclast-activating factor, are secreted, leading to necrosis. Malignant bone pain is classically insidious, with progressive severity over weeks to months. The pain is often described as a focal, constant, deep ache or boring pain without significant radiation. Patients occasionally present with the acute onset of moderate to severe pain after a pathologic fracture. Bone metastases can occur secondary to any solid tumor but are most common in patients with prostate, breast, and lung cancers. In an autopsy series, 85% of patients with these three malignant diseases have bone metastases at the time of death.[12]

EVALUATION

The initial evaluation of bone pain begins with a good pain history and physical examination focused on the sites of pain: Percussion over the bones often identifies areas of point tenderness, a red flag for the diagnosis of a metastatic bone lesion. Particular attention should be paid to patients with pain over a vertebral body because it could be a potential sign of vertebral involvement. Localized back pain is the most common presenting symptom of spinal cord compression and should be evaluated in an expedited fashion. Patients with extensive bone metastases may have myelophthisic anemia secondary to tumor infiltration of the bone marrow, characterized by a leukoerythroblastic peripheral blood smear, or elevated markers of bone turnover such as a high serum alkaline phosphatase.

The initial laboratory evaluation should include a chemistry profile with calcium level, complete blood cell count, and alkaline phosphatase. A clinical suspicion of bone metastases dictates an initial evaluation of the affected area by a plain film. Radiographs often identify a patient at risk for pathologic fracture. Lesions with an

Table 25-1. Liver-Directed Therapy

Modality	Technique	Patient Factors	Risks	Benefits
Surgical resection	Open or laparoscopic approach	Good performance status, able to tolerate major surgery, no other distant disease	Operative morbidity and mortality; post-procedure pain, prolonged recovery	Possibility for cure, best survival outcomes, complete resection
Radiofrequency ablation	Percutaneous friction heat ablation	Unresectable, fewer than 5 lesions, <4 cm in size, surrounded by liver parenchyma, >1 cm from vessels	Post-procedure pain, tract seeding of tumor	Outpatient procedure, no general anesthesia, improved 5-year survival rates for metastatic colon cancer
Cryotherapy	Cold temperature ablation, −190° C	Unresectable, fewer than 5 lesions, <4 cm in size, surrounded by liver parenchyma, >1 cm from vessels	Post-procedure pain, less effective than radiofrequency ablation	Modest survival benefit when combined with systemic therapy
Chemoembolization	Chemotherapy directed into the tumor blood supply	Unresectable primary liver tumors, better outcome with normal hepatic function pre-treatment	Post-procedure pain, fever, nausea, fatigue, acute hepatitis	Minimal systemic toxicity, prolonged survival
Therasphere	Radioactive glass beads	May have multiple liver lesions, fair hepatic reserve, no hepatopulmonary or gastroduodenal shunting	Acute liver toxicity or failure, gastritis or ulcers, pulmonary toxicity if hepatopulmonary shunting exists	Easily administered, minimal discomfort, effective, sparing of normal liver, survival similar to chemoembolization

axial cortical involvement greater than 30 mm indicate an increased risk for fracture, and prophylactic surgical stabilization followed by local radiation therapy should be considered for weight-bearing bones.[13] The most sensitive test to determine the extent of metastatic disease and to characterize (osteolytic or osteoblastic) the lesions is a radionuclide bone scan, although it does not visualize the lesions of multiple myeloma clearly. If a plain film is nondiagnostic, then a bone scan should be performed in most patients at high risk for bone metastases who are experiencing bone pain.

MANAGEMENT

Medical

The treatment of metastatic bone pain lesions is palliative, directed at the patient's tumor and presenting symptoms and the prevention of skeletal complications. Pain secondary to bone metastases is initially treated with medical therapy. First-line analgesic agents for mild skeletal pain include nonsteroidal anti-inflammatory drugs and acetaminophen. If pain control is inadequate, opioids are added to achieve optimal pain control. Antitumor therapy, directed either at the site of metastasis or systemically, may reduce pain and allow dose reductions or discontinuation of analgesics.

The medical management of malignant bone lesions has changed in the era of oral and intravenous bisphosphonates, a class of agents with a variety of actions, most importantly a multifaceted inhibition of osteoclast activity. These agents may improve pain control and delay skeletal complications of metastatic disease, but they do not affect survival. Zoledronic acid is often used because of its potency and ease of infusion (4 mg over 15 minutes). Bisphosphonates are generally well tolerated with unusual acute toxicities of flulike symptoms and bone pain. Patients on prolonged therapy should be monitored for a number of toxicities, including renal impairment, nephrotic syndrome, hypocalcemia, and osteonecrosis of the jaw (ONJ). Patients should be advised to identify and correct dental problems before beginning therapy and avoid dental procedures while receiving intravenous bisphosphonate therapy. A new approach to managing metastatic bone disease recently approved for use by the FDA is the fully humanized monoclonal antibody against RANK-L (Receptor Activator of Nuclear factor κ B ligand), Denosumab, which results in inhibition of osteoclast activity. The drug is administered by subcutaneous injection and was tested in three phase III trials treating over 5,500 patients with multiple myeloma, breast, and prostate cancers with metastatic bone disease. Denosumab proved to be statistically non-inferior to zoledronic acid in delaying the time to the first skeletal related event (SRE) while overall survival, disease progression, and adverse events were similar in the two arms including equal—though rare—risk for osteonecrosis of the jaw.[14-16] Because SREs influence morbidity and possibly mortality, delaying such events also appears to improve health related quality of life.[17]

Additional interventions for the treatment of bone metastases include systemic antineoplastic therapy, radiation therapy, RFA, and surgical fixation. Systemic chemotherapeutic options may exist for some patients with highly responsive cancers, such as breast cancer and testicular cancer. Patients with pathologic fractures of weight-bearing bones may benefit from surgical stabilization, whereas vertebral fractures may be stabilize with vertebroplasty or kyphoplasty.

Radiation

External-beam radiation therapy relieves pain, minimizes further tumor destruction, and prevents or delays pathologic fractures. Although most commonly delivered as multiple fractions, a single, higher-dose fraction (generally 800 Gy) reduces the treatment time necessary and minimizes the overall treatment burden for the patient. A meta-analysis (12 trials, 3508 patients) comparing single-fraction with multifraction radiation treatment of bone metastases demonstrated equivalent reduction in pain (60%), complete pain relief (34%), and toxicity. The necessity for repeated treatment, however, was higher for patients treated with a single-fraction versus multiple fractions, 21.5% versus 7.4%, respectively.[18] The choice of therapy depends on the goals of care and life expectancy.

RFA, an emerging technique for the treatment of bone metastases, introduces a high-frequency current into the tumor bed that induces frictional heating and necrosis. There is significant experience using this technique for the treatment of liver metastases, but data evaluating the effectiveness of RFA for reducing pain from bone metastases are limited. Goetz and colleagues, in a multicenter trial, treated 43 patients with painful osteolytic bone metastases with RFA. Eligible patients were without risk for pathologic fracture, and their lesions were not adjacent to large vessels or the spinal cord. Sustained pain relief was achieved in 95% of patients, with mean pain scores falling from 7.9 to 1.4 ($P < .0005$) over the 24 weeks following treatment.[19] Other small studies confirm these findings, but prospective, randomized data comparing radiation therapy and RFA for more durable outcomes of pain relief, mobility, and post-treatment pathologic fractures are not available.

Surgery

Surgical stabilization can relieve pain and preserve function in patients with unstable vertebral fractures and spinal cord compression and in those with or at risk for pathologic fracture of a weight-bearing or other long bone. Although there are no established criteria, surgical stabilization is generally considered in patients with good functional status (KPS >70), life expectancy longer than 3 to 6 months, and the ability to tolerate major surgery. Surgical risk depends on a variety of patient-related factors, including comorbid cardiopulmonary disease and relative difficulty of the surgical fixation. Prophylactic stabilization procedures are generally less invasive and better tolerated than fixation procedures after a fracture has already occurred. Surgery provides an opportunity to prevent fracture and to preserve ambulation, but it comes with significant potential morbidity and mortality.[20]

Vertebroplasty offers a nonsurgical approach to stabilize a vertebral fracture. The procedure is performed with the patient under conscious sedation with radiographic guidance. Cement is injected into the fractured vertebra to stabilize it, maintain column height, and prevent future nerve impingement. Although data are limited, case reports and a small case series suggest that vertebroplasty can reduce pain rapidly and is safe in conjunction with radiation therapy.[21] Vertebroplasty is contraindicated in patients with spinal cord compression or with a compression fracture with retropulsed fragments.

Radiopharmaceuticals are indicated for the treatment of multiple painful bone metastases in patients with predominantly osteoblastic metastases. These agents work by tracking to binding sites in the bone matrix at the tumor-bone interface and then delivering a therapeutic radiation dose to the local area (Table 25-2). Because these agents are administered systemically, they are appropriate only for patients with multiple painful lesions who are without other options for systemic antineoplastic agents. A Cochrane meta-analysis to evaluate the efficacy of radiopharmaceuticals for metastatic bone pain identified four trials (325 patients with prostate or breast

Table 25-2. Bone-Seeking Radiopharmaceuticals

Drug	Mechanism of Action	Indication	Contraindication
Strontium-89	Calcium homologue tracks to deposition of calcium	Similar for all agents: • Positive bone scan • Bone pain due to cancer • Multifocal disease	Similar for all agents: • Mainly soft-tissue disease • Unifocal bone lesion • Negative bone scan • Significant myelosuppression
Phosphorous-32 (rarely used)	Tracks inorganic phosphorous in the body		
Samarium-153 EDTMP	Phosphonic acid group on carrier molecule, EDTMP, carries agent to areas of newly deposited bone		

EDTMP, Ethylene diamine tetramethylene phosphonate.
Other agents include 186-rhenium, 188-rhenium, and radium-223, but these are not currently approved for use in the United States.

cancer) and demonstrated a small benefit from radioisotopes for the control of bone pain for 1 to 6 months after treatment, without improvement in survival or reduction in the incidence of spinal cord compression. These agents are associated with significant myelosuppression and cost.[22]

Approach to Bowel Obstruction

PRESENTATION

In the majority of patients, the diagnosis of malignant bowel obstruction can be made by history and physical examination. Abdominal distention, nausea, vomiting, crampy abdominal pain, and an absence of flatus and bowel movements are typical presenting symptoms. The colon may take as long as 12 to 24 hours to empty completely; thus, patients with small-bowel obstruction may continue to pass flatus and stool even after the obstruction occurs. The classic complaint is of periumbilical, paroxysmal, crampy abdominal pain. Obstruction should be differentiated from perforation: Peritonitis is suggested by symptoms of focal or diffuse abdominal pain, fever, hemodynamic instability, or peritoneal signs (severe pain with movement, firm abdomen, rebound tenderness, involuntary guarding).

The most common tumors causing malignant bowel obstruction are metastatic ovarian and colon cancers, although any patient with advanced cancer can develop an obstruction, particularly a patient with a history of multiple prior abdominal surgeries or abdominal radiation therapy. In as many as one third of patients, the cause of the obstruction is nonmalignant—that is, secondary to adhesions or other causes. Patients with advanced cancer and malignant bowel obstruction have a short life expectancy, generally measured in weeks.

EVALUATION

The physical examination in patients with obstruction is highly variable: Fever and tachycardia may be signs of a strangulating obstruction or perforation; auscultation may reveal high-pitched, tinkling, or hypoactive bowel sounds and is not generally diagnostic; oliguria and dry mucous membranes are signs of dehydration; tympany on abdominal percussion suggests dilated loops of bowel; rebound tenderness, guarding, pain with light percussion, and abdominal rigidity suggest peritonitis. A rectal examination often detects an empty vault but may demonstrate an obstructing rectal mass or blood.

Plain radiographs of the abdomen and an upright chest radiograph will detect free peritoneal air if perforation is present and the classic dilated loops of bowel with air-fluid levels when obstruction is the cause of the patient's symptoms. The presence of air in the colon or rectum makes a complete obstruction unlikely. In patients with malignant disease, an abdominal CT scan helps to define the extent of the underlying disease and may identify the site of the obstruction. An isolated point of obstruction is potentially reversible with surgical resection. Laboratory evaluation, including chemistry panel and complete blood cell count, will illuminate electrolyte imbalances, dehydration, anemia, acid-base disorders, or signs of secondary infection.

MANAGEMENT

Medical

The management goals for a patient with bowel obstruction in the setting of advanced cancer are to minimize bowel wall edema, to treat and prevent nausea and vomiting, to control pain, to decrease intestinal secretions, and to address end-of-life issues. The initial intervention for patients with a bowel obstruction is nasogastric tube drainage to prevent emesis and to relieve the nausea caused by gastric distention. Occasionally, obstructions remit spontaneously with conservative management: nothing-by-mouth, nasogastric suction, intravenous fluids, and analgesics. Intravenous corticosteroids may minimize bowel wall edema and may partially reverse an obstruction. A Cochrane meta-analysis evaluating dexamethasone, 6 to 16 mg/day, for the treatment of malignant bowel obstruction revealed a trend toward resolution of the obstruction with steroids but no survival advantage.[23]

Pain management is vital for patients with a malignant bowel obstruction. Opioid analgesics are recommended. Patients with a nonfunctioning intestinal tract rely on alternate routes of analgesic administration. Fentanyl transdermal patches, rectal administration of long-acting opioids, and subcutaneous or intravenous opioid administration provide predictable analgesic delivery in the absence of a functioning upper gastrointestinal tract.

Somatostatin analogues, such as octreotide, may provide significant relief of symptoms associated with small bowel obstruction and may be used as first-line therapy in patients who are not surgical candidates. Octreotide reduces gastric acid secretion, inhibits the release of gastrointestinal hormones and therefore decreases intestinal fluid secretion, slows intestinal motility, decreases bile flow, decreases mucus production, and reduces splanchnic blood flow. Furthermore, it inhibits acetylcholine release, resulting in muscle relaxation and reduction in the colicky pain associated with spastic gut activity. These inhibitory effects on peristalsis and gastrointestinal secretions reduce bowel distention, pain, and vomiting. Octreotide is administered by either subcutaneous bolus or continuous infusion. The recommended starting dose is 0.3 mg/day subcutaneously and may be titrated upward until symptoms are controlled; most patients require 0.6 to 0.9 mg/day. Octreotide is expensive, and the cost-to-benefit ratio must be considered, especially for patients who may require prolonged treatment. The main side effects of octreotide are gastrointestinal (nausea, vomiting, abdominal pain), injection site reactions, and hyperglycemia.

Despite aggressive supportive care, a malignant bowel obstruction does not resolve with medical management in most patients with advanced cancer. Without aggressive symptom management, patients with persistent malignant bowel obstructions can develop feculent emesis, intractable pain, and distress.

Interventional

Surgical exploration is the initial treatment of choice for patients with a single site of obstruction, a reasonable quality of life, good performance status, and well-controlled systemic disease. Additionally, for patients who present with a malignant bowel obstruction leading to the diagnosis of cancer, surgery, with or without a diverting ostomy, is standard care. With successful resection of an obstruction point, bowel function may return for an extended period, thus reducing requirements for supportive medications.

A less invasive alternative to surgery is an endoscopically placed colonic stent. Because urgent surgical intervention is associated with a modest risk of morbidity and mortality—16% to 23% and 5% to 20%, respectively—colonic stents are used in patients who are not operative candidates. In surgical candidates, temporary stents may be used for symptom relief before subsequent surgical intervention. Colonic stents provide immediate relief of the obstruction and rapid symptom improvement. Left-sided colon lesions are technically more amenable to stenting. Complications occur in 10% to 20% of cases and include stent migration, pain, bleeding, occlusion, and bowel perforation.[24]

Venting gastrostomy tubes (percutaneous gastric tubes placed into the stomach) relieve intractable nausea, vomiting, and pain by decompressing the stomach and proximal small bowel. They also enable a patient to eat and drink small amounts without symptoms, thus allowing social interactions at mealtime. Oral medications can be administered by clamping the gastric tube for 30 to 90 minutes, thereby allowing some absorption in the stomach and proximal small intestine, although bioavailability of medications in this setting is unpredictable. All patients with advanced cancer and a malignant bowel obstruction, with or without surgical intervention, have a poor prognosis and a high rate of in-hospital mortality.

Approach to Malignant Effusions

PLEURAL EFFUSIONS

Presentation

Malignant effusions are common in patients with cancer. Pleural effusions may manifest insidiously or with severe shortness of breath, depending on the size and speed of accumulation. Pleural effusions produce dyspnea, cough, and pleuritic-type chest pain. Patients often detail progressively worsening shortness of breath, escalating from mild dyspnea on exertion to shortness of breath at rest and orthopnea. Patients may complain of heaviness in the chest and, less frequently, pleuritic chest pain. Physical examination is remarkable for absent or decreased breath sounds and dullness on percussion, typically in the dependent regions of the chest cavity. Although any disease metastatic to the lungs can cause an effusion, more than 75%

Table 25-3. Light's Criteria for Transudative versus Exudative Effusions

Test	Exudate	Transudate
Cytology	Positive	Negative
Cell count	High	Low
Total protein	Pleural: serum ratio < 0.5	Pleural: serum ratio > 0.5
LDH	Pleural: serum ratio < 0.6	Pleural: serum ratio > 0.6
pH	Acidic: <7.3	Basic: >7.3

LDH, Lactate dehydrogenase.
Data from Light RW, Macgregor MI, Luchsinger PC, et al: Pleural effusions: the diagnostic separation of transudates and exudates, *Ann Intern Med* 77:507, 1972.

of malignant pleural effusions are caused by carcinomas of the lung, breast, or ovary or by lymphoma. The median survival of patients with a malignant pleural effusion is 3 months unless effective antineoplastic options are available.[25]

Evaluation

Pleural effusions are easily visualized with standard upright and lateral chest radiographs. Decubitus films identify the fluid as free flowing or not. A CT scan of the chest is useful to evaluate the degree of loculation of the fluid and the status of the underlying malignant disease. A clinically significant pleural effusion of unknown origin is an indication for thoracentesis, generally performed with ultrasonographic guidance. Pleural fluid should be analyzed for cytology, culture, cell count and differential, lactate dehydrogenase, protein, and pH. Malignant effusions are exudates characterized by high lactate dehydrogenase and protein levels and low pH (Table 25-3). The minimum adequate pleural fluid volume for cytologic diagnosis of malignancy is 50 mL. The sensitivity of pleural fluid cytology for the diagnosis of adenocarcinomas rises with three serial thoracenteses to almost 70%, although it is less sensitive for other malignant cell types (e.g., squamous cell carcinoma).

Management

The management of malignant pleural effusions focuses on control of dyspnea, cough, and pain while establishing the overall goals of care and considering therapeutic options.

Medical. Shortness of breath, the sensation of suffocation described by patients, is often relieved with low-dose opioids. In opioid-naïve patients, 2.5 to 5 mg of immediate-release morphine will ease the sensation of dyspnea. Furthermore, when given in anticipation of activity likely to cause dyspnea, opioids are effective for prevention. For patients with persistent anxiety even after relief of acute dyspnea, anxiolytics (e.g., benzodiazepines) are added adjunctively. Supplemental oxygen may ease dyspnea, although there is no correlation between the respiratory rate or the oxygen saturation and the sensation of dyspnea. Increasing the airflow by using a fan directed toward the patient's face may be beneficial. Some evidence suggests that air movement stimulates the trigeminal nerve, which, in turn, has a central inhibitory effect on dyspnea. This may also explain why oxygen, even in the absence of hypoxia, eases dyspnea. Finally, behavioral strategies, including placing the patient in a recumbent position, encouraging slow movements, and preparing for activity with oxygen and opioids, help to reduce symptoms and increase the patient's sense of control.

In addition to relieving dyspnea, the clinician should consider available options for systemic antitumor therapy, especially for chemotherapy-responsive cancers such as breast, testicular, or lung cancer. Symptom control and, in some cases, survival may be improved with chemotherapy. In patients with lung cancer particularly, chemotherapy has been shown to reduce symptoms and improve quality of life even when it does not prolong life.

Drainage. The majority of patients with malignant pleural effusions will require some type of mechanical drainage. Drainage of a pleural effusion may relieve dyspnea, improve function, and reduce medication requirements. Serial thoracentesis is generally not recommended for long-term management because of the increasing incidence of such complications as pneumothorax and loculated fluid collections. In patients whose pleural fluid reaccumulates after therapeutic thoracentesis, more definitive intervention should be considered. Re-expansion pulmonary edema is a rare and potentially fatal complication of thoracentesis, but it does not appear to correlate with the volume of fluid removed.[26]

Interventional. A tunneled pleural catheter (e.g., PleuRx catheter) permits long-term drainage on an outpatient basis and controls the effusion and related symptoms for more than 80% of patients. Patients and families can readily be taught to access the catheter at home and to drain up to 1000 mL of fluid every other day. A tunneled pleural catheter is an option for palliating malignant pleural effusion, both in patients with a good performance status and for those deemed clinical unsuitable for chest tube pleurodesis. The catheter provides the patient with control over the effusion and has been proven safe and effective in the outpatient setting.

Autopleurodesis occurs in approximately 40% of patients by 30 days. Complications from catheters are uncommon and tend to be minor (e.g., local skin infection, catheter occlusion, and skin breakdown), but they can be severe (e.g., pleural fluid infection). Traditional pigtail-type catheters are another option for chronic drainage of pleural effusions. Pigtail catheters are placed percutaneously and curl inside the body cavity, thus holding them in place. These catheters are of a smaller caliber than PleuRx, and autorepositioning in the chest is facilitated as the effusion resolves. When compared with tunneled catheters, however, they have an increased risk of plural and skin infection as well as occlusion.

For patients with recurrent effusions, pleurodesis, either at the bedside via chest tube or with a thorascopic approach with video assistance (VATS), offers long-term control. Chemical pleurodesis acts by inducing an acute pleural injury, resulting in pleural inflammation that, if successful, leads to fibrosis and pleurodesis. Although multiple sclerosing agents are available, sterile talc has become the sclerosant of choice (when compared with bleomycin, tetracycline, mustine, and tube drainage alone) because of cost, availability, and high reported success rates. VATS with talc pleurodesis provides the greatest likelihood of success, although trial results are mixed when comparing VATS with a bedside approach.

A Cochrane systemic review found that VATS-treated patients had a lower effusion recurrence rate (relative risk 1.19; 95% confidence interval, 1.04–1.36) compared with bedside pleurodesis (relative risk, 1.68, 95% confidence interval, 1.35–2.10), but the review was unable to determine differences in toxicity. A phase III trial comparing bedside pleurodesis with VATS showed equivalence with regard to control of the effusion at 30 days (71% vs.78%, respectively) with similar treatment-related mortality. There were more respiratory complications (14% vs. 6%), including respiratory failure (8% vs. 4%), with VATS versus bedside pleurodesis, although VATS-treated patients experienced less fatigue and chest pain.[27,28]

ASCITES

Presentation

Ascites is common in patients with abdominopelvic malignant tumors or metastatic disease to the liver. Ovarian cancer is the cancer most commonly associated with malignant ascites, followed by cancers of gastrointestinal origin. About 50% of patients with malignant ascites present with ascites at the initial diagnosis of cancer. Enlarging abdominal girth; generalized edema; tight-fitting pants; and complaints of early satiety, vomiting, dyspnea when lying flat, weakness, and weight gain suggest the presence of ascites. As the tension in the abdominal cavity rises, pain and shortness of breath increase. With the exception of ovarian cancer, malignant ascites portends a poor prognosis, with a median survival of 5 to 7 months.

Evaluation

Mild to moderate ascites is often difficult to detect on physical examination, and imaging studies may be necessary. Symptomatic ascites is often readily apparent, and imaging, such as an abdominal CT scan, can provide information about tumor bulk, vascular occlusion (e.g., portal vein thrombosis), associated peritoneal or hepatic disease, and the volume of ascites. Diagnostic paracentesis may be helpful to differentiate malignant ascites from other types. Routine fluid analysis includes a cell count and differential, albumin, cytology, and culture (Table 25-4). Peritoneal carcinomatosis accounts for roughly two thirds of patients with malignant ascites. Cytologic testing is positive in nearly 100% of these patients as a result of exfoliation of malignant cells into the ascites. Other causes of malignant ascites include bulky liver metastases and hepatocellular carcinoma with cirrhosis. Chylous ascites from

Table 25-4. Ascites Analysis

Cause of Ascites	Cytology	SAAG	Polymorphonuclear Cell Count (Leukocytes)
Malignant effusion	Positive	<1.1	<250
Cirrhosis	Negative	>1.1	<250
Spontaneous bacterial peritonitis	Negative	<1.1	>250
Right-sided heart failure	Negative	<1.1	<250

$$\text{SAAG, serum} - \text{ascites albumin gradient} = \frac{\text{serum albumin (g/mL)}}{\text{ascitic albumin (g/mL)}}$$

lymphoma is an infrequent cause of ascites and is rarely associated with positive cytologic testing. A neutrophil count greater than 250/mm^3 in the ascitic fluid is suggestive of infection. A serum-ascites albumin gradient (SAAG) of less than 1.1 g/mL is usually thought of as a result of nonportal hypertension etiologies (including malignancies). However, in patients with know cirrhosis, a low SAAG is not useful diagnostically.

Management

The treatment of malignant ascites is aimed at palliation of symptoms and may involve medical therapy, intermittent paracentesis, a semipermanent drainage catheter, or shunt placement.

Medical. The origin of the fluid and the overall goals of care are paramount when considering treatment options. For patients nearing the end of life, relief of pain and shortness of breath may be accomplished with titrated doses of opioids. Nausea is treated with dietary changes (small, frequent meals) and antiemetics, primarily a prokinetic agent (e.g., metoclopramide). Metoclopramide, a dopaminergic antagonist centrally and cholinergic in the gut, is the first-line agent in patients with ascites. It stimulates smooth muscle activity, speeding gastric emptying, and inhibits D$_2$ receptors in the chemoreceptor trigger zone, thus inhibiting nausea centrally. Other antiemetics, such as serotonin antagonists (e.g., ondansetron) and other dopamine antagonists (e.g., prochlorperazine), may be added if needed.

Although malignant ascites is typically resistant to diuretic therapy, an attempt to control the accumulation of ascites with diuretics may be appropriate in patients with signs suggestive of portal hypertension (e.g., a SAAG >1.1 g/dL). Patients with portal hypertension may respond to escalating doses of diuretics in combination with a low-sodium, fluid-restricted diet. Finally, therapies aimed at controlling the underlying malignant disease should be considered in certain patient populations with preserved performance status (KPS >70) and effective antitumor options.

Drainage. Therapeutic paracentesis improves symptoms immediately, is easily performed in an outpatient or home setting, and carries minimal risks. In patients with a low SAAG (<1.1 g/dL), the risk of hemodynamic compromise with large-volume paracentesis (>5 L) is low. Often, fluid reaccumulates rapidly, necessitating repeated large-volume paracenteses for chronic management of the ascites. With repeated large-volume paracenteses, the risk of complications increases, particularly in patients with prior abdominal surgical procedures or peritoneal carcinomatosis, because both conditions predispose to loculated effusions and adherent loops of bowel. Intermittent large-volume paracentesis is appropriate in many patients who require relatively infrequent paracenteses or in those nearing the end of life.

For patients with preserved performance status, an indwelling peritoneal catheter can be considered. Indwelling catheters allow a patient the freedom to drain ascites "as needed" to maintain symptom control. Indwelling catheters are, however, more expensive to place, maintain, and use. The most readily available catheters are pigtail catheters, which use a programmed internal coil to hold them in place. They can be easily inserted in the outpatient setting with minimal risk. Pigtail catheters relieve distention immediately but they are occasionally complicated by catheter-related sepsis, hypotension, and occlusion.[29,30] Tunneled catheters (e.g., PleuRx) are associated with fewer infectious complications than nontunneled catheters and are approved for the management of malignant ascites. Indwelling peritoneal catheters offer a convenient and safe alternative to frequent paracentesis and effectively palliate the symptoms associated with large-volume ascites.[31]

PERICARDIAL EFFUSIONS

Presentation

Pericardial effusions occur in a significant percentage of patients with metastatic cancer. The most common causes are leukemia (69%), melanoma (64%), and lymphoma (24%). Autopsy series report an incidence up to 20%.[32] The effusion is most commonly caused by pericardial metastases, but it may result from direct pericardial tumor invasion or disruption of normal lymphatic drainage.[33] Direct tumor extension to the pericardium occurs from breast, lung, and esophageal cancers. Pericardial effusions may manifest with nonspecific symptoms such as weight loss, fatigue, and nausea. Patients may also present with more severe symptoms of dyspnea on exertion, paroxysmal nocturnal dyspnea, and orthopnea, or with life-threatening cardiovascular shock. As the effusion progresses, patients may develop chest pain, dizziness, and syncope. Pericardial tamponade or constrictive pericarditis manifests with chest pain and dyspnea, and unstable vital signs or shock may also be present.

Pericardial effusions confer a poor prognosis on patients with lung or breast cancer: median survival of 3.2 and 8.8 months, respectively. Patients with hematologic diseases and a malignant pericardial effusion fare better, with a median survival of 17 months.[33]

Evaluation

Pericardial effusions may be suspected on physical examination if the percussed heart border is enlarged, pulsus paradoxus is present, or a flat percussive sound is heard over the lower two thirds of the sternum (Dressler's sign). The effusion is best evaluated with a transthoracic echocardiogram to determine its size, quality, and physiologic significance.

Management

Medical. Many patients with malignant pericardial effusions have vague symptoms related to the slow accumulation of fluid and can be managed with medications directed toward specific symptoms. Supportive medications for dyspnea, nausea, and fatigue are appropriate, such as low-dose opioids, antiemetics, or psychostimulants (e.g., methylphenidate), respectively. Antitumor therapy, if available, may reduce or eliminate the effusion and is particularly effective in patients with hematologic malignant diseases.

Drainage. Pericardiocentesis, in the setting of a hemodynamically significant effusion, relieves tamponade and immediately improves signs and symptoms. However, if left untreated, 90% of malignant pericardial effusions will reaccumulate within 3 months.[34] Pericardial effusions are definitely treated with pericardial sclerosis or surgical decompression. The best recommendation for management of malignant pericardial effusions depends on the patient's anticipated survival and how urgently the intervention is required.

PEARLS AND PITFALLS

- Neurologic symptoms in patients with a history of malignancy (especially lung, melanoma, renal, and breast cancers) should be evaluated quickly and thoroughly.

- Corticosteroids are an important adjunctive therapy for the relief of a variety of cancer-related symptoms, including pain, anorexia, and constitutional symptoms.

- Strong opioids are often required to manage pain in cancer patients and may be used in conjunction with various adjuvant pain relievers.

- Malignant bowel obstruction is a particularly lethal complication of cancer, but consideration should be given to the extent of the illness and the precise cause of the obstruction before ruling out the possibility of surgical intervention.

- The most effective symptom-relieving interventions for cancer patients may be antitumor therapies used in conjunction with palliative medications.

Summary

Patients with cancer face many symptoms and complications from the underlying cancer and its treatment. Aggressive symptom control is vital to maximize quality of life. Only by careful attention to the prevention, evaluation, and treatment of symptoms will patients with cancer receive optimal cancer care.

Patients with malignant disease experience myriad physical symptoms related to the disease and its treatment. Symptoms related to the malignant process should be evaluated completely, and treatment should be directed at the primary cause, if possible. The prognosis varies according to many individual factors and must be carefully considered when making management decisions.

Resources

Berger AM, Shuster JL, Von Roenn JH, editors: *Principles and practice of palliative care and supportive oncology*, ed 3, Philadelphia, 2006, Lippincott Williams & Wilkins.
Journal of Supportive Oncology
    Available at www.supportiveoncology.net.

References

1. Wen PY, Loeffler JS: Overview of brain metastases. In Rose BD, editor: *Up to date 13.3*, Waltham, Mass, 2005, UpToDate.
2. Barnholtz-Sloan JS, Sloan AE, Davis FG, et al: Incidence proportions of brain metastases in patients diagnosed (1973 to 2001) in the Metropolitan Detroit Cancer Surveillance System, *J Clin Oncol* 22(14):2865–2872, 2004.
3. Gaspar L, Scott C, Rotman M, et al: Recursive partitioning analysis (RPA) of prognostic factors in three Radiation Therapy Oncology Group (RTOG) brain metastases trials, *Int J Radiat Oncol Biol Phys* 37(4):745–751, 1997.
4. Markesbery WR, Brooks WH, Gupta GD, Young AB: Treatment for patients with cerebral metastases, *Arch Neurol* 35:754–756,1978.
5. Weissman DE: Glucocorticoid treatment for brain metastases and epidural spinal cord compression: a review, *J Clin Oncol* 6:543–551, 1988.
6. Noordijk EM, Vecht CJ, Haaxma-Reiche H, et al: The choice of treatment of single brain metastasis should be based on extracranial tumor activity and age, *Int J Radiat Oncol Biol Phys* 29:711–717, 1994.
7. Hart MG, Grant R, Walker M, et al: Surgical resection and whole brain radiation therapy versus whole brain radiation therapy alone for single brain metastases, *Cochrane Database Syst Rev* 1:CD003292, 2005.

8. Andrews DW, Scott CB, Sperduto PW, et al: Whole brain radiation therapy with or without stereotactic radiosurgery boost for patients with one to three brain metastases: phase III results of the RTOG 9508 randomised trial, *Lancet* 363:1665–1672, 2004.
9. Zhukovsky DS: Fever and sweats in the patient with advanced cancer, *Hematol Oncol Clin North Am* 16:579–588, viii 2002.
10. Deaner PB: The use of thalidomide in the management of severe sweating in patients with advanced malignancy: trial report, *Palliat Med* 14:429–431, 2000.
11. Adam A: Interventional radiology in the treatment of hepatic metastases, *Cancer Treat Rev* 28:93–99, 2002.
12. Nielsen OS, Munro AJ, Tannock IF: Bone metastases: pathophysiology and management policy, *J Clin Oncol* 9:509–524, 1991.
13. van der Linden YM, Kroon HM, Dijkstra SP, et al: Dutch Bone Metastasis Study Group. Simple radiographic parameter predicts fracturing in metastatic femoral bone lesions: results from a randomised trial, *Radiother Oncol* 69:21–31, 2003.
14. Stopeck AT, Lipton A, Body JJ, et al: Denosumab compared with zoledronic acid for the treatment of bone metastases in patients with advanced breast cancer: a randomized, double-blind study, *J Clin Oncol* 28:5132–5139, 2010.
15. Vadhan-Raj S, Henry D, von Moos R, et al: Denosumab in the treatment of bone metastases from advanced cancer or multiple myeloma (MM): analyses from a phase III randomized trial, *J Clin Oncol* 28(suppl):9042, 2010.
16. von Moos R, Patrick D, Fallowfield L, et al: Effects of denosumab versus zoledronic acid (ZA) on pain in patients (pts) with advanced cancer (excluding breast and prostate) or multiple myeloma (MM): results from a randomized phase III clinical trial, *J Clin Oncol* 28(suppl):9043, 2010.
17. Fallowfield D, Patrick D, Body J, et al: Effects of denosumab versus zoledronic acid (ZA) on health-related quality of life (HRQL) in metastatic breast cancer: results from a randomized phase III trial, *J Clin Oncol* 28(suppl):1025, 2010.
18. Sze WM, Shelley MD, Held I, et al: Palliation of metastatic bone pain: single fraction versus multifraction radiotherapy: a systemic review of randomized trials, *Clin Oncol (R Coll Radiol)* 15:345–352, 2003.
19. Goetz MP, Callstrom MR, Charboneau JW, et al: Percutaneous image-guided radiofrequency ablation of painful metastases involving bone: a multicenter study, *J Clin Oncol* 22:300–306, 2004.
20. Vrionis FD, Small J: Surgical management of metastatic spinal neoplasms, *Neurosurg Focus* 15:E12, 2003.
21. Chow E, Holden L, Danjoux C, et al: Successful salvage using percutaneous vertebroplasty in cancer patients with painful spinal metastases or osteoporotic compression fractures, *Radiother Oncol* 70:265–267, 2004.
22. Roque M, Martinex MJ, Alonso P, et al: Radioisotopes for metastatic bone pain, *Cochrane Database Syst Rev* 4:CD003347, 2003.
23. Feuer DJ, Broadley KE: Corticosteroids for the resolution of malignant bowel obstruction in advanced gynaecological and gastrointestinal cancer, *Cochrane Database Syst Rev* 2:CD001219, 2000.
24. Pothuri B, Guirguis A, Gerdes H, et al: The use of colorectal stents for palliation of large-bowel obstruction due to recurrent gynecologic cancer, *Gynecol Oncol* 95:513–517, 2004.
25. Putnam JB, Jr: Malignant pleural effusions, *Surg Clin North Am* 82:867–883, 2002.
26. Jones PW, Moyers JP, Rogers JT, et al: Ultrasound-guided thoracentesis: is it a safer method? *Chest* 123:418–423, 2003.
27. Shaw P, Agarwal P: Pleurodesis for malignant pleural effusions, *Cochrane Database Syst Rev* 1:CD002916, 2004.
28. Dresler CM, Olak J, Herndon JE 2nd, et al: Phase III intergroup study of talc poudrage vs talc slurry sclerosis for malignant pleural effusion, *Chest* 127:909–915, 2005.
29. Sioris T, Sihvo E, Salo J, et al: Long-term indwelling pleural catheter (PleurX) for malignant pleural effusion unsuitable for talc pleurodesis, *Eur J Surg Oncol* 35:546–551, 2009.
30. Parsons SL, Watson SA, Steele RJ: Malignant ascites, *Br J Surg* 83:6–14, 1996.
31. Courtney A, Nemcek AA, Rosenberg S, et al: Prospective evaluation of the PleurX catheter when used to treat recurrent ascites associated with malignancy, *J Vas Interv Radiol* 19:1723–1731, 2008.
32. Bisel HF, Wroblewski F, Ladue JS: Incidence and clinical manifestations of cardiac metastases, *J Am Med Assoc* 153:712–715, 1953.
33. Cullinane CA, Paz IB, Smith D, et al: Prognostic factors in the surgical management of pericardial effusion in the patient with concurrent malignancy, *Chest* 125:1328–1334, 2004.
34. Vaitkus PT, Herrmann HC, LeWinter MM: Treatment of malignant pericardial effusion, *JAMA* 272:59–64, 1994.

CHAPTER 26

HIV/AIDS

CARLA S. ALEXANDER

Epidemiology	**End-of-Life Issues**
Palliative Approach across the Continuum	Stopping Critical Medications
Unique Family Unit	Life Closure
Teamwork	Time of Death
Advance Care Planning	Self-Care of Providers
Prognosis-Adjusted Management Issues	Cultural Issues and Ritual
	Pearls
Impact of Symptoms	**Pitfalls**
Loss of Viral Control and Threats to Survival	**Summary**
	Impact of International Epidemic on United States

Thirty years of experience with HIV/AIDS has resulted in a new chronic illness for more than 1 million Americans living with ongoing toxicities and a lifespan possibly shortened by premature aging.[1,2] Disease from the human immunodeficiency virus-1 (HIV-1) remains incurable, yet mortality has decreased dramatically and is related to long-term toxicities of therapy or comorbidity such as malignancy or hepatitis C. Previously, a long, unpredictable prodrome preceded death; now death occurs in intensive care units with complications of coexisting diagnoses. Complex antiretroviral therapy is the purview of specialists, but recognition of early illness remains a challenge to all providers; up to 40% of patients with HIV disease are only diagnosed with advanced disease.

HIV/AIDS in the United States remains surrounded by stigma affecting people of color and those in marginalized living situations. Men who have sex with men (MSM remain) at extremely high risk because many young people have not sufficiently learned about or adjusted behaviors to the risk. Twenty-five percent of those carrying HIV-1 are unaware of their own ability to spread disease, and heterosexual contact remains the primary risk factor for women. Although "high-risk" groups exist, such as sex workers and intravenous drug users, any sexually active person is still at risk, and the Centers for Disease Control and Prevention (CDC) implemented an "opt out" testing policy in 2006 to identify those who might be helped by treatment. Integrating palliative approaches can improve quality of life, enhance adherence to combination antiretroviral therapy and other therapies, and address complicated psychosocial issues facing HIV-infected individuals and their families.[3]

Epidemiology

Understanding the epidemiology of HIV disease in the United States is fundamental to being able to plan for the future. Based upon 2007 data from 35 U.S. states and

5 territories, the CDC has calculated that more than 1 million persons are living in the United States with HIV disease (including more than 455,000 with actual AIDS), and more than 56,000 new cases are diagnosed yearly. Although the worldwide epidemic is predominantly female, disease in the United States remains focused (53%–64%, depending on the data set) among MSM. Mortality rates have dropped dramatically, but between 14,000 and 22,000 people continue to die of AIDS annually. The affected population is up to 51% African American, 32% Caucasian, and 17% Hispanic, with prevalence quite high in those living in Pacific Islands. Seventy-two percent of women infected in the United States are heterosexual contacts of either men who have sex with men or intravenous drug users. Death rates are highest for older patients and intravenous drug users.

The epicenter for AIDS in the United States is now in the south (40%), with 29% in the northeast and 20% on the west coast. Ninety percent of those with identified HIV disease are younger than 50, meaning that there will be another peak in deaths from HIV over the next 30 years. If started on optimal therapy at the time of diagnosis, most will live long enough to develop comorbidities such as cancer or end-stage liver disease from hepatitis C or will die of cardiovascular complications and other manifestations of early aging. The current population is likely to develop higher rates of cirrhosis or other end-stage liver disease, prostate and other genitourinary cancers,[4] severe mental illness[5] and neurocognitive disorders, and problems related to osteoporosis.

Someone becomes infected with HIV-1 every 9.5 minutes in the United States, and 36% of those diagnosed may progress to AIDS within 12 months of diagnosis because of delayed diagnosis and complications of opportunistic infections. Thus, providers caring for persons with HIV/AIDS near the end of life are obligated to discuss issues of detection and prevention with loved ones who may have had parenteral or sexual contact with the person. Implications for providers are that HIV remains an infectious illness targeting people who may be marginalized in society and those who are unsuspecting of their diagnosis. Bereavement will continue to be complicated by stigma, recognition of sexual infidelity, and new infectious illness in remaining partners. AIDS may no longer be the primary cause of death, but it continues to pose a subtle threat in populations not yet aware of the diagnosis.

Over the next 10 years, there may be four populations suffering from HIV disease: (1) young people demonstrating usual psychological resistance to managing their chronic illness (similar to diabetes); (2) survivors who are older and "treatment experienced," having lived through a time when many were dying of AIDS; (3) those who have disorganized lives and difficulty remaining in care; and (4) women who have become infected either through intravenous drug use or sexual contact. Each of these will make diverse demands on the health care system. Providers will want to assemble unique approaches to providing support. Those needs near the end of life may differ based on individual ability to participate in care planning.

Palliative Approach across the Continuum

Palliative care, once a critical component of HIV care,[6] is often ignored by providers who believe that once people have access to combination antiretroviral therapy (cART), end-of-life decisions cease to be relevant.[7] However, palliative care remains important in HIV care as in other chronic, life-limiting illnesses. Concurrent palliative care with optimal general treatment throughout the trajectory of illness is clearly

---

Box 26-1. *Domains of High-Quality End-of-Life Care: Patient Preferences*

- Adequate pain and symptom management
- Avoiding inappropriate prolongation of dying
- Achieving a sense of control
- Relieving burden
- Strengthening relationships with loved ones

---

needed for all persons with HIV/AIDS.[8] Symptom recognition and control are paramount, regardless of disease stage. In the United States, people living with HIV historically may have taken sequential single-drug therapy, and although survival may be prolonged, they are plagued by long-term toxicities as well as fear of developing resistance to available therapies. Establishing goals of care is part of good palliative care at all stages of the illness. Having these discussions with patients and their chosen families is also helpful in identifying health care proxies who can assist with decision making at critical junctures involving decisional incapacity. Addressing mental health issues that may also interfere with adherence to cART continues to be critical to successful therapy. Improving skills for communicating serious information (such as negative changes related to management) as well as those for conducting family meetings are essential elements of palliative care that can be woven into ongoing management. Ethical issues faced by patients and families in decision making and spiritual and cultural beliefs are challenges highlighted by the demographics of the U.S. epidemic that can be addressed with palliative skills. More study is needed to evaluate the effectiveness of this type of care across the continuum.

Persons living with advanced disease have improved control of physical symptoms, anxiety, insight, and spiritual well-being when care is provided by home palliative care or inpatient hospice workers.[9] In 1999, Singer and colleagues identified preferred domains of end-of-life care for persons with HIV that are likely to continue to apply (Box 26-1). Families need preparation for impending death of a loved one plus support throughout their mourning and bereavement. HIV providers must recognize that staff are affected deeply when patients do die, because many are young themselves and have not witnessed many deaths from this illness. They are left perplexed and feeling as if there were something more that could have been done (see Box 26-1).

UNIQUE FAMILY UNIT

Given current U.S. epidemiology, providers must clarify with each patient whom he or she considers to be in a significant relationship and who might act on behalf of the patient for making health-related decisions. This must be recorded in the patient record. Stigma continues to play a significant role in how families respond to HIV/AIDS, and providers should be aware that homosexuality may be less acceptable to a family of color than admitting to substance abuse. When substance use is an underlying risk factor, myriad problems ranging from antisocial behavior to complete breakdown of family-of-origin relationships may develop. Mental illness, a common comorbidity, can make identification of a health care proxy challenging. In all families, but perhaps particularly in those with ongoing adjustment, a history of ongoing review of goals of care makes open and honest conversations about end-of-life preferences easier.

TEAMWORK

HIV/AIDS is a complex illness involving multiple body systems and is complicated by psychological and social issues. Patients have a need for personal and family education, support groups, telephone follow-up, and individual counseling sessions with nurses, counselors, or chaplains. Significant numbers suffer from anxiety or depression and risks for neurologic symptoms remain high if not treated. Stigma remains a problem and may worsen in the future given current demographics. For these reasons, it is simply not realistic for one provider to manage this illness without involving other members of an interdisciplinary team, regardless of stage of disease. Team members can provide invaluable assistance and insight.

ADVANCE CARE PLANNING

Discussing serious illness or the end of life is difficult for both clinicians and families. Culturally, many believe that such a discussion itself can hasten death. Having these conversations before being confronted with actual need for decision making removes emotional impact and can ensure that patients receive the best care and support when capacity is diminished or lost. The attitude of the provider plays a role in the patient's ability to discuss these topics. Palliative care teachings described in Chapter 20 provide alternatives to thinking, *There is nothing else we can do.*

Because it is not possible to anticipate every situation one might face near the end of life, patients and families must be encouraged to consider who would take legal responsibility for decision making if the patient were unable to speak for himself or herself. Studies have documented great mistrust among racial and ethnic minorities and medical providers.[10] For this reason, it may be useful to offer group education about end-of-life decision making in large HIV clinics or to have social workers or other clinical counselors available to facilitate this education before actual discussions with the provider. Whatever the mechanism, patients and families fare better during serious illness if these issues are addressed and resolved ahead of time.

Identifying and documenting in the medical record the name and contact information for a health care proxy is essential. If the chosen surrogate is not related by blood or marriage, a well-documented legal designation is the only effective method of ensuring that this person will be respected as decision maker. These issues require time to consider and may need repeated dialogue. Initiating annual discussions regarding "emergency-related" decision making may be a useful technique in practice.

Prognosis-Adjusted Management Issues

Successful management of HIV disease requires an understanding of where the patient is along the continuum of illness. This can be accomplished in consultation with an HIV specialist. It may be useful to think of the illness in five stages based on treatment status:

1. Treatment naïve
2. Initiation and stabilization of cART
3. Stable health maintenance, probably including symptom management
4. New onset of symptoms signifying treatment failure or other disease
5. Lack of viral control or active dying

Table 26-1. Stages of HIV Illness for Purposes of Care and Support

Stage of Illness	Treatment Status	Management Strategy	Specialist Need
1. Treatment naïve	1. Engagement in care with clarification of support system & mental health issues	Clinical stabilization & staging	++++
2. Initiation of cART and viral control	2. Treatment initiation and stabilization, including intensive adherence support	Initiation of cART New symptoms: rule out immune reconstitution syndrome (IRIS)	++++
3. Health maintenance	3. Health maintenance: stable on therapy for >1year	Local management for intercurrent illness with referral back to HIV specialist	++ (phone) Local evaluation
4. Loss of viral Control	4. New onset of symptoms consistent with: • Treatment failure • New disease, such as advanced liver disease (history of hepatitis B or C) or malignancy requiring further evaluation	Clinical stabilization Diagnostic workup Management of cART per HIV specialist	++ (phone) Local evaluation
5. Inability to control HIV or comorbidity	5. Decline, with death expected	Referral for palliative care and/or hospice services; involve HIV specialist	+ Local care; courtesy contact

cART, combined antiretroviral therapy.

Care needs vary based on clinical stage of disease. Asking about available support system, previous attempts at advance care planning, and psychosocial/spiritual beliefs may be helpful in adjusting or creating new goals of care (Table 26-1).

Predicting prognosis is the foundation of good end-of-life care and must be based on history of cART, current markers such as CD4 cell count and viral load, and patient goals of care. In the past, many with HIV/AIDS experienced a gradual deterioration that alerted clinicians to their poor prognosis. Now, with improved medical management, comorbidities or complications of intravenous substance use are often the cause of death. Toxicities such as lactic acidosis can result in very rapid deterioration and death. Box 26-2 lists indicators of a poor prognosis documented in the literature.

The Medicare/Medicaid Hospice Benefits provide home-based care when life expectancy is less than 6 months if the disease runs its normal course. Although this

Box 26-2. *Predictors of Poor Prognosis*

LABORATORY DATA

Persistent CD4+ cell count < 25 cells/mm^3

Persistent HIV RNA > 100,000 copies/mL

Serum albumin < 2.5 g/dL

Lactate level > 10 mmol/L and pH < 7.0

Central nervous system disease (e.g., lymphoma, unresponsive toxoplasmosis, progressive multifocal leukoencephalopathy)

HIV dementia (associated with early death)

Unresponsive lymphoma, visceral Kaposi sarcoma, other progressive malignant disease

Persistent cryptosporidiosis-related diarrhea (>1 month)

Advanced end-organ failure (e.g., liver failure secondary to hepatitis C; cardiomyopathy)

Disseminated and resistant atypical *Mycobacterium avium* complex (MAC) or coccidiomycosis

Resistant wasting (>10% body weight loss)

Adapted from National Hospice Organization: Medical Guidelines for Determining Prognosis in Selected Noncancer Diseases, Arlington, Va, National Hospice Organization, 1996; based on literature before the use of highly active antiretroviral therapy; modified with HRSA treatment guidelines and Bartlett; *CID* 42:1059, 2006; Sevigny JJ, Albert SM, McDermott MP, et al: An evaluation of neurocognitive status and markers of immune activation as predictors of time to death in advanced HIV infection, *Arch Neurol* 64(1):97–102, 2007.

is not a realistic guideline for patients with HIV disease, providers should be aware that these services are available in caring for patients who are deteriorating. One simple way to decide about use of this benefit is to ask yourself, *Would I be surprised if this person died in the next month?*[11] If the answer is no, then it is time to begin discussions with patient and family regarding support needs at home. Social work or palliative care consultation can be helpful.

IMPACT OF SYMPTOMS

Optimal HIV care includes focus on management of side effects and long-term toxicities that negatively impact daily quality of life. Although a symptom may be expressed physically, it can also reflect, or be modified by, emotional, social, and spiritual issues. For example, pain can be complicated by its meaning to the patient who may have a fear of being punished for his lifestyle, or it may bring back memories of a friend who died with unrelieved pain. It can reflect anguish regarding lack of appropriate guardianship for a child or any number of unspoken worries. Without recognizing these modifiers, the symptom in question can be relieved acutely but may recur or seem "out of proportion" to the identified stimulus.

Studies conducted by the AIDS Clinical Trials Group (ACTG) have identified multiple symptoms that plague patients taking cART. Symptom prevalence documented throughout the epidemic demonstrates that the same symptoms worsen quality of life regardless of stage of illness (Table 26-2). An individual patient may have as many as 16 active signs or symptoms at any given time.[12] The ACTG symptom

Table 26-2. Symptom Prevalence

Sign/ Symptom	Fontaine et al (France) (N = 290) (%)	Vogl et al (U.S.) (N = 504) (%)	Matthews et al (U.S.) (N = 3,072) (%)	Fantoni et al (Italy) (N = 1,128) (%)	Karus et al (U.S.) (N = 255) (%)
Fatigue	77	85	68	55	72
Fevers	59	—	51.1	29	14
Hand/foot pain	—	—	48.9	—	38
Nausea	48	—	49.8	22	48
Diarrhea	45	—	51	11	39
Sadness/ Depression	63	82	—	—	47
Sleep problems	62	73.8	—	—	48
Skin problems	37	—	24.3	17	36
Cough	57	60.3	30.4	32	48
Appetite loss (anorexia)	55	—	49.8	34	40
Weight loss	60	—	37.1	—	46
Pain	—	76	29	40	69
Dyspnea	41	62.4	30.4	19	52

Data from Fontaine A, Larue F, Lassauniere JM: Physicians' recognition of the symptoms experienced by HIV patients: How reliable? *J Pain Symptom Manage* 18:263–270, 1999; Vogl D, Rosenfeld B, Breitbart W, et al: Symptom prevalence, characteristics, and distress in AIDS outpatients, *J Pain Symptom Manage* 18:253–262, 1999; Mathews WC, McCutchan JA, Asch S, et al: National Estimates of HIV-related symptom prevalence from the HIV Cost and Services Utilization Study, *Med Care* 38:750–762, 2000; Fantoni M, Ricci F, Del Borgo C, et al: Multicentre study on the prevalence of symptoms and symptomatic treatment in HIV infection: Central Italy PRESINT Group, *J Palliat Care* 13:9–13, 1997; Karus D, Raveis VH, Alexander C, et al: Patient reports of symptoms and their treatment at three palliative care projects servicing individuals with HIV/AIDS, *J Pain Symptom Manage* 30(5):408–416, 2005.

index should be used clinically to document problems facing patients daily, providing an objective picture of each patient,[13] because it has been well documented that providers at all levels fail to recognize either the number or severity of problems experienced by patients. The HIV Cost and Service Utilization Study (HCSUS) showed that number of symptoms may have greater impact on health-related quality of life than CD4+ cell count or measured viral burden.[14] Symptoms such as fatigue are difficult for patients to describe or quantify and require increased efforts by providers to incorporate other team members who might document how these problems impact daily quality of life for patients.[15]

Opportunistic infections, wasting syndrome, and AIDS-related malignancies were hallmarks of early HIV infection. It is useful to associate the level of T-helper cell destruction with specific symptomatic problems (Table 26-3). Constitutional symptoms such as cachexia, anorexia, night sweats, and fevers can occur in persons with

Table 26-3. Infections Correlated with CD4+ Cell Count

CD4+ Cell Count	Infection
>500	Candidal vaginitis
200–500	Pneumococcal disease, herpes zoster, pulmonary tuberculosis, Kaposi sarcoma, oral thrush, cervical cancer, idiopathic thrombocytopenia purpura
<200	*Pneumocystis* pneumonia, miliary and extrapulmonary tuberculosis, wasting, peripheral neuropathy, non-Hodgkin's lymphoma, disseminated histoplasmosis, recurrent bacterial disease (e.g., pyomyositis)
<100	Toxoplasmosis, cryptococcosis, chronic cryptosporidiosis, microsporidiosis, candidal esophagitis
<50	Cytomegalovirus, atypical *Mycobacterium avium* complex (MAC), central nervous system lymphoma, progressive multifocal leukoencephalitis

From Khambaty M: HIV Curriculum. Baltimore, Md, UMSOM Institute of Human Virology.

unrecognized HIV infection or comorbidities such as tuberculosis or hepatitis C. These problems associated with untreated and advanced disease require full assessment by an HIV specialist to determine eligibility for cART. They may occur in patients no longer responsive to treatment because of viral resistance or from having halted therapy. When such symptoms are present, "salvage therapy" may be possible, but it should ideally be determine in consultation with an HIV specialist. Regardless of cause of symptoms, they should be addressed symptomatically while antiretroviral therapy management strategy is being considered.

Side Effects of Antiretroviral Therapy

Symptoms may be caused by HIV disease itself (treated or untreated), by medications used to manage HIV, or by unrelated issues. A recent survey of outpatients taking cART in the United Kingdom showed that patients receiving therapy experience more symptoms than do those who are not being treated.[16] An experienced HIV clinician recognizes that most side effects resolve over 2 to 4 weeks and can offer advice or even other medication to prevent predictable side effects at the time therapy is initiated. These weeks, although brief from the point of view of the provider, may be quite difficult for the patient to tolerate and can be a reason for poor adherence to the regimen. As viral control has improved, side effects have been minimized and dosing regimen is more user friendly. Nevertheless, these agents are a form of chemotherapy and may not be easy for patients to tolerate (Table 26-4).

Xerostomia from direct invasion of salivary glands by HIV was also precipitated by an early antiretroviral drug, didanosine. Although this medication is rarely used now, it accentuates the need for providers using a checklist of possible side effects, because xerostomia is not routinely targeted in history taking but can cause serious consequences for patients who fails to reveal its presence. Likewise, peripheral neuropathy caused by direct invasion of virus or chemical toxicity of medications can be debilitating if unrecognized.

Table 26-4. Side Effects of Frequently Used Antiretroviral Therapy

Drugs	Side Effects
Nucleoside Reverse Transcriptase Inhibitors (NRTIs)	
Abacavir	Hypersensitivity reaction, nausea, malaise
Didanosine (ddl)	Pancreatitis, xerostomia, peripheral neuropathy
Lamivudine (3TC)/ Emtricitabine (FTC)	Negligible, occasional hyperpigmentation of palms and soles
Stavudine (D4T)	Peripheral neuropathy, lipoatrophy, lactic acidosis, steatosis
Tenofovir	Bloating, Fanconi's syndrome (rare)
Zidovudine (AZT)	Headache, anemia, nausea, pigmented nail beds, darkened skin, insomnia, myopathy
Non-nucleoside Reverse Transcriptase Inhibitors (NNRTIs)	
Efavirenz	Vivid dreams, mental status changes, lowers methadone levels, rash
Nevirapine	Rash (15%–30%), hepatotoxicity (fatal)
Etravirine	Rash (9%)
Protease Inhibitors (PIs) (Most with GI distress)	
Lopinavir/ritonavir	Nausea, bloating, diarrhea (15%–25%)
Indinavir	Renal stones, diarrhea, GI distress
Nelfinavir	Diarrhea
Atazanavir	Hyperbilirubinemia, GI distress
Saquinavir	GI intolerance, headache
Amprenavir	Diarrhea, oral paresthesias, rash
Darunavir/ritonavir	Rash
Tipranavir	Hepatotoxicity, intracranial hemorrhage (with head trauma)
Integrase Inhibitor	
Raltegravir	
Fusion Inhibitor	
Enfuviride (T20)	Local induration at injection site, GI, gastrointestinal
CCR5 Inhibitor	
Maraviroc	Postural hypotension, GI distress

GI, Gastrointestinal.
See http://aidsinfo.nih.gov/contentfiles/AA_Tables.pdf; Bartlett www.mmhiv.org.

Symptoms to Target

The 10 most commonly encountered symptoms in the HIV population include fatigue, anorexia, worries or feelings of sadness/depression, pain from multiple parts of the body, shortness of breath (dyspnea) or cough, dry mouth, and problems with sleep. Any provider caring for a person with HIV/AIDS regardless of stage of illness should be able to competently address each of these because they cause significant suffering for the individual when left unrecognized. Pain can affect any body part and requires separate evaluation and management; depression is often overlooked as an independent symptom. These symptoms are also addressed in other parts of this book because they are common to patients with most advanced illnesses.

Box 26-3. *Pain as an Important Symptom*

TYPES OF PAIN IN HIV/AIDS
Headaches
Oral cavity/throat/esophagus
Chest
Abdomen
Genital/rectal
Extremities
Related to diagnostic procedures

Pain

Pain continues to be an important symptom in HIV disease despite improvement secondary to cART (Box 26-3). Management of pain in this population may be complicated by an overlay of substance abuse. It is useful to obtain a baseline pain consultation on any patient. If previous substance abuse is part of the history, tolerance to opioids will exist, and patients may require higher doses for routine management.[17] Long-acting opioids are preferred to eliminate possible "triggers" to addiction experienced with changing drug levels. In the HIV population of persons with previous intravenous drug use, management may be complicated by current methadone treatment; however, pain management must be addressed as an independent problem. There are interactions with antiretrovirals that can lower methadone levels; treatment of pain in these patients is best done in consultation with a pain specialist.

Clinical experience suggests that patients with pain are grateful for attention to this symptom and will not exhibit "drug-seeking" behavior if acceptable symptom control is achieved. The optimal management of pain requires a multidisciplinary team and a systematic approach.

Peripheral neuropathy, the most common pain in HIV disease, can be present during any stage of illness. It may be secondary to HIV invasion or a consequence of earlier thymidine therapy. Treatment should be based on etiology of the pain and may be improved by using an adjuvant anticonvulsant (e.g., carbamazepine or gabapentin) or antidepressant (e.g., nortriptyline or duloxetine) for the neuropathic component in addition to an opioid. When initiated at the same time, adjuvant medication can lower the total dose of opioid. In the past, it was believed that opioids were ineffective for neuropathic pain, but it is now known that this type of pain simply requires higher doses of opioids (Box 26-4).

The syndrome of pseudo-addiction is well described, in which patients report inadequate control of pain when the current dose of medication is no longer clinically effective, reflecting the actual half-life of the medication. Clinicians previously interpreted this as "drug-seeking behavior" until it was recognized that "end-of-dose failure" meant that active effects of the pain medication were related to half-life and might reflect rapid metabolism of the active agent. Thus, loss of symptom control occurs before the next scheduled dose.[18]

Depression

A multisite study documented that 13% to 30% of patients with HIV disease have major depression that had not been diagnosed previously.[19] Antidepressant treatment

Box 26-4. *Principles for Managing Signs and Symptoms*

Believe the patient.
Take a detailed history.
Complete a targeted examination (try to reproduce the symptom).
Obtain any necessary studies for evaluation.
Educate the patient regarding the use of a 0–10 severity scale (0 = none, and 10 = worst possible).
Begin therapy at the time of evaluation to achieve initial control of symptoms.
Use around-the-clock dosing to avoid peaks and troughs, *not* as-needed orders.
Give directions for what to do if the symptom recurs before the next dose of medication is due (i.e., prescribe a breakthrough dose: one sixth of the total daily dose q2h between scheduled doses).
Establish a mechanism to reassess response to therapy within the first hour after treatment if medication is given by mouth and sooner if using the intravenous route.
Repeat the use of the severity scale to assess relief.
Adjust treatment as necessary.

Adapted from Ingham JM, Portenoy RK: The management of pain and other symptoms. In Doyle D, Hanks GWC, McDonald N, editors: *Oxford textbook of palliative medicine*, ed 2, Oxford, UK, 1998, Oxford University Press.

and psychotherapy have been noted to improve ART adherence and reduce sexual risk behaviors in the HIV population and may be related to disease course.[20] A 9-year longitudinal study of 400 HIV-infected men found earlier progression to AIDS in those who were depressed at entry and 67% greater risk of mortality than those without symptoms after 7 years.[21] Given the current epidemiology in the United States, it is important to screen for depression and childhood trauma in patients at all stages of illness.

LOSS OF VIRAL CONTROL AND THREATS TO SURVIVAL

The HIV-1 virus mutates rapidly, hence the need for combination chemotherapy. Resistance has become a major problem in the United States, with some cities having low treatment success rates even after 1 year of use of cART because of transmissible resistant virus. Lack of adherence to therapy throughout the United States is probably the primary reason for such failure at this time. While pursuing active therapy, it is not recommended to continue a failing regimen for an extended period because this increases the likelihood of greater resistance to future agents. For persons without other treatment options, however, there may be no alternative.

Providers must recognize the psychological impact of implementing "salvage therapies" and recognize this as an indicator of poor prognosis and the need to revisit advance care planning. (Hopefully this will have been done when the patient was clinically stabilized; if not, raising it for the first time is necessary.) Life expectancy will likely be prolonged with changes in therapy, but attention to diet, use of antioxidants, and exercise plus other self-care methods will be helpful for both

---

Box 26-5. *Possible Indicators of Clinical Decline in HIV/AIDS*

- Need for more than one attempt at "salvage therapy"
- Occurrence of opportunistic infections
- Patient complains of being tired of taking antiretroviral medications
- Death of a spouse or partner
- Unresponsive depression despite pharmacologic treatment
- Need for monthly or more frequent clinical visits

---

patient and family. Box 26-5 highlights indicators of clinical decline in persons with HIV/AIDS.

Co-Morbidities and Long-Term Toxicities

MSM are at risk for diseases of the genitourinary system and may suffer cardiovascular toxicities. Persons with a history of intravenous drug use are likely to have hepatitis B or C and develop liver toxicity with cART; they may require repeated hospitalizations for infectious complications such as deep abscess or endocarditis. Regardless of risk factors for acquiring HIV, as life expectancy is extended, infected individuals appear to develop more malignancies and have time to suffer from end-organ failure of multiple causes.

Toxicity from thymidine analogues (nucleoside reverse transcriptase inhibitors [NRTIs]) is insidious and progressive; it is related to mitochondrial damage. Early manifestations may be loss of facial fat and muscular wasting, followed by nonspecific anorexia, myalgias, and nausea; finally it becomes fatal with a presentation of unresponsiveness and lactic acidosis. Clinicians must be aware of this syndrome to remove offending agents in time to avert rapid demise in an intensive care setting (Box 26-6).

Attention to symptoms helps to build a trusting patient–provider relationship. Because of expected toxicities, other specialists may be needed to ensure best clinical care, but it is imperative that the managing provider keep patient and family goals of care in sight. Dealing with multiple specialists may distract both patients and providers from substantive issues such as identification of a health proxy or psychospiritual components of care. Primary providers must routinely and specifically ask about patient goals of care and avoid the trap of trying to prolong life without balancing the burden of illness.

Life Expectancy and Changing Causes of Death

The CDC's life table curves for persons diagnosed since 2003 demonstrate little loss of life in the short term. Recent changes to treatment guidelines recommending initiation of cART at higher CD4 cell counts make it likely that this trend will continue. The impact on the number of new cases per year is yet to be determined, but ability to maintain fully suppressed viral replication predicts positive clinical outcomes. Advanced immunosuppression can be overcome if post-treatment CD4+ cell counts rise above 0.200×10^9 cells/L[22] and incidence of AIDS-defining events declines significantly ($P < .001$) after initiation of cART, especially those of viral origin such as Kaposi sarcoma.[23] Persons living with HIV disease now develop

Box 26-6. *Toxicities Associated with Highly Active Antiretroviral Therapy and Prolonged Survival*

INTRAVENOUS DRUG USE
Injection site abscess
Sepsis
Endocarditis
Hepatitis B and C

HIGHLY ACTIVE ANTIRETROVIRAL THERAPY TOXICITY
Anemia (zidovudine)
Peripheral neuropathy (stavudine, didanosine, zalcitabine)
Xerostomia (didanosine)
Rash (nevirapine)
Lipodystrophies (protease inhibitors)
Osteoporosis (?)
Lactic acidosis (thymidine analogues)
Cardiomyopathy (protease inhibitors/abacavir)
Hepatotoxicity (non-nucleoside reverse transcriptase inhibitors)
Hypersensitivity reaction (abacavir) (HLAB*5701 5%–8%)

INFECTIOUS COMPLICATIONS (NONOPPORTUNISTIC)
Recurrent bacterial pneumonias
Liver failure (hepatitis C)
Vaginitis

MALIGNANT DISEASES
Kaposi sarcoma
Cervical cancer (human papillomavirus)
Rectal cancer (human papillomavirus)
Non-Hodgkin's lymphoma
Lung cancer[16] (smoking)

non-AIDS–defining malignancies, osteoporosis, and cardiovascular disease over time. Many with intravenous drug use as a risk factor also have hepatitis C and eventually may opt for liver transplant, putting their families at risk for complex bereavement issues after breaking free from addiction plus HIV disease, then dying from complications of transplant.

As life expectancy increases in persons with HIV/AIDS, there must be a shift to focus on quality of life, skills for coping with stress, decreasing social isolation, and improvement of well-being.[24] In the affected population, mental health issues such as depression, substance abuse, and childhood sexual or physical abuse can impact ability to adhere to therapy and remain in care, and these must be addressed in routine care settings.[25]

Recognition of Clinical Decline

Providers intent on achieving good health and chronic viral suppression in their patients may lose sight of signs that suggest a person living well with HIV disease is actually declining. Although HIV providers routinely monitor weight and immuno-logic parameters, it is possible to overlook general clinical decline unless one has a sense of the patient's overall quality of life. At the same time, the clinical delivery site must have some mechanism for tracking patients who drop out of care, because these may be the ones who are not doing well. Tables 26-2 and 26-3 contain parameters for reviewing patient progress.

Causes of Death

More than 50% of deaths in HIV-infected persons receiving cART are from causes other than AIDS. The French mortality survey of people dying with HIV in 2005 documented only 36% of that year's deaths with an AIDS-related diagnosis, 17% from cancer not related to AIDS or hepatitis, and 15% from liver disease.[26] The DAD study, an 11-cohort prospective study of 23,441 people taking cART that watched for adverse events, recorded 1246 deaths in the first 3.5 years, with 31% AIDS related; 14.5% liver related (primarily intravenous drug use and hepatitis B or C); 11% cardiac; 9.4% non-AIDS malignancies; and 33% other.[27]

End-of-Life Issues

STOPPING CRITICAL MEDICATIONS

As a person nears the end of life, it is useful to consolidate treatment and eliminate unnecessary drugs. Having been constantly prompted to "not miss" medications, it is extremely difficult for persons on cART to stop therapy. Medications used to prevent long-term side effects, such as those to control lipid levels, can be discontin-ued. Those that protect against opportunistic infections might be maintained until the last weeks of life. Providers must be aware of the emotional and psychological trauma of being told that medications taken diligently for years are no longer neces-sary. It is helpful to use wording that implies a need to reduce further toxicity by eliminating certain medications.

Persons living with HIV disease may not have been exposed to multiple deaths from this disease and are unaware of potential benefits of a hospice referral. These programs consider it part of their mandate to assist patients in gradually letting go of unnecessary therapies when death seems likely. It is worth a call to the local hospice program to understand specific entry requirements because support given can be useful for the whole family.

LIFE CLOSURE

Ensuring that patients and families have adequate time to complete end-of-life tasks is the responsibility of a primary care provider. To do this, it is necessary to under-stand what needs to be accomplished before someone can die peacefully in the United States. These tasks can be time consuming and cannot be accomplished quickly. Examples include making a will; arranging guardianship for small children or pets; resolving business issues; possibly making amends with estranged family members; making contact with close relatives who are incarcerated; saying goodbye to family and friends; and dispersing material goods of sentimental value.

Families and professionals alike feel disconcerted approaching the bedside of one who is dying. People who are dying want to know they are loved and will be

---

Box 26-7. *Topics for Families to Discuss with Patients Near*
the End of Life

Thank you for all that you have given me or done for me.
I love you, and your memory will stay alive with me.
Please *forgive me* if I have done anything to offend or hurt you.
I forgive you for any incidents that still concern you.
Goodbye—you have my permission to die. I will be okay, but I will remember you.

Adapted from Byock I: *The four things that matter most: a book about living,* New York, 2004, Free Press.

---

remembered after death. Talking about funny or even sad events, sharing stories and memories, or just sitting quietly are ideal methods for reassuring the dying person that his or her life has been of value and that he or she will be missed. In many cultures and religions, forgiveness is of paramount importance, and providing an opportunity to discuss this issue is welcomed. Conversation may seem uncomfortable at first, but those who are approaching the end of life have little time for superficial discussion and will appreciate meaningful time spent with close family and friends. An experienced provider recognizes that these conversations take time and will initiate the topic when signs begin to suggest deterioration of the patient's condition[28] (Box 26-7).

TIME OF DEATH

End-stage events can arrive with little warning; it is not unusual to see patients with HIV/AIDS admitted, intubated, and dead within hours to days of admission. For this reason, it is even more important to hold conversations regarding end-of-life care well ahead of time. Sudden critical illness is a time when input of a primary care provider is most useful in determining a patient's wishes.

Dying is ultimately a personal event and not a medical problem to be manipulated. Efforts of staff should be to create a safe and private space for the dying person and related family or friends to have time to themselves to adjust to this emotional experience. Cultural beliefs and practices must be respected, and allowing time to complete personal rituals is of utmost importance. Providing information regarding what will happen next with regard to facility policy is useful. Reassuring families and friends that they have provided comfort to the deceased can be helpful in their being able to grieve this loss of a loved one.

SELF-CARE OF PROVIDERS

Changes in long-term outlook for those with HIV disease require a different mentality on the part of providers. Treating HIV is no longer the emergency it once appeared to be, and providers must adapt their own management style. Although persons with HIV disease have historically taken an active role in their own care, shift to chronic illness management entails even more of a shift to patient empowerment and self-management.[29] This has implications for the managing provider and represents need for infrastructure that can respond to the self-care needs of patients. Mental health issues are common in people with HIV/AIDS; now that disease outcomes are better controlled, these issues may become more pressing, with implications for constructing effective referral networks.

Relative to HIV disease, workers have traditionally had difficulty coping with death of patients who are young or near their own age. Karasz and colleagues interviewed 16 physicians in the era since the introduction of combination antiretroviral therapy (cART). They identified core myths that interfere with providers' ability to fulfill the role of comforter and supporter. When patients do not adhere to cART and thus die "unnecessarily," from point of view of the provider, there is a psychological and practical challenge to the provider's concept of being a successful caregiver. Both cognitive and behavioral coping can lead to either positive acceptance or anger and detachment on the part of the provider. This has psychological consequences that may affect care.[30] Providers must be aware of how losses affect them personally. Palliative care acknowledges these challenges and the subsequent need for provider support similar to that needed by members of the family. Studies such as this illustrate the importance of insight and the judicial use of professional support mechanisms. Avoiding self-care activities may result in staff members who are dysfunctional, short tempered, or prone to absenteeism.

CULTURAL ISSUES AND RITUAL

For those experiencing loss either personally or professionally, the emotional response is similar across race, culture, religion, and country of origin, but responses and practices associated with recognition of death and coping with loss vary remarkably. Clinicians must attempt to understand cultural beliefs and practices of each family to assist in grieving. Anger often accompanies the dying process in any culture, and staff must not react to it personally. Quiet listening is an appropriate response for the family.

The AIDS Quilt, which memorializes more than 91,000 individuals who have died of AIDS, would now be more than 51 miles long if individual panels were laid end to end (www.aidsquilt.org). It is a visual reminder and represents the mourning of a society for those who have died as children and young people, thus robbing the survivors of a future with their loved ones. Mourning is often carried on silently by health care providers and workers and can become a source of chronic stress that leads to burnout and decreased effectiveness. The use of ritual is one mechanism to avert this syndrome.

Placing a silk flower on a vacated hospital bed after death, keeping a bulletin board in the staff area with pictures of patients, or creating a routine opportunity for staff members to remember those who have died can help individual workers achieve emotional closure after the death of a patient. Staff members often become surrogate family for patients who have outlived their own support systems.

Grieving losses related to HIV/AIDS can lead to complicated or unresolved grief[31] because coping with multiple deaths in a brief time is not equivalent to that of a single loss. Family members may have other losses to mourn, such as death from drug overdose or murder, in addition to the loss from HIV disease. When one experiences multiple loss, it is best to get counseling support from someone experienced with grief counseling.

PEARLS

- The number of simultaneous symptoms has more impact on quality of life than actual viral load or CD4 cell count.
- Use a checklist for tracking common symptoms; health professionals minimize their impact on quality of life.
- Control of one pain usually unmasks others.
- Loss of the facial fat pad forewarns of mitochondrial toxicity.
- A short course of steroids can stimulate appetite, activity, and well-being in persons with advanced disease.
- Implementing chronic care requires long-term self-care.

PITFALLS

- Not having the opinion of an HIV specialist when trying to predict prognosis
- Avoiding routine discussions, by the calendar, about a patient's desired goals of care
- Not taking into account performance status and wishes of patient when determining prognosis
- Focusing on making a living will when what is needed is a health power of attorney
- Assuming that current staff members can handle a patient's death without debriefing

Summary

AIDS, or acquired immune deficiency syndrome, has been transformed by combination antiretroviral therapy into a chronic illness. Changes in epidemiology in the United States must be considered when designing services for persons with HIV. The palliative approach to care can be integrated during all stages of illness to recognize psychological, emotional, spiritual, and social issues facing persons with this disease. Prognosis is generally based on response to cART. Life expectancy can be normal, but chances of developing comorbidities or advanced toxicities such as early aging are high.

HIV is becoming a comorbidity for other medical illnesses that simply complicates prognosis. The threat of HIV disease is the unexposed side of the proverbial iceberg. New "opt out" testing of multiple populations, such as pregnant women and patients admitted to hospitals (as occurred in the past with use of VDRL testing for syphilis), may identify other populations that can benefit from coordinated use of cART.

Symptom prevalence is high among AIDS patients—some experience up to 16 symptoms at any given time; providers consistently underestimate this. Peripheral neuropathy is the most common pain experienced; both HIV itself and antiretroviral therapies may contribute to this. Comorbidities exist for many AIDS patients, such as hepatitis C among those who acquired HIV through intravenous drug use, and include end-organ failure and malignancies that are related to either HIV or therapy.

Patients with AIDS face many losses as well as ongoing stigma; teamwork and support for the patient's unique family unit is important.

IMPACT OF INTERNATIONAL EPIDEMIC ON UNITED STATES

In 2007, there were 1.8 to 2.3 million deaths worldwide because of HIV/AIDS; more than 1000 people died each day in South Africa alone. Life expectancy decreased in many African countries, dropping from the 50s to 29 years in some countries. Sixty percent of patients in sub-Saharan African hospitals are HIV positive. Deaths from HIV/AIDS in adults and children in the United States increased to 22,000 in 2007. For at least 12 sub-Saharan African countries, death figures are 1.5 to 15 times greater than that, depending on the country. Statistics are hard to come by because of poor record systems, but the point is clear—thousands die daily with little documented care.

Ultimately there has been an impact on care in the United States as providers are attracted to work where there is greater need, taking trained professionals from the HIV workforce. Immigrants continue to enter the United States carrying strains of HIV that require different management skills from those encountered in the early epidemic here. Lessons learned from treatment attempts in African countries show that near-perfect adherence can be achieved at least initially and that this has a positive impact on the course of illness even when patients present late. Palliative care in African countries has a much broader focus, without funding restrictions seen in the United States, although resources remain scarce and such care is very limited.

Additional figures for this chapter can be found online at www.expertconsult.com.

Resources

Alexander CS, Carter KR: Palliative and end-of-life care. In Bartlett JG, editor: *Primary Care of People with HIV/AIDS, 2004 Edition*. USHHS-HRSA HIV/AIDS Bureau, 2004. Available at www.hab.hrsa.gov.

Bartlett JG, Gallant, JE, Pham PA: Medical Management of HIV Infection 2009–2010. Available at www.mmhiv.org.

O'Neill JF, Selwyn PA, Schietinger H, editors: *A clinical guide to supportive and palliative care for HIV/AIDS*, Rockville, Md, 2003, Health Resources and Services Administration.

Workgroup on Palliative and End-of-Life Care in HIV/AIDS: Integrating Palliative Care into the Continuum of HIV Care: An Agenda for Change. Promoting Excellence in End-of-Life Care. University of Montana, 2004. Available at www.promotingexcellence.org/hiv/hiv_report/downloads/hiv_report.pdf.

References

1. 12th European AIDS Clinical Society Conference Abstract PS5/3. Presented November 12, 2009.
2. Deeks SG: Immune dysfunction, inflammation, and accelerated aging in patients on antiretroviral therapy, *Topics in HIV Medicine* 17(4):118–123, 2009.
3. Selwyn PA: Why should we care about palliative care for AIDS in the era of anti-retroviral therapy? *Sex Transm Infect* 81:2–3, 2005.
4. Silberstein J, Downs T, Lakin C, et al: HIV and prostate cancer: a systematic review of the literature, *Prostate Cancer Prostatic Dis* 12(1):6–12, 2009.
5. Meade CS, Kershaw TS, Hansen NB, et al: Long-term correlates of childhood abuse among adults with severe mental illness: adult victimization, substance abuse, and HIV sexual risk behavior, *AIDS Behav* 13(2):207–216, 2009.
6. Selwyn PA, Rivard M: Palliative care for AIDS: Challenges and opportunities in the era of highly active anti-retroviral therapy, *J Pall Med* 6:475–487, 2003.
7. Grady PA, Knebel AR, Draper A: End-of-life issues in AIDS: the research perspective, *J Roy Soc Med* 94:479–482, 2001.
8. Selwyn PA, Forstein M: Overcoming the false dichotomy of curative vs. palliative care for late-stage HIV/AIDS: "Let me live the way I want to live, until I can't," *JAMA* 290:806–814, 2003.
9. Harding R, Karus D, Easterbrook P, et al: Does palliative care improve outcomes for patients with HIV/AIDS? A systematic review of the evidence, *Sex Transm Infect* 81:5–14, 2005.

10. Curtis JR, Patrick DL, Caldwell E, et al: The quality of patient-doctor communication about end-of-life care: a study of patients with advanced AIDS and their primary care clinicians, *AIDS* 13:1123–1131, 1999.
11. Lynne J: Personal communication.
12. Vogl D, Rosenfeld, Breitbart W, et al: Symptom prevalence, characteristics, and distress in AIDS outpatients, *J Pain Symptom Manage* 18:253–262, 1999.
13. Justice AC, Holmes W, Gifford AL, et al: Development and validation of a self-completed HIV symptom index, *J Clin Epidemiol* 54(Suppl 1):S77–S90, 2001.
14. Hays RD, Cunningham WE, Sherbourne CD, et al: Health-related quality of life in patients with human immunodeficiency virus infection in the US: results from the HIV Cost and Services Utilization Study, *Am J Med* 108:714–722, 2000.
15. Corless IB, Voss JG, Nicholas PK, et al: Fatigue in HIV/AIDS patients with co-morbidities, *App Nurs Res* 21:116–122, 2008.
16. Harding R, Molloy T, Easterbrook P, et al: Is antiretroviral therapy associated with symptom prevalence and burden? *Int J STD AIDS* 17:400–405, 2006.
17. Basu S, Bruce RD, Barry DT, et al: Pharmacological pain control for human immunodeficiency virus-infected adults with a history of drug dependence, *J Subst Abuse Treat* 32:399–409, 2007.
18. Weissman DF, Haddox JD: Opioid pseudoaddiction: an iatrogenic syndrome, *Pain* 36:363–366, 1989.
19. Karus D, Raveis VH, Marconi K, et al: Mental health status of clients from three HIV/AIDS palliative care projects, *Palliat Support Care* 2:125–138, 2004.
20. Leserman J: Role of depression, stress, and trauma in HIV disease progression, *Psychosomatic Med* 70:539–545, 2008.
21. Mayne TJ, Vittinghoff E, Chesney MA, et al: Depressive affect and survival among gay and bisexual men infected with HIV, *Arch Int Med* 156:2233–2238, 1996.
22. Anastos K, Barron Y, Cohen MH, et al: The prognostic importance of changes in CD4+ cell count and HIV-1 RNA level in women after initiating highly active antiretroviral therapy, *Ann Intern Med* 140:256–264, 2004.
23. Antiretroviral Therapy Cohort Collaboration: The changing incidence of AIDS events in patients receiving highly active antiretroviral therapy, *Arch Intern Med* 165:416–423, 2005.
24. Vosvick M, Koopman C, Gore-Felton C, et al: Relationship of functional quality of life to strategies for coping with the stress of living with HIV/AIDS, *Psychosomatics* 44:(1)51–58, 2003.
25. Pence BW: The impact of mental health and traumatic life experiences in antiretroviral treatment outcomes for people living with HIV/AIDS, *J Antimicrob Chemother* 63:636–640, 2009.
26. Lewden C, Thierry M, Rosenthal E, et al: Changes in causes of death among adults infected by HIV between 2000 and 2005: the "Mortalité 2000 and 2005" surveys (ANRS EN19 and Mortavic), *J AIDS* 48(5):590–598, 2008.
27. Weber R, Sabin CA, Friis-Moller N, et al: Liver-related deaths in persons infected with the human immunodeficiency virus: the D.A.D. study, *Arch Int Med* 166(15):1632–1641, 2006.
28. Larson DG, Tobin DR: End-of-life conversations, *JAMA* 284(12):1573–1578, 2000.
29. Wagner EH, Austin BT, Davis C, et al: Improving chronic illness care: translating evidence into action, *Health Affairs* 20(6):64–78, 2001.
30. Karasz A, Dyche L, Selwyn P: Physicians' experiences of caring for late-stage HIV patients in the post-HAART era: challenges and adaptations, *Soc Sci Med* 57:1609–1620, 2003.
31. Rando T: *Treatment of complicated mourning*, Champaign, IL, 1993, Research Press.

CHAPTER 27

Heart Failure and Palliative Care

JOSHUA M. HAUSER and ROBERT O. BONOW

An 82-year-old woman who had not been to a physician in over 30 years was admitted to the hospital with fatigue and dyspnea. At home, she had been bedbound for the past two months and only got up to use the bathroom, which caused her dyspnea and panic. During this time, she had also lost 20 to 30 pounds of weight. On physical examination, she had rales half-way up both lung fields and a prominent systolic ejection murmur. An echocardiogram revealed severe systolic dysfunction.

She decided, with her son, that she did not want further intervention or investigation of either her cardiac status or of her weight loss. Upon hearing this, her physician called a palliative care consultation: "I'm not sure why, but I think it will help—she's not really in pain or anything" he said when the palliative care physician talked with him. At the end of the conversation, he added: "And I don't want her to give up."

This case is not an unusual one and it highlights the uncertain role of palliative care for patients with heart failure. Does palliative care have something to offer in this case? Is she giving up? Is her doctor giving up? What are the appropriate treatments for her dyspnea? What other symptoms might she be expected to have? This chapter addresses these questions.

Despite the fact that heart disease is the leading cause of death in the United States, it accounts for a minority of patients in palliative care and hospice programs. According to the latest figures available, cardiovascular disease was the leading cause of death in 2006: it accounted for over 631,00 deaths in the United States, or more than 25.6% of all deaths.[1] Two other diseases which are closely linked to heart disease, cerebrovascular disease and diabetes contribute to another 137,119 and 72,449 deaths

391

annually. In the same year, cancer accounted for over 559,000 deaths or 23.0% of all deaths. By contrast, in 2008 while 11.7% of patients enrolled in hospice had a primary diagnosis of heart disease, 38.3% had a diagnosis of cancer.[2] Compared to the burden in the general US population, cancer is over-represented among patients receiving hospice care and heart disease is under-represented. Given this incongruence, it is likely that many patients who might benefit from palliative care are not receiving it. Although it is likely that there are patients with heart disease who receive palliative care outside of formally being enrolled in hospice, these numbers serve as some objective data concerning the volume of patients formally enrolled in one type of palliative care program.

This chapter discusses the epidemiology of heart failure, the prevalence and treatment of common symptoms in patients with heart failure and ends with a consideration of some of this issues that are particularly challenging for patients with heart failure considering palliative care.

How is Heart Failure Different from Cancer?

Both heart failure and cancer are increasingly viewed as chronic conditions. This view implies that there is usually no specific point at which the illness switches from "treatable" to "terminal" but rather a transition exists and its nature depends on features that include illness severity and patient and family goals of care. The ideas denoted by the terms palliative care, survivorship and rehabilitation are all part of a recognition that optimizing quality of life and functional status can and should go hand-in-hand with disease-directed treatments. Both the Centers for Disease Control (CDC) and the American Cancer Society, for example, have devoted significant resources to educating the public around issues of long-term survival in cancer.[3,4] Multiple stages exist for both heart failure and cancer during which a combination of disease-modifying and symptom-directed or palliative therapies are appropriate. Data from Lunney and colleagues has lent empirical evidence to the chronic and stuttering trajectory of symptoms and care that heart failure patients experience in the last year of life.[5] It is a trajectory that frequently involves multiple exacerbations of symptoms, multiple changes in medications and management strategies and multiple emergency department visits and hospitalizations.

This view of heart failure as a chronic illness may make the transition to palliative care more challenging: Cardiologists and their patients may perceive that continuing advances in drug therapy and cardiac devices will prolong length of life and quality of life, and thus may be less inclined to consider the possibility of treatment failure than oncologists and their patients. As an example, Schoevaerdts and colleagues identified a number of differences between cancer and heart failure that may influence decisions about palliative care:[6] The illness course is often perceived of as fluctuating as opposed to progressive; prognosis is perceived as unpredictable as opposed to predictable; the "terminal phase" of the illness is less clearly delineated; and sudden death is more frequent in the case of heart failure compared to cancer.

In this area of disease perception, there are data to suggest that physicians may view palliative care and heart failure as a challenging combination. In a qualitative study of British physicians including cardiologists, general practitioners and palliative medicine specialists, Hanratty and colleagues[7] found that barriers to developing approaches that integrated palliative care and heart failure fell into three main groups: the organization of health care, the unpredictable course of heart failure, and physicians' understanding of the roles of different specialists and disciplines caring for patients. It is likely that each of these may be a barrier for the optimum delivery of palliative care to patients with heart failure. The authors interpreted their findings to mean that these barriers can lead to late referrals and a lack of complete palliative care for patients with heart failure at multiple stages of their illness.

These differences in disease perception between cancer and heart failure have implications for how physicians care for patients with heart failure. A study by McKinley and colleagues compared care delivered by general practitioners in the last year of life to people who died with cancer and those who died with cardiovascular and respiratory disease.[8] They found that when compared with people who died with cardiovascular and respiratory disease, those who died with cancers were more likely to have had a "terminal phase" of their illness identified by their health care providers and to have been prescribed more palliative (symptom control) medications. At the same time, there were some encouraging similarities in the care of both groups of patients with cancer and with heart disease: both groups had a similar number of specialist consultations, experienced similar continuity of care, had similar levels of comorbid conditions, and were equally likely to die at home.

Data also exist that suggest that patients view the experience of living with (and dying of) heart failure and cancer differently. Murray and colleagues conducted longitudinal in-depth interviews with both groups of patients and found that patients with heart failure generally had less information about and poorer understanding of their condition and prognosis and were less involved in decision making than those with heart failure. While those with cancer more explicitly talked about dying, they found that "Frustration, progressive losses, social isolation, and the stress of balancing and monitoring a complex medication regimen dominated the lives of patients with cardiac failure".[9]

Taken as a group, these studies suggest that both physician and patient perception may present challenges in introducing palliative care into the setting of heart failure.

Epidemiology and Mortality

There are approximately 5.8 million Americans living with heart failure and there are 670,000 new (or incident) cases per year.[10,11] The number of patients discharged from hospitals with a diagnosis of heart failure was more than 1.1 million in 2006.[10] From an economic standpoint, estimates for the direct and indirect costs of heart failure range from $39.2–58 billion a year.[10,12]

In terms of mortality, newly diagnosed heart failure in the community carries a mortality of 24%, 37%, and 75% at 1, 2, and 6 years. For patients with advanced (New York Heart Association [NYHA] class IV) heart failure, the rate of rehospitalization or death is 81% at 1 year. In patients with a left ventricular ejection fraction of less than 25%, NYHA class IV symptoms (for example, dyspnea and angina at rest) for more than 90 days, oxygen consumption of 12 ml/kg or inotropic dependence, mortality is 50% at 6 months. For patients on continuous inotropic support, mortality is 75% at 6 months. Although these numbers parallel the mortality from a number of advanced stage cancers, another key difference for patients with heart failure is the frequency of sudden death: unlike cancer, where deaths may be perceived as following a predictable course, up to one-half of all deaths are sudden.[13]

Guidelines

In the face of the high disease burden that heart failure confers on the population, the consideration of palliative care for these patients has taken on some urgency. In general, the integration of palliative care principles into disease-specific guidelines has been an important step in increasing the presence of palliative care in mainstream medicine for both cancer and non-cancer illnesses. The American Hospice Foundation, for example, has developed such guidelines for cancer and non-cancer illnesses and the National Comprehensive Cancer Network (NCCN) has done so for a range of cancer diagnoses.[14,15] More recently, in cardiology and pulmonary medicine, guidelines issued by both the American College of Chest Physicians[16] and the American College of Cardiology/American Heart Association (ACC/AHA)[17] have addressed palliative strategies within their overall management guidelines. Finally, the Heart Rhythm Society (HRS) in collaboration with the American College of Cardiology, the American Geriatrics Society, the American Academy of Hospice and Palliative Medicine, the American Heart Association, and the European Heart Rhythm Association have developed a consensus statement on the management of ICDs and other implantable devices in patients nearing the end of life. These guidelines lay out clear ethical principles regarding the right of patients and families to withdraw implantable devices and also suggest communication strategies to discuss these decisions.[18]

The newest (2009) ACC/AHA guidelines lay out clear assessment and management strategies for every stage of heart failure. Importantly, these guidelines include a section on "end-of-life considerations in the setting of heart failure." Among the recommendations for patients with end-stage heart failure are areas such as ongoing education for patients and their families concerning prognosis, functional capacity, the role of palliative care, discussion of implanted cardiac defibrillators (ICD) deactivation, coordination of care, and the use of opioids for symptomatic relief. Importantly, the ACC/AHA guidelines also suggest that the use of inotropes and intravenous diuretics may be appropriate for some patients with end-stage heart failure who are receiving palliative care. The issue of inotropes in patients with heart failure in palliative care is discussed later in this chapter.

These recommendations parallel an overall palliative approach to any illness in their attention to symptoms, comprehensive assessment, whole-person care, goals of care, and coordination of care. In addition to these general principles, the ACC/AHA guidelines advise that "aggressive procedures (including intubation and AICDs) within the final days are not appropriate." Although this presents a challenge to our recognized inaccuracies of prognostication,[19] there are generally agreed upon criteria that include decreased to minimal responsiveness, severely compromised functional status and minimal urine output that palliative care physicians routinely use to assess the last days of life. Although some of these signs and symptoms have been shown to be valid and reliable predictors of prognosis in the setting of patients in palliative care with cancer,[20] they have not been subjected to empirical scrutiny in the setting of heart failure. The ACC/AHA guidelines take a broad view of the question of determining when the "end of life is nearing" to include multiple subjective and objective factors, including functional status, oxygen dependence, and echocardiographic evidence of heart failure. In the end, they recommend an individualized approach to care: "Ultimately the decisions regarding when the end of life is nearing reflect a complex interaction between objective and subjective information, emotions and patient and family readiness."

The ACC/AHA guidelines are a comprehensive attempt to gather state-of-the-art evidence for recommendations to clinicians. For many of the recommendations concerning disease-specific treatments, such as the use of angiotensin converting enzyme (ACE) inhibitors and beta blockers, evidence reaches the level of "class A" (data derived from multiple randomized clinical trials or meta-analyses). For all of the recommendations concerning palliative care, however, it is revealing that the level of evidence is "class C" (only consensus, case studies, and standard of care as opposed to data from clinical trials). This suggests that the field may be early in its integration of palliative care. At the same time, it is likely that the types of evidence needed to support some of the palliative interventions may differ from traditional clinical trials for disease-modifying medications.

Another set of guidelines specifically concerning palliative care and heart failure has been issued by a group of cardiologists and palliative care physicians.[21] These guidelines were issued from a consensus conference "convened to define the current state and important gaps in knowledge and needed research on 'Palliative and Supportive Care in Advanced Heart Failure.'" Although they did not formally grade their evidence in the same manner as the ACC/AHA guidelines, they derive their guidelines from expert opinion and review of the medical literature and other guidelines. They identified the need for research on symptom clusters, prognostication, and coordination of care approaches to heart failure as priorities as the fields of palliative care and heart failure become more tightly linked and move forward.

Symptoms

Despite some of the limitations of the empirical evidence behind these guidelines, we do have some data concerning symptoms in patients with heart failure. Two of the largest trials that examined symptoms for patients near the end-of-life include the SUPPORT trial (The Study to Understand Prognoses and Preferences for Outcomes and Risks of Treatments)[22] and the United Kingdom Regional Study of Care of the Dying (RSCD).[23] Each of these studies had a component that assessed symptoms of patients facing the end-of-life and each included patients with heart failure.

In one analysis of the SUPPORT trial that examined elderly patients with heart failure, Levenson and colleagues reported that 60% of patients had dyspnea and 78% had pain. Among those in the hospital, the number in pain was 41%. Notably, these symptoms persisted through the final days of life: patient surrogates reported that 41% of patients were in severe pain and 63% were severely short of breath at some point during the final three days before death.[24] Psychological symptoms, including depression, anxiety, and confusion were all between 10 and 20% in this sample from SUPPORT. In the subsample of patients in the RSCD with heart failure, pain was experienced by 50%, dyspnea by 43%, and low mood and anxiety in 59 and 45% of patients respectively.

Smaller studies of the prevalence of symptoms in patients with heart failure have reported similar results. In a study of patients in one hospital, Jiang and colleagues found that 35% of patients screened positively on the Beck Depression Inventory and 13.9% of patients had a diagnosable major depressive disorder. These numbers have prognostic implications for patients: Jiang's study found that untreated depression in the setting of heart failure is a risk factor for increased mortality.[25] The high symptom burden on patients with heart failure is not just for those who are hospitalized: A study of patients with heart failure in a community-based hospice found a prevalence of pain in 25%, dyspnea in 60%, and confusion in 48%.[26] If anything, these numbers may underestimate the numbers in a general population of home-bound patients with heart failure, as it is likely that these patients were receiving some symptomatic care through their hospice program.

Treatment

STANDARD TREATMENT FOR HEART FAILURE

Heart failure is unlike some illnesses in palliative care because a number of its treatments have quality of life benefits as well as disease-modifying effects. This contrasts with many types of cancer in which the disease-modifying treatments may have deleterious effects on quality of life while also having the potential to increase length of life. For example, two of the cornerstones of treatment for heart failure, laid out in the most recent ACC/AHA guidelines[27] and in recent review articles[28,29] include the use of ACE-inhibitors or angiotensin receptor blockers (ARBs) and beta blockers, both types of medications which have been shown to both improve survival and decrease repeated hospitalizations: i.e., mortality as well as quality of life benefits. Since they have documented effects on quality of life, these medicines should be continued in palliative care. Their use is an important example of how to implement the philosophy that palliative care might include the continuation of disease-modifying therapies as well as comfort-oriented therapies concurrently.

Two other medications for heart failure, diuretics and digoxin, also have effects on quality of life with less clear effects on mortality. Furosemide is the main diuretic for use for patients with fluid overload in the setting of heart failure. Its effects can be potentiated by spironolactone which, when added to a loop diuretic such as furosemide, has been shown to have both mortality and symptomatic benefits and also result in reduced hospitalizations in the setting of heart failure.[30] Although digoxin has been shown to have no effect on mortality,[31] it has been shown in a Cochrane review to have symptomatic benefits in terms of decreased dyspnea and result in fewer repeat hospitalizations.[32] Therefore, these medications should be continued as well.

Intravenous inotropic medications (such as dobutamine or milrinone) may represent a dilemma for many patients, families, and providers. Although these medications have been shown to result in excess mortality in some randomized trials, they have also been shown to decrease hospitalizations and symptoms among patients with end-stage heart failure.[33,34] Recommendations concerning these medications in advanced heart failure management generally includes their use as a "bridge" to cardiac transplantation and as a palliative measure in patients with end-stage heart failure whose symptoms are refractory to other treatments.[35] In the setting of hospice and palliative care, the use of intravenous inotropes may represent a challenges to philosophy of care (Is this treatment "aggressive" or "palliative"?), education (Do we have the resources among our nurses and/or physicians to administer these safely in the home or nursing home setting?), and finances (In the face of the capitated reimbursement that hospices receive, are we able to afford this medication?). Although there are no clear guidelines at this point in time for the use of these medications in the palliative care or hospice context, there are case studies of patients benefiting from their use.[36] As the number of patients with heart failure who elect to be cared for by hospices increases, more and more individual programs and physicians will face this dilemma.

SYMPTOMATIC TREATMENT

The treatments described above directed at the underlying pathophysiology heart failure will frequently have symptomatic benefits. However, in addition to such "disease-modifying" treatments, additional symptomatic treatment may be needed for every patient with heart failure.

DYSPNEA

The key medications for the medical treatment of dyspnea in the setting of heart failure include diuretics and opioids. Wherever possible, treatment directed at the underlying etiology of the dyspnea will help to avoid potential side effects of opioids which can include confusion, somnolence, nausea, and constipation. For example, if dyspnea is due to a pleural effusion, drainage by thoracentesis may be effective temporarily, but these effusions frequently recur. If dyspnea is due to pulmonary edema, furosemide, or another loop diuretic may be effective.

Patients with heart failure may have other causes of dyspnea: when it is due to cardiac ischemia (angina), a nitrate should be used. This can include immediate release sub-lingual nitroglycerin and extended oral or transdermal nitrates when the angina is recurrent and predictable. Patients who get anginal symptoms and dyspnea with a predictable amount of exertion can be counseled to take a nitrate before activity. When dyspnea is due to rapid atrial fibrillation, rate control with digoxin, a beta-blocker, or other agent is appropriate to decrease cardiac workload.

Clinicians also need to be alert to co-morbid non-cardiac conditions in patients with heart failure before ascribing all symptoms to their primary diagnosis. When dyspnea is due to co-existing asthma or chronic obstructive pulmonary disease (COPD), an appropriate symptomatic approach includes inhaled beta-agonists (e.g., albuterol), inhaled steroids (e.g., beclamethasone), or inhaled anti-cholinergic medications (e.g., ipratropium bromide) as well as oral steroids (e.g., prednisone) in the setting of sever illness. In the setting where it is difficult to differentiate between heart failure and COPD as the cause for dyspnea, the measurement of brain natriuretic peptide (BNP) can help to distinguish between the two etiologies and help to direct therapy.[37]

Pneumonia is also common in patients who are debilitated due to heart failure, and its treatment will depend on the patient's overall prognosis and goals of care. There may, for example, be situations in which patients who appear to have a life expectancy of weeks to months develop a pneumonia, and they and their physicians make a decision to treat with either oral or intravenous antibiotics. There may be other times when a patient with heart failure is bedbound and minimally responsive and whose prognosis is likely days, where a candid and sensitive discussion with the patient and his or her family may result in a decision not to use antibiotics, but to emphasize treatments for the symptom of dyspnea alone.

Finally, sleep apnea has been shown to be associated to heart failure and its treatment may help to improve symptoms of fatigue and dyspnea.[38] The formal diagnosis of sleep apnea requires an overnight sleep study in a sleep laboratory. In patients who are homebound, overnight pulse oximetry in the home can sometimes be an alternative. The standard treatment for sleep apnea is the nighttime use of continuous positive airway pressure (CPAP). More recently, a randomized trial has shown some efficacy using acetazolamide as treatment for sleep apnea.[39] Although the use of CPAP is initially difficult for many patients, it is frequently something that they can adapt to and tolerate after continued use. Medical centers with experienced respiratory care programs will have expertise in the adjustment of specific ventilatory settings as well as suggestions to increase patient comfort and tolerance of CPAP.

Although oxygen is commonly used in hospice and hospital contexts, a review found little data to support its use in relieving dyspnea secondary to heart failure,[40] especially when used as the sole treatment for dyspnea. As an adjunct to other symptomatic treatments as described above, its efficacy is less clear. It may hold symbolic value as an example of continued care and attention for the patient and family and therefore, its use, including the possibility that it may contribute to prolonging life, can be discussed openly with patient and family. Patients and families may feel that it is a requirement when they are in the hospital and not be aware that like any other intervention, its use can be considered in terms of overall goals for care for a given patient. Conversely, patients and families may perceive discontinuing oxygen as a sign that the physicians are "giving up" on a patient. Along with the administration of oxygen, patients in the hospital context as well as those being discharged, may be accustomed to having their pulse oximetry measured at regular intervals and oxygen titrated accordingly. As the patient's clinical condition and goals for care change and as symptom relief becomes the primary focus for patients, both the administration of oxygen and the monitoring of it should be re-addressed with patients and their families.

PAIN

Pain is common in patients with heart failure. Most of this pain is actually non-cardiac in origin and stems from co-existing arthritic or musculoskeletal disease.[41] Anginal pain can be treated with nitrates. Other pain in patients with heart failure can be treated with standard doses of opioids according to World Health Organization (WHO) criteria.[42] One should be cautious in patients with renal insufficiency, which is common in patients with advanced heart failure. First, non-steroidal anti-inflammatory (NSAIDs) medications can worsen renal insufficiency. Second, both morphine and hydromorphone (Dilaudid) have metabolites that can accumulate and lead to adverse neuro-excitatory effects including tremors, myoclonus, and more rarely, seizures. Generally, doses should start low and be increased slowly, especially in elderly patients. When neuro-excitatory side effects do occur, one can reduce the opioid dose, rotate opioids, or add a low dose of a benzodiazepine such as clonazepam. Since patients with heart failure are frequently on multiple medications and at risk for polypharmacy, this last approach should be reserved for cases when opioid dose-reduction or opioid rotation are unsuccessful. When the pain has a neuropathic component, treatment with an adjuvant medication, such as a tricyclic antidepressant (e.g., nortriptyline which has fewer anticholinergic side-effects than amitriptyline) or an anti-convulsant (e.g., gabapentin or pre-gabelin) are both effective.

Nonsteroidal anti-inflammatory drugs should generally be avoided because of the risk of renal dysfunction and increased sodium and fluid retention. In patients with co-existing arthritis whose pain has been amenable to NSAIDs, one needs to balance the risks and the benefits of NSAID therapy. A recent review in this area strongly recommended the use of acetaminophen instead of NSAIDs for these reasons.[43] However, in patients whose prognosis may be weeks and who has unacceptable side effects to opioids or to steroids, the use of NSAIDs should be considered.

DEPRESSION

The prevalence of depression ranges from 24 to 42% in patients with heart failure.[44] Predictors of depression in patients with heart failure include living alone, alcohol abuse, perception of medical care being a substantial economic burden, and poor health status.[45] Its presence is associated with increased mortality in patients with heart failure.[46] In addition to being highly prevalent, it is often overlooked in the treatment of heart failure—up to 50% of patients with depression had it go undetected in one study.[47]

An approach to treatment includes counseling interventions and the use of selective serotonin reuptake inhibitors (SSRIs). Tricyclic antidepressants should generally be avoided due to potential cardiotoxic effects. The data concerning counseling and psychological interventions are mixed. A recent review from the Cochrane collaboration concerning depression in the setting of heart failure found that, although there is randomized clinical trial evidence for the effectiveness of counseling in the setting of depression following myocardial infarction, there is no such evidence for patients with heart failure. This review did, however, identify three observational trials suggesting some benefit to counseling.[48] The overall message of these studies is that depression is common, should be screened for, and requires both medications as well as counseling approaches.

We now turn to three topics that of particular importance in heart failure in the palliative care context: resuscitation and automated implantable defibrillators (AICDs), prognosis, and disease management programs.

Resuscitation and Automated Implantable Defibrillators (AICDs)

Twenty years ago, Wachter and colleagues found that do-not-resuscitate (DNR) orders were instituted for 5% of patients with heart failure, 47% of patients with unresectable malignancy, and 52% of patients with AIDS[49] despite similar prognoses. In a more recent trial that analyzed data from the SUPPORT study, Krumholz and colleagues found a low level of preferences for DNR order and a low level of discussions of resuscitation among patients with heart failure: 23% and 25% respectively. This study also found a moderate level of instability among preferences: when answering the same question two months later concerning resuscitation, 14% of patients who initially wanted resuscitation changed their preferences and 40% of those who did not want resuscitation changed their preferences.[50] In a study of homebound elderly patients with heart failure and dementia, investigators found that patients with heart failure were less likely to have a DNR order (62% vs. 91%), less likely to use hospice (24% vs. 61%), and more likely to die in hospital (45% vs. 18%) compared to patients with dementia.[51]

In summary, patients with heart failure appear to exhibit a lower prevalence of having DNR orders than patients with other illnesses. Although these studies cannot answer the question of what is the "correct" number of patients that "should" have DNR orders, the lack of these may be a marker for a lack of discussion about goals of care and prognosis with these patients and their families.

These studies are an important baseline upon which to consider approaches to patients with heart failure and AICDs. The goal of palliative care physicians should not be universal counseling against their use or in favor of their deactivation, but rather an approach that helps patients and families understand the relative benefits and burdens of this intervention at different stages of disease.

AICDs are currently indicated for primary and secondary prophylaxis of life-threatening arrhythmias and sudden death in the setting of heart failure and depressed ejection fraction. The numbers of patients who will be receiving AICDs will undoubt-edly expand significantly as indications for these devices grow.[52] Both conceptual and empirical literature concerning ethical issues in AICDs[53] has been developed and includes issues of when these "should" be deactivated and models for how we discuss these decisions with patients. In 2010, the main professional association of electro-physiologists, the Heart Rhythm Society, issued comprehensive guidelines as well.[54] There are clearly parallels with overall advance care planning discussions and discus-sions about general DNR orders.

But, as with many new technologies, our comfort level with utilizing the technol-ogy clinically may be outpacing out comfort level with communicating about the technology, both its benefits and its burdens. In one empirical study in this area, Goldstein and colleagues examined family members' views of the management of AICDs in end-of-life care.[55] In a retrospective survey of 100 family members of patients who died with AICDs in place, these investigators found that only 8 family members recalled patients receiving a shock from their AICDs in the minutes before death. They also found that these family members reported discussions of possible deactivation in only 27 of 100 cases and often only in the last few days of life. Although this study did not attempt to characterize the optimum time or the optimum structure for such discussions, it provides important baseline information that both shocks for resuscitation and prospective discussions of resuscitation may be uncommon in this group of patients. Nationally, recent data reveals that hospices frequently admit patients (97% of hospices surveyed) with AICDs, these patients are often shocked (58% of the time), and only 10% of hospices have a policy addressing deactivation.[56]

When these investigators began to analyze the barriers to these conversations, they found that although physicians (including cardiologists, electrophysiologists, inter-nists, and geriatricians) thought that these discussions should be part of advance care planning, there "was something intrinsic in these devices" that made them different from other decisions to withdraw therapies: this included their small size, the lack of an outward reminder of the device, and the absence of an established relationship with the patient.[57]

It is likely that these continued discussions will parallel the increasing level of comfort that the ICU community, the palliative care community, and the medical ethics community has had with withdrawal of ventilator support.

Prognosis

One of the often-repeated challenges for applying palliative care principles to heart failure is the issue of prognosis. It is likely not a significant difference when compared with the short length of survival among hospice patients overall: the most compre-hensive trial in this regard among a national sample of Medicare patients showed the hospice length of stay among heart failure patients to be slightly greater than among all hospice patients, regardless of diagnosis: 43.5 days vs. 36.0 days.[58] In a more recent, smaller survey of hospice providers, Goodlin and colleagues found a mean length of stay of 60 days among patients with heart failure in 70 US hospices.[59]

In recent years, investigators have developed more sensitive and better validated models of prognosis for inpatients with heart failure. Fonarow and colleagues used admission blood urea nitrogen (BUN) (43 mg/dl), creatinine (2.75 mg/dl),[60] and systolic blood pressure (115 mm Hg) to identify in-hospital mortality of 20% when all three criteria were met. Lee and colleagues identified clinical criteria to predict one-year mortality of 1–10% for lowest risk heart failure patients of 50–75% for highest risk patients.[61] Both of these studies will help us to prognosticate better in the context of heart failure, but they require us to apply them consistently and use the information to guide care and discussions with patients. It is important to note that both of these recent efforts have studied inpatients who may be more seriously ill and may have more clinical and laboratory data available than in outpatients, who comprise the majority of hospice patients with heart failure.

HOSPICE CRITERIA FOR HEART FAILURE

The National Hospice and Palliative Care Organization (NHPCO) has published criteria for the determination of prognosis in the setting of heart failure and other non-cancer diseases. Although the last update of these criteria was 1996, they do provide a framework for prognostication for patients with heart failure. Since they were issued before some of the studies cited above, they lack some of the more specific prognostic markers that those investigators found. The criteria include "symptoms of recurrent heart failure at rest (including an ejection fraction of 20%)," "optimal treatment" with medications directed at heart failure, and a number of co-morbidities include documented arrhythmias, syncope, previous cardiac arrest, and co-existing cerebrovascular disease.[62]

A study by Fox and colleagues examining the performance of these criteria in a well-defined population from the SUPPORT trial, however, has cast some doubt on the accuracy of these standards.[63] Although not limited to patients with heart failure, this study sheds light on the drawbacks of these overall prognostic criteria for non-cancer illnesses. These authors tested the ability of three levels of criteria (broad, intermediate, and narrow) aimed at providing low, medium, and high thresholds for hospice eligibility based on NHPCO guidelines. Broad inclusion criteria identified the most patients eligible for hospice care, of whom 70% survived longer than 6 months. Intermediate inclusion criteria identified only one third as many patients, of whom 65% survived longer than 6 months. Narrow inclusion criteria identified only 19 patients for inclusion, of whom 53% survived longer than 6 months. They concluded that for seriously ill hospitalized patients with advanced chronic obstructive pulmonary disease, heart failure, or end-stage liver disease, recommended clinical prediction criteria from NHPCO are not effective in identifying a population with a survival prognosis of 6 months or less. An analysis of SUPPORT data cited by Albert and colleagues demonstrated similar difficulties in our ability to prognosticate: among those with a predicted survival of 10% at 6 months, 38% were alive 6 months later.[64]

More recently, Bao and colleagues have developed a four item risk score for prognosticating in the setting of heart failure.[65] They used multivariate logistic regression analysis to identify four independent predictors of 6-month mortality in a cohort of patients aged 70 or above. These included blood urea nitrogen (BUN) of 30 mg/dL or greater, systolic blood pressure less than 120 mm Hg, peripheral arterial disease, and serum sodium less than 135 mEq/L. When they stratified patients into four risk groups based on the presence or absence of these four risk factors, they found six month mortality rates for patients with zero, one, two, or three or more risk factors to be 3.7%, 16.3%, 41.0%, and 66.7%. They interpreted these results as suggesting that a relatively simple risk score might be able to aid in prediction of mortality for patients with heart failure.

The continued attention to prognostic data will be important since as it is currently designed, hospice care is targeted to patients with a high risk of dying at 6 months.

Disease Management Programs

One investigator who studied physician views of palliative care and heart failure identified a disturbing but perhaps not surprising trend: "Care for patients dying with heart failure was described as uncoordinated, with patients going from hospital to community and back again. Repeated admissions to different consultant teams were common, and patients' medical notes were sometimes said to arrive on the wards after the patient had been discharged or died. A picture emerged of poor quality care for the patients and frustration for the doctors."[66] One potential solution to this is the further promotion of disease management programs for patients with heart failure and the more concerted integration of these with palliative care programs. There will be economic challenges to achieving this as currently hospice is reimbursed under a separate Medicare funding stream than home-based cardiology disease-management programs.

Although these programs have generally been distinct from hospice programs, they share certain care processes and care goals with traditional hospice: they usually consist of an interdisciplinary team that pro-actively manages patients at home with the goal of a) improved coordination and continuity of care and b) prevention of inappropriate hospitalization or emergency department use. They generally consist of phone calls or electronic contact with patients on a weekly or more frequent basis to inquire about symptoms such as dyspnea or chest pain and signs such as weight gain or edema and adjust medications (principally diuretics) and physician visits accordingly. Some of these programs have shown mortality benefits as well as reductions in hospitalizations and costs for patients.[67,68,69,70] As palliative care and hospice continues to integrate into the care of patients with heart failure, taking advantage of the both the infrastructure as well as the management techniques of these programs will be a crucial advance.

Conclusion: The Transition

Part of the difficulty in the transition to palliative care or hospice for patients with heart failure is that it is often considered only after the most aggressive treatments have been tried or proposed. For many patients and their families, this makes it a sudden shift in care and goals instead of a smooth transition. It is likely that palliative care principles of symptom management, attention to goals for care, and support for patients and their families may have the greatest impact on quality of life when introduced as early as possible in a patient's management. This will not mean an abandoning of traditional care and management of heart failure, but rather an augmentation of these.

In Jessup's review of heart failure in the *New England Journal of Medicine*, his stepwise management model includes treatments for patients with refractory symptoms such as inotropes, ventricular assist devices, and transplantation. This is a helpful algorithm for physicians. When these fail, the last step is hospice. By definition, this last step clearly includes aggressive means of symptom control and support for patients and their families. But in this sequence of heart failure management, the most symptom-focussed approach comes only after the most invasive, disease-modifying approaches.

As an alternative, increasing numbers of practitioners in the cardiology community and palliative care community are now advocating for early integration of symptomatic care in the management of patients with heart failure just as many in the palliative care community have advocated for the early integration of palliative principles from diagnosis onward.[71,72] Since many of the symptomatic therapies have disease-modifying aspects to them, this integration is all the more crucial.

This sentiment that palliative care is a dramatic, and perhaps unwelcome, alternative to cure, is not isolated to heart failure. As practitioners, we should not necessarily idealize palliative care as "equivalent to" a curative approach because for most patients and families, it is not. But nor should we underestimate its importance. Morgan and Murphy wrote of this sentiment in an editorial concerning the treatment of children with cancer, "In the United States, the need to fight the good fight is idealized and resistance to giving up is continued even in the face of overwhelming odds. The shift in the goal from achieving a cure to making the patient comfortable usually occurs only when all other options have been exhausted, perpetuating the myth that palliative care is second best."[73] For patients with heart failure and their families as well as their health care team, this "fight" may be an important one to engage in, especially in the face of expanding technologies and treatments with clear mortality benefits for heart failure. There are, however, two clinical instincts that need to accompany this fight: One, the integration of palliative care principles from diagnosis on and two, the recognition of when a patient might be better served by re-focusing the goals for such a battle from victory in the form of a "cure" to victory in the form of the best possible quality of life and support we can offer.

References

1. National Vital Statistics Reports: www.cdc.gov/nchs/data/nvsr/nvsr54/nvsr54_13.pdf, 2006.
2. National Hospice and Palliative Care Organization: http://www.nhpco.org/files/public/Statistics_Research/NHPCO_facts_and_figures.pdf.
3. www.cdc.gov/cancer/survivorship/index.htm.
4. www.cancer.org/docroot/HOME/srv/srv_0.asp.
5. Lunney JR, Lynn J, Foley DJ, et al: Patterns of functional decline at the end of life, *JAMA* 289:2387–2392, 2003.
6. Schoevaerdts D, Swine C, Vanpee D: Heart failure [letter], *N Eng J Med* 349:1002–1004, 2003.
7. Hanratty B, Hibbert D, Mair F, et al: Doctors' perceptions of palliative care for heart failure: focus group study, *Br Med J* 325(7364):581–585, 2002.
8. McKinley RK, et al: Care of people dying with malignant and cardiorespiratory disease in general practice, *Br J Gen Pract* 54(509):909–913, 2004.
9. Murray SA, Boyd K, Kendall M, et al: Dying of lung cancer or cardiac failure: prospective qualitative interview study of patients and their carers in the community, *Br Med J* 325:929, 2002.
10. Rogers JG, Rich MW: Management of Advanced Heart Failure. In Berger AM, Portenoy RK, Weissman DE, editors: *Principles and practice of palliative care and supportive oncology*, ed 2, Philadelphia, 2002, Lippincott Williams and Wilkins.
11. http://circ.ahajournals.org/cgi/reprint/CIRCULATIONAHA.109.192667.
12. O'Connell JB: The economic burden of heart failure, *Clin Cardiol* 23(Suppl III):III-6–III-10, 2000.
13. Hauptman PJ, Havranek EP: Integrating palliative care into heart failure care, *Arch Intern Med* 165(4):374–378, 2005.
14. Emanuel L, Alexander C, Arnold RM, et al: Palliative Care Guidelines Group of the American Hospice Foundation: integrating palliative care into disease management guidelines, *J Palliat Med* 7(6):774–783, 2004.

15. NCCN Guidelines: Available at www.nccn.org.
16. Selecky PA, Eliasson CA, Hall RI, et al: American College of Chest Physicians. Palliative and end-of-life care for patients with cardiopulmonary diseases: American College of Chest Physicians position statement, *Chest* 128(5):3599–3610, 2005.
17. Hunt SA, Abraham WT, Chin MH, et al: ACC/AHA 2010 guideline update for the diagnosis and management of chronic heart failure in the adult, *Circulation* 112:1–28, 2005.
18. Lampert R, Hayes DL, Annas GJ, et al: HRS expert consensus statement on the management of cardiovascular implantable electronic devices (CIEDs) in patients nearing end of life or requesting withdrawal of therapy, *Heart Rhythm*, 2010, in press. Available at www.hrsonline.org/Policy/ClinicalGuidelines/ceids_mgmt.cfm.
19. Christakis NA, Lamont EB: Extent and determinants of error in doctors' prognoses in terminally ill patients: prospective cohort study, *Br Med J* 320(7233):469–472, 2000.
20. Stone CA, Tiernan E, Dooley BA: Prospective validation of the palliative prognostic index in patients with cancer, *J Pain Symptom Manage* 35(6):617–622, 2008.
21. Goodlin SJ, Hauptman PJ, Arnold R, et al: Consensus statement: palliative and supportive care in advanced heart failure, *J Cardiac Failure* 10(3):200–209, 2004.
22. SUPPORT Investigators: A controlled trial to improve care for seriously ill hospitalized patients, *JAMA* 274:1591–1598, 1995.
23. Gibbs JSR, McCoy ASM, Gibbs LME, et al: Living with and dying from heart failure: the role of palliative care, *Heart* 88:ii36–ii39, 2002.
24. Levenson JW, McCarthy EP, Lynn J, Davis RB, Phillips RS: The last six months of life for patients with congestive heart failure, *J Am Geriatr Soc* 48(5 Suppl):S101–S109, 2000 May.
25. Jiang W, Alexander J, Christopher E, et al: Relationship of depression to increased risk of mortality and rehospitalization in patients with congestive heart failure, *Arch Intern Med* 161(15):1849–1856, 2001.
26. Zambroski CH, Moser DK, Roser LP, et al: Patients with heart failure who die in hospice, *Am Heart J* 149:558–564, 2005.
27. Hunt SA, Abraham WT, Chin MH, et al: ACC/AHA 2010 guideline update for the diagnosis and management of chronic heart failure in the adult, *Circulation* 112:1–28, 2005.
28. Nohria A, Lewis E, Stevenson LW: Medical management of advanced heart failure, *JAMA* 287(5):628–640, 2002.
29. Jessup M, Brozena S: Heart failure, *N Engl J Med* 348(20):2007–2018, 2003.
30. Pitt B, Zannad F, Remme WJ, et al: The effect of spironolactone on morbidity and mortality in patients with severe heart failure. Randomized Aldactone Evaluation Study Investigators, *N Engl J Med* 341(10):709–717, 1999.
31. The Digitalis Investigation Group: The effect of digoxin on mortality and morbidity in patients with heart failure, *N Engl J Med* 336:525–533, 1997.
32. Hood WB, Jr, Dans AL, Guyatt GH, et al: Digitalis for treatment of congestive heart failure in patients in sinus rhythm, *Cochrane Database Syst Rev* 2004;2:CD002901.
33. Felker GM, O'Connor CM: Inotropic therapy for heart failure: an evidence-based approach, *Am Heart J* 142(3):393–401, 2001.
34. Gheorghiade M, Pang PS: Acute heart failure syndromes, *J Am Coll Cardiol* 53:557–573, 2009, doi:10.1016/j.jacc.2008.10.041.
35. Felker GM, O'Connor CM: Inotropic therapy for heart failure: an evidence-based approach, *Am Heart J* 142(3):393–401, 2001.
36. Rich MW, Shore BL: Dobutamine for patients with end-stage heart failure in a hospice program? *J Palliat Med* 6(1):93–97, 2003.
37. Morrison LK, Harrison A, Krishnaswamy P, et al: Utility of a rapid B-natriuretic peptide assay in differentiating congestive heart failure from lung disease in patients presenting with dyspnea, *J Am Coll Cardiol* 39:202–209, 2002.
38. Kaneko Y, Floras JS, Usui K, et al: Cardiovascular effects of continuous positive airway pressure in patients with heart failure and obstructive sleep apnea, *N Engl J Med* 348:1233–1241, 2003.
39. Javaheri S: Acetazolamide improves central sleep apnea in heart failure: a double-blind, prospective study, *Am J Respir Crit Care Med* 173(2):234–237, 2006.
40. Booth S, Wade R, Johnson M, et al: Expert Working Group of the Scientific Committee of the Association of Palliative Medicine. The use of oxygen in the palliation of breathlessness. A report of the expert working group of the Scientific Committee of the Association of Palliative Medicine, *Respiratory Med* 98(1):66–77, 2004.

Complete references used in this text can be found online at www.expertconsult.com.

CHAPTER 28

Kidney Failure

ALVIN H. MOSS

A textbook on palliative care would not be complete without a chapter on kidney disease. Palliative care is especially appropriate for patients with kidney disease who are undergoing dialysis because of their significantly shortened life expectancy, high symptom burden, and multiple comorbid illnesses. In addition, there is a unique need for advance care planning for these patients because of their dependence on life-sustaining treatment for their continued existence and because, for approximately 25% of these patients, death is preceded by a decision to stop dialysis. As in other populations, pain is undertreated. Research suggests that 75% of patients undergoing dialysis have either untreated or undertreated pain. Treatment of pain in patients with kidney disease is more challenging because of the renal excretion of some opioid metabolites and the development of opioid neurotoxicity. For this reason, codeine, meperidine, morphine, and propoxyphene are not recommended for the treatment of severe pain in patients with kidney disease. The nephrology community has developed a clinical practice guideline on dialysis decision making. The guideline endorses the process of shared decision making in reaching decisions about who should undergo dialysis. It recognizes that the burdens of dialysis may substantially outweigh the benefits in some patients. Almost all patients with end-stage renal disease (ESRD) who stop dialysis die within a month. Research shows that only about half these patients are referred to hospice. This chapter describes the growing interest in the nephrology community of incorporating palliative care into the routine treatment of patients with chronic kidney disease (CKD), particularly for those who receive dialysis.

Relevance of Palliative Care

There is an increasing recognition that skills in palliative and end-of-life care are required for physicians, nurses, and others who treat patients who have ESRD and who are undergoing dialysis. The principal reasons are as follows: First, patients with ESRD who are undergoing dialysis have a significantly shortened life expectancy; they live approximately one fourth as long as age-matched patients without kidney

405

disease. For example, a 70-year-old white man starting dialysis has a life expectancy of 2.8 years, compared with 13.2 years for an age-matched white man in the general U.S. population. The 5-year survival for incident patients undergoing dialysis is only 38%, and the 10-year survival is only 20%.[1] Patients for whom palliative care is unquestionably considered appropriate (e.g., those with cancer and acquired immunodeficiency syndrome) have more than twice the survival rate of patients with ESRD. Approximately 23% of patients undergoing dialysis in the United States die each year. In the United States in 2007, more than 87,000 patients undergoing dialysis died. Approximately 20% of those patients died after the decision was made by the patient or family to stop dialysis. There is an average of 17 deaths per dialysis unit per year. Hence, the death of patients undergoing dialysis is a common experience for health care professionals who treat them.

Second, patients with ESRD have multiple comorbidities and consequently many symptoms. The majority of patients have congestive heart failure and coronary artery disease. Forty-five percent of all new patients undergoing dialysis have diabetes mellitus as the cause of their renal failure. Cardiac disease accounts for 45% of all-cause mortality in patients undergoing dialysis. More than 80% of new patients undergoing dialysis have anemia at the start of dialysis. Peripheral vascular disease is also prevalent in 20% to 45% of new patients depending on the population studied. With better care of cardiac disease, diabetes, hypertension, and cancer, patients are living long enough to develop kidney disease, and older patients with considerable comorbidities who previously would not have survived as long are now starting dialysis. Patients undergoing dialysis have been found to have a mean number of nine symptoms per patient; pain, fatigue, and itching are ranked as most severe by the highest number of patients.

Third, the dialysis population has been growing progressively older. In 2002, the median age for new patients starting dialysis in the United States was 65.1 years. The incidence rates of ESRD are highest in patients 75 years old and older, and they continue to rise in this group. Older patients survive the shortest time on dialysis, and they withdraw from dialysis significantly more often than younger patients.

In consideration of the high symptom burden and the low survival rate for patients undergoing dialysis, leading nephrology organizations such as the American Society of Nephrology (ASN) and the Renal Physicians Association (RPA) have recommended that dialysis units incorporate palliative care into their treatment of patients.[2] Nephrologists have been encouraged to obtain education and skills in palliative care so that they are comfortable addressing end-of-life issues with their patients, and dialysis facilities have been urged to develop protocols, policies, and programs to ensure that palliative care is provided to their patients.[3] Also, dialysis units have been urged to develop a working relationship with local palliative care programs, so patients with ESRD who stop dialysis or patients undergoing dialysis with a nonrenal terminal diagnosis may be referred for palliative care.

Symptom Management

PAIN MANAGEMENT

As in other patient populations, the burden of symptoms for patients undergoing dialysis is inversely associated with their reported quality of life.[4] Pain is the one of the most common symptom reported by patients undergoing dialysis, and several studies have found that approximately 50% of these patients report pain. For

Table 28-1. Recommendations for Opioid Use in Kidney Failure

Safe and Effective	Use with Caution	Do Not Use
Fentanyl	Hydromorphone	Codeine
Methadone	Oxycodone	Meperidine
Morphine		
Propoxyphene		

Adapted from Dean M: Opioids in renal failure and dialysis patients, *J Pain Symptom Manage* 28:497–504, 2004, with permission from the U.S. Cancer Pain Committee.

most patients undergoing dialysis, the pain is musculoskeletal in origin. Smaller numbers of patients have pain related to the dialysis procedure, peripheral neuropathy, peripheral vascular disease, or carpal tunnel syndrome. Less common causes of pain include that from polycystic kidney disease, malignant disease, or calciphylaxis (calcification of cutaneous blood vessels associated with skin necrosis). Three studies have found that pain is undertreated in 75% of patients undergoing dialysis.[5–7] Use of the World Health Organization (WHO) three-step analgesic ladder has been found to be effective in the treatment of pain in dialysis patients.[6] This study and other clinical experience also suggest that application of the WHO analgesic ladder results in effective pain relief for patients undergoing dialysis, and its use has been recommended to nephrologists treating patients with ESRD; however, because their metabolites are renally excreted and active, morphine, codeine, meperidine, and propoxyphene are *not* recommended for use in patients with chronic kidney disease (Table 28-1).[8]

Morphine is the best studied of the opioids used for pain management, and its most common metabolites (including morphine-3-glucuronide, morphine-6-glucuronide, and normorphine) are excreted renally. The clearance of these metabolites therefore decreases in renal failure. Morphine-6-glucuronide is an active metabolite with analgesic properties and the potential to depress respiration. Morphine-6-glucuronide crosses the blood–brain barrier and may have prolonged central nervous system effects because, even though it may be removed by dialysis, it diffuses slowly out of the central nervous system. Morphine-3-glucuronide does not have analgesic activity, but it may cause neurotoxicity manifested by agitation, myoclonus, or confusion. Morphine is 35% protein bound, and it has intermediate water solubility. Studies suggest that morphine is dialyzable to a limited degree. Some clinicians recommend the use of morphine for patients undergoing dialysis but with a decreased dose or an increased dosing interval. A comprehensive review of the use of opioids in renal failure recommended that morphine not be used in patients with kidney disease because it is so difficult to manage the complicated adverse effects of the morphine metabolites.[9]

Codeine is metabolized to codeine-6-glucuronide, norcodeine, morphine, morphine-3-glucuronide, morphine-6-glucuronide, and normorphine. Studies of codeine pharmacokinetics suggest that codeine metabolites would accumulate to toxic levels in a majority of patients undergoing hemodialysis. It is recommended that codeine not be used in patients with kidney failure because of the accumulation of active metabolites and because serious adverse effects have been reported from codeine use in patients with chronic kidney disease.

Hydromorphone is metabolized in the liver to hydromorphone-3-glucuronide as well as to dihydromorphine and dihydroisomorphine. Small quantities of additional metabolites are also formed. All metabolites are excreted renally. The hydromorphone-3-glucuronide metabolite does not have analgesic activity, but it is neuroexcitatory in rats. This metabolite also accumulates in patients with kidney disease. Some studies suggest that hydromorphone is removed with dialysis. It is recommended that hydromorphone be used cautiously in patients stopping dialysis. The parent drug is probably removed by dialysis, but no data exist concerning the removal of the metabolites by dialysis.

On the WHO analgesic ladder, oxycodone is recommended for treatment of both moderate and severe pain. Use of oxycodone in patients with kidney disease has not been well studied. The elimination half-life of oxycodone is lengthened in patients undergoing dialysis, and excretion of metabolites is impaired. Almost all the oxycodone metabolites are inactive. There are anecdotal reports of opioid neurotoxicity when oxycodone has been used in patients with kidney disease. Oxycodone has limited water solubility and 45% plasma protein binding, both of which suggest limited dialyzability. Oxycodone can be used with caution and careful monitoring in patients with chronic kidney disease who are undergoing dialysis.

The WHO analgesic ladder recommends the use of fentanyl for severe pain. Fentanyl is metabolized in the liver primarily to norfentanyl. There is no evidence that any fentanyl metabolites are active. Several studies have found that fentanyl can be used safely in patients with chronic kidney disease. Because 85% of fentanyl is protein bound and fentanyl has very low water solubility, it has negligible dialyzability. Fentanyl is deemed to be one of the safest opioids to use in patients with chronic kidney disease.

The WHO analgesic ladder recommends methadone for severe pain. Approximately 20% to 50% of methadone is excreted in the urine as methadone or as its metabolites, and 10% to 45% is excreted in the feces as a pyrrolidine metabolite. Studies in anuric patients have found that nearly all of methadone and its metabolites doses are excreted in the feces, mainly as metabolites. Methadone metabolites are inactive. Methadone is 89% bound to plasma proteins and has moderate water solubility. These two factors suggest that it is poorly removed by dialysis. No dose adjustments are recommended for patients undergoing dialysis. The use of methadone appears safe in patients with chronic kidney disease and those undergoing dialysis.

Opioids are often used to treat pain or dyspnea at the end of life in patients with chronic kidney disease or who are undergoing dialysis. In the setting of worsening renal function or withdrawal of dialysis, the clinician may be challenged to distinguish uremic encephalopathy from opioid neurotoxicity. Both can cause sedation, hallucinations, and myoclonus. If respiratory depression is also present, it is advisable to stop the opioid until the respiratory depression subsides. If the patient's respiratory rate is not compromised, the opioid can usually be continued, and a benzodiazepine such as lorazepam is added to control the myoclonus. Occasionally, a lorazepam continuous intravenous infusion at 1 or 2 mg/hour is necessary to control the myoclonus.

Although nonsteroidal anti-inflammatory drugs are recommended for use in step 1 on the WHO analgesic ladder, the use of these drugs in patients with chronic kidney disease is contraindicated because of their nephrotoxicity, and their use in patients undergoing dialysis is risky because of the higher frequency of upper gastrointestinal bleeding in these patients. The use of these drugs may also cause loss of residual renal function.

The Mid-Atlantic Renal Coalition and the Kidney End-of-Life Coalition assembled a panel of international experts on pain management in chronic kidney disease and developed an evidence-based algorithm for treating pain in dialysis patients, "Clinical Algorithm and Preferred Medication to Treat Pain in Dialysis Patients," which is accessible on the Internet.[10]

OTHER SYMPTOM MANAGEMENT

Because of their comorbid illnesses, patients undergoing dialysis are among the most symptomatic of any population with chronic disease. In one study[11] of 162 patients undergoing dialysis from three different dialysis units, the median number of symptoms reported by patients was 9.0. Pain, dyspnea, dry skin, and fatigue were each reported by more than 50% of the patients. Of the 30 different symptoms reported by the patients, the 6 most bothersome (starting with the worst first) were as follows: chest pain, bone or joint pain, difficulty becoming sexually aroused, trouble falling asleep, muscle cramps, and itching.

The greater the number of troublesome symptoms reported by patients undergoing dialysis, the lower they rate their quality of life. For this reason, it is very important for clinicians who treat these patients to assess and manage symptoms aggressively. Treatment with erythropoietin therapy in patients undergoing dialysis has led to a correction of the anemia with improved quality of life, decreased fatigue, increased exercise tolerance, and improved overall general well-being. It also has been shown to improve sexual desire and performance in some, but not all, patients undergoing dialysis. Pain from muscle cramps is a common symptom among dialysis patients, especially if they undergo significant fluid removal during dialysis. Decreasing the volume of fluid removed during any given dialysis treatment may lessen cramps. For patients with chronic kidney disease who are not yet undergoing dialysis, decreasing the dose of diuretic often works to eliminate cramps. Patients need to limit their intake of fluids and salt-containing fluids to avoid worsening of edema and fluid overload if diuretic doses are decreased. Benzodiazepines may be helpful for cramps.

Pruritus, or itching, is one of the most common and frustrating symptoms experienced by patients undergoing dialysis. Secondary hyperparathyroidism, increased calcium-phosphate deposition in the skin, dry skin, inadequate dialysis, anemia, iron deficiency, and low-grade hypersensitivity to products used in the dialysis procedure have all been identified as possible contributory factors. In addition to careful management of all these factors, the following interventions have been tried for pruritus with some success: emollient skin creams; phototherapy with ultraviolet B light three times weekly; intravenous lidocaine (100 mg) during dialysis for severe, refractory itching; and thalidomide (100 mg at bedtime; must not be used in pregnant women).

Insomnia is also reported by the majority of patients undergoing dialysis. In obese patients, sleep apnea should be excluded. The patient should also be evaluated for adequacy of dialysis. Avoidance of caffeinated beverages, alcoholic drinks, and naps have all been recommended. If these measures are not effective in improving insomnia, anxiolytic/hypnotics (e.g., zolpidem) or benzodiazepines (e.g., triazolam) are generally safe in patients undergoing dialysis.[12]

Care Planning

ADVANCE CARE PLANNING

Advance care planning is a process of communication among patients, families, health care providers, and other important individuals about the patient's preferred decision maker and appropriate future medical care if and when a patient is unable to make his or her own decisions. Advance care planning has been recognized as particularly important for patients undergoing dialysis for three reasons. First, more than half of all new patients undergoing dialysis are more than 65 years old, and elderly patients are the most likely to withdraw or be withdrawn from dialysis. Second, prior discussions of patients' wishes and completion of advance directives have been shown to help patients undergoing dialysis and their families approach death in a reconciled fashion. Third, unless a specific directive to withhold cardiopulmonary resuscitation (CPR) is obtained (which can be done within the framework of advance care planning), this treatment will automatically be provided, although it rarely leads to extended survival in these patients. For these reasons, clinicians have been encouraged to discuss with their patients the circumstances under which patients would want to discontinue dialysis and forgo CPR and to urge patients to communicate their wishes to their family verbally and through written advance directives.

The benefits of advance directives for patients and families and clinicians are twofold. First, families report that it is easier for them to make a decision to stop dialysis of a loved one if their loved one told them the health states under which he or she would not want to continue treatment. Second, patients undergoing dialysis who discuss and complete written advance directives are significantly more likely to have their wish to die at home respected.

Despite these benefits, the practice of advance care planning, including the completion of advance directives, has not been optimized for patients undergoing dialysis. First, most of these patients do not discuss or complete an advance directive, even though advance directives are particularly important for chronically ill patients with shortened life expectancy who are dependent on life-sustaining treatment for their daily existence. Dialysis units were not included in the U.S. Patient Self-Determination Act list of health care providers who were required to ask patients about completion of advance directives and also provide them with an opportunity to execute an advance directive. Second, even when patients undergoing dialysis complete written advance directives, only one third have indicated to their family the circumstances under which they may want to stop dialysis.[13] This failure to indicate their preferences is disappointing because patients undergoing dialysis do have strong preferences about stopping dialysis and other life-sustaining treatments under certain health states. For example, fewer than 20% of patients undergoing dialysis would want to continue dialysis, have CPR, or be maintained with tube feedings or a ventilator if they had severe dementia or were in a permanent coma.[14] Recognizing these deficiencies, the ASN, the National Kidney Foundation, the RPA, and the Robert Wood Johnson Foundation's ESRD Workgroup on End-of-Life Care have all strongly encouraged dialysis units to provide advance care planning to patients undergoing dialysis and their families and in the process to include a discussion of health states under which patients would want to stop dialysis and other life-sustaining treatments.

In 2008, the Centers for Medicare and Medicaid Services updated the Conditions for Coverage for dialysis facilities. In these updated regulations under Subpart C—Patients' Rights, dialysis facilities are required to inform patients about their rights to complete advance directives and the facility's policy regarding advance directives. In this same section of the updated regulations, the conditions state that the patient has the right to be informed of his or her right to refuse treatment and to discontinue treatment.

Patients undergoing dialysis and their families view advance care planning as a way to prepare for death, relieve burdens on loved ones, strengthen interpersonal relationships, and maintain control over present and future health care. Research with patients undergoing dialysis and families shows that patients prefer to center the advance care planning process within the patient–family relationship rather than the patient–physician relationship. Clinicians who treat dialysis patients should urge them to participate in an advance care planning discussion with their families and should instruct them to tell their families and put in writing health states in which they would not want life-sustaining treatment, including dialysis.

CARDIOPULMONARY RESUSCITATION

There is a low likelihood of benefit from CPR for most patients undergoing dialysis. One 8-year study of the outcomes of CPR in a dialysis population documented an 8% survival to discharge rate after CPR.[15] Other studies have documented similarly poor results. Despite these findings, almost 9 out of 10 patients undergoing dialysis would want to undergo CPR if cardiac arrest were to occur during dialysis or at other times. Patients who have seen CPR on television are more likely to report that they know what it is and that they want it. Because patients undergoing dialysis have an overly optimistic assessment of the outcomes of CPR, clinicians need to educate patients and their families about the risks and benefits of CPR, based on the patient's condition, before asking patients about their preferences. Patients undergoing dialysis often have other comorbid conditions that would also indicate a poor outcome from CPR, even without factoring in the patient's ESRD. Patients undergoing dialysis who do not want CPR are significantly older, have more comorbid conditions, and are more likely to have a living will, be widowed, and live in a nursing home. Black patients undergoing dialysis are six times more likely to want CPR than white patients receiving the same treatment.[16] Ninety-two percent of patients undergoing dialysis who want CPR agree that patients who do not want CPR should have their wishes respected by the dialysis unit. Most important, health care professionals in dialysis units and others who care for patients undergoing dialysis need to educate them about the poor outcomes of CPR so that these patients can make an informed decision about CPR.

DIALYSIS DECISION MAKING

For more than a decade, nephrologists have reported being increasingly asked to dialyze patients for whom they perceive dialysis to be of marginal benefit. At the end of the 1990s, the leadership of the RPA and the ASN assigned the highest priority for clinical practice guideline development to the topic of appropriateness of dialysis for patients. The subsequent guideline, "Shared Decision-Making in the Appropriate Initiation of and Withdrawal from Dialysis," was published in 2000 and provides nine recommendations for the dialysis of patients with acute renal failure and ESRD (Box 28-1). In the context of an expanding dialysis program with an increasing number of patients who have substantial comorbid conditions, the nephrology leadership believed that an evidence-based clinical practice guideline that could assist patients, families, and the nephrology team in making decisions about initiating,

Box 28-1. *Recommendations in the Clinical Practice Guideline: Shared Decision Making in the Appropriate Initiation of and Withdrawal from Dialysis*

RECOMMENDATION 1: SHARED DECISION MAKING

A patient–physician relationship that promotes shared decision making is recommended for all patients with either advanced renal failure (ARF) or end-stage renal disease (ESRD). Participants in shared decision making should involve at a minimum the patient and the physician. If a patient lacks decision-making capacity, decisions should involve the legal agent. With the patient's consent, shared decision making may include family members or friends and other members of the renal care team.

RECOMMENDATION 2: INFORMED CONSENT OR REFUSAL

Physicians should fully inform patients about their diagnosis, prognosis, and all treatment options, including: available dialysis modalities; not starting dialysis and continuing conservative management, which should include end-of-life care; a time-limited trial of dialysis; and stopping dialysis and receiving end-of-life care. Choices among options should be made by patients or, if patients lack decision-making capacity, their designated legal agents. Their decisions should be informed and voluntary. The renal care team, in conjunction with the primary care physician, should ensure that the patient or legal agent understands the consequences of the decision.

RECOMMENDATION 3: ESTIMATING PROGNOSIS

To facilitate informed decisions about starting dialysis for either ARF or ESRD, discussions should occur with the patient or legal agent about life expectancy and quality of life. Depending on the circumstances (e.g., availability of nephrologists), a primary care physician or nephrologist who is familiar with prognostic data should conduct these discussions. These discussions should be documented and dated. All patients requiring dialysis should have their chances for survival estimated, with the realization that the ability to predict survival in the individual patient is difficult and imprecise. The estimates should be discussed with the patient or legal agent, patient's family, and among the medical team. For patients with ESRD, these discussions should occur as early as possible in the course of the patient's renal disease and continue as the renal disease progresses. For patients who experience major complications that may substantially reduce survival or quality of life, it is appropriate to discuss and/or reassess treatment goals, including consideration of withdrawing dialysis.

RECOMMENDATION 4: CONFLICT RESOLUTION

A systematic approach for conflict resolution is recommended if there is disagreement regarding the benefits of dialysis between the patient or legal agent (and those supporting the patient's position) and a member of the renal care team. Conflicts may also occur within the renal care team or between the renal care team and other health care providers. This approach should review the shared decision-making process for the following potential sources of conflict: miscommunication or misunderstanding about prognosis, intrapersonal or interpersonal issues, or values. If dialysis is indicated on an emergency basis, it should be administered while pursuing conflict resolution, provided the patient or legal agent requests it.

RECOMMENDATION 5: ADVANCE DIRECTIVES

The renal care team should attempt to obtain written advance directives from all dialysis patients. These advance directives should be honored.

Box 28-1. *Recommendations in the Clinical Practice Guideline:*
Shared Decision Making in the Appropriate Initiation
of and Withdrawal from Dialysis—cont'd

RECOMMENDATION 6: WITHHOLDING OR WITHDRAWING DIALYSIS

It is appropriate to withhold or withdraw dialysis for patients with either ARF or ESRD in the following situations:
- Patients with decision-making capacity who, being fully informed and making voluntary choices, refuse dialysis or request dialysis be discontinued
- Patients who no longer possess decision-making capacity who have previously indicated refusal of dialysis in an oral or written advance directive
- Patients who no longer possess decision-making capacity and whose properly appointed legal agents refuse dialysis or request that it be discontinued
- Patients with irreversible, profound neurologic impairment such that they lack signs of thought, sensation, purposeful behavior, and awareness of self and environment

RECOMMENDATION 7: SPECIAL PATIENT GROUPS

It is reasonable to consider not initiating or withdrawing dialysis for patients with ARF or ESRD who have a terminal illness from a nonrenal cause or whose medical condition precludes the technical process of dialysis.

RECOMMENDATION 8: TIME-LIMITED TRIALS

For patients requiring dialysis, but who have an uncertain prognosis, or for whom a consensus cannot be reached about providing dialysis, nephrologists should consider offering a time-limited trial of dialysis.

RECOMMENDATION 9: PALLIATIVE CARE

All patients who decide to forgo dialysis or for whom such a decision is made should be treated with continued palliative care. With the patient's consent, persons with expertise in such care, such as hospice health care professionals, should be involved in managing the medical, psychosocial, and spiritual aspects of end-of-life care for these patients. Patients should be offered the option of dying where they prefer, including at home with hospice care. Bereavement support should be offered to patients' families.

Adapted from Renal Physicians Association and American Society of Nephrology: *Shared decision-making in the appropriate initiation of and withdrawal from dialysis*, Washington, DC, 2000, Renal Physicians Association.

---

continuing, and stopping dialysis would be timely and quite beneficial. The guideline recommendations have been widely accepted and endorsed by 10 professional organizations. In addition, the guideline has been cited in numerous publications. It helps physicians and nurses answer the question, Who should be dialyzed? The guideline recommends that shared decision making—the process by which physicians and patients agree on a specific course of action based on a common understanding of the treatment goals and risks and benefits of the chosen course, compared with reasonable alternatives—should be used in making decisions about dialysis. In most cases, the shared decision-making process results in decisions that are individualized to the patient's particular circumstances and preferences. The guideline recognized, however, that limits to the shared decision-making process protect the rights of patients and the professional integrity of health care professionals. The patient has the right to refuse dialysis even if the renal care team disagrees with the decision and wants the patient to undergo dialysis. Similarly, the renal care team has the right to not offer dialysis when the expected benefits do not justify the risks. The guideline also recognizes that there are circumstances in which patients and renal care teams may disagree about decisions to start, continue, or stop dialysis; the guideline recommends process-based conflict resolution in these cases.

The process of shared decision making results in the physician's obtaining informed consent or refusal for dialysis. The treating physician first needs to assess whether the patient has decision-making capacity and is capable of giving informed consent or refusal. For patients with acute kidney injury or ESRD, decision-making capacity may be diminished by uremic encephalopathy, infection, hypoxia, major depression, drug adverse effect, or some other disorder. If the patient lacks decision-making capacity, the physician must have discussions and obtain consent or refusal from the patient's legal agent (e.g., durable power of attorney for health care or health care surrogate, depending on state statutes).

Elderly (75 years or older) patients with stage 4 or 5 CKD constitute a special group for whom the informed consent process regarding initiation of dialysis requires special consideration of the risk-benefit ratio. Because of the significant comorbidities, severe functional impairment, and severe malnutrition of some elderly CKD patients, research shows that nephrologists should not take an age-neutral approach to the management of CKD patients. On the other hand, age alone should not constitute a contraindication to starting dialysis because comorbidity, not age, is the single most important determinant of outcome in dialysis patients. Age and comorbidity are additive in predicting dialysis patient survival. Thus, before placement of arteriovenous access, elderly patients with stage 4 or 5 CKD and significant comorbidities should be specifically informed of the following:

1. Dialysis may not confer a survival advantage.
2. Patients with their level of illness are more likely to die than live long enough to progress to ESRD.
3. Life on dialysis entails significant burdens that may detract from their quality of life.
4. The majority of patients in their condition either die or undergo significant functional decline during the first year after dialysis initiation.
5. The burdens of dialysis include surgery for vascular access placement and complications from the vascular access.
6. They may experience adverse physical symptoms on dialysis, such as dizziness, fatigue, cramping, and a feeling of "unwellness" after dialysis.

Further, patients need to be informed that there will be travel time and expense to and from dialysis, long hours spent on dialysis, and a reduction in the time available for physical activity and meals. Dialysis may entail an "unnecessary medicalization of death" resulting in invasive tests, procedures, and hospitalizations.

In one study, elderly patients with significant comorbidity treated with dialysis as opposed to conservative management were more than four times as likely to die in the hospital as at home and spent 47.5% of the days they survived either in the hospital or at the dialysis clinic.[17] Such patients should be informed that conservative management without dialysis is an acceptable alternative that may better achieve patients' goals of care. Conservative management is still active treatment. It entails advanced care planning; implementation of patients' goals; and management of anemia, bone disease, fluid balance, acidosis, pain, and blood pressure. Multiple studies report a median survival greater than 1 year for patients managed conservatively.[17,18]

The RPA/ASN guideline recommends that a discussion about starting or stopping dialysis should contain an estimate of prognosis, life expectancy, and likely quality of life. Although there is not yet a single mathematical formula to combine all risk factors to provide a numerical estimate of life expectancy (an integrated prognostic model for ESRD patients is in the process of being validated), certain factors identified by multivariate analyses are significant predictors of mortality for patients with ESRD: older age, low serum albumin level, limited functional status, and number and severity of comorbid illnesses (usually measured by the Charlson Comorbidity Index or Index of Coexistence Diseases). The RPA/ASN guideline has a concise review of these most significant predictors. In addition, since the guideline publication, the "surprise" question—"Would I be surprised if this patient died in the next year?"—has been found in multivariate analysis to be a statistically significant predictor of dialysis patient 1-year mortality. Using the surprise question, nephrologists and nurse practitioners classified patients into two groups: a "No, I would not be surprised if this patient died in the next year" group and a "Yes, I would be surprised" group. Patients in the "No" group were found to have odds of dying 3.5 times greater than those in the "Yes" group.[19]

Most nephrologists have encountered patients with poor predicted survival undergoing dialysis who have outlived life expectancy estimates. Thus, a complicating factor is clinical uncertainty. In fact, it is in situations of clinical uncertainty that patients introduce their own extramedical values (e.g., importance of living for an upcoming wedding of family member or a desire to not be a burden on family) to assist in the decision-making process; hence, candor about the uncertainty of the prognosis may encourage shared decision making.[20]

Nephrologists have been urged to consider providing a time-limited trial of dialysis when the treating team and consultants cannot reach a consensus and also when dialysis is indicated but the prognosis is uncertain. The patient's clinical course during the time-limited trial may provide patients and families with a better understanding of dialysis and its benefits and burdens. The trial will also provide the treating team with a more informed assessment of the likelihood that the benefits of dialysis will outweigh the burdens. Surveys of nephrologists have indicated that more than three fourths utilize time-limited trials of dialysis for this purpose and that dialysis is stopped after a trial in only 20% of cases.

Recommendation number 6 of the RPA/ASN guideline identifies patients for whom there is consensus that dialysis should be withheld or withdrawn. In addition to patients who previously indicated that they would not want dialysis or for whom such a decision is made by their appropriate legal agent, dialysis is also not appropriate for patients with irreversible neurologic impairment so profound that they lack signs of thought, sensation, purposeful behavior, and awareness of self and environment. Patients who are permanently unconscious (e.g., those in a persistent vegetative state) or those who are comatose from a cerebral vascular accident fall into this category. In addition, recommendation number 7 identifies two additional groups of patients for whom it is reasonable to consider not providing dialysis. These are patients who have a terminal illness from a nonrenal cause such as cancer and those whose medical condition precludes the patient's cooperation with the technical process of dialysis, such as patients with severe mental retardation or advanced dementia.

For patients for whom dialysis is being withheld or withdrawn, the RPA/ASN guideline recommends a palliative care approach in collaboration with health care professionals who have expertise in managing the medical, psychosocial, and spiritual aspects of end-of-life care. The RPA/ASN guideline recognizes the role of palliative care professionals.

For patients other than those identified in recommendations 6 and 7, there may be conflict about the appropriateness of dialysis. Some may use the argument of medical futility. Strictly speaking, in patients for whom it is possible to conduct dialysis (i.e., they have adequate blood pressure and access to the circulation to enable dialysis), dialysis is not futile because it improves blood chemistry and volume status. Recommendation number 4 of the RPA/ASN guideline recommends a systematic approach for conflict resolution when disagreement about the benefits of dialysis exists between the patient (or his or her legal agent) and members of the treating team. The fair process–based approach for conflict resolution recommended in the guideline was adapted from that proposed by the Council on Ethical and Judicial Affairs of the American Medical Association.[21]

Nephrologists and others who treat patients undergoing dialysis may also be challenged by a patient's request to stop dialysis. To ensure that potentially reversible factors such as depression or family conflict are not responsible for the patient's request, the treating physician needs to consider certain questions before honoring the patient's request (Box 28-2). After a systematic evaluation, if it is determined that the patient has capacity and is making an informed decision to stop dialysis, the patient's decision should be honored. Patients at high risk for withdrawing from dialysis have been identified from research studies; they are more likely to be older, diabetic, and divorced or widowed; to live in a nursing home; and to have a higher comorbidity index.

Once the decision has been made to stop dialysis, patients and families should be informed that death will probably occur in 8 to 12 days and will be caused by uremia resulting from a buildup of toxins and electrolyte disturbances. In 10% of cases, death may take 1 month or longer to occur. The likelihood of a more prolonged dying

---

Box 28-2. *Consideration of Patient Requests to Stop Dialysis*

Consider the following questions when responding to a patient's request to stop dialysis:

1. Does the patient have decision-making capacity, or is the patient's cognitive capacity diminished by major depression, encephalopathy, or other disorder?
2. Why does the patient want to stop dialysis?
3. Are the patient's perceptions about the technical or quality-of-life aspects of dialysis accurate?
4. Does the patient really mean what he or she says, or is the decision to stop dialysis made to get attention, help, or control?
5. Can any changes be made that could improve life on dialysis for the patient?
6. Would the patient be willing to continue dialysis while the factors responsible for the patient's request are being addressed?
7. Has the patient discussed his or her desire to stop dialysis with significant others such as family, close friends, or spiritual advisors? What do they think about the patient's request?

Table 28-2. Management of Patients Who Withdraw from Dialysis

Fluid overload	Salt and fluid restriction and/or use of ultrafiltration without diffusion to remove fluid
Pain	Methadone or fentanyl*
Nausea	Haloperidol, metoclopramide, or prochlorperazine
Dyspnea	Methadone or fentanyl*
Hiccups	Chlorpromazine or baclofen
Myoclonus	Clonazepam or lorazepam
Agitation/restlessness	Haloperidol or lorazepam
Excessive secretions ("death rattle")	Glycopyrrolate or scopolamine
Seizures (occur in only 10% of cases)	Diazepam or phenytoin

*Half-life is short, so use as a continuous infusion.

course depends on the extent of the patient's residual renal function as reflected by daily urine output. Patients and families should be informed that death from uremia is usually a comfortable and peaceful one in which the patient becomes increasingly somnolent and then dies. Patients who have decided to stop dialysis should be referred to a palliative care program, and the dialysis team should adopt a palliative care approach to patient care. It is important to determine where the patient would like to die and whom the patient would like to be with during the dying process. Medications and measures useful to treat the common symptoms and signs that result from dialysis withdrawal are listed in Table 28-2.

Despite the recommendations of the ASN, the RPA, and the Robert Wood Johnson Foundation's ESRD Peer Workgroup on End-of-Life Care, hospice utilization by patients undergoing dialysis in the United States is very low. In a 2001 to 2002 cohort study of these patients, the United States Renal Data System reported that only 13.5% of patients undergoing dialysis died with hospice, about half the national average for the percentage of patients dying with hospice, and fewer than half (42%) of the patients who withdrew from dialysis and for whom death was expected within 1 month received hospice care. The low referral rate to hospice appears to result from at least two factors: physician practice patterns and a lack of knowledge about hospice on the part of patients undergoing dialysis and families. The latter may be the result of a widespread lack of understanding of the life-limited nature of ESRD and the failure of the multidisciplinary team members to talk to patients undergoing dialysis and their families about end-of-life issues. It also appears that many hospices may not want to accept such patients unless they discontinue dialysis. Medicare regulations allow patients undergoing dialysis to continue dialysis and receive the Medicare hospice benefit, provided the patient's terminal diagnosis for hospice is not related to kidney disease. The National Hospice and Palliative Care Organization in the United States is conducting programs to educate hospices that continuation of dialysis for patients in this situation is not a violation of the hospice philosophy, but instead affords terminally ill patients undergoing dialysis the opportunity to receive pain and symptom management, to initiate advance care planning, and to receive support for themselves and their families during the final stages of their lives.

Box 28-3. *Components of a Dialysis Unit Palliative Care Program*

1. Palliative care focus
   - Educational activities, including dialysis unit in-service training
   - Quality improvement activities, including morbidity and mortality conferences
   - Use of the "Would you be surprised if this patient died within the next year?" question to identify patients appropriate for palliative care
   - Collaboration with local palliative care programs to coordinate a smooth transition to end-of-life care
2. Pain and symptom assessment and management protocols
3. Systematized advance care planning
4. Psychosocial and spiritual support to patients and families, including the use of peer counselors
5. Terminal care protocols that include hospice referral
6. Bereavement programs for families that include memorial services

---

In October 2004, the CMS added a question about hospice utilization to the CMS-2746 ESRD Death Notification Form.

The Robert Wood Johnson Foundation's ESRD Peer Workgroup on End-of-Life Care recommended that dialysis units and large dialysis provider organizations establish palliative care programs in individual dialysis units. A comprehensive dialysis unit palliative care program has multiple components (Box 28-3); it is easiest to introduce them incrementally. Palliative care consultants and hospice personnel can help dialysis units implement palliative care programs. Dialysis units and hospices working collaboratively can help to ensure quality end-of-life care for patients undergoing dialysis.

PEARLS

- The 5-year survival rate for incident patients undergoing dialysis is 38%, just over half that of incident patients with cancer (70%).

- Hospices are underutilized by patients undergoing dialysis. Only one in five of these patients die with hospice, compared with the national average of one in three.

- Even though patients who stop dialysis have 1 month or less to live, only 60% receive hospice services at the end of life.

- When a patient stops dialysis, it is highly likely that the patient will die within 8 to 12 days. Almost all patients undergoing dialysis who stop dialysis die within 1 month.

- Because they do not have active renally excreted metabolites, fentanyl and methadone are the safest drugs to use for severe pain in patients with kidney disease.

- Collaboration with hospices can help dialysis units implement a palliative care program and appropriately refer patients for hospice care at the end of life.

PITFALLS

- Only one third of patients undergoing dialysis who complete a living will and a medical power of attorney indicate the circumstances under which they would want to stop dialysis. Studies show that patients undergoing dialysis are most comfortable indicating the health states (e.g., severe dementia or permanent coma) under which they would want to forgo dialysis, mechanical ventilation, CPR, and tube feeding.

- Advance directives are completed by fewer than 50% of patients undergoing dialysis. Dialysis units were not included on the list of health care providers in the Patient Self-Determination Act that were required to ask patients about advance directives, but the 2008 CMS Conditions for Coverage require dialysis units to have a policy with regard to advance directives and to inform patients of their policy.

- Almost 9 out of 10 patients undergoing dialysis indicate that they would want CPR even though CPR results in survival to discharge in fewer than 10% of patients undergoing dialysis. Patients who have seen CPR on television are significantly more likely to report that they know what it is and to indicate that they want it. Education of patients and families on the topic is needed.

- Dialysis is often requested by families of patients with a very poor prognosis. Significant predictors of early mortality for ESRD patients are age, serum albumin level, functional status, comorbid illnesses, and a "no" response to the surprise question. A fair process–based approach for resolving conflicts with families over the provision of dialysis is described in the RPA/ASN Clinical Practice Guideline, "Shared Decision-Making in the Appropriate Initiation of and Withdrawal from Dialysis."

Summary

There is a growing commitment among the leadership in the nephrology community to enhance end-of-life care for patients undergoing dialysis. It is highly likely that palliative care for patients undergoing dialysis will be significantly improved over the next decade as nephrologists and palliative care consultants apply the knowledge and skills discussed in this chapter.

Note: In October 2010 the Renal Physicians Association released a second edition of the clinical practice guideline, *Shared Decision-Making in the Appropriate Initiation of and Withdrawal from Dialysis.* Based on the multiple articles on renal palliative care published since the first edition in 2000, this guideline makes even stronger recommendations for the incorporation of palliative medicine principles in to the care of dialysis patients.

Resources

Chambers EJ, Germain M, Brown E, editors: *Supportive care for the renal patient,* Oxford, UK, 2004, Oxford University Press.

End-Stage Renal Disease Peer Workgroup of the Robert Wood Johnson Foundation's Promoting Excellence in the End-of-Life Care National Program: Completing the Continuum of Nephrology Care. http://promotingexcellence.org/esrd/

Renal Physicians Association and American Society of Nephrology: *Shared decision-making in the appropriate initiation of and withdrawal from dialysis,* Washington, DC, 2000, Renal Physicians Association.

Renal Physicians Association and American Society of Nephrology: Position Statement on Quality Care at the End of Life. 2002.
www.renalmd.org/members_online/members/c_rpapolicies.cfm
Kidney End-of-Life Coalition website.
www.kidneyeol.org

References

1. United States Renal Data System: *USRDS 2009 annual data report: atlas of chronic kidney disease and end-stage renal disease in the United States*, Bethesda, Md, 2009, National Institutes of Health, National Institutes of Diabetes and Digestive and Kidney Diseases.
2. Renal Physicians Association and American Society of Nephrology: *Shared decision-making in the appropriate initiation of and withdrawal from dialysis*, Washington, DC, 2000, Renal Physicians Association.
3. Renal Physicians Association and American Society of Nephrology: Position Statement on Quality Care at the End of Life, 2002. Available at www.renalmd.org/members_online/members/c_rpapolicies.cfm.
4. Kimmel PL, Emont SL, Newmann JM, et al: ESRD patient quality of life: symptoms, spiritual beliefs, psychological factors, and ethnicity, *Am J Kidney Dis* 42:713–721, 2003.
5. Davison SN: Pain in hemodialysis patients: prevalence, cause, severity, and management, *Am J Kidney Dis* 42:1239–1247, 2003.
6. Barakzoy AS, Moss AH: Efficacy of the World Health Organization analgesic ladder to treat pain in end-stage renal disease, *J Am Soc Nephrol* 17:3198–3203, 2006.
7. Bailie GR, Mason NA, Bragg-Gresham JL, et al: Analgesic prescription patterns among hemodialysis patients in the DOPPS: potential for underprescription, *Kidney Int* 65:2419–2425, 2004.
8. Moss AH, Holley JL, Davison SN, et al: Core curriculum in nephrology: palliative care, *Am J Kidney Dis* 43:172–185, 2004.
9. Dean M: Opioids in renal failure and dialysis patients, *J Pain Symptom Manage* 28:497–504, 2004.
10. Mid-Atlantic Renal Coalition: Clinical Algorithm and Preferred Medications to Treat Pain in Dialysis Patients. Available at www.kidneyeol.org/painbrochure9.09.pdf. Accessed on December 15, 2009.
11. Weisbord S, Fried L, Arnold R, et al: The prevalence, severity, and importance of physical and emotional symptoms in chronic hemodialysis patients, *J Am Soc Nephrol* 16:2487–2494, 2005.
12. Germain M, McCarthy S: Symptoms of renal disease: dialysis-related symptoms. In Chambers EJ, Germaine M, Brown E, editors: *Supportive care for the renal patient*, Oxford, UK, 2004, Oxford University Press, pp 75–94.
13. Holley JL, Hines SC, Glover J, et al: Failure of advance care planning to elicit patients' preferences for withdrawal from dialysis, *Am J Kidney Dis* 33:688–693, 1999.
14. Singer PA, Thiel EC, Naylor CD, et al: Life-sustaining treatment preferences of hemodialysis patients: Implications for advance directives, *J Am Soc Nephrol* 6:1410–1417, 1995.
15. Moss AH, Holley JL, Upton MB: Outcome of cardiopulmonary resuscitation in dialysis patients, *J Am Soc Nephrol* 3:1238–1243, 1992.
16. Moss AH, Hozayen O, King K, et al: Attitudes of patients toward cardiopulmonary resuscitation in the dialysis unit, *Am J Kidney Dis* 38:847–852, 2001.
17. Carson RC, Juszczak M, Davenport A, et al: Is maximum conservative management an equivalent treatment option to dialysis for elderly patients with significant comorbid disease? *Clin J Am Soc Nephrol* 4:1611–1619, 2009.
18. Murtagh FEM, Marsh JE, Donohoe P, et al: Dialysis or not? A comparative survival study of patients over 75 years with chronic kidney disease stage 5, *Nephrol Dial Transplant* 22:1955–1962, 2007.
19. Moss AH, Ganjoo J, Sharma S, et al: Utility of the "surprise" question to identify dialysis patients with high mortality, *Clin J Am Soc Nephrol* 3:1379–1384, 2008.
20. Michael DM, Moss AH: Communicating prognosis in the dialysis consent process: a patient-centered, guideline-supported approach, *Adv Chronic Kidney Dis* 12:196–201, 2005.
21. Council on Ethical and Judicial Affairs, American Medical Association: Medical futility in end-of-life care, *JAMA* 281:937–941, 1999.

CHAPTER 29

Gastrointestinal Malignancies

MAXWELL T. VERGO, REGINA M. STEIN, and AL B. BENSON III

Gastrointestinal malignancies are the most commonly diagnosed cancers in the world. Before any management decisions are made with this patient population, it is critical to understand the patient's expected overall survival (Table 29-1), potential further antineoplastic therapy that may be available, the amazing variability of each tumor's biology, and how all these features and other factors result in the intent of the therapy (curative vs. palliative or something in between). Care must be individualized to the patient and not to the statistics. For example, it is possible to find a patient with metastatic pancreatic cancer alive years after the diagnosis or, alternatively, a patient with metastatic neuroendocrine tumor who only survives months after their diagnosis despite aggressive chemotherapy.

Because patients' symptoms vary widely and are often exacerbated by tumor-directed therapy as well as disease progression, those caring for patients with gastrointestinal malignancies must be cognizant of each malignancy's and each treatment's unique manifestations and their effect on the patient's quality of life. This chapter provides approaches to palliative management, including antineoplastic therapy, of patients with various advanced gastrointestinal cancers. The National Collaborative Cancer Network (NCCN), listed in Resources at the end of this chapter, provides more detailed information about each malignancy discussed.

421

Table 29-1. Summary of Median Overall Survival for Each Gastrointestinal Malignancy

Cancer	Median Overall Survival for Advanced Disease (with Treatment)
Gastric[2]	8–10 months
Neuroendocrine[8]	>5 years
Hepatocellular[11]	6–8 months
Pancreatic[15,16]	6 months
Colorectal[23,24]	2+ years
Esophageal[28,29]	8–10 months

Gastric Cancer

BACKGROUND

Gastric cancer remains one of the most common forms of cancer worldwide, as well as one of the most deadly.[1] In the United States, patients present more than half the time with symptoms of weight loss, abdominal pain, and dysphagia[2] but unfortunately the majority of patients have disease too advanced to receive curative therapy. Cancers that affect the gastroesophageal junction (GEJ) are included in this classification. Histologically, squamous cell carcinoma is felt to be more chemosensitive and radiosensitive than adenocarcinoma. In recent years, there has been a rapid rise in GEJ adenocarcinoma.

ROLE OF CHEMOTHERAPY

Chemotherapy has a definitive role in the palliative care of advanced gastric cancer patients with a good performance status. In patients with metastatic disease, chemotherapy regimens not only offer a doubling of survival (3–4 months vs. 8–9 months) compared with best supportive care but also appears to delay the time to deterioration of functional status and quality of life.[2]

COMMON PALLIATIVE CARE ISSUES

Abdominal pain in this population could be caused by peritoneal carcinomatosis (even if there is no evidence of it on imaging) and/or gastric distention, called malignant gastroparesis. Pain associated with increased hiccups, early satiety, and relieved by vomiting occurs with and may be the first suggestion of malignant gastroparesis. Peritoneal carcinomatosis pain tends to respond to anti-inflammatory agents, including steroids (e.g., Decadron 4–16 mg PO/IV every morning) or nonsteroidal anti-inflammatory drugs (NSAIDs), either alone or given as an adjuvant to opioids.[3] Mechanical relief of malignant gastroparesis can be achieved with prokinetic therapy aimed at improving dysfunctional gastric motility. Metoclopramide (Reglan), a dopamine antagonist that sensitizes gastric tissue to the effects of acetylcholine, at doses of 5 to 20 mg PO/IV every 6 hours around the clock, improved pain, nausea, and vomiting, reduced the use of other antiemetics, and even led to weight gain compared with placebo. In addition, erythromycin stimulates motilin receptors at a dose of 150 to 250 mg PO every 8 hours and has been shown to be as effective as Reglan.[4]

Radiation therapy should be considered in patients who present with bleeding that is refractory and significant; dysphagia (usually GEJ cancers); or pain that is refractory to systemic management.[2] An option for relieving dysphagia in patients who are not good radiation candidates is the placement of an esophageal self-expanding metallic stent (SEMS). These stents give almost immediate relief of dysphagia in 86% to 100% of patients, leading to improved quality-of-life scores.[5] Generally, smaller diameter stents are favored, despite an increased need for further intervention as a result of stent migration or recurrent or refractory dysphagia when compared with larger diameter stents (42% vs. 13%), because of the increased risk of hemorrhage (2%–14%), perforation (2%–6%), fistula, and chest pain (15%–27%) with the larger stents.[5] Stents that cross the GEJ have a 30% chance of causing gastroesophageal reflux symptoms; if this occurs, consideration of a proton pump inhibitor would be warranted.[5] Endoscopic stent placement should be done by an experienced interventional gastroenterologist.

At select centers, two other options exist for patients who have a recurrence of cancer after radiation therapy (and are unable to safely get more) or who are unable to tolerate radiotherapy: neodymium yttrium aluminum garnet (Nd:YAG) laser therapy, ideal for accurate and localized coagulation, and photodynamic therapy. Photodynamic therapy (PDT) uses an intravenous photosensitizer (called porfimer in the United States) and an endoscopic nonthermal laser for ablation. In a prospective, randomized controlled trial of these two therapies in 236 patients, although they were of similar efficacies for relieving dysphagia, PDT worked better for larger lesions (>8 cm) and for lesions in the upper and mid-esophagus and was better tolerated (termination of treatment 3% for PDT and 19% for Nd:YAG).[6]

Gastric outlet obstruction can also occur in this population if the malignancy involves the distal portion of the stomach. This tends to cause almost immediate postprandial vomiting, but symptoms can be quite similar to malignant gastroparesis. Options for treating this symptom include creation of a gastrojejunostomy, placement of a SEMS, or placement of a venting gastrostomy tube, which is similar to a feeding gastrostomy tube but used solely to decompress the stomach. A recent systemic review of the literature comparing gastrojejunostomy with SEMS revealed similar success and complication rates; however, although gastrojejunostomy yielded fewer recurrent obstructive symptoms compared with SEMS (1% vs. 18%), it was associated with a longer hospital stay (164 days vs. 105 days). SEMS may be best for patients with shorter life expectancies, but gastrojejunostomy may be best for patients with longer life expectancies if they are able to tolerate this procedure.[7] Venting gastrostomy tubes should be considered for patients not amenable to SEMS placement, but caution should be taken if there is a large burden of ascites or peritoneal carcinomatosis, which increases the potential technical difficulty of the procedure. Because of the availability of SEMS, gastrojejunostomy, and venting gastrostomy tubes to relieve symptoms, partial gastrectomy procedures for patients with metastatic disease should only be performed by the surgeon on a case-by-case basis.

Neuroendocrine Tumors

BACKGROUND

Carcinoid tumors are the most common neuroendocrine tumors of the gastrointestinal tract, but they are quite rare in terms of overall gastrointestinal malignancies.

Carcinoid tumors are generally well differentiated and therefore are comparatively less aggressive than small-bowel adenocarcinomas. In patients with metastatic disease, a 70% 5-year survival rate has been reported.[8] Approximately 90% of patients presenting with symptomatic carcinoid tumors have advanced disease with liver metastases, even though some patients will have normal imaging. It is also worth noting that islet cell carcinoma falls in the category of neuroendocrine tumors; even though it does not produce carcinoid syndrome, it can secrete a hormone that causes symptoms such as excessive insulin.

ROLE OF CHEMOTHERAPY

The first-line therapy in malignant, metastatic neuroendocrine tumors is a somatostatin analogue, which acts by specifically binding to the somatostatin receptors commonly expressed on these tumors. These receptors can be measured using an imaging study called an OctreoScan, which can be helpful in determining the utility of a somatostatin analogue in these patients. Although historically this therapy was used almost exclusively in patients with carcinoid syndrome and was purely for symptom management, recently it has been recognized that using octreotide, a somatostatin analogue, in all patients with advanced neuroendocrine tumors may delay progression of disease by more than a year.[8] If somatostatin analogues fail to control the disease, other options include the addition of interferon, traditional chemotherapy agents, and new agents that target cell signaling pathways.

COMMON PALLIATIVE CARE ISSUES

Carcinoid syndrome is a collection of symptoms that results from secretion of excessive serotonin and other biologically active amines and generally is a consequence of metastatic disease that involves the liver. The syndrome is often associated with flushing, diarrhea, abdominal cramping, wheezing, fatigue, and heart disease as a result of carcinoid infiltration, and the syndrome can significantly impact a patient's quality of life. Carcinoid syndrome can be significantly improved with initiation of somatostatin analogue therapy, usually octreotide long-acting release (LAR) 20 to 40 mg subcutaneously every 2 to 4 weeks. In approximately 50% of patients, treatment with this single agent provides a response duration ranging from 3 to 60 months.[9] In refractory carcinoid syndrome, octreotide continuous infusion pump or other somatostatin analogues can be considered, as well as more aggressive therapy, including chemotherapy and targeted agents (noted in the previous section) and liver-directed therapies as listed next.

An emerging strategy for maintaining disease control and improving symptoms associated with neuroendocrine tumors has been liver-directed therapy.[10] This can be with transarterial chemoembolization (TACE), which involves infusing chemotherapy and embolizing material locally to the tumor via the hepatic arterial system, or radioactive beads infused via the hepatic arterial system.

Causes of abdominal pain secondary to neuroendocrine tumors that should be considered include stretching or irritation of the hepatic capsule, mesenteric ischemia from compression of vessels with mesenteric masses or lymph nodes, and bowel obstruction. Stretch or irritation of the hepatic capsule responds well to anti-inflammatory management with NSAIDs or steroids (e.g., Decadron 4–16 mg IV/PO every morning).[3] Because of the relatively lengthy survival of most patients with neuroendocrine tumors, if pain from vascular compromise or bowel obstruction is amenable to surgical intervention, this should be strongly considered.

Hepatocellular Carcinoma

BACKGROUND

Hepatocellular carcinoma is the leading cause of cancer death worldwide, with a median overall survival of around 8 months. The main risk factor for the development of hepatocellular carcinoma remains hepatocellular injury resulting from chronic liver disease or cirrhosis. Caring for these patients can be challenging for several reasons, including potential underlying substance abuse issues (which may have been the reason for their chronic liver disease), morbidity associated with their underlying liver disease, and altered clearance of medications, including opioids. The current mainstay of therapy for cure is surgery (resection or liver transplant), or loco-regional control can be achieved with percutaneous ablation, transarterial chemoembolization, or radioactive beads. However, only about 30% to 40% of patients present at an early enough stage to consider these techniques.[11]

ROLE OF CHEMOTHERAPY

Traditional chemotherapy has not been effective in advanced hepatocellular carcinoma, but recently a targeted molecular agent, sorafenib, has been shown to improve survival by a median of 3 months for those with good liver function (e.g., those with a Child-Pugh score of class A). No quality-of-life assessments were performed, but about 37% of patients discontinued sorafenib because of adverse effects, and the most common symptoms of any grade were diarrhea (55%), hand-foot syndrome (21%), rash (19%), and weight loss.[11] Palliative clinicians caring for patients receiving this therapy should pay attention to these side effects and discuss potential dose modifications or other supportive care with the oncologist.

COMMON PALLIATIVE CARE ISSUES

A retrospective study of 991 patients with hepatocellular carcinoma in a hospital-based hospice ward in Taiwan demonstrated that the most common symptoms at admission were pain, fatigue, weakness, anorexia or vomiting, peripheral edema, cachexia, and ascites.[12] Pain is likely to be from stretching or irritation of the hepatic capsule but can also result from bulky retroperitoneal adenopathy that causes stretching of the retroperitoneal cavity. Therefore, treatment with potent anti-inflammatory medications (e.g., steroids and/or NSAIDs) is appropriate before the addition to an opioid to limit adverse effects from the latter.[3] However, because of the thrombocytopenia in this population and high rate of potential bleeding varices, caution should be taken with use of NSAIDs.

Caution should also be used with opioid administration because of liver dysfunction and potential decreased clearance, as well as the potential for renal dysfunction from hepatorenal syndrome. Generally, start with lower doses and titrate slowly. In patients with decompensated liver failure, avoid using long-acting formulations (including transdermal patches) and use immediate-release preparations as needed until the steady-state dynamics are evident. Opioids metabolized by glucuronidation (e.g., morphine, hydromorphone) are preferred to those metabolized by the cytochrome P450 (CYP) system (e.g., fentanyl, methadone, oxycodone) in patients with liver dysfunction because the half-life is more predictably related to liver function measured by bilirubin, prothrombin time, albumin, presence of ascites, or encephalopathy.[13] Monitor for neurotoxicity from the opioids and opioid byproducts, especially from glucuronidated byproducts of morphine and hydromorphone, which

Table 29-2. Summary of Opioid Metabolism and Dosing Recommendations

Opioid	Liver Metabolism	Ascites Accumulation	Renally Cleared	Dosing Recommendation in Liver Failure
Morphine	Glucuronidation	Yes	Yes	Lower starting doses and dosing intervals (q6–8h)
Hydromorphone	Glucuronidation	Yes	Yes	Lower starting doses and dosing intervals (q6–8h)
Fentanyl	CYP system	No	Yes	Avoid long-acting transdermal preparation
Methadone	CYP system	No	Minor	Hepatitis C virus increases clearance
Oxycodone	CYP system	Yes	Yes	Immediate release same half-life as sustained release formulation

CYP, Cytochrome P450.

can be exacerbated by renal failure, leading to myoclonus, confusion, sedation, and even seizure. See Table 29-2 for a summary of opioid metabolism, as well as recommendations for dosing.

Obstructive jaundice can result from biliary tree invasion or intrahepatic duct compression. Endoscopically placed, expandable metal stents can provide minimally invasive, effective palliation of jaundice and obstructive symptoms. Cholestasis-induced pruritus should be managed with bile acid–binding agents (cholestyramine 30 minutes before breakfast and 30 minutes after breakfast, as well as at noon, titrated up to a maximum of 32 g/day), but refractory symptoms can be managed with rifampin 150 to 600 mg/day or opioid receptor antagonists.[13] Pruritus (as well as other symptoms such as anorexia) may be mediated by increased endogenous opioid production; blocking this effect with opioid receptor antagonists poses a possible solution, but endogenous opioid withdrawal has been reported despite patients being opioid naïve. Therefore, the recommendation is to start with a continuous infusion of naloxone at a dose of 0.002 µg/kg/min and titrating up to 0.2 µg/kg/min, followed by naltrexone orally 12.5 mg twice daily, titrated to response (usually 25 mg twice daily).[13] Because of the difficulty of titrating intravenous naloxone, another strategy is to start with naltrexone 25 mg PO daily and titrate to twice a day dosing if there is no effect.[14] Acetaminophen and NSAIDs should not be given concurrently with naltrexone because this may increase liver toxicity.[13]

Fever can develop as a result of central tumor necrosis and is treated with a combination of antipyretics and corticosteroids. Appropriate workup for other infectious causes, including spontaneous bacterial peritonitis, is indicated if appropriate for the patient's goals of care.

See Chapter 25 for more information on management of ascites, which can be critical in patients with hepatocellular carcinoma.

Pancreatic Cancer

BACKGROUND

Only about 15% to 20% of patients with pancreatic cancer will be candidates for surgical cure, but even these patients have only about a 30% chance of 5-year survival. Median survival for metastatic pancreatic cancer patients is approximately 6 months.[15,16]

ROLE OF CHEMOTHERAPY

Gemcitabine (Gemzar) is the standard therapy for treating patients with metastatic pancreatic cancer. It is important to note that this was the first chemotherapy approved by the Food and Drug Administration (FDA) based on data showing an improved quality of life as opposed to survival improvement. Gemcitabine showed a clinical benefit response (50% reduction in pain intensity, 50% reduction in analgesic consumption, or 20-point Karnofsky Performance score improvement, all for 4 weeks) in about one fourth of patients, with only a minimal survival benefit.[15] Tarceva (Erlotinib) has shown an additional survival benefit of weeks, but its improvement in quality of life has not been assessed and it comes with adverse effects such as diarrhea, rash, and fatigue.[16] Lastly, a combination of oxaliplatin, irinotecan, and 5-fluorouracil called FOLFIRINOX has shown improved overall survival of 5 to 6 months in carefully selected patients with metastatic disease compared with Gemzar, but with a significantly increased adverse effect profile (see Colon Cancer section for common side effects of these agents). Interestingly, patients receiving FOLFIRINOX maintained their global quality-of-life scores for much longer than those receiving Gemzar.[17]

COMMON PALLIATIVE CARE ISSUES

Pain is present in up to 90% of patients with locally advanced or metastatic pancreatic cancer. Pain in patients with advanced pancreatic cancer may be from malignant gastroparesis, peritoneal carcinomatosis, or celiac plexus invasion, especially for tumors in and around the head of the pancreas. Pain from malignant gastroparesis and peritoneal carcinomatosis was covered in the Gastric Cancer section. Pain from celiac plexus invasion usually is unremitting, radiates to the back and across the upper abdomen in a bandlike fashion, and can be characterized as both sharp and achy. Often this diagnosis is made simply by radiographically establishing that the tumor is proximal to the celiac plexus, without any other obvious cause of the pain.

Medical management of celiac plexus pain usually requires the combination of an opioid and a neuropathic pain agent. Neuropathic agents, including gabapentin (starting at 100 mg every 8 hours and titrating by 100 mg every 3 days to effect, up to 3600 mg/day), pregabalin (starting at 50 mg orally every 8 hours, titrated up to 150 mg orally every 8 hours), or the tricyclic antidepressants (nortriptyline or amitriptyline starting at doses of 25 to 50 mg orally at bedtime, titrated every 2 to 3 days up to a maximum of 150 mg/day), are recommended.[18] Generally, gabapentin is titrated first, with addition of a tricyclic antidepressant if optimal control is not achieved. In addition, pregabalin can be substituted for gabapentin if pain persists on these regimens. In terms of the optimal opioid, there is no clear standard, but methadone may be a rational choice given its additional NMDA (N-methyl D-aspartate) receptor antagonism, which may play a role in neuropathic pain syndromes.[19]

If the combination of an opioid and at least one or two neuropathic agents does not adequately control pain or if there are dose-limiting adverse effects from the pain regimen, a celiac plexus nerve block should be considered. An interventional gastro-enterologist injects a neurolytic solution directly into the celiac plexus, or the injection is administered percutaneously by an interventional radiologist. In a double-blind, randomized control trial, celiac plexus nerve block significantly improved pain intensity compared with the control group (14% vs. 40% of patients reporting pain levels of greater than 5 out of 10 at one or more follow-up appointments; $P = 0.005$) but did not significantly decrease the opioid requirement or improve the quality of life.[20]

Other symptoms are commonly encountered in patients with advanced pancreatic cancer. Obstructive jaundice caused by cancers of the head of the pancreas can lead to significant pruritus from the jaundice, fevers from cholangitis, and a disturbing yellow complexion. Therefore, it is recommended to alleviate the obstruction with stent placement by an experienced interventional gastroenterologist if possible. Lastly, anorexia-cachexia syndrome and fatigue are quite common in people with pancreatic cancer, with approximately 80% of patients displaying symptoms at diagnosis.[21] Anorexia-cachexia syndrome consists of a loss of appetite, involuntary weight loss (especially despite adequate nutrition), and fatigue. Refer to Chapter 9 for further information on anorexia-cachexia syndrome and fatigue.

Colon Cancer

BACKGROUND

Only prostate, lung, and breast cancers had a higher incidence and more deaths than colon cancer in 2008. Approximately 20% of all colorectal patients are found to have metastatic disease at diagnosis, and approximately 20% to 30% of patients who are initially diagnosed with stage III colorectal cancer will be found to have metastatic disease despite receiving adjuvant chemotherapy.[22] It should be noted that colorectal cancer with oligometastatic disease to the liver or lung is still considered curable in some circumstances.[23]

ROLE OF CHEMOTHERAPY

Without systemic chemotherapy, patients with metastatic colon cancer have a life expectancy of 5 to 6 months, compared with a median overall survival of approximately 2 years for patients treated with a combination of agents that include 5-fluorouracil and leucovorin, oxaliplatin, irinotecan, bevacizumab, and cetuximab.[24,25] In patients who undergo chemotherapy, attention must be aimed at controlling the potential toxicity related to chemotherapy.[26]

Oxaliplatin can cause acute neurotoxicity symptoms such as muscle cramping, sensitivity to cold (importantly, laryngospasm to cold, which can feel like choking), and other odd neurologic symptoms, as well as a chronic peripheral stocking-and-glove-pattern sensory neuropathy, usually at cumulative doses of more than 750 mg/m². Intravenous infusion of 1 g magnesium sulfate and 1 g calcium gluconate in 100 mL 5% dextrose in water (D_5W) over 30 minutes before and after oxaliplatin administration reduces the risk of significant chronic neuropathy (grade 2 or more) by approximately 50% compared with placebo, but only significantly reduces the risk of muscle cramps in cases of acute neurotoxicity.[27] Irinotecan can cause diarrhea that is life threatening if not treated urgently.

An aggressive treatment guideline has been established (Figure 29-1) that recommends loperamide 2 mg every 4 hours as a first-line treatment, loperamide 2 mg every 2 hours (up to 16 mg per day) plus an antibiotic as a second-line treatment, and finally discontinuing loperamide 48 hours if unsuccessful with use of alternative anti-diarrheal agent such as octreotide 100 to 150 μg every 8 hours or deodorized tincture of opium 10–15 drops in water every 3–4 hours for refractory or severe cases, in addition to intravenous fluids and a workup to look for infections.[28,29]

Cetuximab can cause a severe acneiform-type rash all over the body, which is usually successfully prevented, in our experience, with doxycycline 100 mg orally twice daily and alclometasone dipropionate (Aclovate) cream. Bevacizumab is generally well tolerated, with a side effect profile consisting of blood clots, bleeding, hypertension, and proteinuria, as well as infusional allergic reactions. Lastly, 5-fluorouracil can lead to oral mucositis, anemia, and diarrhea, which can impact patients' quality of life.

In a randomized controlled trial of 200 patients receiving chemotherapy who developed oral mucositis, salt and soda (1 teaspoon table salt, 1 teaspoon baking soda, and approximately 500 mL tap water), chlorhexidine solution, and "magic mouthwash" (see Esophageal Cancer) were all equally effective in treating mucositis, although a systemic review found that chlorhexidine was associated with tooth discoloration and alteration in taste, limiting its utility.[30,31]

COMMON PALLIATIVE CARE ISSUES

Abdominal pain can be the result of a partial or complete obstruction, peritoneal carcinomatosis, or intestinal perforation that leads to generalized peritonitis. Tenesmus may be the result of a locally advanced lesion encroaching on the pelvic nerves, leading to a neuropathic pain syndrome, especially in patients with rectal or low sigmoid cancers. Treatment of tenesmus may require combination of strong opioids with neuropathic agents, but there is evidence that in refractory cases neurolysis of the superior hypogastric nerve may alleviate symptoms.[3]

In metastatic disease, resection of the primary tumor is indicated in all patients with obstructive symptoms or other problems such as refractory anemia, tumor hemorrhage, or perforation. If the patient is not an appropriate surgical candidate, palliative radiation can be performed to control bleeding. In addition, if the patient is not a reasonable surgical candidate but has obstructive symptoms, consideration for a colonic stent by an experienced interventional gastroenterologist would be appropriate. In some cases, patients receive a stent instead of undergoing surgery, despite being a reasonable surgical candidate, if chemotherapy is scheduled to start soon, with the expectation that it will reduce the tumor burden. See Chapter 25 for more information on malignant bowel obstructions.

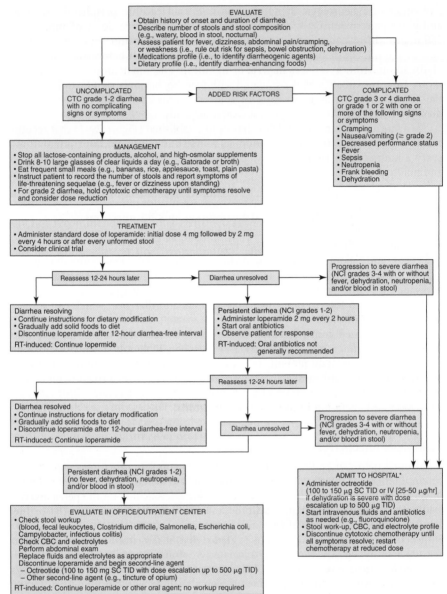

Figure 29-1. Algorithm for treatment of treatment-induced diarrhea. *For radiation-induced diarrhea and select patients with CID, consider aggressive outpatient management unless the patient has sepsis, fever, or neutropenia. CBC, Complete blood cell count; CID, chemotherapy-induced diarrhea; CTC, common toxicity criteria; IV, intravenous; NCI, National Cancer Institute; RT, radiotherapy; SC, subcutaneous; tid, three times a day. *(Adapted with permission from Grothey A, Nikcevich DA, Sloan JA, et al: Evaluation of the effect of calcium and magnesium (CaMg) on chronic and acute neurotoxicity associated with oxaliplatin: results from a placebo controlled phase III trial, J Clin Oncol 27(Suppl):S15, 2009 (suppl; abstr 4025).)*

Esophageal Cancer

BACKGROUND

At diagnosis, nearly 50% of patients have advanced disease that extends beyond the primary tumor. Five-year survival in patients with advanced esophageal cancer is 15% to 20% despite aggressive chemoradiation therapy in appropriate cases. Squamous cell carcinoma is felt to be a more favorable histologic diagnosis compared with adenocarcinoma, but no survival differences have been established in clinical trials.[32]

ROLE OF CHEMOTHERAPY

If the cancer is not metastatic, then serious consideration of combined chemoradiation (with 5-fluorouracil and cisplatin) is warranted because it appears to improve survival compared with radiation alone (27% vs. 0% at 5 years).[28] Unfortunately, in patients with metastatic esophageal cancer, chemotherapy does not appear to improve survival, but the hope is to help control the disease and prevent or delay development of symptoms. Chemotherapy regimens resemble those used in gastric cancer.[33]

COMMON PALLIATIVE CARE ISSUES

Dysphagia is a common presenting symptom and clearly impacts a patient's quality of life. This symptom is managed, as discussed in the Gastric Cancer section, with radiation therapy or stent placement. It should be noted that brachytherapy—placement of radioactive beads into the tumor itself—has not been shown to improve dysphagia symptoms and have fewer complications compared with external beam radiation, so its role at this time is unclear.[34]

Pain in patients getting radiation therapy can be multifactorial; causes include infection (*Candida* esophagitis), radiation esophagitis, and stomatitis from chemotherapy. Radiation esophagitis is managed with a combination of local therapies and systemic opioids. Use of local therapies is limited to topical anesthetics (2% viscous lidocaine), antacids (magnesium aluminum hydroxide), topical antihistamine (diphenhydramine), liquid opioids, and coating substances such as sucralfate. A double-blind, randomized controlled study found only a trend toward improved symptom management when sucralfate was added to the combination of lidocaine/magnesium aluminum hydroxide/diphenhydramine, compared with the latter combination alone.[35] Although no studies exist evaluating topical viscous morphine use in patients with esophagitis, a study comparing it to "magic mouthwash" (a combination of lidocaine, magnesium aluminum hydroxide, and diphenhydramine) in patients with oral mucositis found that the topical viscous morphine group needed one third less supplemental analgesia, reported severe pain ratings for 3 fewer days, and better tolerated the treatment.[36] Given minimal systemic absorption, the proposed mechanism of action was local upregulation of mu-opioid receptors on inflamed mucosal surfaces. Lastly, palifermin is a recombinant human keratinocyte growth factor that is given intravenously. It has been shown to prevent severe mucositis in bone marrow transplant patients after they have received conditioning chemotherapy regimens (63% vs. 98%; $p < 0.001$). Studies investigating its use in other malignancies are scarce, but it appears to have the ability to decrease duration and intensity of mucositis in the setting of chemotherapy and radiotherapy.[37]

PEARLS

- Gastrointestinal cancers each have unique symptoms and quality-of-life issues that must be addressed to effectively palliate these patients.
- Chemotherapy is generally a useful palliative measure in advanced gastrointestinal malignancies, but the patient must have an acceptable performance status to gain benefit (out of bed more than 50% of the day).
- In nonsurgical candidates with a poor overall prognosis, consideration of stents for upper or lower gastrointestinal obstruction should be strongly considered. Patients not amenable to this intervention should be considered for a venting gastrostomy tube.
- Symptoms of anorexia-cachexia syndrome, fatigue, celiac plexus pain syndrome, gastric distention, peritoneal carcinomatosis, radiation esophagitis, carcinoid syndrome, liver capsular stretch, pruritus, tenesmus, and fever all have therapies that can potentially improve a patient's quality of life.

PITFALLS

- Care should be taken when dosing and titration of opioids in patients with hepatocellular carcinoma and decompensated liver failure.
- There is a need for well-designed clinical studies to guide symptomatic management of gastrointestinal cancer patients.
- A patient's treatment and goals-of-care recommendations should not be based on a statistical prognosis without a full multidisciplinary team discussion and a personalized prognosis is reached.
- It is critical to address advanced care planning early in patients with advanced disease.

Summary

Gastrointestinal malignancies are common, and almost all the care given to these patients with advanced disease is palliative in nature. Practitioners must not only understand treatments that improve progression-free and overall survival but also be prepared to manage the symptoms resulting from the malignancy or treatments to prevent unnecessary patient suffering. Given the number of different interventions and procedures, as discussed throughout the course of this chapter, optimal patient care entails a multidisciplinary team including surgeons, interventional radiologists, radiation oncologists, interventional gastroenterologists, palliative medicine specialists, and medical oncologists.

Resources

National Collaborative Cancer Network
   www.nccn.org
National Cancer Institute
   www.cancer.gov
American Cancer Society
   www.cancer.org
CANCERcare
   www.cancercare.org
World Health Organization
   www.who.int

References

1. Garcia M, Jemal A, Ward EM, et al: *Global cancer facts & figures 2007*, Atlanta, 2007, American Cancer Society.
2. Catalano V, Labianca R, Beretta GD, et al: Gastric cancer, *Crit Rev Oncol Hematol* 71:127–164, 2009.
3. Shaiova L: Difficult pain syndromes: bone pain, visceral pain, and neuropathic pain, *Cancer J* 12:330–340, 2006.
4. Donthireddy KR, Ailawadhi S, Nasser E, et al: Malignant gastroparesis: pathogenesis and management of an underrecognized disorder, *J Support Oncol* 5:355–363, 2007.
5. Lambert R: Balancing the benefits and risks of esophageal stenting in the palliation of malignant dysphagia, *J Support Oncol* 6:275–276, 2008.
6. Javle M, Ailawadhi S, Yang GY, et al: Palliation of malignant dysphagia in esophageal cancer: a literature-based review, *J Support Oncol* 4:365–373, 379, 2006.
7. Jeurnink SM, van Eijck CH, Steyerberg EW, et al: Stent versus gastrojejunostomy for the palliation of gastric outlet obstruction: a systematic review, *BMC Gastroenterol* 7:18–27, 2007.
8. Rinke A, Müller HH, Schade-Brittinger C, et al: PROMID Study Group. Placebo-controlled, double-blind, prospective, randomized study on the effect of octreotide LAR in the control of tumor growth in patients with metastatic neuroendocrine midgut tumors: a report from the PROMID study group, *J Clin Oncol* 27:4656–4663, 2009.
9. Toumpanakis C, Garland J, Marelli L, et al: Long-term results of patients with malignant carcinoid syndrome receiving octreotide LAR, *Aliment Pharmacol Ther* 30:733–740, 2009.
10. O'Toole D, Ruszniewski P: Chemoembolization and other ablative therapies for liver metastases of gastrointestinal endocrine tumours, *Best Pract Res Clin Gastroenterol* 19:585–594, 2005.
11. Llovet JM, Ricci S, et al: SHARP Investigators Study Group. Sorafenib in advanced hepatocellular carcinoma, *N Engl J Med* 359:378–390, 2008.
12. Lin M, Wu P, Tsai ST, et al: Hospice and palliative care for patients with hepatocellular carcinoma in Taiwan, *Palliat Med* 18:93–99, 2004.
13. Davis M: Cholestasis and endogenous opioids: liver disease and exogenous opioid pharmacokinetics, *Clin Pharmacokinet* 46:825–850, 2007.
14. Terra SG, Tsunoda SM: Opioid antagonists in the treatment of pruritus from cholestatic liver disease, *Ann Pharmacother* 32:1228–1230, 1998.
15. Rothenberg ML, Moore MJ, Cripps MC, et al: A phase II trial of gemcitabine in patients with 5-FU-refractory pancreas cancer, *Ann Oncol* 7:347–353, 1996.
16. Moore MJ, Goldstein D, Hamm J, et al: Erlotinib plus gemcitabine compared with gemcitabine alone in patients with advanced pancreatic cancer: a phase III trial of the National Cancer Institute of Canada Clinical Trials Group, *J Clin Oncol* 25:1960–1966, 2007.
17. Conroy T, Desseigne F, Ychou M, et al: Randomized phase III trial comparing FOLFIRINOX versus gemcitabine as first-line treatment for metastatic pancreatic adenocarcinoma: final analysis results of the PRODIGE 4/ACCORD 11 trial. ASCO Annual Meeting, Oral Abstract Session, 2010.
18. Paice JA: Mechanisms and management of neuropathic pain in cancer, *J Support Oncol* 1:107–120, 2003.
19. Mannino R, Coyne P, Swainey C, et al: Methadone for cancer-related neuropathic pain: a review of the literature, *J Opioid Manag* 2:269–726, 2006.
20. Wong GY, Schroeder DR, Carns PE, et al: Effect of neurolytic celiac plexus block on pain relief, quality of life, and survival in patients with unresectable pancreatic cancer: a randomized controlled trial, *JAMA* 291:1092–1099, 2004.
21. Uomo G, Gallucci F, Rabitti PG: Anorexia-cachexia syndrome in pancreatic cancer: recent development in research and management, *J Pancreas Online* 7:157–162, 2006.
22. American Cancer Society: *Colorectal cancer facts & figures, 2008–2010*, Atlanta, 2008, American Cancer Society. Available at www.cancer.org.
23. Berri RN, Abdalla EK: Curable metastatic colorectal cancer: recommended paradigms, *Curr Oncol Rep* 11:200–208, 2009.
24. Grothey A, Sugrue MM, Purdie DM, et al: Bevacizumab beyond first progression is associated with prolonged overall survival in metastatic colorectal cancer: results from a large observational cohort study (BRiTE), *J Clin Oncol* 26:5326–5334, 2008.
25. Van Cutsem E, Köhne CH, Hitre E, et al: Cetuximab and chemotherapy as initial treatment for metastatic colorectal cancer, *N Engl J Med* 360:1408–1417, 2009.
26. Eng C: Toxic effects and their management: daily clinical challenges in the treatment of colorectal cancer, *Nat Rev Clin Oncol* 6:207–218, 2009.

27. Grothey A, Nikcevich DA, Sloan JA, et al: Evaluation of the effect of calcium and magnesium (CaMg) on chronic and acute neurotoxicity associated with oxaliplatin: results from a placebo controlled phase III trial, *J Clin Oncol* 27(suppl; abstr 4025):15s, 2009.

28. Benson AB, 3rd, Ajani JA, Catalano RB, et al: Recommended guidelines for the treatment of cancer treatment-induced diarrhea, *J Clin Oncol* 22:2918–2926, 2004.

29. Kornblau SM, Benson AB, 3rd, Catalano R, et al: Management of cancer treatment-related diarrhea: Issues and therapeutic strategies, *J Pain Symptom Manage* 19:118–129, 2000.

30. Dodd MJ, Dibble SL, Miaskowski C, et al: Randomized clinical trial of the effectiveness of 3 commonly used mouthwashes to treat chemotherapy-induced mucositis, *Oral Surg Oral Med Oral Pathol Oral Radiol Endod* 90:39–47, 2000.

31. Potting CM, Uitterhoeve R, Op Reimer WS, et al: The effectiveness of commonly used mouthwashes for the prevention of chemotherapy-induced oral mucositis: a systematic review, *Eur J Cancer Care (Engl)* 15:431–439, 2006.

32. Cooper JS, Guo MD, Herskovic A, et al: Chemoradiotherapy of locally advanced esophageal cancer. A long-term follow-up of a prospective randomized trial (RTOG 85-01), *JAMA* 281:1623–1627, 1999.

33. Shah MA, Schwartz GK: Treatment of metastatic esophageal and gastric cancer, *Sem Oncol* 31:574–587, 2004.

34. Sur RK, Donde B, Levin VC, et al: Fractionated high dose rate intraluminal brachytherapy in palliation of advanced esophageal cancer, *Int J Radiat Oncol Biol Phys* 40:447–453, 1998.

35. Meredith R, Salter M, Kim R, et al: Sucralfate for radiation mucositis: results of a double-blind randomized trial, *Int J Radiat Oncol Biol Phys* 37:275–279, 1997.

36. Cerchietti LC, Navigante AH, Bonomi MR, et al: Effect of topical morphine for mucositis-associated pain following concomitant chemoradiotherapy for head and neck carcinoma, *Cancer* 95:2230–2236, 2002.

37. Barasch A, Epstein J, Tilashalski K: Palifermin for management of treatment-induced oral mucositis in cancer patients, *Biologics* 3:111–116, 2009.

CHAPTER 30

Neurodegenerative Diseases

JEFF MYERS and ANITA CHAKRABORTY

Neurodegenerative diseases (NDs) encompass an array of distinct illnesses with unique clinical manifestations, management strategies, and disease courses. Three specific diseases have been chosen for this chapter in an effort to demonstrate the diverse range of both disease characteristics and patient and family experiences with ND: amytrophic lateral sclerosis (ALS), Parkinson's disease (PD), and multiple sclerosis (MS). For each disease, unique aspects of care are highlighted and principles of symptom control and palliative care are outlined and reviewed.

Key clinical and epidemiologic characteristics of ALS, PD, and MS are summarized in Table 30-1.[1-3] The presentation for ALS is most often a progressive loss in motor function; of these three diseases ALS has by far the lowest incidence, despite a tremendous volume of literature addressing the associated complex care needs.[1] Particularly for individuals older than age 80, PD is a relatively common disease in which the loss of dopaminergic neurons in the brain clinically manifests with both motor and nonmotor impairments.[1] Multiple sclerosis most commonly presents in young adults and is an autoimmune inflammatory disease characterized by multifocal plaques of demyelination throughout the central nervous system.[1]

Common Elements of Care

Despite wide variation in the clinical manifestations of ND, certain key elements are common to most ND patients and should be integrated as part of standardized care.

Table 30-1. Key Clinical and Epidemiologic Characteristics of Three
Neurodegenerative Diseases

	Amyotrophic Lateral Sclerosis (ALS)	Parkinson's Disease (PD)	Multiple Sclerosis (MS)
Prevalence	6/100,000	160/100,000	30–80/100,000
Male-to-Female ratio	1.6:1	1.5:1	1:3.2
Pathophysiology	Progressive degeneration of anterior horn cells and upper and lower motor neurons	Loss of dopaminergic neurons in substantia nigra	Idiopathic inflammation of the central nervous system characterized by demyelination and axonal degeneration
Mean age at diagnosis	47–52 (familial) 58–63 (sporadic)	60–70	18–35
Diagnostic tests	Clinical diagnosis and electromyography	Clinical diagnosis	Clinical diagnosis, supplemented by magnetic resonance imaging of brain and spinal cord; sensory evoked potential testing; and cerebrospinal fluid analysis
Mean survival from time of diagnosis	3–5 years	Normal life expectancy	Life expectancy 6–7 years less than normal
Disease-modifying agents	Riluzole (prolongs survival by 3 months)	None	Beta-interferons Mitoxantrone Glatiramer acetate
Signs/symptoms at presentation	Weakness Spasticity Cramps Fasciculations	Bradykinesia Rigidity Rest tremor Postural instability	Optic neuritis Paresthesias Limb weakness Impaired coordination
Signs/symptoms in advanced disease	Dysphagia Respiratory failure Sialorrhea Pain	Dysphagia Levodopa induced movement disorders Sialorrhea	Spasticity Pain Bowel/bladder dysfunction Fatigue Depression
Clinical course	Progressive	Progressive	Relapsing-remitting Primary progressive Secondary progressive

ADVANCE DIRECTIVES/GOALS OF CARE

Patients in general have difficulty initiating discussions regarding goals for their care. Despite a general awareness of the incurable nature of ND, it remains particularly uncommon for these patients to identify a substitute decision maker or have in place a formal advance directive.[4] It is therefore incumbent upon interprofessional teams to provide guidance regarding advance directive completion and ensure that discussions addressing patient goals are a part of routine clinical assessment. The goals of an individual patient may change over time, highlighting the critical importance of consistent revisiting and ongoing documentation.

KEY DECISIONS

Given the progressive nature of ND and the eventual likelihood of both dysphagia and respiratory insufficiency, patients commonly face key decisions relating to corresponding clinical interventions. Patients and families often carry strong beliefs and values related to these decisions, and the interprofessional team must ensure timely, consistent, and effective communication and education. Team members should remain aware that cognitive impairment is a common feature of ND that must influence the timing of all discussions concerning key decisions and goals of care. In subsequent sections addressing management of specific symptoms, current evidence regarding impact on quality of life and survival for nutritional and respiratory interventions will be outlined.

Nutritional Support

The presence of key clinical features determines the level of urgency for discussions related to the insertion and use of a percutaneous gastrostomy tube (PGT). Potential indications include acceleration of weight loss, frequent choking, and/or impaired quality of life because of stress surrounding eating.[5] The aim of PGT use should not be to prevent aspiration, as PGT use is itself associated with this risk.[6] Overall safety of PGT insertion can be gauged by respiratory function, and in particular by forced vital capacity (FVC), because procedural risks increase when FVC is less than 50% of the predicted value.[5]

Respiratory Support

Symptoms suggestive of respiratory insufficiency include breathlessness, sleep disturbances, appetite loss, excessive fatigue, and daytime sleepiness.[7] Despite limited sensitivity, FVC is widely used to assess respiratory insufficiency because symptoms often correlate with values less than 50% of the predicted value. Both nocturnal oximetry and sniff nasal inspiratory nasal pressure (SNIP) are more sensitive tools to evaluate respiratory insufficiency.[3] However, any symptom or sign of respiratory insufficiency should prompt discussions with patients and their caregivers regarding the potential use of noninvasive positive pressure ventilation (NIPPV) and mechanical ventilation (MV).

Clinicians are strongly encouraged to initiate discussions addressing these key decisions early in the course of illness. Even in the absence of symptoms, early discussion and decision making is, in general, welcomed by patients and families and not associated with a loss of hope or distress.

Interprofessional Care and Collaboration

Given the complex needs of ND patients and their families, it has been proposed that dedicated interprofessional teams may be better suited to ensure that care is comprehensive and coordinated. In addition, improvements in both quality of life and survival have been demonstrated in the setting of care delivered by an interprofessional team.[8]

ROLE OF PALLIATIVE CARE

Although involvement of palliative care has been associated with improvements in overall quality of life for patients with ND, it remains unclear which specific elements of care should routinely be provided by clinicians with palliative care expertise.[9] To provide comprehensive care to patients with ND and their families, it is necessary to identify the primary palliative care competencies required of individual interprofessional team members. Secondary and tertiary palliative care expertise should be accessed if the clinical and symptom needs of patients are complex and unresponsive to primary level interventions.

With the intent of addressing myths regarding palliative care, interprofessional team members, including neurology clinicians not from the palliative care team, should be encouraged to label symptomatic interventions as "palliative in nature"—that is, not intended to modify disease. If consistent, these efforts support an increased understanding that palliative care occurs throughout the ND trajectory and is not "saved" for end of life.

The following are suggested specific roles for palliative care (possibly palliative care specialists, depending on the setting) in the care of ND patients and families:

1. *Direct care.* Palliative care clinicians can address the complex physical and psychosocial symptom issues of ND patients and provide end-of-life care.
2. *Patient/team experience.* Early identification to the patient of palliative care expertise as an integral component of the team enables education of patients and families regarding the possible current and future role for specialist palliative care clinicians.
3. *Advocacy.* Advocacy may include participation and/or facilitation of institutional policy development addressing advanced care planning, national policy development regarding long-term mechanical ventilation, or laws related to physician-assisted suicide.

Given the trajectory and often complex symptom burden ALS patients experience, many advocate for the involvement of palliative care expertise soon after diagnosis.[7] In contrast, PD and MS continue to be considered more chronic in nature, resulting in a less clarity regarding appropriate integration of palliative care expertise.

Symptom Management

The disease-related symptom burden impacting the daily experience of ND patients may lead to substantial distress and, for many, an unacceptable quality of life. Efforts to support a greater emphasis on patient-centered care have led many institutions to integrate the routine use of valid and reliable symptom severity screening tools. Tools targeted for ND patients can serve as a starting point for further dialogue, have the potential to identify physical and psychosocial symptoms before reaching a severe or crisis level, and support the development of targeted symptom management strategies.

SIALORRHEA

Sialorrhea (drooling) may feature prominently in ND, with reported rates of 50% and 70% to 80% in patients with ALS and PD, respectively.[10,11] Sialorrhea typically develops secondary to dysphagia or weakness of orofacial muscles, such that the normal volume of daily saliva production (1.5 L/day) manifests as drooling. Sialorrhea negatively impacts quality of life both physically (e.g., irritation of perioral skin, worsening dysarthria) and psychosocially (e.g., embarrassment, isolation). Treatment strategies are directed at decreasing the volume of saliva produced and summarized in Table 30-2. Anticholinergics are the most common class of medication used in the management of ND-related sialorrhea. Despite efficacy, significant adverse effects (e.g., delirium) may limit the use of these medications for ND patients with cognitive impairment.

SPASTICITY AND CRAMPS

Spasticity, or increased muscle tone, is a manifestation of upper motor neuron dysfunction and is a symptom commonly encountered in both ALS and MS. Patients typically complain of stiffness, immobility, involuntary spasms, joint contractures, and pain.[1]

Occupational therapy and physiotherapy team members play a critical role in the management of spasticity through individualizing appropriate stretching and range-of-motion exercises, splints, and orthotics.[12] Aggressive treatment of spasticity is critically important because the level of severity for any given patient directly

Table 30-2. Treatment Strategies for ND-Related Sialorrhea

Treatment	Comments
Nonpharmacologic	
Manual suction	May cause agitation in end-stage disease
Chest physiotherapy with postural drainage	
Incentive spirometry	
High-frequency chest wall oscillation	Effective in cystic fibrosis; no evidence specific to ALS
Mechanical insufflation/exsufflation	Recommended by ALS practice parameter (6)
Pharmacologic	
Glycopyrrolate (0.5 mg PO bid or tid)	
Scopolamine (1 patch every 3 days)	
Amitriptyline (10–150 mg qd)	Also indicated to treat pseudobulbar affect and depression
Atropine 1% eye drops (1–3 drops q4h)	
Interventions	
Botulinum toxin (10,11)	Maximum response at 4 weeks; duration of action up to 4 months; may cause transient dysphagia
Radiation to parotid and/or submandibular glands (10)	Duration of action up to 6 months; may cause xerostomia

ALS, Amyotrophic lateral sclerosis; ND, neurodegenerative disease.

Table 30-3. Management of ND-Related Spasticity

Treatment	Comments
Nonpharmacologic	
Moderate exercise	
Pharmacologic	
Baclofen (10–40 mg tid)	Can cause weakness and fatigue
Tizanidine (2–8 mg tid)	Can cause weakness and fatigue
Dantrolene (50–100 mg qid)	
Clonazepam (0.5–1.0 mg tid)	
Gabapentin (300–900 mg tid)	Can cause weakness and fatigue
Cannabinoids (THC) (5–10 mg/day)	
Interventions	
Botulinum toxin (14)	Specific to MS
Intrathecal baclofen (13)	For intractable spasticity

MS, Multiple sclerosis; ND, neurodegenerative disease.

correlates with an ability to both transfer and ambulate. Although uncommon, refractory spasticity may be treated with a continuous intrathecal baclofen infusion. Efficacy has been demonstrated in a small cohort of ALS patients with no reported neurologic morbidity or mortality.[13] Therapeutic interventions for spasticity are summarized in Table 30-3.

Muscle cramps are a manifestation of lower motor neuron dysfunction and are commonly encountered in patients with ALS. Relief may be obtained with physical therapy (e.g., passive stretching and massage) or quinine (400 mg/day).[1]

MOTOR COMPLICATIONS IN PARKINSON'S DISEASE

Motor complications in PD comprise a group of aberrant movement phenomena that typically emerge after 5 to 7 years of levodopa therapy.[2] Long-term levodopa therapy can result in drug-induced dyskinesias (involuntary choreiform movements involving the head, trunk, and limbs), dystonias (sustained or repetitive involuntary muscle contractions), and motor fluctuations.[1] Specific motor symptoms include the following:

- "Wearing-off": Increasingly shorter duration of therapeutic benefit following each dose of levodopa; associated with reemergence of Parkinsonian symptoms
- "On-off" fluctuations: Unpredictable and abrupt fluctuations in motor state from times of symptom control ("on") to times of worsening Parkinsonian symptoms ("off")
- Hypokinesis/akinesis: Near immobility associated with "off" periods of dopaminergic treatment
- Dyskinesias/dystonias: Abnormal involuntary movements that may be choreic (typical during "on" periods) or dystonic (can occur during either "on" or "off" periods)
- "Freezing": Near akinesis when initiating walking, turning, or ambulating past visual barriers

The general management of motor symptoms in advanced PND involves levodopa dose adjustments and initiation of adjuvant medications. Specific strategies include the following:

- Fractionate levodopa dosing (lower, more frequent doses)
- Addition of a dopamine agonist (e.g., bromocriptine, pergolide, pramipexole, ropinirole)
- Addition of a catechol-O-methyltransferase (COMT) inhibitor (e.g., entacapone, tolcapone)
- Addition of a monoamine oxidase-B inhibitor (e.g., selegiline, rasagiline)
- Addition of amantadine

"Freezing" is poorly responsive to increases in dopaminergic medication but may respond to sensory stimulation and assisted devices.[1] For advanced motor symptoms poorly responsive to conventional management techniques, parenteral apomorphine (a powerful dopamine agonist) is indicated.[14] In addition, surgical interventions such as deep brain stimulation of the subthalamic nucleus and unilateral pallidotomy can be effective in treating refractory motor complications.[14]

NONMOTOR COMPLICATIONS IN PARKINSON'S DISEASE

Unlike motor complications, symptoms associated with nonmotor complications in PD do not respond to adjustments in dopaminergic therapy.

Autonomic Dysfunction. Common symptoms of autonomic dysfunction include urinary dysfunction and orthostatic hypotension. Symptoms such as urinary frequency and urgency, nocturia, and urge incontinence may be treated with oxybutynin (5 mg two or three times daily) and/or tolterodine (1–2 mg twice daily).[2] These agents have not been specifically studied in PD, however, and may worsen cognitive symptoms.

Postural Hypotension. Management strategies include reassessment of antihypertensive medications, if applicable, and the addition of agents such as midodrine (2.5 mg two to three times daily) and/or fludrocortisone (0.1 mg two or three times daily).[14]

PAIN

In the setting of nonmalignant disease, pain is in general poorly assessed and undertreated. Additionally, the evidence base from which to guide treatment decisions is sparse. A recent Cochrane review examining the medical management of pain in ALS failed to identify any randomized controlled trials or quasi-randomized trials.[15]

Physical weakness, debilitation, and impaired mobility serve as potential sources for pain in the setting of ND.[1] Patients affected by upper motor neuron (UMN) dysfunction resulting in spasticity or lower motor neuron dysfunction (LMN) resulting in weakness present with symptoms of musculoskeletal pain such as stiffness and contractures. General principles for the assessment and treatment of pain should be applied. The expert recommendations of occupational therapy and physiotherapy professionals are essential components of a comprehensive management plan. Pharmacologic management typically begins with agents such as acetaminophen, nonsteroidal anti-inflammatory drugs (NSAIDs), and muscle relaxants. If adequate relief is not achieved with nonpharmacologic techniques in combination with nonopioid analgesics, the introduction of opioids should be considered in accordance with the World Health Organization (WHO) guidelines.[1]

Unlike ALS and PD, pain is a well-described clinical entity for patients with MS. Estimates of pain prevalence in MS range from 29% to 86%, with both neuropathic and nociceptive-somatic pain syndromes having been described. Examples of nociceptive pain include painful tonic spasms, musculoskeletal back pain, and headache.[16] The most common types of neuropathic pain include dysthetic extremity pain, trigeminal neuralgia, and Lhermitte's sign (a transient sensation related to neck movement). Although no efficacy trials have compared various analgesics, options include anti-epileptics (gabapentin and pregabalin), NSAIDS, opioids, tricyclic antidepressants (TCAs), and antispasmodic agents (see Spasticity and Cramps).[16] In a recent consensus guideline, cannabinoids were positioned as second-line agents, given the lack of randomized controlled trials and concerns regarding long-term safety.[17] In the setting of refractory pain, interventional pain management strategies such as nerve blocks have also been reported to be effective.[17]

BREATHLESSNESS

Progressive respiratory muscle weakness in patients with ND may eventually result in the sensation of breathlessness. This can occur with exertion or at rest and can initially present with a history suggestive of nocturnal hypoventilation—that is, disordered sleep and daytime fatigue.

Although routine clinical screening and assessment of breathlessness (including both history and investigations) can support decision making regarding future interventions, management of the symptom itself should not be delayed. Specific strategies are outlined in Table 30-4.

Table 30-4. Management of ND-Related Breathlessness

Treatment	Comments
Nonpharmacologic	
Oxygen therapy	Only use in setting of symptomatic hypoxia (possibly exacerbates hypercapnia)
	Limited evidence for efficacy regardless of underlying cause
Pharmacologic	
Opioids	Dosing and titration similar to dosing and titration for pain
	If chronic, consider routine dosing
Benzodiazepines	Overall lack of evidence for efficacy
	Assess for co-morbid anxiety disorder (benzodiazepine use may be appropriate)
Interventions	
NIPPV	Must be used 4 consecutive hours in a 24-hour period
	Strong evidence for improvements in and maintenance of quality of life
	Some evidence for improving survival
	Patients with bulbar disease less likely to tolerate
Mechanical ventilation	Some evidence for improving survival
	Possibly effective in maintaining quality of life
	Substantial caregiver burden must be considered

ND, Neurodegenerative disease; NIPPV, noninvasive positive pressure ventilation.

Table 30-5. Assessment and Management of ND-Related Dysphagia

Screening/Assessment	General Comments
Clinical nutrition and speech-language assessment at time of diagnosis and each subsequent visit	Nutritional status has been shown to be an independent risk factor for survival.
Weight, diet history, body mass index, swallowing safety should each be monitored	Outcome of assessment should focus on clinically relevant parameters, such as activity limitation, participation restriction, and health-related quality of life.
Video fluoroscopy and fiberoptic endoscopic evaluation as indicated	
Interventions	
Nonpharmacologic interventions	Include dietary counseling and education regarding modification of food/fluid consistency and swallowing techniques.
Nasogastric tube (NGT)	PGT probably prolongs survival in ALS patients.
Percutaneous gastrostomy tube (PGT)	No evidence clarifying impact of PGT use on quality of life for ND patients in general.

ALS, Amyotrophic lateral sclerosis; ND, neurodegenerative disease.

CONSTIPATION

Constipation can be a significant and uncomfortable experience for ND patients.[1] Assessment of both stool frequency and possible incontinence should be routinely assessed, particularly in patients taking medications with constipation as a known side effect. Regular constipation protocols should guide management.

DYSPHAGIA

With ND progression, swallowing difficulties can substantially impact the lives of patients and families. The time required for the process of eating a meal may gradually increase, and the ability to safely swallow may lessen to the point where the patient is at high risk for aspiration.[5] Table 30-5 summarizes the key elements of care associated with dysphagia, including current evidence related to specific interventions.

INSOMNIA

Sleep disturbances are common in patients with ND and require meticulous exploration of related details (e.g., a comprehensive list of all contributing factors, such as pain, discomfort, restlessness, mood, secretions, and breathlessness) to establish targeted and effective management plans. This must include an assessment for both REM behavioral disorder (RBD) and restless leg syndrome (RLS), because each may be an early feature of PD (1). In general, management strategies for ND-related insomnia are largely determined by individual contributing factors, such as pain management, caregiver support, and use of NIPPV. Pharmacologic strategies for common ND-related sleep disturbances are outlined in Table 30-6.

Table 30-6. Pharmacologic Management of ND-Related Insomnia

	Pharmacologic Agent	Comments
ALS	Amitriptyline, zolpidem	
PD	Quetiapine, clonazepam	If nightmares occur, initiate clonazepam.
RBD	Clonazepam, melatonin	RBD is worsened by anticholinergics, selegiline, and dopaminergic medications; low-dose clonazepam should be used.
RLS	Dopamine agonists (pramipexole, pergolide) Benzodiazepines Gabapentin Valproic acid	There is a high prevalence in patients with multiple sclerosis (especially patients with severe pyramidal and sensory disability). Low doses of dopamine agonists should be used. (Note the possible side effect of rebound phenomenon.)

ALS, Amyotrophic lateral sclerosis; MS, multiple sclerosis; ND, neurodegenerative disease; PD, Parkinson's disease; RBD, REM behavior disorder; RLS, restless leg syndrome.

FATIGUE

Fatigue is a common and often untreated symptom in patients with ND. Prevalence ranges for PD and MS patients are 35% to 55% and 70% to 90%, respectively.[18,19] With a complex and multifactorial etiology, fatigue is often present at the time of diagnosis and is specifically identified by one third of ND patients as the worst and most distressing symptom of their disease.[19]

A major challenge in the management of fatigue is a lack of consistently effective therapeutic interventions. Nonpharmacologic options to manage fatigue include structured energy conservation strategies and regular exercise programs. Specifically for MS patients, fatigue is often exacerbated by heat; therefore, avoidance of hyperthermia and initiation of cooling therapies are important management strategies.[20] Although evidence is limited, possible pharmacologic interventions include stimulants (e.g., methylphenidate and modafinil); in addition, specifically for MS, amantadine is often introduced at doses of 100 to 200 mg daily.[20]

Signs and symptoms of sleep disorders and nocturnal insomnia are key features of the clinical assessment for fatigue in ND patients because appropriate diagnosis and treatment of underlying conditions may impact the severity of fatigue experienced.

IMPAIRED COMMUNICATION

Neuromuscular impairment of the tongue and mouth muscles may result in progressive difficulties in the ability to form words. The result is often tremendous frustration and social isolation. For patients with ALS, loss of communication is rated as one of the worst aspects of the disease.[1] Over time, decline in language function is a common feature of cognitively impaired ND patients, which may further compound communication difficulties. Interprofessional team members must consistently demonstrate a strong commitment to identifying ways of addressing communication difficulties to patients and families.

Communication should be routinely assessed every 3 to 6 months by a speech-language therapist.[5] Management strategies include augmentive/alternative communication systems (e.g., writing, hand signals, letter boards, word lists, electronic devices such as gaze communication systems).[3] Recent efforts to develop systems that allow brain electrical currents to directly control computers have shown encouraging results.[5]

COGNITIVE IMPAIRMENT

Table 30-7 summarizes characteristics and management strategies for common forms of ND-related cognitive impairment. Compensatory strategies (e.g., the use of

Table 30-7. ND-Related Cognitive Impairment

ND Cognitive Impairment	Characteristics	Management	Comments
Frontotemporal dementia (FTD)	Occurs in 5% of ALS patients; presents as personality changes, poor insight, irritability, impaired verbal fluency, and deficits in executive functioning.	Trazodone and SSRIs may control behaviors but do not impact cognition; if signs of nocturnal hypoventilation occur, consider NIPPV.	Currently no efficacy data exist for donepezil, rivastigmine, galantamine, or memantine.
PD-related dementia	Occurs in 40%–50% of patients as impairment in attention, memory, and executive and visuospatial functions; behavioral symptoms such as affective changes, hallucinations, and apathy are common.	Pharmacologic management includes donepezil and rivastigmine.	
PD-related psychosis	Occurs in 40% of patients with end-stage PD and typically manifests as visual hallucinations and/or delusions.	Pharmacologic treatments include donepezil, rivastigmine, clozapine, and quetiapine.	Clozapine carries the risk of agranulocytosis. Olanzapine is not recommended.
MS-related cognitive deficit	Occurs in 40%–65% of patients as impairments in memory, attention, and concentration.	Disease-modifying agents (e.g., interferon) modestly improve cognition. Donepezil and SSRIs can also be effective.	Severity of cognitive impairment does not appear to be correlated with level of physical disability.

ALS, Amyotrophic lateral sclerosis; MS, multiple sclerosis; ND, neurodegenerative disease; NIPPV, noninvasive positive pressure ventilation; PD, Parkinson's disease; SSRI, selective serotonin reuptake inhibitor.

Table 30-8. Pharmacologic Management of ND-Related PBA, Depression, and Anxiety

Pharmacologic Agent	Comments
Amitriptyline 10–50 mg/day	Also indicated for sialorrhea
Nortriptyline 25–150 mg/day	For use in depression; studies mostly address PD patients
Desipramine 75–200 mg/day	For use in depression; studies mostly address MS patients
Fluoxetine 20–40 mg/day	
Sertraline 25–100 mg/day	Minimal drug interactions
Citalopram 10–20 mg/day	Minimal drug interactions
Ecitalopram 10–20 mg/day	Minimal drug interactions

ALS, Amyotrophic lateral sclerosis; ND, neurodegenerative disease; PBA, pseudobulbar affect; PD, Parkinson's disease.

memory aids) serve as primary nonpharmacologic interventions for all forms of cognitive impairment.[1]

PSEUDOBULBAR AFFECT

Pseudobulbar affect (PBA), or involuntary emotional expression disorder (IEED), is a syndrome of pathologic laughing and crying often experienced by both ALS and MS patients. An incidence of 10% has been reported for MS; severity of PBA symptoms are often a reflection of disease trajectory.[1] Treatment options for PBA are outlined in Table 30-8. Phase III clinical trials examining the role of dextromethorphan in the treatment of PBA are currently underway.

PSYCHOSOCIAL SYMPTOMS

Psychosocial elements of care in ND patients are often complex and require particular attention and focus. ND-related quality of life correlates more strongly with measures of suffering, depression, and hope or hopelessness than with physical state.[21] Controlling for age, disease severity, and time since diagnosis, shorter survival times and higher rates of mortality have been reported for patients with high levels of hopelessness, depression, and distress.[21]

A summary of recommendations for management of the psychosocial symptoms of ND patients is provided in Box 30-1.

Mood Disorders and Hope

The prevalence of major depression in patients with ALS is between 9% and 11%, and rates of anxiety are reported to be as high as 30%.[21] Several studies have demonstrated that the presence of depression does not correlate with level of physical disability. Although depression and anxiety occur in approximately 40% of patients with advanced PD, mood disorders continue to be under-recognized and under-treated.[22] Significantly higher than in the general population, the prevalence of depression in patients with MS ranges from 15% to 50%.[20] Although conclusive evidence is lacking, it has been speculated that neuroimmunologic factors may contribute to depressive symptoms in MS.

> **Box 30-1.** *Management of Psychosocial Symptoms in Neurodegenerative Disease*
>
> Recommendations for management of the psychosocial symptoms associated with neurodegenerative diseases, such as mood disorders, a desire to hasten death, and desire-to-die statements, include the following:
> - Routinely screen for mood disorders and treat accordingly.
> - Screening for depression and anxiety is not an adequate screen for a desire for hastened death.
> - Explicit conversations regarding a desire to hasten death are necessary.
> - Team members must be prepared to respond to a desire-to-die statement.
> - Be aware that a desire-to-die statement may not represent a desire to hasten death.
> - Remember that desire for hastened death may fluctuate over time and may often not extend to an actual desire for suicide or euthanasia.

When a diagnosis of depression or anxiety is made, standard psychological interventions (supportive therapy, cognitive behavioral therapy) and medications should be initiated. In general, selective serotonin reuptake inhibitors (SSRIs) and TCAs tend to be medications of choice; however, specific selection should be individualized and determined based on presence of accompanying symptoms (e.g., agitation, pseudobulbar affects) and potential antidepressant side effects (see Table 30-8).

Currently, no controlled studies have examined the role of antidepressant medications specifically in the ALS population, and treatment recommendations are largely based on consensus guidelines.

For patients with PD, trials examining SSRI efficacy in the setting of depression demonstrate improvements in depressive symptoms and no exacerbation of extrapyramidal symptoms (EPS). Citalopram, escitalopram, and sertraline demonstrate the lowest potential for drug interactions and therefore may be reasonable first choices in patients taking PD medications. Specific to PD-related depression and anhedonia, treatment may include pramipexole (a dopamine agonist).[1]

Although few studies have examined the management of depression in MS patients, some evidence supports the use of SSRIs, TCAs, cognitive behavioral therapy, and group psychotherapy.[20] Special consideration must be given to MS patients treated with interferon-beta. Previously thought to induce depression, recently it has been shown that interferon-beta is of concern only for patients with a baseline history of depressive symptoms.[20]

Hopelessness is a psychological construct now known to be distinct from and not necessarily associated with depression. Hopelessness is independently related to suicidality, the desire for hastened death, and the willingness to consider assisted suicide.[23] Predictors of hopelessness are most often existential in nature. For patients with ALS, neither severity nor length of illness has been shown to be predictors of hopelessness.[24]

Desire for Hastened Death

Compared with patients living with other chronic illnesses, particular attention should be paid to those with ND with respect to the presence of a desire to hasten death. As a neurodegenerative disease progresses, patients are less able to work, engage in pleasurable activities, care for themselves, and communicate.[25,26] These together constitute a substantial loss of autonomy, and it is not uncommon for patients to seek a sense of control over dying as a means to mitigate any loss in a sense of self.

Compared with other chronic diseases, many reports indicate ND patients are at greater risk for experiencing desire for hastened death.[25,26] The relationship among depression, hopelessness, and a desire for hastened death is complex. Given that hopelessness and depression are two different constructs with differing predictors, it has been suggested that when they are present simultaneously, a desire for hastened death is mutually reinforced.[23]

For patients with MS, severity of depression is the single most important factor associated with a desire to hasten death.[26] Screening for depression, however, does not adequately identify patients with this desire because only one third of patients with depression report a desire to hasten death.[26] It has been recommended that explicit discussions regarding this issue must occur. For patients with PD, up to one third will experience desire to hasten death.[25] More so than physical PD-related variables, the presence of comorbid psychiatric conditions in patients is more likely to lead to a desire for hastened death.

Physician-Assisted Suicide

Much attention has been paid to patients who make the request of health care professionals to assist them in ending their life. In most parts of the world, physician-assisted suicide is illegal. In Oregon, one of three states in the United States where physician-assisted suicide is currently legal, 56% of patients with ALS would consider it. In the Netherlands, where physician-assisted suicide is also a legalized act, one in five patients with ALS die as a result of either voluntary euthanasia or physician-assisted suicide.[27] Patients who choose a physician-assisted death do not differ from those who do not with respect to socioeconomic demographics, level of pain, despair, fear, or anger.[27] In addition, greater than average suffering and lack of palliative care do not contribute to decisions around seeking physician-assisted death.

Given that physician-assisted suicide is not legal in most jurisdictions, desire-to-die statements from ND patients warrant careful attention and open, sensitive communication. The clinician's initial response to a desire-to-die statement made by a patient is a critical opportunity to explore meaning, rather than simply dismissing the statement by citing legalities. Seeking to understand the meaning behind a desire-to-die statement is crucial to formulating a professional response and appropriate intervention. The dialogue is iterative in nature, and a focus on implementation of care plans such as advance directives should be maintained.

End-of-Life Care

Although the interface between chronic care and palliative care in ND continues to evolve, at present little is known about end-of-life experiences for these patients and their families. Perspectives offered by bereaved caregivers of PD patients have identified certain distressing symptoms for patients and families, which include difficulty eating, difficulty communicating, pain, and suffering.[28] One large retrospective study looking at deaths in ALS patients reported that the vast majority died peacefully.[29] In this same study, symptoms found to be distressing included breathlessness, fear and anxiety, pain, insomnia, and choking.[29] Studies comparing end-of-life care in PD and ALS patients that report symptoms of breathlessness and difficulty eating were more common and severe in ALS, whereas confusion was more commonly experienced in PD.[28] Duration of hospice care was significantly shorter in PD patients; however, overall intensity of suffering, as determined by caregivers, was comparable between the two patient populations.[28]

PEARLS

- Interprofessional teams providing care to specific ND patient populations should determine the relevant care decisions that will at some point need to be addressed by the patient and family and incorporate these "key conversations" as part of routine care.

- Advance directives, substitute decision makers, and care goals should be well documented and made available to all care providers.

- Effective physical and psychosocial symptom management must be a central component of care for all ND patients and families.

- Palliative care as a field should define for itself specific roles regarding direct patient care, professional education, and advocacy.

- Given the complex nature of the ND patient and family experience, future research in ND-related symptom management should explore alternative and innovative treatment modalities, including such things as music, art, and pet therapy.

PITFALLS

- Appropriate and targeted support of families and caregivers is a crucial element of care for ND patients. A study of ALS caregivers revealed that primary caregivers spend a median of 11 hours per day caring for patients, with time requirements being significantly higher for patients who are mechanically ventilated.[30] Examining ALS patient-caregiver couples, burden and depression were found to increase significantly over a 9-month period in caregivers while quality of life measures in patients remained stable.[30]

- Demands on informal caregivers often increase as patients transition from the chronic to the terminal phase of illness. Caregivers of patients with PD feel significantly burdened in providing end-of-life care. At least one third will feel poorly prepared to cope with the stress of caregiving and meet the patient's physical needs, as well as handle emergencies.[28]

Summary

Patients and families facing the diagnosis of a neurodegenerative disease require a communicative and proactive interprofessional team willing to anticipate, discuss, and aggressively manage the uniquely challenging physical and psychosocial symptoms and experiences.

Resources

A variety of resources for caregivers can be found via the following websites:
www.als.ca/_caregivers.aspx
www.pdcaregiver.org/
mssociety.ca/en/help/services.htm

References

1. Elman L, Houghton D, Wu G, et al: Palliative care in amyotrophic lateral sclerosis, Parkinson's disease and multiple sclerosis, *J Palliat Med* 10(2):433–457, 2007.
2. Rao S, Hofmann L, Shakil A, et al: Parkinson's disease: diagnosis and treatment, *Am Fam Physician* 74:2046–2054, 2006.
3. Phukan J, Hardiman O: The management of amyotrophic lateral sclerosis, *J Neurol* 256:176–186, 2009.
4. Chahine L, Malik B, Davis M: Palliative care needs of patients with neurologic or neurosurgical conditions, *Euro J Neurol* 15:1265–1272, 2008.
5. Andersen P, Borasio G, Dengler R, et al: EFNS task force on management of amyotrophic lateral sclerosis: guidelines for diagnosing and clinical care of patients and relatives, *Euro J Neurol* 12: 921–938, 2005.
6. Miller R, Jackson C, Kasarskis E, et al: Practice parameter update: the care of the patient with amyotrophic lateral sclerosis: drug, nutritional, and respiratory therapies (an evidence-based review), *Neurology* 73:1218–1226, 2009.
7. Radunovic A, Mitsumoto H, Leigh P: Clinical care of patients with amyotrophic lateral sclerosis, *Lancet Neurol* 6:913–925, 2007.
8. Chio A, Bottacchi E, Buffa C, et al: Positive effects of tertiary centres for amyotrophic lateral sclerosis on outcome and use of hospital facilities, *J Neurol Neurosurg Psychiatry* 77:948–950, 2006.
9. Liao S, Arnold R: Attitudinal differences in neurodegenerative disorders, *J Palliat Med* 10(2):430–432, 2007.
10. Stone C, O'Leary N: Systematic review of the effectiveness of botulinum toxin or radiotherapy for sialorrhea in patients with amyotrophic lateral sclerosis, *J Pain Symptom Manage* 37(2):246–258, 2009.
11. Molloy L: Treatment of sialorrhea in patients with Parkinson's disease: best current evidence, *Curr Opin Neurol* 20:493–498, 2007.
12. Lewis M, Rushanan S: The role of physical therapy and occupational therapy in the treatment of amyotrophic lateral sclerosis, *NeuroRehab* 22:451–461, 2007.
13. McClelland S, Bethoux F, Boulis N, et al: Intrathecal baclofen for spasticity-related pain in amyotrophic lateral sclerosis: efficacy and factors associated with pain relief, *Muscle Nerve* 37:396–398, 2008.
14. Goetz C, Poewe W, Rascol O, et al: Evidence-based medical review update: pharmacological and surgical treatments of Parkinson's disease: 2001 to 2004, *Mov Disord* 20:523–539, 2005.
15. Brettschneider J, Kurent J, Ludolph A, et al: Drug therapy for pain in amyotrophic lateral sclerosis or motor neuron disease, *Cochrane Database Syst Rev* 16(3):CD005226, 2008.
16. Kenner M, Menon U, Elliott DG: Multiple sclerosis as a painful disease, *Int Rev Neurobiol* 79:303–321, 2007.
17. Pollmann W, Feneberg W: Current management of pain associated with multiple sclerosis, *CNS Drugs* 22:291–324, 2008.
18. Henze T: What's new in symptom management, *Int MS J* 14:22–27, 2007.
19. Lou JS: Fatigue in amyotrophic lateral sclerosis, *Phys Med Rehabil Clin N Am* 19(3):533–543, 2008.
20. Ziemssen T: Multiple sclerosis beyond EDSS: depression and fatigue, *J Neurol Sci* 277:S37–S41, 2009.
21. McLeod J, Clarke D: A review of psychosocial aspects of motor neuron disease, *J Neurol Sci* 258:4–10, 2007.
22. Reijnders JS, Ehrt U, Weber WE, et al: A systematic review of prevalence studies of depression in Parkinson's disease, *Mov Disord* 23(2):183–189, 2008.
23. Rodin G, Lo C, Mikulincer M, et al: Pathways to distress: the multiple determinants of depression, hopelessness, and the desire for hastened death in metastatic cancer patients, *Soc Sci Med* 68(3):562–569, 2009.
24. Fanos J, Gelinas D, Foster R, et al: Hope in palliative care: from narcissism to self-transcendence in amyotrophic lateral sclerosis, *J Palliat Med* 11(3):470–475, 2008.
25. Nazem S, Siderowf A, Duda J, et al: Suicidal and death ideation in Parkinson's disease, *Mov Disord* 23(11):1573–1579, 2008.
26. Turner A, Williams R, Bowen J, et al: Suicidal ideation in multiple sclerosis, *Arch Phys Med Rehabil* 87:1073–1077, 2006.
27. Veldink J, Wokke J, Van Der Wal G, et al: Euthanasia and physician-assisted suicide among patients with amyotrophic lateral sclerosis in the Netherlands, *N Eng J Med* 346(21):1638–1644, 2002.
28. Goy E, Carter J, Ganzini L: Neurologic disease at the end of life: caregiver descriptions of Parkinson's disease and amyotrophic lateral sclerosis, *J Palliat Med* 11(4):548–554, 2008.
29. Mandler RN, Anderson FA, Miller RG, et al: The ALS patient care database: insights into end-of-life care in ALS, *ALS* 2:203–208, 2001.
30. Gauthier A, Vignola A, Calvo A, et al: A longitudinal study on quality of life and depression in ALS patient-caregiver couples, *Neurology* 68:923–926, 2007.

CHAPTER 31

Principles of Palliative Surgery

PETER ANGELOS and GEOFFREY P. DUNN

Palliative Philosophy, History, and Definitions	**Special Topics**
Goals of Palliative Surgery	Do Not Resuscitate Orders in the Operating Room
	Advanced Care Planning
Palliative Surgery by All Surgeons	Futility
Cancer and Palliative Surgery	**Responding to Perioperative Suffering**
Procedure Selection and Patient Assessment	**The Role of Research**
	Pearls
Complications and Outcomes Measures	**Pitfalls**
	Summary

> *"I hope we have taken another good step [gastrectomy] towards securing unfortunate people hitherto regarded as incurable or, if there should be recurrences of cancer, at least alleviating their suffering for a time."*
> —THEODOR BILLROTH, MD, 1881[1]

The old adage "a chance to cut is a chance to cure" is often used to characterize the primary motivation and attitude of most surgeons. Despite the commendable goal of cure, the statement does not acknowledge that much of surgical care is for the equally commendable purpose of palliation. In the following pages, the tactics and strategy of palliative surgery are examined in the context of surgical palliative care when the goals of care transition from cure to palliation. Next, the long tradition of palliative surgery in surgical history is reviewed. Subsequently, the evolving definition of palliative surgery and the application of its goals in different disease settings is demonstrated. Measurement of outcomes for palliative surgery is examined. The ethical issues surrounding operating on patients who have a "do not resuscitate" (DNR) order is considered, along with the importance of communicating well with patients and families in palliative surgical situations. Finally, the challenges to conducting palliative surgical research are reviewed.

Palliative Philosophy, History, and Definitions

Much of medical care reflects the widespread expectation of the curative model of disease. According to this model, the goal of medicine is to cure disease, where "cure" is understood as "the eradication of the cause of an illness or disease [or] the ... interruption and reversal of the natural history of the disorder".[2] Patients commonly

451

assume this model when they seek the assistance of a physician. Many physicians, in fact, believe that cure should be the primary goal of all medical or surgical interventions. As appealing as such an approach may seem initially, the curative model pushes physicians to focus on the disease rather than on the patient. The disease focus emphasizes analytic and rationalistic thinking that favors objective facts and empirical knowledge over subjective issues.[3] Such an approach to medical care suggests that physicians have little to offer when cure is not possible. As such, the curative model provides an unacceptably narrow conception of medical and surgical care.

In contrast to the curative model, the palliative model focuses far more on the patient than on the disease or illness itself. The palliative model aims to control symptoms, relieve suffering, and reestablish functional capacity.[4,5] All these goals are directly related to how the patient experiences the illness. As such, the patient and his or her circle of family and immediate community become central to the palliative model of medicine, and subjective assessments by patients are of critical importance. Although the strict dichotomy between the curative model and the palliative model is somewhat artificial, these opposing approaches emphasize different aspects of the interaction between physician and patient.

Because it stresses the patient's experience of illness and disease, the palliative model provides a better conceptualization of the central tenets of the surgeon–patient relationship. Every surgical intervention is grounded in an analysis of the risks and benefits of the operation for the particular patient. There can be no meaningful general discussion of the risks and benefits of an operation with a patient. For such a discussion to be meaningful, the surgeon must help patients consider the individual risks and benefits of the particular operation for themselves. The analysis of risks and benefits of an operation are necessarily specific to a particular patient. In fact, one cannot really understand benefits without a particular patient to define what will be of benefit to him or to her. For these reasons, the palliative model is more closely associated with the relationship between surgeons and patients, even though much of surgical thinking about intervention is still currently focused on cure.

Palliative surgery is a topic of recent interest, but in historical context it is the presumption of curative surgery that is recent. Although many surgeons consider cure the usual goal of most operations, this development is recent. Before the last century and a half, illness and disease expressed themselves through signs and symptoms. There was no basis for conceptualizing a disease apart from the symptoms that it caused a patient. As such, surgery was firmly grounded on procedures that were thought to alleviate symptoms. Bloodletting, cauterization, amputations, and extractions of bladder stones are all examples of common surgical procedures from ages past.[6,7] None of these procedures are curative, yet at one time they were thought to help in the alleviation of symptoms.

Surgery frequently continues to be directed at palliation rather than at cure. In recent decades, the explosion of cardiac surgery to treat coronary artery disease is certainly palliative surgery.[7] Patients with angina are operated on to diminish or eliminate the symptoms of coronary artery disease. Coronary artery bypass grafts are not curative operations. This procedure does nothing to alter the disease process of atherosclerotic narrowing of the coronary vessels, and there is little or no effect on longevity, but quality of life is much improved. The status of peripheral vascular surgery is similar in that the operations seek to find alternate routes around blocked or narrowed arteries. These surgical procedures are designed to be palliative, but they are never curative.

In transplant surgery, for example, the replacement of a failed kidney with a new donor kidney does not cure the underlying cause of the renal failure. The new kidney may be seen as a cure for end-stage renal disease; however, the operation does nothing to alter the disease process that led to the renal failure. Other common examples of palliative surgical procedures are the increasingly common laparoscopic fundoplication procedures to treat gastroesophageal reflux disease and the common bariatric surgical procedures for morbidly obese patients. Both operations aim to improve problematic symptoms and quality of life, and perhaps to palliate, but not to cure the underlying cause of illness.

All these examples should emphasize the fact that although surgeons may tend to think of their procedures as leading to cure, most surgical procedures over the last several hundred years were, at best, palliative. The focus on curative surgery is a phenomenon of the last few decades, even though many procedures still have a strong element or sole goal of palliation. In fact, cancer surgery provides one of the few examples in which an operation may help lead to a cure of a disease.

An important feature of defining palliative surgery as aiming to relieve symptoms is that it has implications for how success and failure are defined. Palliative surgery is directed at alleviating symptoms rather than curing disease. However, the term *palliative surgery* has had conflicting definitions in the past. The fundamental conflict lay in an understanding of what was being mitigated—disease or symptoms. Easson and colleagues[8] suggest that palliative surgery in oncology has been defined in three distinct ways relative to the extent of resection possible:

1. Surgery to relieve symptoms, with knowledge in advance that all the tumor cannot be removed
2. Resection with microscopic or gross residual tumor left in situ at the end of the procedure
3. Resection for recurrent or persistent disease after primary treatment failure

Miner has expanded the definition of palliative surgery for cancer to include quality of life considerations in addition to relief from burdensome symptoms: "a procedure used with the primary intention of improving quality of life or relieving symptoms caused by the advanced malignancy. The effectiveness of a palliative intervention should be judged by the presence and durability of patient-acknowledged symptom resolution".[9]

Based on this description, a failed curative operation will not necessarily become a palliative operation. A noncurative operation is not a palliative operation. In the realm of cancer surgery, one must be especially careful to distinguish a noncurative resection from an operation that has been designed and performed as a method of relieving the patient's symptoms. Some procedures are both curative and palliative, others are neither curative nor palliative, and yet others are palliative but not curative. For example, if a patient has obstructing colon cancer and carcinomatosis, resection could certainly be palliative even though it is not curative. However, if a patient has a localized low rectal carcinoma that is resected but the margins are found to be positive, this procedure becomes part of a diagnostic process and possibly part of a treatment plan, but it is neither curative nor strictly palliative.

When considering whether to proceed with a palliative operation, the surgeon must carefully assess what symptoms the operation may be able to palliate. As with any surgical intervention, a careful assessment of risks and benefits to the patient must be undertaken. This consideration requires the surgeon to assess the patient's symptoms and then, with the patient's input, consider whether the symptoms can be alleviated by an operation. As a general rule, localized symptoms are more amenable to palliative surgical intervention than systemic symptoms. Patients are often more willing to accept higher risks of morbidity and mortality if the potential benefit is cure, but each individual case is different and requires that the surgeon and patient communicate about the risks and potential benefits of the procedure.

Patients must fully understand the goals of an operation before they consent to the procedure. If the goal is palliative resection of bleeding gastric carcinoma, the patient should not expect that curative resection will be the outcome. Sometimes if curative resection is not possible, a palliative operation will be performed. For example, in patients with obstructing jaundice from cancer of the head of the pancreas, most surgeons plan a palliative choledochojejunostomy if a potentially curative pancreaticoduodenectomy is not possible. In such a situation, it is important for the patient to understand the likelihood of a curative resection relative to the possible nonoperative means of alleviating symptoms.

It is also important for patients to understand the potential time frame for palliation. For example, it may be very significant for a patient to know that the alleviation of symptoms from an operation would be expected to last for a few weeks rather than for a few months. If a patient has a short life expectancy, then the longer hospital stay may offset the benefit of a palliative procedure. Similarly, the appeal to a patient of a palliative procedure may diminish if there is a high risk that the patient will not survive until discharge from the hospital.

These considerations demonstrate that it is essential for surgeons to understand the patient's goals when any intervention is considered. To give recommendations about what procedure is best for a patient with a potentially incurable disease, the surgeon must first fully understand the patient's goals so the benefits of the procedure can be suitably assessed. Pathologists, for instance, routinely evaluate the outcome of the procedure by the extent of residual cancer, but a palliative procedure can be deemed a success only relative to the patient's goal for alleviation of symptoms.

The previously conflicting definitions of palliative surgery are indicative of the need for a comprehensive philosophy of surgical care that addresses the needs of the seriously and incurably ill beyond a repertoire of procedures. Palliative surgery is only a component of the armamentarium available to the surgeon working in the broad context of surgical palliative care. Surgical palliative care describes the appropriate context in which palliative surgery occurs. Not all patients with life-limiting illness who are under surgical care will undergo surgery, yet their needs with respect to relief of suffering and promotion of quality of life will require the unique expertise and experience of a surgeon. Surgical palliative care is defined as the treatment of suffering and the promotion of quality of life for seriously or terminally ill patients under surgical care.[10]

Goals of Palliative Surgery

In determining whether a palliative operation should be performed, the surgeon and patient should consider how the procedure would benefit the patient. Many different procedures may be performed related to multiple different organ systems, yet the procedures can be broadly categorized as directed toward four general symptom-related goals: local control of disease; control of pain; control of other disturbing symptoms; and other goals related to the relief of suffering.

A mastectomy to remove a fungating breast carcinoma that is performed on a patient with distant metastases is an example of a palliative procedure directed solely at control of local disease symptoms. Although the operation will not cure the disease, it may alleviate major problems associated with the local extension of the tumor through the skin.

The well-proven benefits of celiac plexus block for unresectable pancreatic carcinoma illustrate how a palliative procedure can be directed specifically at alleviation of pain.[11]

The broadest categories of palliative procedures are those directed at control or alleviation of disturbing symptoms other than pain. Procedures such as bypasses to relieve intestinal or vascular obstructions, tumor resections to control bleeding, and drainage of pleural effusions to alleviate dyspnea are all important palliative measures that are directed at alleviating diverse, specific symptoms.[12]

Sometimes other goals are met by palliative procedures. For example, the placement of a feeding jejeunostomy tube may allow parenteral nutrition that could facilitate a patient's discharge from the hospital.

Palliative Surgery by All Surgeons

The most recent American College of Surgeons (ACS) Statement of Principles of Palliative Care (Box 31-1) is an important document that seeks to define the manner in which palliative care is integral to the comprehensive care of all surgical patients.[13]

Box 31-1. *American College of Surgeons' Statement of Principles of Palliative Care*

Respect the dignity and autonomy of patients, patients' surrogates, and caregivers.

Honor the right of the competent patient or surrogate to choose among treatments, including those that may or may not prolong life.

Communicate effectively and empathetically with patients, their families, and caregivers.

Identify the primary goals of care from the patient's perspective, and address how the surgeon's care can achieve the patient's objectives.

Strive to alleviate pain and other burdensome physical and nonphysical symptoms.

Recognize, assess, discuss, and offer access to services for psychological, social, and spiritual issues.

Provide access to therapeutic support, encompassing the spectrum from life-prolonging treatments through hospice care, when they can realistically be expected to improve the quality of life as perceived by the patient.

Recognize the physician's responsibility to discourage treatments that are unlikely to achieve the patient's goals, and encourage patients and families to consider hospice care when the prognosis for survival is likely to be less than a half-year.

Arrange for continuity of care by the patient's primary or specialist physician, thus alleviating the sense of abandonment patients may feel when "curative" therapies are no longer useful.

Maintain a collegial and supportive attitude toward others entrusted with care of the patient.

Adapted from American College of Surgeons: Statement of principles of palliative care, *Bull Am Coll Surg* 20:34–35, 2005.

All surgical textbooks contain descriptions of the techniques utilized for these numerous palliative procedures. However, it is critical for the surgeon to apply those techniques in a manner that best benefits individual patients. To do so, the surgeon must think broadly of the impact that the procedure will have on the patient's symptoms.

Because virtually any surgical intervention may be palliative for some patients, every surgeon must be fully competent in how to make decisions about palliative surgery. Unlike internal medicine, which has defined palliative care as a specialty, all surgeons must be able to apply the techniques of their particular anatomic area of expertise to the goal of palliation of patient's symptoms. Although surgeons should consult appropriate palliative care specialists to aid in the treatment of their patients, every surgeon should be prepared to apply surgical techniques to palliate symptoms. Indeed, part of the skill of surgery is to make intraoperative decisions to allow the greatest relief of patients' symptoms.

CANCER AND PALLIATIVE SURGERY

As noted earlier, palliative procedures are found in virtually every aspect of surgery. Much attention in surgical palliation is appropriately directed toward treating the terminally ill patient with cancer. This group of patients is particularly challenging to treat because of the inherent stresses suffered by patients, caregivers, and families when a patient is nearing the end of life. Although these stresses have always been present, the issues have become more problematic in recent decades for several reasons.[14] First, physicians have more life-prolonging options to offer patients, although many of these options do not alleviate symptoms. Second, because social changes have increased the importance of shared decision making, physicians are required to become better at communicating with patients about the patient's values and interests, to determine what will benefit the patient. Finally, with the increasing mobility of modern society, few patients have long-standing relationships with their primary care physicians, let alone with their surgeons. As a result, surgeons must seek to understand the values and interests of their patients rapidly, to help them decide how best to palliate the disease processes.

In caring for patients with cancer near the end of their lives, physicians must be sure that patients and families are fully cognizant of the goals of specific interventions. Because so much care in the early phases of cancer is directed toward eradicating the disease, patients and families are sometimes hesitant to focus on interventions that can diminish symptoms. When a decision is made to pursue a palliative operation in a terminally ill patient with cancer, the patient and family may harbor unreasonable expectations that the intervention will not only alleviate symptoms but also extend life. Care must be taken to ensure that the patient, family members, and physicians all understand that the intervention is designed to improve symptoms. In such situations, informed consent requires a discussion of the various possibilities related to both curative and palliative goals.

Procedure Selection and Patient Assessment

In any situation in which the decision is made to proceed with a palliative operation, a careful assessment of the risks and benefits of the procedure and the characteristics and expectations of the patient/family must be undertaken. The three main determinants for selecting a procedure include: (1) the patient's symptoms and personal goals; (2) the expected impact of the procedure on quality of life, function, and prognosis (time; and (3) the prognosis of the underlying disease (time and functional decline expectations).[15] When the benefits of an operation are potential cure, the risks a patient is willing to take may be quite large. However, when the benefit is alleviation of some of the patient's symptoms, the risks must be careful compared with the proposed benefit. Additional considerations for selection of a procedure include an assessment of the reconstruction and rehabilitation requirements; the surgeon's personal characteristics, such as efficient versus slow, empathic versus "technician," experienced versus inexperienced; expectation of intraoperative difficulties (e.g., adhesions); and the availability of nonsurgical means to achieve palliation. When there are both surgical and nonsurgical options for alleviating symptoms, the nonsurgical approach should often be favored unless the nonsurgical option has greater anticipated side effects. In some situations, the possible benefits of the palliative operation to the patient may be so very low that the surgeon will decide that the procedure should not be performed. One may come to such a conclusion when there is a small chance that the procedure will alleviate the patient's symptoms or when the patient is so critically ill that the operation itself would likely cause death. This situation is summarized by the assessment that a patient is "too sick for surgery." There is no sound ethical argument to operate on a patient who will certainly not survive the operation, and surgeons should not feel obligated to undertake such procedures.[16] In contemplating a palliative surgical procedure, the surgeon must be mindful of the danger of unchallenged benevolence as he or she balances the moral imperative to help with the ethical imperatives of nonmaleficence and beneficence—that is, the need to "do something" even if of doubtful benefit—stemming from the surgeon's (or family's) own fear of powerlessness.[17]

Complications and Outcomes Measures

Until the previous decade, outcomes after palliative surgery were usually reported in terms of mortality and morbidity. Other previous outcome measures focused narrowly on a specific endpoint such as ability to discontinue nasogastric suction after operation for bowel obstruction. This type of outcome measurement could not predict an improved quality of life. Recently, several outcomes measures have been proposed for the assessment of palliative surgical intervention for symptomatic cancer patients. Complicating this assessment is the expected transient increase in symptoms stemming from the operation itself—such as incision pain, postoperative ileus, and delirium—and future symptoms emerging from the underlying disease process.

The Palliative Surgery Outcome Score (PSOS), introduced by McCahill and colleagues,[18] is expressed as a ratio of symptom-free, nonhospitalized days to the number of postoperative days, up to 180 days. For patients who live less than 180 days after operation, the days survived are used as the denominator. "Symptom-free" refers to the symptom treated and to the absence of major postoperative complications. "Hospitalized" indicates days hospitalized for the palliative procedure and any additional days required for monitoring and treatment of postoperative complications. Based on patient/family follow-up interviews, it was determined that a score of 0.7 or greater on a scale of 0 to 1 indicated the procedure resulted in good to excellent palliation. Patients with a survival of less than 180 days had significantly lower PSOS scores in this study, which underscores the importance of accurate prognostication as part of the consent process before undergoing surgical palliation.

Special Topics

DO NOT RESUSCITATE ORDERS IN THE OPERATING ROOM

Because palliative surgery is often contemplated for patients with incurable diseases who are near the end of life, many of these patients have DNR orders. It is therefore important to consider what a DNR order really means and the impact it has on operative interventions.

DNR refers to a decision to withhold cardiopulmonary resuscitation (CPR) from a patient. When a patient has been suitably included in the decision to write a DNR order, it is a means of extending a patient's autonomous decision making so the patient can specifically opt out of the presumed consent for CPR in the hospital. Thus, DNR orders can be seen as grounded in the principle of respect for patient autonomy.[19]

Although the writing of DNR orders seems to be increasing and they are widely accepted in hospitals,[20] problems remain when a patient with a DNR order has surgery. DNR orders in the operating room and during the perioperative period are problematic for several reasons. First, there is a clear precedent for a patient's previous hospital orders to be seen as irrelevant in the specialized environment of the operating room. This assumption is partly reflected in the common practice of writing a new complete set of orders after a patient leaves the operating room. Second, the relationship between "resuscitation" and providing general anesthesia is complex. Because general anesthesia often involves intubation, positive-pressure ventilation, paralysis, and fluid resuscitation, it often becomes difficult to determine where the administration of anesthesia ends and resuscitation begins.[21] Third, pulmonary or vascular compromise in the operating room and during the perioperative period is more readily reversible than in other situations. As a result, it is very difficult for surgeons and anesthesiologists to start an operation that could precipitate a patient's death if they are forbidden to try to resuscitate the patient.

For the reasons noted, many hospitals have adopted policies that do not allow a patient to enter the operating room unless all DNR orders are rescinded, at least for the operation. However, such an all-encompassing approach seems inappropriately to limit the autonomy of patients who may have very thoughtful and clear reasons for retaining their DNR order even in the operating room. Some have argued that patients should not be deprived of having their autonomous choices respected just because they need an operation. Furthermore, even if surgery with a DNR order is riskier than surgery without one, patients are allowed to choose riskier procedures or to reject beneficial ones.

How can this dilemma be settled? In 1991, Cohen and Cohen suggested an approach called "required reconsideration" that has subsequently been endorsed by the ACS and the American Society of Anesthesiologists.[22] It is described as "an individualized policy of required reconsideration by which patients and their responsible caregivers would reexamine DNR orders before surgery whenever possible".[23] According to this approach, the involved physicians and the patient must agree on a definition of "resuscitation." Once this is agreement is reached, the parties must consider whether withholding resuscitation will compromise the patient's basic objectives. Finally, the positions taken must be clearly communicated so caregivers, patient, and family fully understand the plan for resuscitation in the operating room. This agreement should also be documented in the medical record.

Two hypothetical cases help to illustrate how required reconsideration can be valuable in considering requests for DNR orders in the operating room. Consider the case of a patient with advanced gastric lymphoma who is admitted with pneumonia. The patient requested a DNR order at the time of admission because she has no desire to receive further chemotherapy, and if her heart stops, she does not want CPR. Although she does not want CPR if cardiac arrest occurs in the operating room, she would possibly seek operative intervention if she were to develop a life-threatening gastrointestinal hemorrhage. Such a request is consistent with the patient's basic goals of care. If the parties agree, for example, that the DNR order should be restricted to actual cardiac arrest in the perioperative period, this could be documented in the chart, and the operation should proceed.

In contrast, consider a case in which an 80-year-old man with rectal carcinoma and extensive local disease is scheduled for a pelvic exenteration. He requests a DNR order be in effect before and during surgery and states that he hopes to die in his sleep while in the operating room. If the patient confides that he agrees to the operation and hopes that the surgery and anesthetic will kill him, then this is clearly a very different type of situation. Surgery should not be used as a pretext for desired passive euthanasia. When considering the issues of required reconsideration, a clear discrepancy can be detected between the goals of the operation as understood by the patient in contrast to the goals as understood by the anesthesiologist and surgeon. In this case, the surgeon and anesthesiologist would be justified in opposing the patient's reason for the DNR order in the perioperative period and should instead prompt a reassessment of the patient and the goals and care plan.

ADVANCED CARE PLANNING

When a patient has a palliative operation, it is important that the patient, family, and caregivers fully understand the goals of the intervention. In addition, when the discussion about the palliative operation occurs, the physician should also explore the patient's wishes regarding future decision making. In other words, if the patient is able to participate in the decision to have a palliative operation, the surgeon should take this opportunity to explore the patient's choices about what decisions he or she would prefer if he or she became unable to make autonomous choices. This attempt to identify advance directives may help to alleviate problems in the future. If these discussions are pursued while the patient is able to participate, the family may benefit greatly in the future should the patient be unable to participate in the decision-making process. Although it is sometimes difficult to discuss with a patient what he or she would want done if the palliative operation does not go well, it is certainly preferable to have those discussions with the patient rather than with surrogates who may not fully understand the patient's wishes.

FUTILITY

Sometimes discussions about palliative surgery involve the question whether there is even a role for surgery when the likelihood for success is very low. In some circumstances, these discussions revolve around the concept of futility. The argument often proceeds as follows: "Physicians need not provide futile care. Any intervention that is an exercise in futility should not be provided even if the patient wants it." The flaw in this line of thinking is the assumption that futility is an objective determination.

The attempt to make futility an objective concept was proposed by Schneiderman and colleagues. These authors defined a treatment as futile if empirical data showed the treatment to have a less than 1 in 100 chance of success.[24,25] According to this definition, if an operation has a less than 1 in 100 chance of providing palliation, a surgeon would not be obligated to perform such a palliative operation. As appealing as it may initially be to make such decisions into empirical facts, there are problems with the attempt to make such decision making dependent on empirical data. First, do we really need to see that something does not work 100 times in a row to conclude that it will not work the next time? Such an assumption seems to ignore how physicians use clinical judgment to make decisions. Second, and more important, to determine whether an operation will benefit a patient, the physician must consider the patient's values. Benefit cannot be defined theoretically, but rather relative to a particular patient with specific goals. As Truog and colleagues suggested, "It is meaningless to say that an intervention is futile; one must always ask, 'Futile in relation to what?'"[26] Thus, rather than trying to define an operation as futile, one should attempt to determine whether it will lead to realistically possible benefits that are sought by the patient. In other words, surgeons must use the concept of a risk-to-benefit analysis for a specific patient in which the patient's values define what will be of benefit to him or her.

Responding to Perioperative Suffering

Surgeons should be cognizant of the significant suffering associated with any surgical intervention, whether curative or palliative. However, for the reasons noted in this section, many patients are at greater risk for potential suffering when they face a palliative, rather than a curative, operation. The suffering that patients endure with surgery can be broadly categorized as mental, physical, social, and existential. Mental suffering may be preoperative (e.g., anxiety about the procedure and what to expect) or postoperative (e.g., postoperative confusion or delirium from narcotic pain medication). Mental suffering is perhaps best addressed preoperatively by the surgeon's careful descriptions of what to expect from the procedure. Postoperative mental suffering can best be addressed by a high degree of sensitivity to the anguish that such confusion can cause patients.

Care of physical suffering has seen the most dramatic improvements in recent decades. Surgeons should strive to reduce physical suffering through intraoperative choices, such as avoiding a nasogastric tube if it is not necessary or considering a gastrostomy tube if the nasogastric tube is likely to be needed for a long period. Whenever possible, postoperative pain medication should be given intravenously rather than intramuscularly. Allowing patients to administer their own analgesia with a patient-controlled analgesia device can also decrease physical suffering and the dependence on nurses to administer the medication.

Social suffering may be related to the disability of the postoperative period and the resulting role changes or financial hardships. Surgeons can help to alleviate these issues by preoperative discussions and preparation of patients regarding what to expect after surgery. In the postoperative period, a sensitivity to social suffering should lead surgeons to inquire about these issues with their patients and to consult appropriate support personnel as needed.

Existential suffering relates to the big questions patients may have regarding an operation, such as, "Will I die on the table?" Although the likelihood that a patient will have existential suffering is clearly dependent on the patient's overall medical condition and the operation being undertaken, most patients have some similar concerns even if they do not fully express them to their physicians. Surgeons can best alleviate such existential suffering by encouraging patients to be open about their concerns and to ask questions.

All the parameters noted here are often more serious in patients who undergo palliative surgical procedures. When facing a palliative operation, the patient may have heightened anxiety about the surgical procedure and may be more susceptible to postoperative confusion or delirium. Furthermore, with fewer reserves for physical recovery, many patients have the potential for greater physical suffering. Finally, if patients are near the end of life, social and existential concerns may be further heightened. Surgeons must be prepared to address these issues when palliative surgery is being considered.

The Role of Research

Palliative surgery is quite different from a failed curative operation. Because the goals of a curative operation are so very different from the goals of most palliative procedures, the effectiveness of palliation must be studied specifically and separately from studies of the optimal curative procedures. Thus, a clinical trial designed to determine which intervention leads to the highest cure rate would rarely shed light on the question of which intervention would be most likely to lead to optimal palliation of symptoms.

To determine which approaches provide the best palliation, surgeons must explore these questions with the same rigor that has been used to explore optimal curative resection strategies. Because the success of palliative surgery is relative to the patient's symptoms, data are much more subjective than those considered for curative trials. This situation leads to more complex end points that are often more difficult to assess. In addition, it is difficult to obtain funding for palliative clinical trials because the end points are not the usual ones of disease-free survival or longevity. Furthermore, because palliative surgery is commonly done near the end of life, a subject who has consented to participate in a research protocol may soon lose the capacity to give consent. These issues suggest the importance of developing and completing carefully designed palliative surgical trials. Surgeons will be able to determine the optimal palliative procedures for many diseases only after such trials have been completed.

PEARLS

- Much surgery is palliative; it is often appropriate for people near the end of life and for the chronically ill.
- Palliative surgery is a core part of surgical palliative care, a fundamental aspect of surgical practice.
- Measure the quality of palliative surgery by the reduction in suffering and improvement of quality of life.
- Impeccable perioperative symptom management is essential and should include all domains of suffering: physical, mental, social, and spiritual.

PITFALLS

- Measuring the quality of palliative surgery by technical aspects alone is too limited. Technical quality is necessary but not sufficient.

- Omitting discussions with the patient and family about goals of care is risky. They may accept interventions they do not really want or need.

- Barring all patients with a DNR order from surgery is unethical. Use the required reconsideration approach so the DNR order applies to, for example, cardiac arrest but not palliative surgery.

- Research that uses designs and outcome measures that fail to reflect palliative surgery goals will misguide practices. Select designs and outcome measures that take palliative care approaches into account.

Summary

In the previous pages, we have explored many of the central issues of palliative surgery. We have sought to show the tradition of surgical palliation in the history of surgery and how surgical palliation can be so very important to a patient's well-being. Although surgeons have not always been at the forefront of the development of palliative care as an important component of comprehensive care, the American College of Surgeons has taken a leadership role in teaching surgeons the importance of palliative care in surgery. The most recent ACS Statement of Principles of Palliative Care (see Box 31-1) is an important document that seeks to define the manner in which palliative care is integral to the comprehensive care of all surgical patients (11). Although much of the foregoing discussion has focused on the patient with cancer at the end of life, a review of the ACS Principles of Palliative Care will readily show that palliative care is essential throughout the course of a patient's illness. Surgeons need to be prepared to intervene to improve a patient's symptoms and to alleviate the suffering of patients in all stages of illness and disease. Surgeons must understand that appropriate preoperative discussions with patients and families, intraoperative decision making, and postoperative attention to patient needs can optimize the alleviation of suffering.

Resources

Milch RA, Dunn GP: The surgeon's role in palliative care, *Bull Am Coll Surg* 82:14–17, 1997.
Dunn GP: The surgeon and palliative care: an evolving perspective, *Surg Oncol Clin North Am* 10:7–24, 2001.
Angelos P: Palliative philosophy: The ethical underpinning, *Surg Oncol Clin North Am* 10:31–38, 2001.
Easson AM, Asch M, Swallow CJ: Palliative general surgical procedures, *Surg Oncol Clin North Am* 10:161–184, 2001.
Krouse RS: Advances in palliative surgery for cancer patients, *J Support Oncol* 2:80–87, 2004.
Wagman LD, editor: Palliative surgical oncology, *Surg Oncol Clin N Am* 13(3):401–554, 2004.
Dunn GP, editor: Surgical palliative care, *Surg Clin N Am* 85(2):169–398, 2005.

References

1. Billroth T: Open letter to Dr. L. Wittelshofer, by Prof. Th. Billroth, Vienna, Feb. 4, 1881, *Wiener Medizinische Wochenschrift* 31(1):162–166, 1881.
2. Pellegrino ED, Thomasma D: *Helping and healing*, Washington, DC, 1997, Georgetown University Press.

3. Fox E: Predominance of the curative model of medical care: a residual problem, *JAMA* 278:761–763, 1997.
4. Angelos P: The ethics of interventional care. In Dunn GP, Johnson AG, editors: *Surgical palliative care*, New York, 2004, Oxford University Press, pp 33–38.
5. Dunn GP: Introduction: Is surgical palliative care a paradox? In Dunn GP, Johnson AG, editors: *Surgical palliative care*, New York, 2004, Oxford University Press, pp 3–15.
6. Zimmerman LM, Veith I: *Great ideas in the history of surgery*. Baltimore, 1961, Williams & Wilkins.
7. Dunn GP, Milch RA: Introduction and historical background of palliative care: where does the surgeon fit in? *J Am Coll Surg* 193:324–328, 2001.
8. Easson AM, Asch M, Swallow CJ: Palliative general surgical procedures, *Surg Oncol Clin North Am* 10:161–184, 2001.
9. Miner T: Palliative surgery for advanced cancer. Lessons learned in patient selection and outcome assessment, *Am J Clin Oncol* 28:411–414, 2005.
10. Dunn GP: Surgical palliative care. In Cameron JL, editor: *Current surgical therapy*, ed 9, Philadelphia, 2008, Mosby Elsevier, pp 1179.
11. Lillemoe KD, Cameron JL, Kaufman HS, et al: Chemical splanchnicectomy in patients with unresectable pancreatic cancer: a prospective randomized trial, *Ann Surg* 217:447–455, 1993.
12. Ng A, Easson AM: Selection and preparation of patients for surgical palliation. In Dunn GP, Johnson AG, editors: *Surgical palliative care*, New York, 2004, Oxford University Press, pp 16–32.
13. American College of Surgeons, Committee on Ethics and Surgical Palliative Care Task Force: Statement of principles of palliative care, *Bull Am Coll Surg* 20:34–35, 2005.
14. Angelos P: End of life issues in cancer patient care, *Tumor Board* 4:17–27, 2000.
15. Dunn G, Martensen R, Weissman D, editors: *Surgical palliative care: a resident's guide*, Chicago, 2009, American College of Surgeons, pp 136.
16. American College of Surgeons, Committee on Ethics and Surgical Palliative Care Task Force. Statement of principles of palliative care, *Bull Am Coll Surg* 20:34–35, 2005.
17. Hofmann B, Håheim LL, Søreide JA: Ethics of palliative surgery in patients with cancer, *Br J Surg* 92:802–809, 2005.
18. McCahill LE: Methodology for scientific evaluation of palliative surgery, *Surg Oncol Clin N Am* 13:413–427, 2004.
19. Beauchamp TL, Childress JF: *Principles of biomedical ethics*, New York, 1979, Oxford University Press.
20. Jonsson PR, McNamee M, Campion EW: The "do-not-resuscitate" order: a profile in its changing use, *Arch Intern Med* 148:2373–2375, 1988.
21. Truog R: Do-not-resuscitate orders in the operating room, *Anesthesiology* 74:606–608, 1991.
22. Cohen CB, Cohen PJ: Do-not-resuscitate orders in the operating room, *N Engl J Med* 325:1879–1882, 1991.
23. Truog R: Do-not-resuscitate orders in the operating room, *Anesthesiology* 74:606–608, 1991.
24. Schneiderman LJ, Jecker NS, Jonsen AR: Medical futility: its meaning and ethical implications, *Ann Intern Med* 112:949–954, 1990.
25. Schneiderman LJ, Jecker NS, Jonsen AR: Medical futility: response to critiques, *Ann Intern Med* 125:669–674, 1996.
26. Truog RD, Brett AS, Frader J: The problem of futility, *N Engl J Med* 326:1560–1564, 1992.

CHAPTER 32

Dementia

JENNIFER M. KAPO

Dementia	Decision Making
Prognosis	Caregiving
Pharmacologic Management	Pearls
	Pitfalls
Pain Assessment	

This chapter focuses on the specialized knowledge needed in providing end-of-life care to older patients with dementia.

Dementia

Dementia is a progressive, chronic, and incurable neurodegenerative disorder that results in suffering and loss as patients develop impairments in memory, judgment, language, behavior, and function. Multiple types of dementia have been defined, but Alzheimer's is the most common type, followed by vascular dementia. The prevalence of dementia increases with age from roughly 1% in persons 60 to 65 years old to approximately 40% in persons 85 years old. The current U.S. population of patients with dementia is roughly 4 million and is projected to increase 10-fold, to approximately 40 million, in the next 40 years. Worldwide, the elderly population with dementia is projected to increase from 25 million in the year 2000 to 114 million in 2050. Patients with dementia are increasingly receiving palliative care for other life-limiting diagnoses, although many die without benefiting from these services. The palliative care specialist therefore needs to be proficient in providing care to patients with early stages of dementia, as well as to patients with advanced dementia who enroll in hospice care with a primary diagnosis of dementia.

Prognosis

The failure to recognize dementia as an incurable and progressive disease may result in inadequate end-of-life care, including delayed referral to hospice.[1] However, it is challenging to determine accurate prognosis in dementia. Prognosis guidelines focus on functional indicators for people with Alzheimer's disease. For example, the Functional Assessment Staging Scale (FAST) describes the progression of functional decline in patients with dementia in a series of seven stages. In a validation study of

464

the FAST staging system, patients who reach stage 7 (language limited to several words and dependence in all activities of daily living [ADLs]) have a prognosis of less than 1 year. Based on the results of this study, the loss of the ability to ambulate (stage 7c) is particularly indicative of a prognosis of less than 1 year, and it is included as a criterion for hospice enrollment in guidelines for noncancer diagnoses from the National Hospice and Palliative Care Organization.[2] A recent study describes additional criteria that may more accurately identify patients with dementia who have a prognosis of 6 months or less.[3] Data was analyzed from the Minimal Data Set, a federally mandated, standardized assessment that was collected on admission and quarterly for every nursing home resident. The following significant mortality risk factors for nursing home residents diagnosed with dementia were demonstrated: a decline in ADLs, a secondary diagnosis of cancer, congestive heart failure, dyspnea and oxygen requirement, aspiration, weight loss, and age greater than 83 years. A mortality risk index score based on these data was derived that stratifies patients into degrees of risk of 6-month mortality. This study also suggests that hypoactive delirium is a marker of poor prognosis in dementia. Of note, this was a study of patients who were recently admitted to a nursing home, so the results may not be applicable to a wider population. Similarly, in a review of the medical records of hospice-dwelling patients with dementia, age, anorexia, and the combination of nutritional and functional impairment were associated with shorter survival times.[4]

As discussed earlier, it may be possible to identify characteristics that predict poorer prognosis in people with dementia. In addition, acute illness that requires hospitalization may also be associated with poor prognosis. A study of patients with dementia who were admitted to the hospital with a diagnosis of hip fracture or pneumonia found that more than half the patients died within the 6-month postdischarge period.

Pharmacologic Management

In addition to providing information about diagnosis and prognosis, palliative care physicians may need to provide information about treatment options. In the early stages, families and patients often seek guidance regarding potential pharmacologic treatments for dementia. All acetylcholinesterase inhibitors are thought to have similar efficacy.[5] Although a modest benefit was seen in about 30% to 40% of study subjects, the benefit to an individual patient may be difficult to recognize clinically. Therefore, families need to be counseled that, although these medications may slow the progression of the dementia and may result in minimal improvement in functional status, behavior, and memory, it is unlikely that they will significantly improve the patient's cognition. The side effect profile of the acetylcholinesterase inhibitors, including anorexia, nausea, and weight loss, may be particularly burdensome for older patients, who often have decreasing oral intake. There are very few data to describe efficacy in end-stage dementia. Memantine, an N-methyl-D-aspartate receptor antagonist, was approved by the U.S. Food and Drug Administration in 2004 for the treatment of moderate to severe dementia. It was shown (by Mini-Mental State Examination) to decrease the rate of cognitive decline modestly in patients with moderate to severe dementia.[3,5] Some clinicians believe that combining memantine with an acetylcholinesterase inhibitor may benefit some patients. However, further research is required before this regimen is made standard practice. Vitamin E, at high doses of 1000 IU twice daily, was shown to delay the time to nursing home placement as well as the time to impairment in ADLs in patients diagnosed with Alzheimer's disease. However, more recent data suggest a possible trend toward an increase in overall mortality in patients who take high doses of vitamin E, and therefore the risks and benefits of this treatment need to be carefully weighed.

Determining the appropriate time to discontinue dementia-specific medications is a complicated decision. Medication cessation may result in a full spectrum of family response, from significant psychological distress to great relief. The data on efficacy of these medications in severe end-stage dementia are very limited. There may be some benefit of these medications for behavior apart from cognition,[5] so discontinuation may raise concerns of worsening behavioral problems. Moreover, one study suggests that stopping acetylcholinesterase inhibitors and then resuming usage at a future date may result in decreased responsiveness to the medication. Regardless, concerns about side effects, the considerable cost, and perceived prolongation of poor quality of life may lead many clinicians to advise and families to decide to discontinue the therapy, particularly for patients near the end of life and for whom Alzheimer's dementia is the terminal diagnosis.

Psychiatric and behavioral problems are common in dementia. Palliative care providers who care for patients with dementia can play an important role by offering guidance about these problems to families and caregivers. Depression is common throughout the course of dementia, but it may be easier to recognize in the early stages when patients are better able to communicate and express some insight into their experience. In later stages, behavioral problems such as visual and aural hallucinations, paranoia, agitation, and restlessness are common and occur in up to 80% of patients. Patients may also exhibit physical or verbal aggression and sexually inappropriate behaviors.

For acute changes in behavior, the first step should be to assess for potential delirium with a focused assessment to rule out a reversible medical condition such as fecal impaction or medication adverse effect. After ruling out a reversible cause, the initial management should focus on nonpharmacologic modifications, especially decreasing external stimuli and encouraging family visits or the use of a sitter. Strategies to control behaviors include the creation of a safe, physical home environment, distraction and redirection from sources of anxiety, the identification of nonstressful activities (i.e., day care, groups), and the use of calming, sensory experiences such as aromatherapy, soothing sounds, or touch.[6] There are several well-referenced reviews on treatments for behavioral problems in dementia. However, few randomized, controlled trials have been conducted that substantiate efficacy.[6]

Antipsychotic medications are the main agents used to treat dementia-associated agitation and behavioral problems. These antipsychotic drugs are generally divided into two groups based on side effect profile: typical (e.g., haloperidol) and atypical (e.g., risperidone).

The atypical antipsychotics also have a role in controlling agitated behavior. Several placebo-controlled studies have shown efficacy of the atypical antipsychotic medications risperidone and olanzapine in controlling aggressive behaviors and psychosis in patients with moderate to severe dementia, with virtually no extrapyramidal side effects or tardive dyskinesia. Head-to-head comparisons of haloperidol and risperidone show no difference in efficacy or side effects in the treatment of delirium. Sedation is a notable side effect for all antipsychotic medications, and the development of parkinsonism may limit their use. In addition, the Food and Drug Administration has issued a warning of a possible increased risk of stroke in older people who take any antipsychotic. Recent data also suggest that haloperidol and the atypical antipsychotics are both associated with increased mortality.[7] The atypical antipsychotics (olanzapine in particular) may also predispose diabetic patients to hyperglycemia. Although important considerations, concern for these side effects may not be as relevant for patients close to the end of life or for those cases in which the primary goals are to decrease the severity of behavioral problems and caregiver burden. Given these potential adverse effects, however, it is important to review a patient's need for antipsychotics periodically and to consider discontinuing or decreasing the medications, if possible.[6] This is of particular importance when caring for patients in nursing homes. Since the passage of the Omnibus Budget Reconciliation Act in 1987 in the United States, physicians must document the indication for the use of all such psychotropic medications in the nursing home setting, as well as intermittent attempts to wean the dose. A systematic review of the pharmacologic treatment of neuropsychiatric symptoms of dementia suggests guidelines for the best therapeutic strategy.[8] Second-line and third-line classes of drugs, including benzodiazepines and anticonvulsants, are discussed in this review.

Pain Assessment

Assessing symptoms can be challenging in patients who have difficulty verbalizing their needs. Clinicians must therefore pay close attention to nonverbal signs. Several scales can be used to assess the nonverbal, behavioral signs of pain. One useful scale is the Checklist of Non-verbal Pain Behaviors, which includes six pain-related behaviors: vocalizations, grimacing, bracing, verbal complaints, restlessness, and rubbing.[9] This scale was tested on 88 cognitively impaired and cognitively intact older adults who were hospitalized with hip fractures. No differences were identified in the pain-related behaviors of the cognitively impaired and intact patients, and the pain-related behaviors correlated with verbal reports of pain. Another pain scale is the Hurley Hospice Approach Discomfort Scale, which evaluates nine behaviors such as tense body language and frightened expressions. This scale was originally tested longitudinally in 82 nursing home residents with advanced Alzheimer's disease. The traditional signs of facial grimacing were accurate for the presence of pain but not pain intensity. Physician assessment of pain has been found to be accurate in mildly to moderately demented patients but less accurate in severely demented people. Data also suggest that caregivers tend to underestimate the severity of pain.

Many patients with dementia can express that they are experiencing pain, and most are able to complete a pain assessment instrument. Such instruments can be helpful in the initial evaluation of pain, as well as in follow-up assessment. In addition to their own assessment, clinicians may need to use multiple assessment tools and caregiver input to assess pain.

Documented changes in behavior and delirium, whether more disruptive or withdrawn, should prompt a thorough pain assessment as part of the routine assessment for an acute medical illness or unmet needs (e.g., need for toileting or feeding). In these cases, analgesics should be used on a trial basis when history and physical findings suggest a cause of pain. The American Geriatric Society guidelines for the management of chronic pain in older persons endorse this strategy.[10] Depending on the likely source of pain, a trial of opioids or nonsteroidal anti-inflammatory drugs may be beneficial. Such use of analgesics should be reassessed frequently to ensure that medications are not being used for sedative side effects in the absence of pain.[9]

Decision Making

Palliative care physicians and other health care professionals can play an important role by addressing advance care planning and discussing goals of care with patients and families early in the disease course. For example, a randomized, controlled trial that involved palliative care consultations for patients with advanced dementia showed that the intervention group was significantly more likely to have a palliative care plan on discharge (23% vs. 4%) and more likely to decide to forgo medical interventions (e.g., intravenous fluids).[11] In another study, proactive involvement of an inpatient palliative care service decreased intensive care unit length of stay for patients with dementia, reduced nonbeneficial interventions, and increased the identification of poor prognosis and "do not resuscitate" goals. Because the patient's cognitive status will eventually decline, it is of prime importance to assist with the timely discussion of advance directives and to facilitate completion of appropriate paperwork as early as possible. It is also consistent with the overall goal of honoring the patient's wishes.

Patient-centered care is a major goal of palliative medicine. The determination of a patient's ability to make decisions is fundamental to respecting his or her wishes. Certainly, at some point in the progression of dementia, a patient will no longer be able to make decisions. However, physicians should recognize that a person with dementia may still be able to make some decisions. Demented patients often still want to participate in their care. In one study, 92% of patients with mild to moderate dementia indicated that they wanted to be involved in treatment options, and most of their caregivers supported this decision. Much of the focus of research and effort in this area is on the capacity to consent to treatment. *Decision-making capacity* is defined as the clinical determination that a patient is able to understand the risks and benefits of a specific medical decision, to appreciate that these risks and benefits apply to their personal care, to reason the choice to be made, and to communicate that choice. Determining capacity is essential to determining who should make a treatment decision for the patient, and it affects the relation of the physician to family members.

People with dementia may still participate in decision making, even if they need assistance in that process. Using three assessment instruments, one study showed that most mildly to moderately demented patients had acceptable decision-making capacity based on the domains of understanding, appreciation, reasoning, and choice. Although mean performance for subjects was lower than that of controls on all the instruments, most subjects were still in the normal range for each domain. Capacity is specific to the level of decision making, and a patient may still retain the ability to make decisions at a simpler level (e.g., refusing a urinary catheter), even when he or she is not able to decide a more complex matter (e.g., neurosurgery).

The distinction between competency and decision-making capacity is important. Whereas *competency* is a legal term in which an individual retains their legal rights, *decision-making capacity* reflects a person's ability to demonstrate understanding of a central issue and the options; to appreciate the consequences and offer reasons; and to voice a decision about a specific situation at a specific time. Thus, a person may be competent (in that a judge has not appointed a conservator or guardian) but may not have reasonable decision-making capacity as determined by a licensed physician, psychiatrist, or psychologist. Impairment of capacity may be temporary, such as resulting from delirium or depression. In these situations, the stability of the decisions and their consistency with prior expressed wishes become key pieces of information. Loss of competency is relatively permanent, until a court gives the individual his or her rights back.

Caregiving

Those who care for demented patients at the end of life face considerable challenges. These challenges include management of the disturbing behavioral problems described earlier and the inability to stop the relentless and severe functional and cognitive impairments that worsen over time. Many caregivers provide care for their loved one for years and incur both personal and financial costs. A recently published study characterizes family caregiving for demented patients at the end of life. In this study, more than half the caregivers spent 46 hours or more weekly assisting with ADLs and independent ADLs, and more than half reported that they provided care 24 hours a day. Another study reports that 75% of hours spent caring for patients with dementia are provided by family caregivers. It is not surprising that caregivers of demented patients are at increased risk for medical and psychiatric disease, and possibly even death. In addition, many families of patients with dementia suffer significant financial losses, including the value of caregiving time, the caregiver's lost income, out-of-pocket expenditures for formal caregiving services, and caregivers' excess health costs.[12]

A growing body of evidence describes the morbidity and mortality of caring for chronically ill, functionally impaired persons, including those who are not demented. The burdens of serious illness clearly extend to families and friends. A study that analyzed the effects of caregiving reported that 34% of patients who needed 24-hour care were cared for by the family, 20% of families experienced a major life change (e.g., a child did not go to college), and 12% reported a family illness that was attributable to the stress of caring for family member.[13] Studies have found that caregivers have an increased risk of clinical depression and anxiety and decreased use of preventive health measures. Finally, troubling data suggest that caregivers with unmet needs are more likely to consider euthanasia and physician-assisted suicide.

PEARLS

- Palliative care providers play an important role in educating patients and families to understand that dementia is a progressive, ultimately fatal disease.
- Antipsychotic medications are the main pharmacologic agents used to treat dementia-associated agitation and behavioral problems when non-pharmacologic interventions fail.
- Assessing pain and other symptoms can be challenging in patients with advanced dementia who have difficulty verbalizing their needs. Clinicians must therefore pay close attention to nonverbal behavioral signs.

PITFALLS

- The failure to recognize dementia as an incurable and progressive disease may result in inadequate end-of-life care, including delayed referral to hospice.

Resources

Alzheimer's Association
  www.alz.org
American Academy of Hospice and Palliative Medicine
  www.aahpm.org
National Hospice and Palliative Care Organization
  www.nhpco.com
National Family Caregiver's Association
  www.thefamilycaregiver.org

References

1. Volicer L: Hospice care for dementia patients, *J Am Geriatr Soc* 45:1147–1149, 1997.
2. Luchins DJ, Hanrahan P, Murphy K: Criteria for enrolling dementia patients in hospice, *J Am Geriatr Soc* 45:1054–1059, 1997.
3. Mitchell SL, Kiely DK, Hamel MB, et al: Estimating prognosis for nursing home residents with advanced dementia, *JAMA* 291:2734–2740, 2004.
4. Schonwetter RS, Han B, Small BJ, et al: Predictors of six-month survival among patients with dementia: an evaluation of hospice Medicare guidelines, *Am J Hosp Palliat Care* 20(2):105–113, 2003.
5. Trinh NH, Hoblyn J, Mohanty S, Yaffe K: Efficacy of cholinesterase inhibitors in the treatment of neuropsychiatric symptoms and functional impairment in Alzheimer disease: a meta-analysis, *JAMA* 28:210–216, 2003.
6. Sutor B, Rummans T, Smith G: Assessment and management of behavioral disturbances in nursing home patients with dementia, *Mayo Clin Proc* 76:540–550, 2001.
7. Schneider LS, Dagerman KS, Insel P: Risk of death with atypical antipsychotic drug treatment for dementia: meta-analysis of randomized placebo-controlled trials, *JAMA* 294:1934–1943, 2005.
8. Sink KM, Holden KF, Yaffe K: Pharmacological treatment of neuropsychiatric symptoms of dementia: a review of the evidence, *JAMA* 293:596–608, 2005.
9. Feldt KS: The checklist of nonverbal pain indicators (CNPI), *Pain Manage Nurs* 1:13–21, 2000.
10. AGS Panel on Chronic Pain in Older Persons: The management of chronic pain in older persons, *J Am Geriatr Soc* 46:635–651, 1998.
11. Ahronheim JC, Morrison RS, Morris J, et al: Palliative care in advanced dementia: a randomized controlled trial and descriptive analysis, *J Palliat Med* 3:265–273, 2000.
12. Prigerson HG: Costs to society of family caregiving for patients with end-stage Alzheimer's disease, *N Engl J Med* 349:1891–1892, 2003.
13. Emanuel EJ, Fairclough DL, Slutsman J, et al: Assistance from family members, friends, paid care givers, and volunteers in the care of terminally ill patients, *N Engl J Med* 341:956–963, 1999.

CHAPTER 33

Pulmonary Palliative Medicine

HUNTER GRONINGER and J. CAMERON MUIR

The symptoms that derive from pulmonary disease processes account for a large percentage of referrals to palliative care practices. Although most of these cases involve malignant lung disease, more than 7% of palliative care referrals are for primary pulmonary diseases such as chronic obstructive pulmonary disease (COPD), interstitial lung diseases, and acute respiratory distress syndrome.[1] These diseases are uniformly chronic, progressive, and debilitating, thus mandating that comprehensive care of these patients includes a solid understanding of palliative methods.

This chapter outlines how palliative care can be applied to patients who suffer from a primary pulmonary disease. COPD receives the most attention because of its relatively high prevalence.

Pathophysiology of Dyspnea

The symptoms of dyspnea are comprehensively addressed elsewhere in this text. However, for the purposes of discussing COPD disease and other primary pulmonary disease processes here, a brief description is given of the pathophysiology of dyspnea as encountered in the palliative care of the patient with pulmonary disease. A common definition of *dyspnea* is an unpleasant or uncomfortable sensation of breathing or a sensation of breathlessness.

As a qualitative symptom, characterizations of dyspnea may vary widely among patients with different disease processes or even among individuals with similar, underlying cardiopulmonary diseases. In a manner similar to generating a differential diagnosis for chest pain, the clinician may find that different adjectives help to uncover the origin of the patient's dyspnea. Several studies that examined patients' descriptors of dyspnea have demonstrated that feelings of "chest tightness" and "increased work of breathing" may be more strongly associated with asthma, whereas "suffocation" and "air hunger" are more consistent with COPD or congestive heart failure.[2]

The origins of dyspnea are complex at best. Many details of the underlying pathophysiology have yet to be described, particularly the neural pathways that contribute to generating a sensation of breathlessness. Additionally, correlating the symptom onset with a specific underlying stimulus can be quite difficult for both clinician and researcher. For example, in a given patient with metastatic lung cancer, is the dyspnea the result of tumor compression of the bronchi, the malignant pleural effusion, the pulmonary embolism, existential anxiety, or a combination thereof? Chapter 15 provides a more detailed discussion of the pathophysiology of dyspnea. Here, we consider three major mechanisms through which dyspnea manifests itself in COPD: chemoreceptors, mechanoreceptors, and the sensation of respiratory effort.[2]

Both peripheral and central chemoreceptors are thought to play a role in evoking dyspnea, although it is not always clear exactly how this occurs. Normal subjects and patients suffering from pulmonary diseases complain of dyspnea while breathing carbon dioxide (CO_2). Conversely, many patients, especially those suffering from COPD, have baseline elevations of the partial arterial pressure of CO_2 ($PaCO_2$) at rest without experiencing breathlessness.[3] Similarly, although hypoxia is commonly thought to contribute to dyspnea (it is known to stimulate respiration via chemoreceptors), many dyspneic patients are not hypoxic. Furthermore, in those who are hypoxic, correction often only partially alleviates the symptom.[3]

Mechanoreceptors in the upper airways may explain the benefit that many pulmonary patients receive when they sit next to an open window or a fan. Several studies have suggested that vibration of mechanoreceptors in the chest wall may improve dyspnea in normal subjects and in patients with COPD.[3] In the lung, epithelial irritant receptors contribute to bronchospasm, whereas unmyelinated C-fibers in the alveolar walls respond to pulmonary congestion.[2] Interestingly, many patients with COPD exhibit dynamic airway compression, as evidenced by an improvement in breathlessness from pursed-lip breathing. One study described such an improvement when patients with COPD who did not normally breathe in such a manner were taught how to do so. However, the degree to which each of these mechanisms contributes to dyspnea is unclear and is likely relatively specific to the individual patient.

Finally, one's sense of respiratory effort—the conscious awareness of the activity of the skeletal muscles—seems to play a part as well. This effort is related to the ratio of pressure generated by the respiratory muscles to the maximum pressure generated by the muscles. Evidence indicates that most of this sense derives from simultaneous activation of the sensory cortex at the initiation of the motor cortex to breathe.[2] A stimulus that increases the neural drive to breathe (either when the respiratory muscle load is increased or when the muscles become fatigued) will increase this ratio and therefore the sense of effort, as seen in patients with neuromuscular disorders such as amyotrophic lateral sclerosis or myasthenia gravis.[2]

Unfortunately, although we understand many of the mechanisms that contribute to dyspnea, no one mechanism has been linked to a single disease process. It is more likely that dyspnea in a patient with pulmonary disease is multifactorial. For example, a patient with COPD may experience breathlessness from airway hyperinflation leading to weakened diaphragmatic muscle curvature and inspiratory muscle fibers, acute or chronic hypoxia, hypercarbia, mechanical compression of the airway, or increased dead space requiring increased minute ventilation.[4] The clinician must bear in mind such pathophysiologic complexity when caring for the patient with advanced pulmonary disease processes because effective palliative management usually requires multiple approaches, both pharmacologic and nonpharmacologic. The next section introduces possible interventions for symptom palliation in the patient with COPD. As yet, no published data describe when to begin palliation of COPD with opioids or benzodiazepines. Traditional primary care and pulmonary specialty practice tend to begin these agents when the disease is far advanced and more "conservative" therapies have proven to be of only marginal benefit. Concern about opioid and benzodiazepine side effects is often cited as the primary reason for the delay in initiation of these therapies.[5]

Primary Disease Management

Representing the majority of pulmonary diseases for which many data are available regarding palliative management and referrals to hospice and palliative care, the major focus of this chapter is palliative management of COPD. In 1997, COPD affected 10.2 million U.S. residents; in 1998, it accounted for between 15% and 19% of hospitalizations in the United States.[6] It is the fourth leading cause of death in the world.[7] This section reviews approaches to primary disease treatment, as well as emerging pharmacologic and nonpharmacologic palliative techniques for managing the symptoms of COPD (primarily dyspnea).

It is important to underscore the distinction between the goals of treating the primary disease ("curative" or "disease modifying") and relieving symptoms associated with a given disease, so-called palliative therapy. The *Merriam-Webster Dictionary* suggests that *palliation* is "treatment aimed at lessening the violence of a disease when cure is no longer possible".[8]

Primary disease management of COPD includes prescribed combinations of short- and long-acting bronchodilators, corticosteroids, and oxygen, as well as nonpharmacologic interventions such as pulmonary rehabilitation and preventive measures such as influenza and pneumococcal vaccinations. Treatment regimens must be designed specifically for each patient based on responses to medications. No drug or drug combination has been shown to modify the progressive decline of the disease process itself. Therefore, although the foregoing framework is often useful, in the management of COPD the distinctions between disease modifying and palliative are particularly blurred or overlapping. Generally, the success of pharmacologic and nonpharmacologic management strategies has been evaluated in terms of improvement in pulmonary function tests, exercise capacity, and symptoms. Established guidelines are readily available.[7] A summary of interventions is provided in Table 33-1. The primary focus here is on symptom control and a review of the evidence surrounding various traditional pharmacologic and nonpharmacologic interventions.

BRONCHODILATORS

Bronchodilators (ß$_2$-agonists, anticholinergics, methylxanthines) tend to be the first-line interventions in attempts to improve dyspnea in the patient with COPD. The ß$_2$-agonists and anticholinergics may be delivered in short- or long-acting compounds and in inhaled forms (ß$_2$-agonists are also manufactured in oral formulations, but these are not frequently used in adults). Short-acting bronchodilators can improve symptoms rapidly and can be administered on a scheduled basis for consistent control. For stable disease (i.e., not acute symptom management), the regular

Table 33-1. Pharmacologic and Nonpharmacologic Interventions Applicable to Managing Symptoms in Chronic Obstructive Pulmonary Disease

Drug/Intervention	Curative	Disease Modifying	Longevity Modifying	Palliative
Lung transplant	X			
β_2-Agonists		X		X
Anticholinergics		X		X
Methylxanthines		X		
Corticosteroids				X
Oxygen			X	X
Opiates (systemic)				X
Opiates (nebulized)				(Unclear if any benefit)
Benzodiazepines				X

use of long-acting formulations has been reported to be more effective than short-acting bronchodilators, and once- or twice-daily dosing promotes improved compliance. These drugs are, however, more expensive (Table 33-2).[7] Inhaled forms (via metered-dose inhaler or nebulizer) are typically better tolerated and have fewer side effects, but they require additional patient and caregiver education for correct administration. The results of this education have demonstrated important benefit, however.[9]

For the stable patient with COPD, short-acting ß2-agonists or short-acting anticholinergics should be administered at intervals of 4 to 6 hours for symptom improvement beginning at mild stages of disease (forced expiratory volume in 1 second [FEV$_1$]/forced vital capacity [FVC] < 70; FEV$_1$ = 80% predicted, with or without symptoms at baseline).[7] A Cochrane meta-analysis examining patients with a predicted FEV$_1$ of 60% to 70% studied the scheduled administration of inhaled short-acting ß2-agonists for 7 days to 8 weeks and demonstrated that regular use of inhaled short-acting ß2-agonists for at least 7 days improved breathlessness scores.[10] Long-acting bronchodilators should be reserved for those with moderate to severe COPD (i.e., FEV$_1$/FVC < 70; FEV$_1$ = 80% predicted, with or without symptoms).[7] Long-acting ß2-agonists have also been associated with slight decreases in breathlessness.[11] In one study, the administration of salmeterol, 50 µg twice daily, resulted in significant improvement in health-related quality of life scores versus placebo. Interestingly enough, 100 µg twice daily did not have the same effect.[12] Administration of the long-acting anticholinergic tiotropium bromide also demonstrated statistically significant improvement in dyspnea compared with placebo, as well as better dyspnea relief compared with salmeterol.[13]

Methylxanthines (most commonly theophylline) remain third-line agents, given their relatively wide side effect profile and narrow therapeutic windows. Patients with COPD who were more than 60 years old who took a long-acting formulation of theophylline exhibited wider interpatient variability and fluctuation in serum drug concentration.[14] Therefore, careful and frequent drug level monitoring is essential.

Table 33-2. Common Pulmonary Medications: Mechanism, Dosing, Costs, and Route of Administration

Drug Class	Drug Name	Mechanism and Dosing Interval	Cost
β-agonists	Albuterol (generic)	Short acting (q4–6h)	$30 (inhaler)
	Metaproterenol (Alupent)	Short acting (q4–6h)	$56 (inhaler)
	Pirbuterol (Maxair)	Short acting (q4–6h)	$95 (autoinhaler)
	Albuterol (Ventolín)	Short acting (q4–6h)	$36 (inhaler)
	Terbutaline (generic, Brethine)	Intermediate (q6–8h)	$31 (oral, subcutaneous, intravenous)
	Albuterol (Proventil)	Intermediate (q6–8h)	$38 (inhaler)
	Levalbuterol (Xopenex)	Intermediate (q6–8h)	$65 (inhaler)
	Formoterol (Foradil)	Long acting (q12h)	$97 (inhaler)
	Salmeterol (Serevent)	Long acting (q12h)	$98 (inhaler)
Anticholinergics	Ipratropium (generic)	Short acting (q4–6h)	$34 (inhaler)
	Ipratropium (Atrovent)	Intermediate (q6–8h)	$77 (nebulized)
	Tiotropium (Spiriva)	Long acting (q24h)	$120 (inhaler)
Inhaled steroids	Triamcinolone (Azmacort)	Intermediate (q6–8h)	$90 (inhaler)
	Flunisolide (AeroBid)	Long acting (q12h)	$75 (inhaler)
	Fluticasone (Flovent)	Long acting (q12h)	$92 (inhaler)
	Beclomethasone (QVAR)	Long acting (q12h)	$74 (inhaler)
	Budesonide (Pulmicort)	Long acting (q12–24h)	$148 (inhaler)
Combination	Combivent, DuoNeb (Albuterol/Ipratropium)	Short acting (q4–6h)	$74 (inhaler)
	Advair (Fluticasone/Salmeterol)	Long acting (q12h)	$148 (inhaler)

CORTICOSTEROIDS

Inhaled corticosteroids do not modify progressive decline in FEV_1. Thus, they are not disease-modifying agents but rather purely palliative in symptom relief (dyspnea and congestion). Steroids may be appropriate for symptom management in patients with severe ($FEV_1 < 30\%$ predicted) to very severe ($FEV_1 < 50\%$ predicted) COPD.[7] This treatment may decrease the frequency of exacerbations, and it does improve respiratory symptoms and decrease utilization of hospital resources for respiratory management.[15] Withdrawal of inhaled corticosteroids has been shown to increase the frequency of exacerbations.[16] The combination of inhaled corticosteroids and a long-acting ß₂-agonist demonstrated greater efficacy in controlling respiratory symptoms than did the combination of a short-acting anticholinergic and ß₂-agonist.[17]

Courses of intravenous or oral corticosteroids are commonly employed during COPD exacerbations and work best in those patients with a strong inflammatory component to the disease; these systemic formulations have been repeatedly demonstrated to shorten recovery time from a COPD exacerbation. One randomized, controlled trial found inhaled budesonide to be as efficacious as oral prednisolone in patients hospitalized for COPD exacerbations.[18] However, long-term courses of oral corticosteroids have not been shown to be of benefit in symptom management, and there is an increased risk of proximal myopathy that adversely affects respiratory mechanics and management of oral secretions. Other deleterious effects of long-term corticosteroid use are osteopenia, fat redistribution, diabetes, decreased immune function, and increased infection. Systemic corticosteroids are not recommended for long-term use in COPD.[7]

OXYGEN

Oxygen remains a mainstay in the management of COPD and other chronic lung diseases. Benefits of long-term oxygen use in patients with COPD include improvements in hemodynamics, hematologic characteristics, exercise capacity, lung mechanics, and mental state. More importantly, oxygen increases survival, a truly disease-modifying increase in survival.[7] In general, therapy should be initiated in patients with very severe COPD—that is, patients with either (1) arterial partial pressure of oxygen (PaO_2) lower than 55 mm Hg or oxygen saturation (SaO_2) less than 88% or (2) PaO_2 lower than 60 mm Hg or SaO_2 less than 89% *and* pulmonary hypertension, evidence of congestive heart failure, or secondary polycythemia.

With regard to symptomatic management, however, strong evidence that supports the long-term use of oxygen remains somewhat elusive; it is not clearly "palliative." Although investigators do record changes in physiologic variables with oxygen use, many studies have not employed dyspnea assessments. Confounding this is the issue that few studies are randomized, controlled trials, and most studies involve small patient numbers. A summary from the Association of Palliative Medicine Science Committee regarding patients with COPD advises the following:

1. There is currently equivocal evidence for the use of long-term oxygen at rest for palliation of dyspnea.
2. Oxygen may be appropriate for decreasing breathlessness associated with exercise.
3. The effect of oxygen on quality of life during ambulation cannot be predicted a priori by patient characteristics.[19]
4. Short-term therapy during exacerbations of dyspnea or during ambulation and exercise may be useful in patients with COPD.[19]

OTHER MODES OF PRIMARY DISEASE MANAGEMENT

Other pharmacologic modifiers used in the management of the patient with COPD include leukotriene inhibitors, chemokines, inhibitors of tumor necrosis factor-a, and phosphodiesterase inhibitors. Each of these drug classes may subsequently be shown to contribute to disease improvement in COPD and to palliative relief of breathlessness. At this time, however, no clear evidence exists to support the routine use of these medications for the palliation of COPD symptoms.

Symptom Management

OPIATES

Opiates are the mainstay of palliative management of dyspnea in COPD. Opiates decrease the ventilatory response to exercise, hypoxia, and hypercarbia. It is possible that they decrease the sensation of breathlessness by decreasing respiratory effort.

Intermittent dosing of opioids has been studied in patients with COPD. Most of these studies enrolled relatively small numbers of patients, administered study drug and placebo orally, and utilized exercise testing as a means of measuring improvement in dyspnea. Although one meta-analysis of nine studies demonstrated significant heterogeneity in study results, it nevertheless appears evident that systemic opiate administration improves breathlessness in patients with COPD.[20] Notably, four of the nine studies measured arterial blood gas tensions before and after treatment; three of these studies found no significant difference. In the one study that did find a difference, using dihydrocodeine in multiple-dose exercise testing, $PaCO_2$ never rose more than 40 mm Hg, and PaO_2 did not change significantly.[21]

The benefits of scheduled or sustained-release opiates are less clear in patients with COPD who require more than intermittent dosing of opiates for relief. There have been even fewer trials investigating these methods and dosing of drug administration, and these trials have tended to demonstrate mixed results. For example, one study employed 30 or 60 mg of dihydrocodeine or placebo administered three times daily; compared with placebo, a benefit was found in the 30-mg group but not in the 60-mg group.[21] The same confounding results ring true for sustained-release opiates. In a randomized, double-blind, crossover trial, sustained-release morphine was shown to have no benefit over placebo in breathlessness scores and was actually associated with decreased exercise tolerance.[5] However, in a similarly designed study, 4 days of sustained-release morphine provided improved dyspnea scores and improved sleep as compared with placebo.[22] Therefore, whereas sustained-release opiates are a mainstay of clinical palliative care practice, with seemingly positive benefit, the data are still unclear regarding whether scheduled or sustained-release opiates will prove beneficial for management of dyspnea in patients with COPD.

Clinicians continue to examine alternative routes of administering opiates. Nebulization of morphine or fentanyl is of interest to many investigators because of possible benefits localized to lung parenchyma and neuromusculature and less risk of the side effects that are associated with systemic administration (most commonly constipation and nausea). In spite of numerous trials, meta-analyses still suggest that nebulization of morphine has no role in relief of dyspnea,[20] and although several researchers are now turning their attention to nebulized fentanyl, no study has yet investigated the role of this agent in COPD. Finally, epidural opiate administration may eventually prove an additional route for symptom relief in COPD, as shown by one uncontrolled trial of nine patients who gained relief of breathlessness with epidural methadone.[23]

BENZODIAZEPINES

Benzodiazepines can be useful in palliating dyspnea. Typically, they are initially administered on an as needed dosing schedule and then scheduled when necessary.

Although benzodiazepines are often used for symptom management in palliative care patients (anecdotally, with significant success in patients with dyspnea), few studies have examined the role of benzodiazepines in patients with COPD. One study examined the effect of alprazolam on exercise capacity and dyspnea and found no significant difference between intervention and placebo.[24] Further research is needed to understand better the role of benzodiazepines in this setting.

As a corollary, the prevalence of anxiety is quite high among patients with COPD, and as many as 34% of patients meet the criteria for either generalized anxiety disorder or panic disorder, a rate at least three times that of the general population.[25] Certainly, anxiety negatively affects the lives of these patients, especially in terms of functional status, mental health function, and bodily pain perception.[25] However, benzodiazepines are not recommended for routine treatment of anxiety in patients with COPD, given the concern for decreased respiratory drive and worsened exercise tolerance. Several small studies have suggested that buspirone,[26] sertraline,[27,28] or nortriptyline[29] should be used for the pharmacologic management of anxiety. Non-pharmacologic management strategies include cognitive behavioral therapy and pulmonary rehabilitation.[25]

End-of-Life Care

Despite aggressive research and advances in therapy during the second half of the 20th century, the fact remains that COPD is still a disease marked by inexorable decline and increasingly frequent hospital admissions to treat exacerbations, often requiring extensive periods of ventilator support. Nevertheless, relatively few data have been gathered and incorporated into management guidelines for end-of-life treatment of these patients.[30] One study demonstrated that patients with terminal COPD experience a poorer quality of life, more unaddressed psychological and emotional distress, and less social support compared with patients with inoperable non–small cell lung cancer.[31] Another study found that patients with COPD desire more education than those with cancer or AIDS about the disease process, including what they may experience in the dying process, and information on advanced care planning.[32]

Such findings underline the need for overall improved communication with, and multidisciplinary support for, patients who are terminally ill with COPD. In a recent retrospective survey of 399 British patients who died of COPD, the investigators found that during the last year of life for these patients, 41% either left the house less than once a month or never left, 47% were hospitalized at least twice, 67% died in the hospital, and only 63% knew that they could die.[33] Clearly, these findings exemplify the need for more extensive palliative care services.

In the last days of life, it is common for patients with COPD to experience progressive dyspnea that proves refractory to bronchodilators, corticosteroids, and oxygen. As hypoxia and hypercarbia worsen, patients may become delirious and more anxious. In an attempt to manage these symptoms, hospice and palliative care physicians typically titrate opioids and benzodiazepines for comfort, sometimes at the expense of responsiveness. In these situations, the goal of therapy should remain the alleviation of symptoms rather than sedation. As indicated by the studies cited earlier, it is essential to provide education as well as comprehensive support to the patient and family throughout the dying process.

PEARLS

- Pulmonary disease processes (excluding malignant diseases) constitute more than 7% of palliative care referrals. Most of these referrals are for management of symptoms associated with COPD.

- For patients with COPD, the mainstay of symptom palliation remains similar to treatment during disease exacerbations: bronchodilators (especially anticholinergics and ß$_2$-agonists), oxygen, and short courses of corticosteroids.

- Additional palliation of dyspnea can be achieved with the use of opiates. Current data recommend administration of short-acting rather than long-acting preparations. However, normative palliative practice tends to favor long-acting preparations to improve adherence and compliance when a stable dose of short-acting opiate has been determined.

- As yet, there is no consensus about precisely when in the disease course patients with chronic, degenerative pulmonary disease processes should be referred for palliative care. Where palliative care consultants exist, most pulmonary and critical care physicians have found that early consultation and collaboration with palliative care support are beneficial.

PITFALLS

- There is no proven benefit to the extended use of corticosteroids for COPD palliation.

- Currently, there is only anecdotal evidence to support use of benzodiazepines for palliation of dyspnea.

- Data are insufficient to support the development of palliative care algorithms for COPD. There is, however, a tremendous opportunity for collaboration between pulmonary and palliative care specialists to build this literature.

Summary

This chapter has introduced strategies for managing symptoms in patients who suffering from pulmonary disease and has focused primarily on COPD. No data are available at this time to indicate definitely when patients with chronic, progressive lung disease should be referred to palliative care specialists. However, in the natural course of such diseases, most available therapies are, indeed, palliative (see Table 33-2). Within the category of primary disease management or disease-modifying therapy, inhaled ß-agonists, oxygen, and anticholinergics are beneficial. For primary symptom relief (pure palliation), ß-agonists, anticholinergics, oxygen, systemic opiates, and benzodiazepines have been shown to provide some benefit, although data are limited. Thus, both the general practitioner and the pulmonary specialist should be acquainted with various approaches to addressing chronic and recurring symptoms of dyspnea and anxiety. Given the prevalence of the symptom of dyspnea and the paucity of data regarding its palliative management, clearly more research is needed to improve care for patients with pulmonary manifestations of a variety of diseases.

Resources

End of Line/Palliative Care Research Center: Fast Fact and Concept 027: Dyspnea at End-of-Life
   www.eperc.mcw.edu/fastFact/ff_027.htm

World Health Organization: Management Plan for COPD
    www.who.int/respiratory/copd/management/en/

References

1. Connor SR, Tecca M, LundPerson J, et al: Measuring hospice care: The National Hospice and Palliative Care Organization National Hospice Data Set, *J Pain Symptom Manage* 28:4, 2004.
2. Manning HL, Schwartzstein RM: Pathophysiology of dyspnea, *N Engl J Med* 333:23, 1995.
3. Manning HL, Mahler DA: Pathophysiology of dyspnea, *Monaldi Arch Chest Dis* 56:4, 2001.
4. Mahler DA: Dyspnea relief, *Monaldi Arch Chest Dis* 59:3, 2003.
5. Poole PJ, Veale AG, Black PN: The effect of sustained-release morphine on breathlessness and quality of life in severe chronic obstructive pulmonary disease, *Am J Respir Crit Care Med* 157:1877–1880, 1998.
6. Mannino DM: COPD: epidemiology, prevalence, morbidity and mortality, and disease heterogeneity, *Chest* 121:121–126, 2002.
7. Global Initiative for Chronic Obstructive Lung Disease: Global strategy for the diagnosis, management, and prevention of chronic obstructive pulmonary disease: executive summary 2005. GOLD-A Collaboration of the National Heart, Lung, and Blood Institute, National Institutes of Health, USA, and the World Health Organization Washington DC & Geneva. Available at goldcopd.com/Guidelineitem.asp?l1=2&l2=1&intId=996. Accessed February 12, 2007.
8. Merriam-Webster's Collegiate Dictionary, ed 11, New York, 2003, Merriam-Webster.
9. Song WS, Mullon J, Regan NA, Roth BJ: Instruction of hospitalized patients by respiratory therapists on metered-dose inhaler use leads to decrease in patient errors, *Respir Care* 50:8, 2005.
10. Ram FSF, Sestini P: Regular inhaled short acting b2 agonists for the management of stable chronic obstructive pulmonary disease: Cochrane systematic review and meta-analysis, *Thorax* 58:580–584, 2003.
11. Appleton S, Poole P, Smith B, et al: Long-acting beta2-agonists for chronic obstructive pulmonary disease patients with poorly reversible airflow limitation, *Cochrane Database Syst Rev* 3CD001104, 2006.
12. Jones PW, Bosh PK: Quality of life changes in COPD patients treated with salmeterol, *Am J Respir Crit Care Med* 155:4, 1997.
13. Gross NJ: Tiotropium bromide, *Chest* 126:1946–1953, 2004.
14. Armijo JA, Sanchez BM, Peralta FG, et al: Pharmacokinetics of an ultralong sustained-release theophylline formulation when given twice daily in elderly patients with chronic obstructive pulmonary disease: monitoring implications, *Biopharm Drug Dispos* 24:165–171, 2003.
15. Lung Health Study Research Group: Effect of inhaled triamcinolone on the decline in pulmonary function in chronic obstructive pulmonary disease, *N Engl J Med* 343:26, 2000.
16. Van der Valk P, Monninkhof E, van der Palen J, et al: Effect of discontinuation of inhaled corticosteroids in patients with chronic obstructive pulmonary disease, *Am J Respir Crit Care Med* 166:1358–1363, 2002.
17. Donohue JF, Kalberg C, Emmett A, et al: A short-term comparison of fluticasone propionate/salmeterol with ipratropium bromide/albuterol for the treatment of COPD, *Treat Respir Med* 3:173–181, 2004.
18. Maltais F, Ostinelli J, Bourbeau J, et al: Comparison of nebulized budesonide and oral prednisolone with placebo in the treatment of acute exacerbations of chronic obstructive pulmonary disease, *Am J Respir Crit Care Med* 165:698–703, 2002.
19. Booth S, Anderson H, Swannick M, et al: The use of oxygen in the palliation of breathlessness: a report of the expert working group of the Scientific Committee of the Association of Palliative Medicine, *Respir Med* 98:66–67, 2004.
20. Jennings AL, Davies AN, Higgins JPT, et al: A systematic review of the use of opioids in the management of dyspnoea, *Thorax* 57:939–944, 2002.
21. Woodcock AA, Johnson MA, Geddes DM: Breathlessness, alcohol and opiates, *N Engl J Med* 306:1363–1366, 1982.
22. Abernethy AP, Currow DC, Frith P, et al: Randomised, double blind, placebo controlled crossover trial of sustained release morphine for the management of refractory dyspnoea, *Br Med J* 327:1288, 2003.
23. Juan G, Ramon M, Valia JC, et al: Palliative treatment of dyspnea with epidural methadone in advanced emphysema, *Chest* 128:3322–3328, 2005.
24. Man G, Hsu K, Sproule B: Effective of alprazolam on exercise and dyspnea in patients with chronic obstructive pulmonary disease, *Chest* 90:832–836, 1986.
25. Brenes GA: Anxiety and chronic obstructive pulmonary disease: prevalence, impact, and treatment, *Psychosom Med* 65:963–970, 2003.

26. Argyropoulou P, Patakas D, Koukou A, et al: Buspirone effect on breathlessness and exercise perfor-mance in patients with chronic obstructive pulmonary disease, *Respiration* 60:216–220, 1993.

27. Smoller JW, Pollack MH, Systrom D, et al: Sertraline effects on dyspnea in patients with obstructive airways disease, *Psychosomatics* 39:24–29, 1998.

28. Papp LA, Weiss JR, Greenberg HE, et al: Sertraline for chronic obstructive pulmonary disease and comorbid anxiety and mood disorders, *Am J Psychiatry* 152:1531, 1995.

29. Borson S, McDonald GJ, Gayle T, et al: Improvement in mood, physical symptoms, and function with nortriptyline for depression in patients with chronic obstructive pulmonary disease, *Psychosomatics* 33:190–201, 1993.

30. Mast KR, Salama M, Silverman GK, et al: End-of-life content in treatment guidelines for life-limiting diseases, *J Palliat Med* 7:750–752, 2004.

31. Gore JM, Brophy CJ, Greenstone MA: How well do we care for patients with end stage chronic obstructive pulmonary disease (COPD)? A comparison of palliative care and quality of life in COPD and lung cancer, *Thorax* 55:1000–1006, 2000.

32. Curtis JR, Wenrich MD, Carline JD, et al: Patients' perspectives on physician skill in end-of-life care: differences between patients with COPD, Cancer, and AIDS, *Chest* 122:356–362, 2002.

33. Elkington H, White P, Addington-Hall J, et al: The health-care needs of chronic obstructive pulmonary disease patients in the last year of life, *Palliat Med* 19:485–491, 2005.

CHAPTER 34

Pediatric Palliative Care

STEPHEN LIBEN

The Who, How, What, When, and Where of Pediatric Palliative Care	**Symptom Management**
	Pearls and Pitfalls
Communication with Children and Families	**Summary**

Many of the skills required of general medicine physicians in the day-to-day care of patients are the same as those needed for specialist palliative care. Knowing how to communicate, appreciating the meaning of illness and suffering, and assessing and treating pain and other symptoms are a few examples of the clinical competencies required by physicians in both general and specialist practice. Just as the spectrum of clinical competencies that make up general medical practice overlaps with competencies required in palliative care for adults, the core skills required in adult palliative care overlap with those required for the palliative care of children. Although the general foundations of palliative care apply to both adults and children (e.g., appreciating the importance of care of the whole person, in body, mind, and spirit) and many medical treatments in pediatric palliative care are based on their success in adults (e.g., pharmacologic management of many symptoms), there are important differences in palliative care for children. Although other chapters in this textbook cover areas of care that apply equally to children and adults, this chapter will focus on areas where pediatric palliative care is distinct from adult palliative care.

The Who, How, What, When, and Where of Pediatric Palliative Care

Smaller numbers of children die compared with adults. In the United States, approximately 55,000 children 19 years of age or younger die per year, compared with 2.3 million adults.[1] Although precise statistics are not known, many children in developed (or richer) countries die in hospitals. For a medium-sized pediatric hospital of 150 to 200 beds, about 100 to 150 children may be expected to die per year. This means that health care workers in a pediatric hospital can expect two deaths per week, yet it has only recently been recognized that the needs of these dying children and their families require specialized knowledge and increased attention.[2] Medical advances have resulted in the current high cure rate of approximately 85% for pediatric cancers, but the fact remains that 15% of such children still die. The relative paucity of pediatric deaths compared with adult deaths, coupled with the cultural taboos surrounding death in general, combine to make the experience of a child's death a rarity for most people, including health care professionals. A hundred years ago, most families would have had at least one child die, and most physicians would have seen children die as part of their regular practice. Because most pediatric deaths in richer nations now occur in tertiary care hospitals, there are few professionals with experience and training in meeting the needs of the children who do die. The wider cultural milieu in which we live where all deaths are seen as a tragedy that could be avoided "if we just tried harder and had more technology" is amplified in pediatrics where the goal (implicitly or explicitly) is to have all children survive until adulthood This understandable goal often presents, however, as an expectation ("he/she can't die!") both by health care workers and by parents. If the unspoken goal is only cure, then death will always be seen as a failure. Much of the work in pediatric palliative care is the reframing of death from a failure to an inevitable part of life, including for some children.

Children die of a larger number of causes than do adults. Adult palliative care services have historically been oncology based, although it is recognized that other illnesses that lead to death in adults would also benefit from the principles of palliative care. The most common causes of death in children are age dependent[3]:

- Infants birth to 1 year: Congenital anomalies, prematurity, and sudden infant death syndrome
- Children age 1 to 14 years: Accidental and nonaccidental trauma, cancer, congenital abnormalities, and "other"
- Older children and adolescents age 15 to 19 years: Trauma (including suicide), cancer, and congenital abnormalities such as cardiac disease

Unlike the adult population in which cancer and cardiovascular disease make up a large percentage of the major causes of death, there exists a wide range of often rare diseases that lead to death in children. Although cancer is a common cause of death for adults, it is responsible for only 4% of deaths in childhood.[1]

Large numbers of rare and often poorly understood disorders result in death in children, including rare inborn errors of metabolism and genetic syndromes. For many of these causes of death, little is known about the natural history of the disease and its optimal management, including how to best provide symptom control. For these children, the best way to manage the illness is to apply general principles of pediatric care together with the general principles of palliative care. Another way of answering the question "What is pediatric palliative care?" is to answer that it takes the best practice from general pediatric medicine and combines it with the specialized knowledge of adult palliative care (Case Study 34-1).

Many children who might benefit from palliative care live with illnesses that have an unpredictable time course, which varies from a short-term illness that quickly leads to death to complex chronic diseases that may evolve over years. For complex chronic diseases, the time course may not only be long, spanning years, but may also be unpredictably intermittent in the need for acute and palliative care. For example, a child with severe cerebral palsy and a seizure disorder may be stable for years and then present suddenly with life-threatening aspiration pneumonia that may or may not become a fatal episode. At such times of intermittent crises, it is helpful if a

---

CASE STUDY 34-1

A 4-month-old boy was found to have profound weakness and resulting respiratory failure resulting from a rare, inherited form of congenital myopathy about which there was a lack of information in the medical literature. After much discussion about quality of life and possible outcomes, his parents agreed to placement of a tracheostomy tube, initiation of mechanical ventilation, and placement of a percutaneous gastrostomy tube. The child then lived in the hospital for 2 years, during which time his quality of life was maximized with in-hospital music therapy, regular volunteers assigned to his care, massage therapy, a regularized daily schedule, and personalization of his room. He then developed severe weakness with resulting skin breakdown and many pulmonary infections. His parents, together and in discussion with medical staff, came to accept that his quality of life had deteriorated to the point that he was suffering daily because of his worsening, irreversible illness. After discussions with their religious leaders and the hospital staff, his parents decided to allow him to die at home by removing the ventilator.

The hospital-based pediatric palliative care program had been introduced to the child and family at an early stage for help with symptom control and for anticipatory guidance. The roles and involvement of the pediatric palliative care team evolved as needed at different points in the child's illness trajectory. The initial role of the team was to establish a therapeutic relationship with his parents and to support the health care staff (e.g., intensive care unit staff and surgeons) in the many discussions that occurred at different decision-making points. As his care evolved toward the end of life, the pediatric palliative care team became more directly involved in planning for how end-of-life care would be transferred to the home, including how the child would be taken off the ventilator.

---

management plan has been prepared in advance, including thinking through the kinds of interventions that may or may not be desired for that particular child (e.g., decisions about whether to provide mechanical ventilation). The life-threatening crisis may evolve into an end-of-life situation, or the crisis may resolve and the child may once again require high levels of supportive and rehabilitative care, including access to supportive services for the handicapped (e.g., seating programs, antispasticity programs, multispecialist care). In this way, pediatric palliative care is often not a smooth transition from health to ill health, but rather an intermittently required service that may need to move in and out of a child's care plan as needs evolve. It is always helpful to plan ahead by initiating early discussions about how palliative care may be helpful if and when a life-threatening crisis occurs rather than waiting for the crisis to manifest. Evaluations of the child and family that occur between crises have the advantage of assessing the child when he or she is at the best level of function and offer the opportunity for families to reflect on discussions and take the time needed to come to important decisions about care planning.

Even in places where pediatric home palliative care is available, many children who die do so in hospitals. Most children who are able to make a choice prefer to die at home, if possible. There are several possible explanations for why many children still die in hospitals despite their preference to be at home. These include unpredictability—it is often not possible to know when a critical illness is actually a fatal event as opposed to one from which the child may recover; the lack of availability of home pediatric palliative care services; and the need of many parents to feel that everything possible was done to help avoid the death of their child, including the use of medical technologies that are possible only in a hospital. Pediatric and neonatal intensive care units are common locations of pediatric deaths; because these deaths are a frequent occurrence, many units have their own individualized palliative care and bereavement programs. In some centers, hospitals have set up palliative care rooms that allow families to remain together in a more homelike environment than is typically found in a hospital setting. Unlike adult palliative care, there are rarely entire wards in pediatric hospitals dedicated to palliative care. For the most part, pediatric palliative care programs have developed as consultant services (as opposed to primary care services) to help support the primary caregivers in other pediatric specialties. For example, in-hospital palliative care programs may follow children on different speciality wards as care is concurrently delivered with another pediatric subspecialty, such as respirology for patients with cystic fibrosis and neurology for children with severe cerebral palsy. Not surprisingly, some evidence indicates that instituting the supports necessary to provide services in the home results in larger numbers of children who then do die at home instead of at the hospital.[4] In contrast to the United Kingdom, where large numbers of specialized pediatric hospice centers are already in operation, few adult hospices in North America will admit a child for terminal care. For a dying child and his or her family, the ideal situation is to be able to offer them as many options as possible, including the opportunity for care to alternate among hospital, home, and hospice as needs and situations change.

Communication with Children and Families

Communication is the cornerstone on which pediatric palliative care skills and competencies are based. Developing the ability to communicate effectively and compassionately with others in highly emotional situations is learnable with a combination of specific cognitive skills coupled with experientially based learning (in the moment, on the job). Such reflection in action and on action is a process that requires skilled mentors and periods of time in actual clinical practice. Communication (or, in other words, *connection* with others) is both the biggest challenge in this work as well as its greatest reward. Knowing you have made a positive difference in this work comes from a deep knowing that you have in some way made a caring, compassionate connection with others, regardless of the final outcome of the illness.

Addressing the meaning of hope is a common and challenging task for children, parents, and professionals. The difficult question is sometimes asked directly ("How can we maintain hope in the face of our child's death?") or indirectly ("What do we do now?," "How can we go on?," "What is the point of anything?"). These questions speak to the need to maintain hope and the struggle to find meaning in the tragic loss that is the death of a child. In the face of such questions (which may be unspoken for some), the role and challenge for the pediatric palliative care professional is to assist in reframing what hope can be when a cure is no longer possible. For example, it can be comforting to know that other families have found a way to maintain hope by shifting from hope for cure to hope for a meaningful life or hope for a peaceful death. A starting point for the health care professional is to recognize his or her own need to maintain hope and to find meaning in the work that he or she does. *Hoping* is understood to be distinct from *wishing*. Hope is the understanding that things will somehow be all right, no matter what the outcome. Wishing may be another way to deny reality and is the insistence that, despite the facts, the outcome will somehow "magically" be different. A practical approach to hope is as follows:

1. Be mindful that at times loss of hope may be part of the process. Accepting that hope can at times be lost may relieve the sense of failure that can add to suffering.
2. Understand that "being with" people and things the way they are in this moment is sometimes not only all there is "to do" but is sometimes paradoxically everything that is needed. "Don't just do something, sit there" is a call to "being with" that holds the potential for reducing suffering.
3. Facilitate the process that leads to a shift from hoping for cure, to hoping for quality of life, to hoping that death will be as comfortable as possible or to finding meaning.
4. Create the conditions that allow for the possibility of maintaining hope and finding meaning by optimizing physical comfort and providing care in the best possible setting (e.g., in the home when it is desired and possible).

Understanding children's developmental concepts of death is important in helping guide the content and timing of communication with ill children and their siblings. It is now understood that even very young terminally ill children are often aware that they are dying, despite efforts their parents may have made to keep that information from them.[5,6] The following is an approximate guide to how children understand death at different ages:

- Very young children, younger than 3 years: These children are mostly preverbal, with their needs focused on immediate physical gratification and emotional security. Their major concerns are often physical comfort and to not be separated from their parents.
- Early childhood, age 3 to 6 years: These children lack appreciation of core concepts of death. At this stage, many fears result from misunderstanding the core concepts of death and may be alleviated by explanation and discussion. These concepts include the following:
  Irreversibility: Death is permanent, and the dead cannot be made alive again.
  Universality: Death happens to everyone, not just old people or those who become sick.
  Nonfunctionality: Being dead means that you do not have to breathe, or eat, or maintain other body functions.
  Causation: "Bad" people are not the only ones who die, and wishing death on someone cannot magically cause his or her death. It is important for siblings to understand this because they may have wished their brother or sister "dead" at some time in the past and now wonder whether that wish is coming true.
- Middle childhood, age 6 to 12 years: At this age children begin to understand the concepts of irreversibility, universality, nonfunctionality, and causation. They may, however, believe that death is caused mostly by external forces such

as accidents, although they are beginning to understand that it also occurs via internal (illness) causes.

- Adolescence, older than 12 years: Adolescents may have a disconnect between their factual understanding of the core concepts of death and simultaneous magical thinking that it still cannot happen to them (e.g., risk taking is common at this stage).

Many of the children who require palliative care are either preverbal because of their young age or nonverbal because of their underlying illness. Although communication does occur through nonverbal means, there are many instances in which a lack of cognitive ability limits the child's ability to comprehend and be an active partner in decisions about treatment. In adult palliative care, even if an adult becomes nonverbal, there is still a previous lived experience of the person to help guide decision making. In contrast, young children with little lived experience depend on proxy decision makers. It is often the parents, as proxy decision makers, who make major decisions for and about their children. One challenge in pediatric palliative care is to help parents make decisions that respect what is in the best interests of their child versus those decisions that may help to alleviate their own legitimate suffering. When it is difficult to separate the nonverbal child's suffering from that of the parents, it can be helpful to reframe the situation by asking parents to try to interpret what their child may be "telling" them in actions as opposed to in words. For example, parents may interpret repeated life-threatening episodes as meaning that their child is telling them that he or she is "ready to go" and may find some solace in knowing that they have found a way to "listen" to the nonverbal messages their child is sending.

Communication with verbal children includes, but is not limited to, involving children in their own treatment decisions, listening for their preferences about the way they wish to live, and offering them the opportunity to create lasting memories for the bereaved (e.g., memory books, pictures, bequeathing cherished toys, making personalized music recordings, and paintings). The opportunity to express themselves creatively and nonverbally need not be limited to specialists in expressive therapies; simply offering crayons and paper with the instruction to "make any picture you like" and then asking the child to explain what he or she drew can be very helpful in better understanding what the child is thinking.

It is an axiom in pediatric palliative care that the unit of care is both the child and family, with the definition of family meant to include any loved one who is significant to that child. Communicating with parents, siblings, and extended family can be a challenge and will depend on the particulars of each family. Encouraging parents to include siblings in appropriate discussions and involving siblings in care may serve to improve the long-term function of the bereaved sibling.[7]

Offering ideas about how to share meaning even in uncertain times can be helpful. For example, when a child is near the end of life, families may feel stressed by trying to time important celebrations in this unpredictable situation. It can be suggested that other families in similar situations have chosen to have the event (e.g., a birthday or holiday celebration) as soon as possible and then to repeat it on the actual calendar date if the child continues to do well.

Symptom Management

Most children's pain and many other physical symptoms can be managed with the application of current accepted therapeutic interventions.[8] It remains a distressing fact that many children still have unrelieved pain and symptoms because proven, effective symptom management techniques are not applied.[9] Fears and misunderstandings that have kept pain relief withheld from children include not recognizing the following:

1. Children and neonates feel pain and respond to both pharmacologic and nonpharmacologic management.
2. The use of opioids to manage pain in children is safe and effective when given in age- and weight-appropriate doses by the least invasive route.
3. Behavioral, cognitive, and other nonpharmacologic techniques to reduce pain can be both safe and effective.

Good pain management begins with a pain assessment. Whenever possible, pain assessment should be based on the child's self-report. For the infant and very young nonverbal child, various pain scales may be useful in particular situations (e.g., the COMFORT scale used in an intensive care setting). In clinical practice, pain in infants and young children is most often assessed by a combination of physiologic parameters (e.g., heart rate), behavioral observation (e.g., observation of facial grimacing), and parental report. Children around the ages of 4 to 7 years can use self-report scales. One such scale, the Bieri faces scale, has a pictorial scale of six faces, and the child is instructed to point to the face that shows how much pain (or "oowie" or "boo-boo") the child is having. For children older than about age 7 years, a standard 0 to 10 (or 0 to 5) numeric scale can be used. For older nonverbal or cognitively impaired children, practical pain assessment is usually dependent on a combination of physiologic, behavioral, and parental report parameters similar to that used in preverbal infants. With this population of handicapped children, it is often the parents who are aware of even subtle changes in the physical and psychological states of their children. One potential pitfall is the mistaken extrapolation of the use of physiologic parameters (e.g., heart rate) to assess chronic pain. Chronic pain is often not associated with the kinds of physiologic and behavioral changes that are typically seen with acute pain. One practical approach to pain management in nonverbal children is the following: When in doubt about whether pain is present, a trial of an analgesic medication can be given, and its effects on the child's behavior can be observed.

Procedure-related pain is a common cause of significant suffering in children (when treatment may be more painful than the disease). Pharmacologic pain management (e.g., the use of topical analgesics such as topical anesthetic gels coupled with systemic short-acting sedatives and analgesics) and concomitant nonpharmacologic techniques are very effective in reducing procedure-related pain in children. Some examples of easily applied nonpharmacologic techniques include the following:

- Discuss the child's preferences about who should be present during the procedure; a trusted adult or a parent may be very helpful. Be sure to prepare the adult for exactly what to expect.
- Distraction: Pop-up books, blowing bubbles, movies, and small portable toys with motion can be used.
- Offering choices: Offer the choice of right or left hand for placement of intravenous lines.
- Physical measures: These include light touches and the application of cold.
- Reading a story or having a parent sing a favorite song is another technique.

- Guided imagery and guided relaxation are powerful techniques to help alleviate procedure-related pain. To be effective, these techniques require specialized training and expertise.

Most pain in children can be successfully managed with a stepwise approach as advocated by the World Health Organization (WHO) analgesic ladder, which has been adapted for pediatrics (see Chapter 7). In rare instances, pain may be refractory, and the use of invasive techniques (e.g., epidural blocks) or high doses of sedating medications may be required. Special considerations in the use of opioids and coanalgesics in children include the following:

1. Regular pain should be treated with regularly (not "as needed") scheduled medications (by the clock). As needed rescue doses should be added in case of breakthrough or intermittent pain.
2. The oral route (by the mouth) is always the first choice. Intramuscular injections are painful and should be avoided. Alternate routes to oral administration include subcutaneous and rectal routes, as for adults. Because children have smaller dose requirements, many standard rectal doses are too large, and specially prepared suppositories can sometimes be used. Many children with cancer already have a permanent intravenous port that may be accessed in emergencies, but for care at home, continuous intravenous infusions are technically difficult and the subcutaneous route is often used instead. For older children, a patient-controlled analgesia pump may be used, although caution should be used if the parents were taught to use the pump on demand. Transdermal fentanyl patches must be used with caution by experienced personnel and are appropriate only in children who are not opioid naive.
3. An approach to mild, moderate, and severe pain should begin with the WHO analgesic ladder (see Chapter 7).
4. In the first 6 months of life, opioids are more likely to cause respiratory depression, and this risk mandates more careful monitoring and lower initial doses (start with 25% of the usual pediatric per kilogram opioid dose).
5. The initial dose of opioid medication is only a guide, and some children may need lower or higher doses to achieve pain control.
6. Adjuvant medications include coanalgesics that allow for lower opioid doses and therefore fewer opioid side effects. Adjuvants are often used for their desirable side effects (e.g., sedation). Some of the more common adjuvants include the following:
   - Corticosteroids such as dexamethasone used as an appetite stimulant and coanalgesic, particularly in bone pain and in headaches caused by increased intracranial pressure
   - Stimulants such as methylphenidate in opioid-induced somnolence or for short-term treatment of depression
   - Tricyclic antidepressants such as amitriptyline for neuropathic pain
   - Anticonvulsants such as phenytoin and gabapentin for neuropathic pain
   - Benzodiazepines such as lorazepam for muscle spasticity and as sleep aides
   - Neuroleptics such as chlorpromazine for delirium or nausea
   - Antispasmodics such as baclofen for muscle spasticity

Management of symptoms other than pain in pediatric palliative care is based on the same principles as in adult palliative care. In other words, the benefits of interventions are weighed against the risks of side effects for each symptom and each person. Dyspnea is often responsive to directing a gentle flow of air to the face with a small fan, positioning to prevent aspiration of secretions, and use of systemic opioids to relieve the sensation of breathlessness. The usefulness of oxygen in treating dyspnea is uncertain in children. One way to decide on the possible utility of oxygen in a particular patient is to use a brief trial of oxygen (if available) to assess whether it reduces breathlessness. One caveat is to avoid gauging the success or failure of oxygen by its impact on oxygen saturation alone because oxygen saturation is not necessarily correlated with the sensation of dyspnea. In the event of a sudden episode of anxiety related to the rapid onset of dyspnea, rectal diazepam may provide a good first-line, at-home treatment that can easily be taught to parents. Airway secretions are often problematic in children who have neurologic disorders, and suctioning and the use of oral drying agents such as glycopyrrolate have been used with some effectiveness. The recent use of botulism toxin injection into the salivary glands holds promise as a possible new treatment for excessive saliva.

Difficult decisions about artificial feeding and hydration commonly manifest as ethical issues in pediatric palliative care. The decision to provide nasogastric feedings that are commonly used in the care of ill neonates requires an individualized approach and a careful consideration of the possible benefits versus burdens of treatment. In many circumstances, it is appropriate to initiate a trial of nasogastric feedings for a short period. As in adult palliative care, there is little evidence to suggest that hydration makes the patient feel more comfortable, and equating hydration with comfort may lead to the ineffective and deleterious use of intravenous hydration in a dying child. There may be advantages to less fluid intake for a child in the terminal stages of illness, including decreased airway secretions and decreased urination, both of which may serve to increase comfort.

Constipation is a common symptom that requires proactive treatment with stool softeners and stimulants and, at times, suppositories or enemas. It is important to recognize the phenomenon of paradoxical diarrhea that may result from overflow constipation. Nausea may be more disturbing to the patient than vomiting and can be treated with both centrally acting medications (e.g., ondansetron) and motility agents (e.g., metoclopramide).

Seizures are common in pediatric palliative care, given the significant numbers of children who have underlying neurologic disease. A practical approach for any child at risk for a seizure (e.g., in the case of a brain tumor) is to ensure that doses of rectal diazepam are available in the home and that parents are comfortable administering it in case of need.

Bleeding is often a concern because of chemotherapy-related thrombocytopenia, but it is rarely life-threatening. The use of intermittent blood and platelet transfusions to maintain energy levels and to decrease the risks of bleeding episodes requires individualized judgments based on the availability of transfusions and the effects of coming in to the hospital for children who are otherwise at home and have a short life expectancy.

Skin care issues are important and should be addressed to avoid bedsores and ulcers, which are difficult to treat once they become severe. The use of specialized weight-distribution mattresses, air beds, and careful positioning is important in preventing bedsores, especially for children who are cared for at home.

Most parents look outside traditional medicine for possible alternatives to treat their ill child. It is important for health care professionals to be open to parental use of complementary or alternative treatments and to ask about the use of such therapies because some treatments may be dangerous (e.g., high potassium supplements in a child with renal failure).

PEARLS AND PITFALLS

- Caring for children means being able to appreciate and understand the spectrum of differing needs (of mind, body, and spirit) from birth through adolescence.

- Pediatric palliative care should be partnered with curative therapies long before all attempts at cure have been exhausted.

- The goal of pediatric palliative care is to make the most of whatever time the child has left, and, as such, the focus is mostly on how to live well rather than on dying.

- In the face of uncertainty about the presence of pain in a nonverbal child, one practical tool is to use a therapeutic trial of an analgesic and then observe for changes in behavior that may signal the need for regular analgesics.

- As with pain, a limited trial of therapy is often the only way to assess the effectiveness of a therapy for any given patient and may include such interventions as nasogastric feedings for questions about hunger and oxygen for dyspnea.

- The death of a child is one of the most stressful life experiences, and the void it leaves for the bereaved remains inadequately understood.

Summary

Pediatric palliative care comprises a diverse population with a wide variety of often rare diseases for long and unpredictable periods. Communication is a core skill needed to help children with life-limiting illness and their families, and it requires competencies that include nonverbal assessments and proxy decision making. Pediatric palliative care clinicians aim to ensure that these children and their families have the best quality of life possible under very difficult circumstances by managing painful and unpleasant symptoms as much as possible, offering choices about where and how care is to be delivered, and, perhaps most importantly, recognizing that being with children and families as they live through the end of a child's life is both a duty and a privilege that can make a difference.

Resources

Goldman A, Hain R, Liben S, editors: *The Oxford textbook of palliative care for children*, Oxford, UK, 2006, Oxford University Press.

Hilden J, Tobin DR, Lindsey K: *Shelter from the storm: caring for a child with a life-threatening condition*, New York, 2003, Perseus Publishing.

Initiative for Pediatric Palliative Care (IPPC)
    www.ippcweb.org

Kuttner L: *Making Every Moment Count [video]*, 2004, National Film Board of Canada.
    www.nfb.ca

Storey P, Knight CF, editors: *American Academy of Hospice and Palliative Medicine: Hospice/palliative care training for physicians: a self study program.* In *UNIPdAC 8: The Hospice/Palliative medicine approach to caring for pediatric patients*, New York, 2003, Mary Ann Liebert Publishers.

References

1. National Center for Health Statistics Deaths: Final data for 1999, *Nat Vit Stat Rep* 49:1–15, 1999. Available at www.cdc.gov/nchs/data/nvsr/nvsr49/nvsr49_08.pdf.
2. McCallum DE, Byrne P, Bruera E: How children die in hospital, *J Pain Symptom Manage* 20:417–423, 2000.
3. Institutes of Medicine: *When children die: improving palliative and end-of-life care for children and their families*, Washington, DC, 2003, National Academies Press, pp 41–66.
4. Liben S, Goldman A: Home care for children with life-threatening illness, *J Palliat Care* 14:33–38, 1998.
5. Bluebond-Langner M: *The private worlds of dying children*, Princeton, NJ, 1978, Princeton University Press.
6. Sourkes BM: *Armfuls of time: the psychological experience of the child with a life-threatening illness*, Pittsburgh, 1995, University of Pittsburgh Press.
7. Lauer ME, Mulhem RK, Bohne JB, Camitta BM: Children's perceptions of their sibling's death at home or hospital: the precursors of differential adjustment, *Cancer Nurs* 8:21–27, 1985.
8. World Health Organization: *Cancer pain relief and palliative care in children*, Geneva, 1998, WHO.
9. Wolfe J, Grier HE, Klar N, et al: Symptoms and suffering at the end of life in children with cancer, *N Engl J Med* 342:326–333, 2000.

CHAPTER 35

Palliative Care in the Intensive Care Unit

LAURA A. HAWRYLUCK

The primary goal of intensive care medicine is to attempt to save lives by supporting and normalizing physiology as much as possible during an acute life-threatening illness. Since the inception of critical care medicine in the 1960s, technological advances, innovations in therapeutics, and a greater understanding of life-threatening illnesses have resulted in significant improvements in morbidity and mortality. As a result, the practice of critical care medicine has also evolved. Although most people are still admitted with acute illnesses or an acute deterioration of a chronic illness, the improvement in the ability to sustain life has resulted in more prolonged stays in the intensive care unit (ICU) for many patients, as well as a greater incidence of secondary complications that may be life-threatening in and of themselves. Those who do survive often have significant short- and long-term changes in quality of life.

Decisions to admit patients to the ICU, to continue or withdraw treatments, are inherently challenging because of scientific uncertainty and limited abilities to accurately predict individual's outcomes. ICU teams struggle to weigh both medical criteria (e.g., need for ventilatory and/or hemodynamic support, the likelihood of survival and morbidity) and non-medical criteria (e.g., patient wishes, values and goals, cultural and religious beliefs), and how each should best factor into any decision-making. Critical teams have defined inappropriate treatment as care that

493

involves the use of considerable resources without a reasonable hope that the patient will recover to a state of relative independence or ability to interact with their environment.[1] While pain and suffering are not essential to the definition, they make such situations particularly distressing to clinicians.[1] In a recent study, 87% of physicians and 95% of nurses in Canadian ICUs have reported providing care they felt was inappropriate or futile at least once in the year prior to being surveyed[2] and, in another study, 73% acknowledged frequently agreeing to admit patients for whom they saw intensive care as futile.[3] Many studies support that provision of such care places significant demands on ICU resources. While the ethics sections of Canadian, American and European Critical Care Societies position statements describe the appropriate use of critical care services,[4-6] these fall short of meeting the pressing need of front-line clinicians to answer the fundamental question, *"Just because I can, should I?"*

The difficulties in decision making are further enhanced by patients and families generally not having a clear understanding of what life-sustaining treatments and ICU care entail[2,7] and what is realistic in terms of outcomes. Most decisions are made by responding to questions such as "Would you want to go on life support?" and "Would you want everything done?"—questions that persist in clouding decisions, that do not meet ethical and legal standards of informed consent, and ones that may even contribute to devaluing palliative care or any health care that doesn't strive to "do everything" to maintain life. Decisions are often needed when patients are already severely ill and in times of crisis. Many patients and families cite religious and cultural reasons for insisting on life support even when their faith groups do not mandate treatment plans of life at all costs.[8,9] Often patients are incapable and medical teams must ask surrogate decision makers (SDMs) to decide high-stakes, complicated issues during emotional and stressful times. In one study only 50% of patients' family members, acting as surrogates, understood the information regarding diagnosis, prognosis, and treatment.[10] Participation in such decision making often results in significant psychological symptoms among family members.[10] Consideration of individual values, goals, and, ultimately, perspectives of quality of life; cultural and religious beliefs; concepts of dignity and suffering; and benefits and burdens are crucial to ensure that individual patients' values and beliefs are respected. Yet these concepts may never have been discussed with surrogates.

Many people fear needing ICU care under any circumstances. Others fear being kept in a state of bare existence, and some fear being restored only to an unacceptable quality of life after surviving a life-threatening illness. Such fears have been the driving force behind advanced care planning initiatives and legislation to mandate that patients have a voice in their own health care. Unfortunately, only 10% to 20% of people complete an advance care plan.[11] In the large SUPPORT study, 77% of patients did not discuss their resuscitation preferences by third day in hospital and 58% did not want to talk about preferences.[12] In a recent Canadian study, only 34% of seriously ill patients had discussed cardiopulmonary resuscitation (CPR) with their physician and 37% did not wish to discuss resuscitation status. Twenty-five percent did not want any information on CPR.[13] When asked, most physicians and surrogates are mistaken about patient preferences.

At the same time, the current reality is that one in five U.S. residents will die in an ICU.[14] Research reveals that 11% of Medicare recipients spend more than 7 days in intensive care during the last 6 months of life.[15] Such care may be appropriate if it is consistent with the patient's goals and has the ability to restore a person to some acceptable quality of life, even if only for a short time. However, the numbers of patients receiving intensive interventions are large—and many are not benefiting nor expected to benefit from such care—and the numbers are expected to increase as our population ages. Life in the ICU is continuously and precariously in balance with death on a day-to-day basis and even on a moment-to-moment basis. Caring for dying patients and their families is very much integral to the practice of intensive care medicine, yet palliative care in the ICU poses its own set of unique challenges.

Negotiating Goals of Care

The need for admission to the ICU usually occurs with little warning of the drastic illness and resultant changes in a person's life. Initial goals of ICU care are always to resuscitate, stabilize, and try to save the life of the critically ill patient. The course of critical illness, in spite of all the extensive monitoring and available diagnostic testing, often remains unpredictable. Although the ICU team hopes for steady improvements after the initial resuscitation efforts, deteriorations can be unexpected and profound. Subsequent recovery, if it occurs, is never fast.

To meet ethical and legal standards of informed consent before ICU care is initiated, health care providers must clearly:

1. Explain why potentially life-sustaining treatments/critical care services may be indicated
2. Explain what is entailed in the provision of ICU care, including intubation, ventilation, central and arterial lines, inotropic and vasopressor medications, artificial nutrition, communication challenges, monitoring devices, likelihood of benefit, and potential material risks
3. Explore and explain how these treatments would fit in the context of wishes, values, beliefs, and goals and facilitate development of realistic treatment goals
4. Engage in a separate detailed discussion of CPR in the event of cardiac arrest because the need for CPR is distinct from need for life support and outcomes are markedly different and worse should a cardiac arrest occur
5. Recommend whether or not potentially life-sustaining treatments and CPR should be provided and explain the reasoning behind such recommendations
6. Answer any questions from the patient or their SDM
7. Document the discussions, recommendations, and treatment plans in the patient's chart

Ideally these detailed discussions should occur when a patient is relatively healthy, long before he or she needs ICU care and should involve the patient's surrogate decision maker. Health care providers are either not well trained or may feel uncomfortable engaging in these discussions. When patients and surrogates also don't want to discuss these difficult topics, problems often ensue, with some patients or proxies refusing treatments that could help and others, including sometimes providers, insisting on treatments that will not work or have a very slim chance of restoring any kind of quality of life either in the short or long term.

Once admitted to an ICU, many severity of illness scores (e.g., Acute Physiology and Chronic Health Evaluation [APACHE], Sepsis-Related Organ Failure [SOFA]) have been developed to help improve prognostication. Such scores enable the characterization of patient populations, the ability to audit and compare outcomes, and the ability to stratify for research studies and to quantify resource needs. These scores have limitations, however. The patient population from which they were derived may not apply in all situations of critical illness, the data needed to calculate the score may be unwieldy, collection errors may occur, and the model may not reflect advances in critical care medicine. These scoring systems were developed to predict outcomes for *populations*, not individual patients. Their accuracy in predicting survival for an individual patient is not as reliable or precise.[16] These scoring systems do have value, however, because most intensive care specialists tend to overestimate mortality, and these estimates ultimately influence decisions to withdraw treatment.[17] It has been shown that intensive care specialists are more accurate in their predictions than primary team physicians though, who tended to overestimate the probability of favorable outcomes.[18]

Although another goal of life-sustaining interventions, be they mechanical ventilation or inotropes or vasopressors, is to alleviate symptoms such as dyspnea and pain, the interventions themselves may be a source of significant discomfort and have the potential to cause secondary acute life-threatening complications. These complications, usually infectious or ischemic, may arise after the original illness is cured and can ultimately be fatal. Critically ill patients are "asked" to endure distressing symptoms, including anxiety (68%), depression (40%–70%), fear (54%), pain (52%–75%), discomfort from the endotracheal tube (60%), discomfort from the nasogastric tube (48%), nightmares and hallucinations (31%–74%), dyspnea (33%), insomnia (13%), and thirst (10%). Critically ill patients have described extreme fear, inner tension, and a sense of isolation, all of which can be increased by seemingly small events. Most patients rate these symptoms as moderate to severe in intensity.[19,20] Many survivors report symptoms of posttraumatic stress disorder which may be alleviated if SDMs and family members keep a diary or record of daily events in the patient's life that can be reviewed and discussed in the future. Awareness of such sources of discomfort, asking patients about their experiences, and working with them to alleviate distress as much as possible are crucial to the quality of life of all critically ill patients.

Quality-of-life considerations are viewed as increasingly important in caring for critically ill patients as medical experience treating such patients grows. Whether it's getting patients to a chair, encouraging and helping them to decorate their room with personal mementos and photographs, taking them on excursions to bright patient care areas in the hospital or even outside, having volunteers read to them, or having them watch movies or interact with family via webcams and email, such experiences can help patients deal with their illness and need for life support. Tailored physiotherapy, prevention of muscle wasting and general deterioration in physical condition, occupational therapy, and speech therapy can not only improve their chances of survival but also their sense of well-being in particular in long stay situations. High quality patient-centered care means that many ICU teams are increasingly creative in their efforts to recognize and respect the uniqueness of each person and to give patients some control at a time when it may appear they have little or none.

Regular discussions and revisions of the goals of care as needed are an absolute necessity to ensure that the wishes, values, beliefs, and goals of individual patients are continually respected *and* that treatment goals remain realistic as the patient journeys with critical illness in face of either illness progression, response or lack of response to treatment, or development of secondary complications. Research has revealed that 81.2% of SDMs preferred shared decision making with the physician caring for the patient, 14.8% preferred to leave all decisions to physicians, 23.8% preferred the physician to make final decision after considering their opinion, and only 0.5% wanted to make decisions alone.[21] Unfortunately, an overemphasis on patient autonomy has contributed to failures to develop realistic treatment goals and, hence, to the provision of inappropriate treatment. Medical considerations—of whether treatments will potentially lead to a cure; whether they can prevent, slow, or reduce the progression of illness; and whether potential benefits outweigh harms—should be used to achieve balance and define the limits of such autonomy. Limits to autonomy occur when the rights of one patient infringe or risk infringing on rights of another to access critical care services, which are a limited resource in many hospitals and in many countries. Some personal factors may be less obvious but may also result in limits to individual autonomy: these may result from depletion of family financial or emotional resources such that family members life opportunities are significantly undermined.

Each member of the multiprofessional ICU team can play an invaluable role in improving communication, evaluating response to treatments, developing ongoing treatment plans, providing support, and facilitating such decision making, whether with the patient or with a surrogate. The ICU team has an obligation to ensure that information it communicates is generally consistent. To this end, any intrateam conflict and any conflicts with referring medical or surgical teams should be resolved without ensnaring the patient or family. Furthermore, it is not uncommon for people to choose different words to communicate the same thing, and at times it may seem that different messages are being conveyed. Encouraging patients and families to seek clarification can help prevent confusion and conflict.

All good efforts notwithstanding, conflicts are unfortunately common in the ICU setting.[22] In studies describing conflicts in the care of patients with prolonged ICU stay, nearly a third of patients had conflicts associated with their care. Of these, 48% to 57% of conflicts were between the ICU team and family members, and 31% to 48% occurred between ICU team members.[22,23] The most common types of conflicts arise around decisions regarding whether to withdraw or withhold treatment.[23,24] Most ICU teams work closely with bioethicists, social workers, and pastoral care providers who may be invaluable in helping resolve conflicts. Trials of therapy with preset clear goals and timeframes that everyone can agree on may also be a useful strategy. Intractable conflicts result in substantial use of medical and legal resources and are emotionally and psychologically draining for all those involved. The effects on families can be profound and include increased stress, anxiety, grief, complicated bereavement process, and difficulties in future interactions with the health care system. Conflicts are also sources of frustration, secondary intrateam and interteam conflicts, and staff burnout.[24] To circumvent such conflict situations, physicians may err on the side of caution by continuing life-sustaining interventions, even if treatment is believed to be against the patients' wishes[24] (Box 35-1). Whether this approach is appropriate or not is a source of debate within critical care medicine.

> ### Box 35-1. *Consequences of Conflict*
>
> Reestablishing goals and any subsequent conversations with patients, surrogate decision makers, and team members can be draining and time consuming and lead to escalation of conflict. Other consequences of conflict include the following:
> - Refusal of potentially beneficial treatments
> - Demands for treatments deemed inappropriate
> - Decreased quality of patient care as patient and surrogate interactions are increasing avoided or care interventions come to be considered as meaningless
> - Decreased emotional and psychological support to patients and surrogate decision makers
> - Lack of resources to care for others who could benefit from ICU treatments
> - Recourse to legal means to resolve conflict
> - Staff burnout

Moving to a Palliative Treatment Plan

It is often difficult to determine the optimal timing of the switch from a predominantly curative approach (when pain and symptoms are treated, just not as the main goal of therapy) to a predominantly palliative approach (when survival is no longer possible or even desired and the main goal of therapy is pain and symptom control). The knowledge of the invariably rocky nature of any critical illness; the problems in prognosticating; conflict within and among health care team members and with patients and surrogates; religious and cultural beliefs; and patient, surrogates and even health care teams' wishes to keep going even in the face of diminishing chances of survival, and the hope—realistic or otherwise—that things will improve, are all factors in such decisions. This being said, decisions to limit treatment occurs relatively quickly, with the median time from ICU admission to the first decision to limit treatment 2.8 days (range, 0.6–9.8).[8]

Decision Making with Critically Ill Patients

Communicating with intubated patients is particularly difficult and one of the most frustrating problems for patients and health care providers alike. Options include lip reading (difficult because the endotracheal tube and tape used to stabilize it at the mouth inhibit the formation of words), use of the alphabet boards (to spell out messages), word or picture boards, and writing (also challenging with arterial and intravenous lines in place, as well as the edema and the generalized weakness and fatigue that often accompany critical illness). Studies have shown that very few patients are able to communicate with the health care team at the time of decision making regarding withholding or withdrawing life support.

To participate in any decision-making process to consent to or refuse treatment, patients must first be capable; that is, they must have the ability to understand treatment options, risks, and benefits and must be able to appreciate how such options will affect them in view of their life goals, values, and beliefs. The challenges in communicating with intubated patients can make capacity assessments very difficult but not impossible. Few critically ill patients are actually capable, though, because severe illness, medications, delirium, and lack of sleep all combine to reduce their ability to participate in decision making. A patient's recall of previous conversations and ability to concentrate may be reduced. As in other settings, capacity may be variable, and decisions may change from one day to the next. The challenge in the ICU is to ensure that changes in decision making are real and are not clouded by confusion, "transient" emotional states, or incapacity. In particular, when a patient requests withdrawal or withholding of life support, he or she must clearly understand the consequences, and consistency of such decisions over time is important.

Second, patients must be informed. An additional challenge is to explain life-sustaining interventions in sufficient depth to facilitate decision making. Patients with borderline capacity may be able to understand and appreciate some but not all of this complex information. Because the stakes can be very high, it is crucial to be absolutely certain of a patient's capacity before engaging him or her in any decision making and to be crystal clear about the consequences of any decisions made. Indeed, when dealing with the discomforts inherent in life-sustaining interventions, many patients request withdrawal of such therapies only to change their minds when they are informed that without such therapies they will die.

Although decision making with critically ill patients is rare, when it is possible, a specific set of communication skills is needed. Information must be conveyed in a very clear, complete, and consistent way, with frequent checks of understanding. Unlike in other settings, the health care provider will, by necessity, have to do most of the talking to make the process easier on the patient. Careful attention is needed, therefore, to ensure that the patient is an active participant, that he or she understands the information, is not having treatment goals dictated by the health care team (though sometimes these goals will be dictated by critical illness and failure to respond to treatments), and agrees with any recommendations. The ICU team has to have a clear picture of and stay focused on what the patient needs to know, compared with what would be nice to know, without becoming overly paternalistic. In general, the following information must be conveyed:

1. An explanation of the illness that brought the patient to the ICU, treatments, and response to treatment to date, including implications for future treatment goals
2. Life-sustaining interventions in use, whether more would need to be added, and what they can and cannot potentially achieve
3. The current and future realistic goals of therapy, taking into account patient values, beliefs, and wishes
4. What needs to be done to try to achieve these goals and the chances of success
5. The alternatives, including palliative treatment plans
6. Repeat discussion of CPR and whether it would be appropriate to attempt should the need arise
7. Recommendations and the reasons for recommendations regarding the future course of therapy, including that of withholding or withdrawing life-sustaining interventions

Although some of this information may have been discussed in prior conversations, it is important to recapitulate, even briefly, when facing major decisions. Expressing empathy while trying to be clear and brief can be especially challenging (Box 35-2). Everyone present, including the patient and family members, should be made aware that interruptions for questions or clarifications are expected at any time.

> ### Box 35-2. *Decision Making with Capable Critically Ill Patients*
>
> Agree on a convenient time, decide who will be present, and make participants as comfortable as possible in the intensive care unit room by ensuring as much privacy as the environment will permit. The following steps will help ensure a successful meeting.
> * State the purpose of the meeting.
> * Explain the meeting format.
> * Recapitulate the current stage of illness and explain goals and current life-sustaining interventions.
> * Give information in small, clear, straightforward, and simple chunks, and check frequently for understanding.
> * Be supportive and sensitive to emotional, psychological, cultural, and spiritual needs, especially fear and a sense of isolation.
> * Avoid giving inappropriate hope and avoid the inappropriate destruction of hope.
> * Avoid euphemisms. If the expected outcome of a decision is death, the patient needs to be told as gently and empathetically as possible, but it must be clear.
> * Be patient when and if questions arise.
> * Move the discussion into the future: Where do we go from here?
> * Ask how these treatment options would fit with the patient's values, wishes, goals, and beliefs.
> * Encourage broader family and ICU team participation in discussions.
> * Facilitate the development of realistic goals, and make a recommendation regarding future treatment plans, including trials of therapy.

Health care teams need to be prepared and committed because facilitating decision making is going to take time, and the communication process may be frustrating for all involved.

If the patient consents, the family should also be present during these discussions. Although the family can offer tremendous support, when the news is bad, they may also require significant support themselves. Moreover, a natural desire to shield the patient may also exist and risk hindering discussions. Having the family present while the patient is gently informed and options are discussed can help ease their anxiety and can facilitate future discussions and expression of emotions and support.

Because critically ill patients are rarely capable, though, the burden of trying to grasp the severity of illness and the prognosis and then to consent to or refuse the proposed treatment plans usually rests with the surrogate, who is most often a member of the family.

Decision Making with Surrogates

The role of a surrogate is very difficult because the surrogate is usually a family member or someone who is very close to the patient. On the one hand, surrogates have to deal with myriad emotions engendered by seeing their loved one in a state of profound illness. On the other hand, they have to find a way through these emotions to understand the illness, the life-sustaining interventions used, and the treatment options, and to be able to participate in decision making with the health care team. The decision-making standard is not what the surrogate would want; rather, it is what the patient would want if still able to speak for himself or herself. These two concepts may not agree. The lack of an advance directive or of some prior indication from the loved one results in significantly increased stress levels. In addition, surrogates and families often have difficulty eating and sleeping and are commonly physically and emotionally exhausted. Different coping styles may lead to misunderstandings, hurt, and intrafamily conflicts. Depending on the level of critical care required and the resources available, surrogates may have to travel great distances to be with their loved one. In these situations, their support network may be fragmented or lacking altogether. Even if a surrogate is designated as sole decision maker, he or she often involves the rest of family in any decisions. For these reasons, the ICU team must regard the patient and the entire family as a unit of care.

Not surprisingly, the prevalence of anxiety and depression in family members is high: 69.1% and 35.4%, respectively. Significant symptoms of at least one—anxiety or depression—are seen in 84% of spouses and 72.7% of family members of critically ill patients.[10] Factors that increase anxiety include the absence of prior chronic disease in the patient, a spousal relationship, female gender, the absence of regular meetings with the ICU team, the absence of a quiet room for such meetings, and a desire for or actual professional psychological help. Factors that increase symptoms of depression are younger patient age, a spousal relationship, female gender, the lack of a meeting room, and the provision of seemingly conflicting information. When faced with decisions to withdraw life support, the stress is increased greatly, and symptoms of posttraumatic stress may persist 6 months later.[10,25]

Overall family satisfaction with the care received by the patient in the ICU is high (84%), and most (77%) are satisfied with their role in the decision-making process. There appears to be a direct correlation between satisfaction with care and role in the decision-making process.[26,27] Family satisfaction also increases with the provision of greater amounts of information, with the amount or level of care received, and in proportion to the degree of respect and compassion shown to the patient and family member. However, studies have also shown that ICU family meetings often fail to meet the needs of families. Many ICU teams will ask SDMs, "What do you want us to do?" without making recommendations regarding initiating, continuing, or withdrawing treatments based on discussions of treatment goals and likelihood of success. Such questions place the decision-making burdens on SDMs and do not promote the shared decision-making concept that these SDMs value.

Even though the decisions to withdraw life support are weighty, one study revealed that these meetings are relatively short (32 minutes [SD, 14.8 minutes; range, 7–74 minutes]), and the average time allocated to listening to the family speak was only 29% (SD, 15%; range, 3% to 67%). As the proportion of time spent listening to the family increased, so did the family's satisfaction.[28,29] Allowing the family greater time to speak does not increase the duration of the meeting, a finding that ICU teams need to be aware of because quality of care can be easily improved even when time is in short supply. Although the total meeting time was not associated with family satisfaction, other studies have shown that meetings that last longer than 10 minutes are associated with increased understanding. There appears to be a need for families to identify and speak with the physician "in charge," usually the staff intensive care specialist, because they look to this individual for comfort, information, and reassurance. Failure of the staff physician to establish such a relationship may be perceived as a sign of a lack of caring.[10,28,29]

Misunderstandings and forgetting or mixing up information are common, and repeated explanations may be required over the course of several meetings. In practice, some family members appear to become fixated on the data generated by the ICU, sometimes without really understanding them. Sometimes improvements in one number are sufficient to generate false hope for survival among family members. Focusing on a few laboratory results, the fraction of inspired oxygen, or hemodynamic parameters on the monitor, may not provide an accurate picture of the course of illness or its prognosis. In these situations, gently explaining the limitations of such an approach and refocusing on the larger picture can be very helpful. Families also need to be reassured that any pain and distressing symptoms will be alleviated and that comfort will be ensured no matter what decisions are made.

In the end, the approach to meeting with a surrogate is not all that different from meeting with a capable patient (Box 35-3). Three important added dimensions are: facilitating communication between family members and their critically ill loved one,

---

Box 35-3. _Decision Making with Surrogates_

Choose a convenient time and ensure that all who need or want to be present are there.
- Introduce the ICU team members, and establish the relationships of all present.
- State the purpose of the meeting.
- Explain and recapitulate; avoid euphemisms. Clarify any misconceptions and miscommunications.
- Explore previously expressed patient values, goals, and beliefs, and explore concepts of patient's best interests _and_
- Discuss potential future goals of therapy and trials of therapy.
- Acknowledge the difficulties of the substitute's situation, normalize the experience, and be supportive and sensitive to emotional, psychological, cultural, and spiritual needs. Be prepared to explain that different coping styles are not a sign of lack of caring.
- Pay particular attention to the needs of younger children (if any). Additional resources may be needed—consider consulting pediatric ICU or children hospitals' Child Life programs to develop your own resources for grief and bereavement in children.
- Encourage and respond to questions, either during the meeting or those that arise later, in an open and clear way.
- Explain to the best of your knowledge the experience of the patient while in the ICU. Acknowledge times of distress if they occurred, and explain how pain and symptoms will be alleviated and comfort ensured no matter what decision is taken.
- Encourage all relevant family members and ICU team members' involvement during the meeting.
- Place decision making into a shared team framework.
- Address potentially hidden issues such as anger, blame, or guilt they may be experiencing toward the patient, the team, or themselves.
- Facilitate the development of realistic goals, and make a recommendation regarding future treatment plans.
- Facilitate conversations among and between family members and the critically ill patient. Encourage them to speak and to express love and support.

facilitating communication among family members, and alleviating the burden of decision making as much as possible by acknowledging how difficult the tasks are and placing decisions into a shared decision-making model. Even if the critically ill patient is unconscious, encouraging the family to talk to their loved one, to express emotions, to resolve any conflicts and misunderstanding, and to provide support is important because this approach can often help to improve their own abilities to cope in the days ahead.

Pain and Symptom Management

Pain and other distressing symptoms are very common in the ICU. Recognizing them and evaluating the response to treatment are challenging: Difficulties in communication and decreased levels of consciousness resulting from critical illness and medications often lead to reliance on facial expressions and nonspecific physiologic parameters such as tachycardia or bradycardia, tachypnea with accessory muscle use, and hypertension or hypotension. In view of these inherent difficulties, it is concerning that most health care providers fail to recognize or underestimate the severity of the patient's pain and distress.[30,31] Others refused to administer more medications when asked, for fear of exacerbating hemodynamic instability and causing respiratory depression. Yet, in the ICU, hemodynamics can be supported with increasing doses of inotropes or vasopressors, and fears of respiratory depression have repeatedly been shown to be unfounded. Even when the goal is curative, it is unacceptable not to alleviate pain and distress even if doing so means increasing the amount of support required. Certainly, based on the current literature, the need for concerted efforts to improve pain and symptom control using nonpharmacologic and pharmacologic means in the ICU is undeniable.

In the ICU, continuous infusions of narcotics and sedatives are used to alleviate pain and symptoms caused by the illness itself, to allow the assumption of greater control of respiratory function with mechanical ventilation, and to decrease the discomforts inherent in being on life support. Intermittent bolus doses of medications are used to supplement the infusions in anticipation of and in response to interventions that would be expected to increase pain and suffering. The use of continuous infusions results in better pain control and lower total doses of medication overall, yet many patients do require moderate to high doses of opioids and sedatives. In multisystem organ failure, these medications and their metabolites can accumulate, resulting in very prolonged sedation and decreased levels of consciousness, leading some to recommend daily interruptions in such therapy when treatment goals are curative.

In the last hours of life, though, when life support is being withdrawn, the ICU team has to be prepared to quickly manage dyspnea, pain, and any other signs of distress. Knowledge of the difficulties in assessing and subsequently treating pain and suffering is important, and the current literature indicates that the lack of success in doing so effectively in survivors seems to suggest a need to err on the side of being more aggressive in palliating such symptoms in dying patients. The one-to-one nurse-to-patient ratio is a great advantage in ensuring that patients are continuously assessed and medications are given quickly when needed. Still, it is important for physicians to take an active role in reassessing the patient's comfort during this time when at all possible. Anticipation and understanding of the effects of withdrawing life support, the frequency of reevaluation, and the immediate availability of the team should result in the ICU's being a leader in palliating symptoms at the end of life and ensuring comfort during the dying process.[32]

Sedated patients are usually too ill to be "woken up" to speak to family members one last time. This can be a significant source of distress for the family and should be gently explained. In practice, if the patient is receiving continuous infusions of medications, these are continued and increased as required. Those patients not receiving infusions may have them started: Such infusions will provide a baseline level of comfort, and many nurses find it easier and less disruptive to the family during this time to provide any needed boluses through the infusion pumps rather than through a syringe. Intravenous boluses of opioids, sedatives, or both are usually needed as the ventilator is withdrawn (see earlier). Boluses may also be given every 5 minutes for any signs of pain, dyspnea, agitation, or anxiety. When boluses are given, the infusions may also be increased to maintain symptom control. Infusions should not be increased without bolus dosing: The time to reach steady state from an increase in the infusion rate alone and hence for the patient to perceive any benefit is far too long. To achieve comfort, most patients are sedated into unconsciousness. In the current literature, such a practice may be viewed as terminal sedation, a practice some have questioned as being euthanasia in disguise. In the ICU, continuous infusions of opioids and sedatives while a patient is dying are simply a continuation of that way in which pain and distress are managed on a daily basis and constitute, without question, palliative care.

The amount of narcotics and sedatives required is variable and may be quite high. Doses given may be 5- to 10-fold higher than during the curative phase of treatment. The amount of medication needed depends on the level of distress and is different for each patient.[30,31,33] The patient's baseline requirements of narcotics and sedatives before the withdrawal process also determine both the amount needed for bolus doses and the total dose. The average dose of morphine is 16 to 20 mg/hour and 7.5 mg/hour of lorazepam equivalents from 1 hour before ventilator withdrawal to the time to death.[32,34] The range in other studies was 0.5 to 350 mg/hour morphine and 0.5 to 95 mg/hour midazolam. Patients will require more if they have become tolerant to such drugs during their ICU stay. No hastening of death has been seen in relation to doses of opioids or sedatives. Any difference has, in fact, been inverse: higher doses result in increased time to death.

The *principle of double effect* permits the administration of analgesics and sedatives to alleviate the dying patient's distress, even though such administration could hasten his or her death. Although the current literature emphasizes that the intent must be symptom alleviation, and even seems to refute that any hastening actually occurs, fears still exist that the administration of opioids and sedatives may shorten the time to death. The principle of double effect was given legal sanction in a U.S. Supreme Court decision that stated if the intent in administering analgesics and sedatives is clearly to palliate, physicians do not need to fear being charged with murder or assisting suicide. Fears of being misunderstood—of having an intent to palliate mistaken for an intent to kill—are currently exacerbated by debates and articles in the medical literature in which the legalization of euthanasia is promoted by misappropriating the principle of double effect to diminish the fundamental and very real differences in intent that exist between the practices of palliation and euthanasia.[33] An unintended consequence may be to increase the reluctance on the part of health care providers to administer adequate analgesia and sedation and thus risk undertreating their dying patients. For these reasons, consensus guidelines clarifying palliative care in the ICU, distinguishing it from assisted death, and ongoing efforts to build understanding between medical and legal groups may continue to improve the quality of end-of-life care.[33]

Withholding and Withdrawing Life-Sustaining Interventions

At least 70% of deaths in the ICU follow decisions to withhold or withdraw life support. Withholding and withdrawing are believed to be ethically and, for the most part, legally equivalent. In practice, the two do not feel the same. By the time a decision to withdraw life support has been reached, the relationship among the patient, family, and team may be more established, and the withdrawal is more emotionally difficult. Additionally, withdrawal decisions in general have a more acute, direct, and profound effect on the need to realign hope from that of survival to that of a peaceful death.

Including patient wishes, recommendations to withhold or withdraw life support are also based on the intensive care specialist's and team's assessment of the likelihood of surviving the current acute illness, the likelihood of long-term survival, premorbid cognitive function, patient age, length of ICU stay, and quality of life both before and after the course in ICU. It is well recognized that physicians' assessments of likelihood of survival and quality life are influenced by their own prior experiences and by their ethical, moral, cultural, and religious beliefs. Such inherent differences can result in considerable variability in their recommendations regarding withholding or withdrawing life support. Other factors idiosyncratic to intensive care specialists and their practice environment also come into play: the years since graduation, the location and number of beds in the ICU, and their assessment of the likelihood that they would withdraw life support in comparison with their colleagues. Such variability can be a source of considerable distress both for other members of the involved health care teams and for families. Intensive care specialists need to be conscious of these disparities in practice and must work together to ensure more consistent decision making to improve the quality of end-of-life care provided.

Although the increasing focus on patient autonomy and rights has led to a shared decision-making model, intensive care specialists still make unilateral decisions to withhold or even to withdraw life-sustaining interventions if such interventions won't work. However, unilateral withholding or withdrawing of life support outside of these circumstances without knowledge of the patient's goals or discussion with the patient or surrogate, or when death is not imminent, is troubling because such decisions are prone to bias. If life support is only prolonging the dying process, the standard of care would be to withdraw or withhold such interventions with the surrogate's consent. In cases when life support is serving only to prolong the dying process but the surrogate objects to its withdrawal and the conflict cannot be resolved, intensive care specialists, bioethicists, and the courts are split over whether unilateral withdrawal is acceptable. The standard would be to continue life support until conflict can be resolved through (1) ongoing discussions and perhaps with help of bioethicists, social workers, pastoral care, or a second opinion; (2) trials of therapy with preset goals; or (3) legal means. Courts have repeatedly shown respect for medical judgment regarding appropriate treatments as long as such judgment was based on sound clinical reasoning and was not biased or discriminatory. To date, many courts have, however, been unwilling to make decisions that would result in the death of a patient whose wishes are unknown, and rulings have supported the families' wishes to continue life support.[35] Though critical care clinicians are often frustrated by legal decisions that may draw distinctions that seem arbitrary and devoid of clinical sense, they themselves have to improve their consistency in use of life-sustaining treatments to better educate and guide courts in future.

The first therapy to be withheld is usually cardiopulmonary resuscitation. In view of the very poor survival rates after cardiac arrest in critically ill patients, instituting a Do Not Resuscitate (DNR) order is an understandable and appropriate first step. Subsequent withholding decisions involve instituting limits to levels or numbers of inotropes, to escalations in ventilator settings, or limiting the introduction of new life-sustaining interventions such as dialysis. Placing such limits has been translated into Do Not Escalate (DNE) orders on patients' charts. Such orders may be vague to other team members, especially for team members who were not present during the family meeting. To ensure clarity, DNE orders should be followed by a detailed explanation of what treatments are not to be escalated and what is still considered acceptable. Decisions to withdraw life-sustaining interventions are usually the last to be made.

After decisions are made to withdraw life support, variability exists in what is withdrawn and how. Therapies most likely to result in a more immediate death, those whose withdrawal will not increase pain and distress, those that have been more recently instituted, and those that are more invasive, expensive, and scarce are usually the first to be discontinued. For patients receiving multiple life-sustaining interventions, withdrawal may be sequential or simultaneous. It is not known whether one method of withdrawal is better than another, nor can such a question ever be answered. The most important goal is that the patient be kept comfortable no matter how the withdrawal is accomplished and no matter the length of time the patient survives.

How to Withdraw a Ventilator

With the foregoing considerations in mind, inotropes and vasopressors are simply turned off without being weaned. Most commonly, the ventilator is quickly weaned in stages. The fast, stepwise approach allows the team to control and quickly alleviate any signs of dyspnea, agitation, or distress with a combination of opioids and benzodiazepines, because these medications have known synergistic effects, and antipsychotics (such as haloperidol) especially if delirium is present. Initial bolus doses of an intravenous opioid (usually morphine or fentanyl) and a benzodiazepine (usually midazolam or lorazepam) are commonly given, and infusions of these medications are increased in anticipation of increased dyspnea as the ventilatory support is decreased. If the patient is already sedated with propofol, it may be used instead of benzodiazepines. The ventilatory support is then decreased, and further bolus doses are administered and infusions are increased as required. Once the patient appears comfortable, further reductions in support are made. The speed of weaning the ventilator varies based on patient comfort and the experience and practice of the ICU physician and bedside nurse and the respiratory therapist. In general, if the ventilator is to be weaned, a guiding principle is that it should occur as fast as possible to avoid prolonging the dying process and as slowly as required to ensure comfort. In practice, withdrawal of ventilatory support generally occurs over a period of 10 to 30 minutes.

Many patients who undergo withdrawal of mechanical ventilation are extubated. Removal of the endotracheal and nasogastric tubes and of all the accompanying tape eliminates more sources of discomfort. It has added the benefit of allowing the family to get closer and to see the face of their loved one finally unencumbered once again. An oral airway may be required to maintain the airway and to prevent choking. Secretions in the posterior pharynx may become audible and can be decreased with anticholinergic agents such as scopolamine, given intravenously to ensure absorption. Extubation is sometimes dreaded by ICU team members, in particular the bedside nurse and respiratory therapist, because of fears of causing the patient distress or dyspnea. A physician presence during extubation is important because it can help ensure that any signs of distress are quickly treated, and he or she can also provide emotional support to the bedside nurse, respiratory therapist, and family, for whom extubation may be seen as the final moment of withdrawal.

If the patient has an excessive amount of secretions and requires very frequent suctioning or if he or she is in florid pulmonary edema or having hemoptysis, extubation is probably not a good choice; in these situations, anticholinergic agents are usually insufficient, and patients can be helped by suctioning through the endotracheal tube. Patients who are pharmacologically paralyzed and, hence, are unable to breathe at all without ventilatory support should not have mechanical ventilation completely withdrawn and should definitely not be extubated because these acts will directly and immediately cause death.[32] The difficulty is that sometimes in the presence of multisystem organ failure, metabolites can accumulate; therefore, these drugs take a long time to wear off, and the effect cannot always be reversed. In these situations, the fraction of inspired oxygen can be reduced to room air, and the level of assist and the respiratory rate can be significantly decreased. However, programming a minimal respiratory rate and level of assist from the ventilator must always be provided. Complete withdrawal of a ventilator and extubation of a pharmacologically paralyzed patient, who is unable to breathe, is not condoned.[32] An added challenge is that pharmacologic paralysis eliminates the usual signs of distress, such as facial grimacing and respiratory effort. Ensuring comfort in a paralyzed patient as ventilatory support is reduced requires greater reliance on following hemodynamic parameters and erring on the side of being liberal with narcotics and sedatives.

The ways in which the ventilator is withdrawn and whether or not the patient is extubated have not been associated with any differences in time to death, the families' perceptions of comfort, or the use of narcotics. Most families who have been through this process believe that their loved one was totally or very comfortable during the withdrawal and had a good death. Once life support is withdrawn, however, the time to death is out of the control of the ICU team and may be difficult to predict. Patients receiving extensive support may die within minutes, sometimes before life support is removed in its entirety. Others may take hours, days, or weeks to die. Palliative care is crucial no matter how long a patient survives. Although patients may be kept in the ICU after life support is withdrawn, they may be transferred to other hospital wards if their death is expected to be more prolonged. Palliative care teams can greatly ease this transition and ensure the highest quality of ongoing care.

The Last Hours

Whenever the transition is made in primary goals from cure to palliation, efforts must be made to ensure therapeutic coherence. Therapies aimed at curative plans should be stopped, and only those aimed at palliating symptoms should be continued. Many therapies and all diagnostic tests are no longer indicated. This is one aspect of end-of-life care in the ICU that needs serious improvement: All blood work, radiology, and medications not required to provide comfort should be discontinued.

Some have suggested and found success with end-of-life care protocols designed to bring some standardization to the withdrawal process and to serve as a reminder of what needs to be done. It is hoped that any need for protocols would subsequently diminish as their components become integrated into the team's standard care. Although such protocols may help to improve the quality of care, they should never replace the sharing of humanity so needed at this time. Others have suggested formally involving palliative care teams in the care of dying ICU patients. These efforts have also succeeded in improving end-of-life care in some studies. Palliative care teams need to understand the effects of withdrawing life support and adapt their practice to meet the acuity of pain and symptom management in the ICU.

Some patients, SDMs, and families may request withdrawal of life support at home. Although this can pose some logistical challenges for ICU teams, it may be possible to honor such requests. Each ICU team needs to consider their resources, consider collaborating with palliative care teams and services, and figure out if it is possible to ensure that the patient can be effectively palliated at home and if the human resources exist to make withdrawal at home possible given the circumstances.

Caring for the Family

An important part of providing quality palliative care in the ICU during the withdrawal process is to explain to the family what is happening. Death in the ICU has been portrayed in the media as one of the worst possible situations anyone could ever experience. The common phrase "pulling the plug" leads many to picture an abrupt removal of interventions that were instituted to alleviate distress in the first place. Hence, families commonly fear a death filled with pain, dyspnea, and suffering. Requests for euthanasia are not uncommon at this time and generally are a reflection of such fears. Explicit, clear, and straightforward explanations of how each life-sustaining intervention in use will be stopped, how pain, dyspnea, and any other signs of distress will be assessed and palliated, how the family can help, and how they can be with their loved one are absolute necessities. The ICU team should offer gentle and straightforward explanations of the changes the family will observe in their loved one, changes that will occur in both the patient's hemodynamics and respiratory patterns. Families need reassurance that any signs of distress will be quickly alleviated, that changes are a normal part of the dying processes, and that the team will ensure that their loved one will not suffer during this time. Families need to be clear that the ICU team will not abandon them and that no matter how long their loved one survives after the withdrawal, he or she will be kept comfortable. Family members should be encouraged to ask questions and to express their fears. Grief and bereavement information, including the phone numbers and websites of organizations that may help SDMs and family members cope with their loss, may be very helpful resources to give once the patient has died. Particular attention should be paid to the needs of children, in creating memories and legacies, in explaining death and dying, and in helping them cope during and after the death. Adult ICUs may ask for help from either local children's hospitals' palliative care or Child Life programs or pediatric ICUs to develop grief and bereavement resource kits targeting different age groups. Such toolkits may be very helpful in teaching the ICU team and family members how to help children cope with loss.

In the last days or hours, some ICUs are able to accommodate the family by designating a room to their private presence with the patient, limiting interruptions by staff, and even allowing a spouse to sleep next to the patient in a bed drawn up for the purpose. Efforts should be made to respect any wishes for ceremonies or religious and cultural rituals during and after death. Providing the family with emotional, psychological, and spiritual support and listening to and addressing their concerns throughout this time are crucial to providing high-quality end-of-life care. Support after the death of a loved one, help with funeral arrangements, and resources and information on locally available bereavement supports are also valued.

PEARLS

- Inform the patient and family early on that many health care teams will be involved in the care of a critically ill patient, and explain that this may cause communication challenges because different people may use different words to convey the same message.

- Make it clear to families that the course of critical illness can be unpredictable and that, although the initial hopes and efforts are for survival, life and death are precariously balanced in the ICU.

- Share humanity in the midst of technology: Ask about the patient as a person, and normalize the experience as much as possible by acknowledging the severity of illness, its accompanying emotions, and the complexities of decision making.

- Health care providers have an ethical, professional, and legal obligation to involve patients who are capable in the decision-making process, no matter how difficult such conversations may be.

- Place decisions in the context of goals, values, and beliefs, and discuss short-term and long-term quality-of-life implications as best they can be predicted.

- Ensure that treatment options, their risks and benefits, and the consequences of any decisions are crystal clear.

- Never forget that life-sustaining interventions can both cause and alleviate pain and distress. Ensure that such symptoms are evaluated and promptly treated throughout the course in the ICU.

- Remember that trials of therapy with preset, agreed-upon goals may help ease the burden of decision making on patients, surrogates, and health care teams.

- Be prepared to re-discuss patient's values, beliefs, and treatment goals and whether these are realistic as critical illness evolves.

- Ensure that treatment plans, patient and family goals, concerns, fears, and means of coping are communicated to all members of the health care team.

PITFALLS

- Using the technologic environment to distance oneself from the patient as a person. Although this is an understandable coping mechanism, it can hinder the ability to provide high-quality end-of-life care.

- Failing to clarify consequences of decisions to ensure agreement with the proposed treatment plan or to spare the patient or family grief and suffering.

- Failing to engage in decision making with a patient in the rare situation when he or she is capable of doing so, to avoid difficult conversations that involve death and dying and to spare patients distressing decisions, especially when decisions involve withholding or withdrawing life-sustaining interventions.

- Failing to prepare families (and patients, if they are capable) about what to expect as the patient dies when life-sustaining interventions are withdrawn.

- Failing to explain how pain and distress will be palliated during the withdrawal process.

- Failing to return to the bedside during the withdrawal of life-sustaining interventions to ensure that symptoms are well palliated, to support the family, and to support the ICU team.

- Failing to provide initial bereavement support and information on how additional support can be obtained, if needed, after the patient's death.

- Forgetting the invaluable roles of other team members in helping to communicate with patients and families, facilitating decision making, resolving conflicts, providing emotional and spiritual support, and ensuring comfort.

Summary

Few other fields in medicine have endeavored as much as critical care medicine to improve the quality of care they provide at the end of life. Death in the ICU should not be feared any more than, and perhaps even less than, death in other settings. Certainly great improvements have been made in the last 4 decades, but there is still a need for more. Ongoing education is needed to ensure that all members of the ICU team are taught to communicate clearly and empathically with patients and families, to negotiate the goals of treatment, and to evaluate and manage pain and distress. Efforts are still needed to legitimize research and assign funding for research at the crossroads of critical and palliative care. Future research to identify ongoing problems, develop outcome measures, assess the success or failure of improvement initiatives, and translate this knowledge into practice is the only way to ensure that the level of care provided to those who are dying is as high as that provided to those who will survive.

Resources

Braun KL. In Braun KL, Pietsch JH, Blanchette PL, editors: *Cultural issues in end of life decision-making*, Thousand Oaks, Calif, 2000, Sage Publications.
Danjoux MN, Lawless B, Hawryluck L: Conflicts in the ICU: perspectives of administrators and clinicians, *Intensive Care Med* 35(12):2068–2077, 2009.
Curtis JR, Rubenfeld GD: *Managing death in the ICU: the transition from cure to comfort*, Oxford, UK, 2001, Oxford University Press.
Ian Anderson Continuing Education Program in End of Life Care
www.cme.utoronto.ca/endoflife

References

1. Sibbald R, Downar J, Hawryluck L: Perceptions of "Futile Care" among caregivers in ICUs, *Can Med Assoc J* 177(10):1201–1208, 2007.
2. Palda VA, Bowman KW, McLean RF, et al: "Futile" care: Do we provide it? Why? A semistructured, Canada-wide survey of intensive care unit doctors and nurses, *J Crit Care* 20:207–213, 2005.
3. Vincent JL: Forgoing life support in western European intensive care units: the results of an ethical questionnaire, *Crit Care Med* 27:1626–1633, 1999.
4. Canadian Critical Care Society: Critical Care Unit/Program/Dept Statement of Service and Admission and Discharge Policy, www.canadiancriticalcare.org/cccs/AdmDschTransPolicy.doc, 2000.
5. Society of Critical Care Medicine: Guidelines for ICU Admission, Discharge and Triage, www.sccm.org/professional_resources/guidelines/table_of_contents/Documents/ICU_ADT.pdf, 1999.
6. Thompson BT, Cox PN, Antonelli M: Challenges in end-of-life care in the ICU: statement of the 5th International Consensus Conference in Critical Care, Brussels, Belgium, April 2003: Executive summary, *Crit Care Med* 32:1781–1784, 2004.
7. Heyland DK, Frank C, Groll D, et al for the Canadian Researchers at the End of Life Network: Understanding cardiopulmonary resuscitation decision making: perspectives of seriously ill hospitalized patients and family members, *Chest* 130:419–428, 2006.
8. Sprung CL, Cohen SL, Sjokvist P, et al: End-of-life practices in European intensive care units: the Ethicus Study, *JAMA* 290:790–797, 2003.
9. Vincent JL, Heyland DK, Frank C, et al: Cultural differences in end-of-life care. Understanding cardiopulmonary resuscitation decision making: perspectives of seriously ill hospitalized patients and family members, *Crit Care Med* 29(Suppl 2):N52, 2001.
10. Pochard F, Azoulay E, Chevret S, et al for the French FAMIREA group: Symptoms of anxiety and depression in family members of intensive care unit patients: ethical hypothesis regarding decision-making capacity, *Crit Care Med* 29(10):1893–1897, 2001.
11. Faber-Langendoen K, Lanken PN: Dying patients in the intensive care unit: forgoing treatment, maintaining care, *Ann Intern Med* 135:1091–1092, 2001.
12. Teno J, Lynn J, Wenger N, et al: SUPPORT Investigators. Advance directives for seriously ill hospitalized patients: effectiveness with the patient self-determination act and the SUPPORT intervention. Study to Understand Prognoses and Preferences for Outcomes and Risks of Treatment, *J Am Geriatr Soc* 45:500–507, 1997.
13. Heyland DK, Frank C, Groll D, et al: for the Canadian Researchers at the End of Life Network: Understanding cardiopulmonary resuscitation decision making: perspectives of seriously ill hospitalized patients and family members, *Chest* 130:419–428, 2006.
14. Angus DC, Barnato AE, Linde-Zwirble WT, et al: Robert Wood Johnson Foundation ICU End of Life Peer Group: Use of intensive care at the end of life in the United States: an epidemiological study, *Crit Care Med* 32:638–643, 2004.
15. Mularski RA, Osborne ML: End of life care in the critically ill geriatric population, *Crit Care Clin* 19:789–810, 2003.
16. Herridge MS: Prognostication and intensive care unit outcome: the evolving role of scoring systems, *Clin Chest Med* 24:751–762, 2003.
17. Rocker G, Cook D, Sjokvist P, et al: for the Level of Care Study Investigators, Canadian Critical Care Trials Group: clinician predictions of intensive care unit mortality, *Crit Care Med* 32:1149–1154, 2004.
18. Barrera R, Nygard S, Sgoloff H, et al: Accuracy of predictions of survival at admission to the intensive care unit, *J Crit Care* 16:32–35, 2001.
19. Pochard F, Lanore JJ, Bellivier F, et al: Subjective psychological status of severely ill patients discharged from mechanical ventilation, *Clin Intensive Care* 6:57–61, 1995.
20. Rotondi AJ, Chelluri L, Sirio C, et al: Patients' recollections of stressful experiences while receiving prolonged mechanical ventilation in an intensive care unit, *Crit Care Med* 30:936–937, 2002.
21. Heyland DK, Cook DJ, Rocker GM, et al: Decision-making in the ICU: perspectives of the substitute decision-maker, *Intensive Care Med* 29(1):75–82, 2003.
22. Studdert DM, Mello MM, Burns JP, et al: Conflict in the care of patients with prolonged stay in the ICU: types, sources, and predictors, *Intensive Care Med* 29:1489–1497, 2003.
23. Breen CM, Abernethy AP, Abbott KH, et al: Conflict associated with decisions to limit life-sustaining treatment in intensive care units, *J Gen Intern Med* 16:283–289, 2001.
24. Danjoux MN, Lawless B, Hawryluck L: Conflicts in the ICU: perspectives of administrators and clinicians, *Intensive Care Med* 35(12):2068–2077, 2009.
25. Tilden VP, Tolle SW, Nelson CA, Fields J: Family decision-making to withdraw life-sustaining treatments from hospitalized patients, *Nurs Res* 50:105–115, 2001.

26. Heyland DK, Rocker GM, O'Callaghan CJ, et al: Dying in the ICU: perspectives of family members, *Chest* 124:392–397, 2003.

27. Heyland DK, Tranmer JE: Measuring family satisfaction with care in the intensive care unit: the development of a questionnaire and preliminary results, *J Crit Care* 16:142–149, 2001.

28. McDonagh JR, Elliot TB, Engelberg RA, et al: Family satisfaction with family conferences about end of life care in the intensive care unit: increased proportion of family speech is associated with increased satisfaction, *Crit Care Med* 23:1484–1488, 2004.

29. Rocker GM, Heyland DK, Cook DJ, et al: Most critically ill patients are perceived to die in comfort during withdrawal of life support: a Canadian multi-centre study, *Can J Anaesth* 51:623–630, 2004.

30. Whipple JK, Lewis KS, Quebbeman EJ, et al: Analysis of pain management in critically ill patients, *Pharmacotherapy* 15:592–599, 1995.

31. Wilson WC, Smedira NG, Fink C, et al: Ordering and administration of sedatives and analgesics during the withdrawal and withholding of life support from critically ill patients, *JAMA* 267:949–952, 1992.

32. Brody H, Campbell ML, Faber-Langendoen K, Ogle KS: Withdrawing intensive life sustaining treatment: recommendations for compassionate clinical management, *N Engl J Med* 336:652–657, 1997.

33. Hawryluck L, Harvey W, Lemieux-Charles L, et al: Consensus guidelines on analgesia and sedation in dying PICU patients [abstract], *Crit Care Med* 27:A83, 1999.

34. Chan JD, Treece PD, Engelberg RA, et al: Narcotic and benzodiazepine use after withdrawal of life support: association with time to death? *Chest* 126:286–293, 2004.

35. Luce JM, Alpers A: End of life care: what do the American courts say? *Crit Care Med* 29(Suppl): N40–N45, 2001.

Further Reading

36. Burt D: The Supreme Court speaks: not assisted suicide but a constitutional right to palliative care, *N Engl J Med* 337;1234–1236, 1997.

CHAPTER 36

Emergency Medicine and Palliative Care

TAMMIE E. QUEST

The emergency department (ED) cares for people with conditions all along the spectrum of illness and injury: Those with chronic, progressive illness and those with acute illness; those with and those without good support systems. Although the primary role of the ED is to care for the critically ill and injured, many patients and families with nonemergency, urgent needs are nonetheless in crisis. The ED serves as a vital access point for medical care for people who are suffering, and it is a way station for those in need of crisis intervention.

Understanding the Emergency Department Model

PERSPECTIVES FOR NON–EMERGENCY DEPARTMENT PROVIDERS

Evaluate and treat, admit or discharge—this is the mantra of the ED clinician. Patients with palliative care needs present to the ED for an array of reasons, often crisis driven; their symptoms or pain may have escalated or perhaps the caregiver has panicked. Exceptional symptom management and procedural skills are critical in the ED. A fundamental understanding of how most EDs operate and knowledge of common barriers to palliative care are important first considerations.

Triage

After a visit to the ED, a clinician or relative may reasonably ask: Why was my patient with cancer and uncontrolled pain in the waiting room of the ED for hours before being seen? How quickly a patient's needs are met is one factor in the minimization of suffering. EDs serve a unique role in our society as a 24-hour safety net for the

513

suffering, the underserved, and those with limited social or economic resources to access primary care. This is true of palliative care as well as other types of care. That said, ED overcrowding is well described across the world and is best documented in the United States, Britain, Canada, and Australia. Overcrowding results in long patient waits at a time of crisis for them.

When patients arrive in the ED, they undergo triage. *Triage* means "to sort and allocate aid on the basis of need." The general purpose of a triage system is to classify patient presentations in a way that determines the potential for deterioration and the urgency with which evaluation by a physician or nurse is needed. This is typically done using a combination of factors that includes a patient's appearance, vitals signs, and underlying conditions that present a possibility of threat to life. Under established emergency triage systems, patients who present with mild to moderate exacerbations of chronic illness are triaged to lower priority and therefore often have longer ED waits. Common triage systems generally assign patients who have no immediate threat to the respiratory or cardiac system to a semiurgent or nonurgent level. This results in potentially very long waiting room times and can cause discomfort to the patient and family. For instance, under the Canadian Triage and Acuity Scale, a patient with moderate to severe pain (4 to 7 on a scale of 0 to 10) would have a time-to-physician wait of more than 1 hour, and a patient with constipation would be triaged at the lowest triage priority level (level 5) with an "ideal" wait time of up to 2 hours before even being assessed by a nurse.

Health care professionals who interact with the ED should be aware of the resource constraints and priorities of the emergency setting and should not confuse this with a lack of caring by emergency personnel. Because the focus is on rapid identification of life threats, stabilization of vital signs, and airway management, relief of physical symptoms distress may sometimes take a lower priority than is desirable. Psychosocial aspects of a patient's needs may also not be adequately explored and may even be detailed only if they relate to the triage decision.

Environmental and Systems Barriers

The setting of the ED typically lacks both privacy and the extended spiritual and psychosocial resources that would be more readily available to patients and families in the inpatient or outpatient setting. When available, these resources are typically crisis oriented. The significant time pressure, general lack of privacy and seating, and high level of noise and distractions make the ED environment especially challenging. In the emergency setting, a practitioner must often forego his or her vision of optimal palliative care to meet the patient and family in the midst of crisis. Because of the never-ending stream of patients, the essential focus is on disposition: Where does this patient need to go next? Emergency providers are in search of critical pieces of history, physical findings, laboratory tests, or radiography that determine the disposition—admit, discharge, or transfer.

How to Assist Emergency Personnel

Emergency physicians and nurses are required to make pressing decisions in an environment of information deficits. Time constraints allow for very little time per patient, yet the doctor and nurses are expected to decide the vital next steps for the patient. Actively calling the ED staff, responding to them rapidly (by phone or in person), and letting the ED providers know what to expect are extraordinarily useful. Referring clinicians can be especially helpful if they are familiar with and explicitly communicate a patient's previously stated goals of care or treatments preferences because this knowledge can aid in targeting the correct disposition.

PERSPECTIVES FOR EMERGENCY MEDICINE CLINICIANS

Bedside Rapid Trust Building

In view of the dynamics and workings of an ED, it is important to build trust rapidly, but this can be a particularly difficult task. ED patients with a variety of diagnoses have identified several factors as important for building trust, specifically the following:

1. Being treated as an individual
2. Not having reason to see the clinician as someone who is too busy to see them
3. Having reason to expect clinicians' compassion at the bedside
4. Clinician sensitivity and concern
5. Having reason to expect clinician honesty
6. Having open discussion about treatment options
7. Having confidence that the patient's interests come first

Surprisingly, factors rated as less important for trust building included the patient's perception of the clinician's competence, the clinician's expression of hopefulness or empathy, and the clinician's ability to use laymen's terms.[1] To foster this trust and to honor these considerations, special trust building skills are necessary. Some key skills are suggested in Table 36-1.

Table 36-1. Rapid Trust Building in the Emergency Department

Emergency Department Provider Should:	Suggestions/Script
Avoid seeming too busy	Lean over the gurney and maintain eye contact when no chair is available.
Use nonrushed body language	Hold the patient's hand during the initial contact/discussion.
Be compassionate at the bedside	Maintain eye contact.
Use affirmative phrases that acknowledge the patient is human, not a number	"With so many distractions in the emergency department, I know it is difficult to discuss things ... but you have my full attention now."
	"This can be a difficult setting to get your needs met, but we will do our best."
	"If I am called away suddenly, it is not because your problem is not important, and I will be back as soon as I can."
Show sensitivity and concern	"I know it is hard to speak with a perfect stranger regarding these issues, but it is how I can help you best."
Be honest	"I want to be honest with you regarding how long things will take ..."
	"I want to be honest with you regarding what I see happening, even if it is difficult to talk about."
Use open discussion regarding treatment options	"Based on what I know medically, this is what the options are ... this is what I would recommend."
Keep the patients' interests beyond all others	"I am most concerned with what is right for you."

Revealing the True Effectiveness of Cardiopulmonary Resuscitation

Patients, surrogates, and providers alike may be misinformed about the effect of cardiopulmonary resuscitation (CPR) on a chronic medical condition. Resuscitations should not be described in gruesome or gory terms, but families should be aware of the facts of CPR, including those that pertain to futility when this is relevant. Perhaps influenced by what can be seen on television, the overwhelming majority of laypersons feel that CPR is effective. Because 75% of patients on television survive initial resuscitation and 67% survive until discharge, this view is understandable.[2,3] In spite of the stress and pressure that exist in the ED and in discussions of CPR, when providers talk to patients and families, they should acknowledge the difficulty of talking about the outcomes of CPR and not avoid the conversation. Studies have shown that patients in the ED are willing to hear news of a life-threatening illness.[4]

Core Palliative Care Skills in the Emergency Setting

Core skills in the ED setting include global prognostication, recognition of sentinel ED presentations, noninvasive management of an impending cardiorespiratory arrest, noninvasive management of respiratory failure, management of severe uncontrolled pain, family-witnessed resuscitation, and death disclosure. All these skills require excellent, rapid communication and trust building.

"BIG PICTURE" PROGNOSTICATION

Consider the case of an 85-year-old man with stage IV lung cancer who presents in respiratory failure with no advance care plan regarding resuscitation. How should the emergency provider advise the patient and family regarding CPR without knowing the details of the patient's history and treatments?

Many patients and families with palliative care needs have limited understanding of their prognosis and do not have advance care plans. Because of the information deficit, the emergency provider will not be able to easily estimate life expectancy but can more accurately define "the big picture." For example, the typical patient with cancer who is on a dying trajectory and who presents with a new urinary tract infection may recover from the infection but will still have terminal cancer after the infection is treated. If this information is communicated directly to patients and families, they may elect to treat the symptoms associated with the infection but not the infection itself, and may regard the infection as a natural opportunity to die. A corresponding decision may be made to forgo resuscitation attempts. If the patient and family still need to fully realize that the patient will still have cancer even if resuscitation is successful, this is an important "big picture" communication that will allow an optimal decision for all concerned.

Important steps in rapid prognostication include the following:

1. Define the chronic, progressive, life-limiting illness.
2. Define the "new event."
3. Communicate the global prognosis—the "big picture": *Treatment of the new event will not reverse the chronic illness.*

SENTINEL EMERGENCY DEPARTMENT PRESENTATIONS THAT INDICATE THE ONSET OF ACTIVE DYING

Some sentinel presentations suggest terminal decline in a patient with chronic, progressive illness and signal that an important decision point may have arrived. Sentinel presentations include:

- The inability to eat or drink
- Generalized weakness
- A new illness or injury that would require major intervention (e.g., acute myocardial infarction, fracture, intracranial hemorrhage)
- Last hours of living

Such presentations should alert the ED clinician to the potential need for hospice, inpatient palliative care service, or preparation for a death in the ED. Patients often present with a new constellation of symptoms that are related to the natural progression of the underlying disease.

The progressive inability to eat or drink and generalized weakness may signal progression of illness with or without an acute underlying event. The inability to take nutrition or reaching a point of critical weakness is often a pivotal point for families and caregivers. The ED response is typically to initiate artificial hydration and search for an underlying cause. What should be considered at that juncture is whether the search for a precipitating diagnosis is helpful in view of the relevant risks, benefits, and alternatives. Some patients and families are not willing to undergo invasive testing or painful procedures to give a name to, or even to attempt to reverse the course of, a new illness. Although an artificial feeding device may be appropriate in some cases of inability to eat or drink, patients and proxy decision makers should be empowered to decline these types of interventions if they wish to do so.

Patients who present with progressive, life-threatening, terminal illness may present with a clinical constellation that could potentially be treated with acute surgical or medical interventions (e.g., an orthopedic or neurosurgical operation). Clarification of the goals of care coupled with the global prognosis are key elements to discuss with the patient and family to guide ED clinical decision making. The ED provider should formulate a "big picture" prognosis (perhaps in conjunction with the specialist), assess the range of goals for the patient, followed by recommendations for interventions or therapies.

Patients who present within the last hours of living special attention. These signs include: includes marked weakness, inability to swallow, loss of the ability to close the eyes, skin mottling, tachycardia, and neurologic dysfunction. Signs of imminent death deserve special attention. For these patients, if not yet clarified, the issues of life-sustaining therapies in the event of natural death, such as CPR, must be addressed. A proactive assessment of goals of care may avoid unwanted and futile resuscitations. When cardiovascular collapse can be anticipated within hours or days, proactive discussions should be attempted if relevant plans and physician orders regarding interventions at the end of life are not already in place. In patients with cancer, for example, studies have shown the survival to hospital rate of CPR to be 0% when clinicians anticipate that a patient with cancer may experience cardiopulmonary arrest for which the clinical course could not be interrupted by life sustaining therapies.[5] Even though the provision of nonbeneficial interventions is upsetting to emergency providers, studies show that providers will perform cardiopulmonary support even when they are sure it will not change the outcome because they fear litigation, anger, and criticism by the patient or family.[6] Ultimately, this is generally not helpful for providers, patients, or families.

NONINVASIVE MANAGEMENT OF SEVERE RESPIRATORY FAILURE

Conversations about resuscitation with patients at high risk for pulmonary decompensation, such as those with chronic obstructive pulmonary disease and congestive heart failure, often revolve around invasive or noninvasive supportive airway management. Emergency physicians should ask patients with chronic obstructive pulmonary disease or congestive heart failure about their desires for supportive ventilatory therapies such as endotracheal intubation and noninvasive (NIV) airway management. NIV is an increasingly common modality in the emergency setting as a safe and effective rescue therapy that may serve as a bridge. NIV may represent an intermediate step to endotracheal intubation, but it may also help to avoid endotracheal intubation altogether[7,8] when time is needed to try therapies that may need several hours or days to become effective (e.g., antibiotics, bronchodilators). Additionally, NIV can buy time when critical conversations need to be held. When the issue of resuscitation has never been discussed or no conclusion has been reached, NIV can give the provider and patient or surrogates time to stabilize the patient, gather surrogates, and discuss the potential risks, benefits, and recommendations of more invasive airway management and even cardiopulmonary resuscitation in the event of cardiac arrest. NIV can also temporarily relieve dyspnea during the period when other palliative therapies for breathlessness or terminal dyspnea are being initiated. Candidates for NIV should be hemodynamically stable, conscious, alert, and cooperative, even though fatigued (increased respiratory rate, use of accessory muscles, paradoxical breathing, or the subjective feeling of being tired). Patients commonly excluded from a trail of NIV include those who wish no type of artificial support to extend life and those who are obtunded, uncooperative, lack a gag reflex, or are hemodynamically unstable.[9] Failure to improve within 30 minutes of NIV signals the possible need for either endotracheal intubation or a decision to provide only medical management of symptoms. These are decisions that should be considered in the context of a discussion of goals of care. When NIV is used, the patient should still receive pharmacologic and nonpharmacologic therapies to relieve dyspnea.

RAPID MANAGEMENT OF SEVERE PAIN

Emergency physicians frequently treat pain and other symptoms. Like other specialists, they often undertreat pain and may not use a full range of therapies for symptoms other than pain.

Many emergency providers use a single standard 0.1 mg/kg morphine dose without frequent reassessment and without considering that some patients are opiate naive and others patients may be opiate tolerant.[10] ED physicians and staff may be unfamiliar with how to calculate equianalgesic dosing for opiates, and especially they may be unfamiliar with the use of methadone for pain control. Many patients present at the ceiling of analgesia provided by oral acetaminophen with opiate preparations. Although some protocols exist for rapid titration of pain control in opiate-exposed patients, it is unknown how frequently these algorithms are used. Several dosing strategies for cancer pain have been described, but there is less research with opiate-naive patients in the emergency setting. Several published protocols for patients with

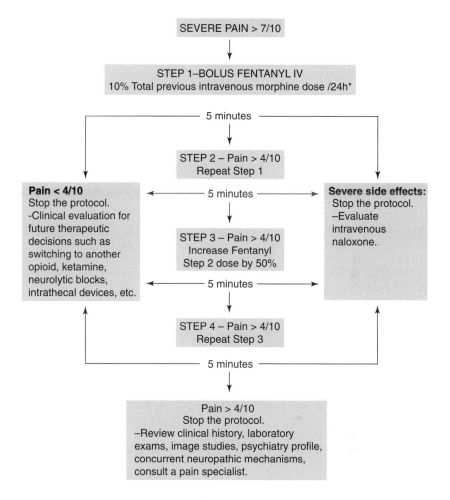

Figure 36-1. Rapid titration with fentanyl. *(From Soares LG, Martins M, Uchoa R: Intravenous fentanyl for cancer pain: A "fast titration" protocol for the emergency room, J Pain Symptom Manage 26:876–881, 2003.)*

cancer in the emergency setting include rapid titration protocols with morphine or fentanyl[11,12] (Figures 36-1 and 36-2). However, there are no published articles on short stays in the ED in which patients are transitioned from intravenous to long-acting oral opiates.

ED patients who have improvement of severe uncontrolled pain and who are discharged from the ED in less than 24 hours (which is typical) should be discharged with intermediate-release preparations of an oral opiate in the equivalent dose of the intravenous preparation received in the ED. They should be instructed on how the dose can be titrated by the patient or family so the dose is safely limited by patient

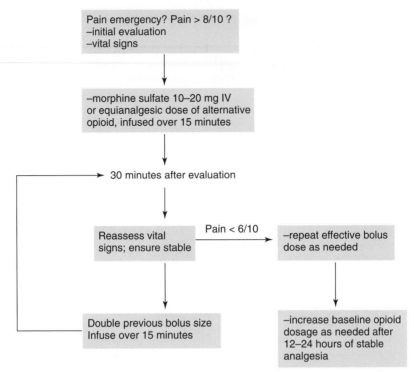

Figure 36-2. Rapid titration with morphine. *(From Hagen NA, Elwood T, Ernst S: Cancer pain emergencies: a protocol for management,* J Pain Symptom Manage *14:45–50, 1997.)*

somnolence to avoid respiratory depression. Careful attention should be paid to the appropriate opiate choice for patients with renal or hepatic insufficiency.

In general, when patients come to the ED from a palliative care environment, ED providers may be hesitant to administer analgesics for fear of causing respiratory depression. These fears should be acknowledged, and the proper educational support should be given to ED staff so patients do not suffer needlessly.

FAMILY-WITNESSED RESUSCITATION

In the event of cardiac arrest, most patients will die nonetheless. Although still controversial, review of the available evidence suggests that inviting the family to be present (with support and supervision) during the resuscitation effort may be of benefit for survivors and patients.[13] Few protocols have been published regarding family-witnessed resuscitation, but studies of this topic support the following conclusions:

1. Most family members would prefer to be given the option to be with the patient at the time of death during the resuscitation efforts.
2. Although such experiences are painful and emotionally draining, they may assist the family in the bereavement period.
3. Although doctors and nurses are sometimes initially reluctant, most soon become convinced of the value of family involvement.
4. A multidisciplinary approach should be used to develop a protocol.

Box 36-1. *Family-Witnessed Resuscitation*[21]

GUIDELINES FOR ESTABLISHING A FAMILY-WITNESSED RESUSCITATION PROTOCOL
- Multidisciplinary team
- Address fears and concerns of staff
- Protocol to address:
  How many family members?
  Key staff needed to be present
  Roles and responsibilities of staff
  Follow-up plan for family and staff
  Training of family facilitator (RN, SW, Chaplain)

IMPLEMENTATION
- Specific area for family
- Obtain consent of the physicians for family to watch
- The family facilitator helps and monitors family

Providers' attitudes may represent a barrier to having the family in the resuscitation area. Providers are concerned that family involvement could cause distress for survivors, interfere in the resuscitation, intimidate the team, bring greater pressure to prolong the code, and cause anxiety in calling an end to the procedure. Physicians are more likely than nurses to oppose having survivors in the resuscitation area.[14] Physicians-in-training are the most resistant and the most concerned that family presence could have a negative impact on patient care or could prove to be a negative experience.

Successful family-witnessed resuscitation requires appropriate preparation and training of the care team to increase receptiveness to the concept and practice of survivor participation (Box 36-1). Medical and nursing staff should discuss the impact of having family members present during resuscitation attempts before bringing a spouse or other family member into such an emotional situation. Advance role playing by resuscitation team members in a number of situations is recommended by hospitals. Resuscitation team members should be sensitive to the presence of family members during resuscitative efforts. One team member should be assigned to answer questions, provide support, clarify information, and offer comfort to family members. Ideally, quality monitoring procedures should be used to assess adherence to prescribed procedures, family and health professional satisfaction with the process, and close monitoring for adverse effects. As part of a systematic evaluation for symptoms of unresolved grief or depression, follow-up assessments should elicit family members' accounts of both positive and negative effects of the witnessed resuscitation attempt.

DEATH DISCLOSURE

Although there are various methods to inform families of a sudden death, some core considerations apply.[15-17] Most family survivors who experience a formal death disclosure in the emergency setting have not been a part of a family-witnessed resuscitation protocol because, in such a case, notification is typically done at the bedside. Delivering the news of death to a surviving family member can be devastating, whether or not the patient was expected to die. It can also be stressful for hospital and prehospital care providers. For both, the difficulty is increased because no relationship exists with the family and there is heightened anxiety about what kind of news is coming. Depending on the culture, a provider may go to meet the family and be asked "Is he or she alive or dead?" before the provider has had a chance to speak. A critical difference in the emergency setting is that the provider should take a leading role in delivering the news of death without using the "tell me what you know" approach because that approach typically does not help the survivors hear or accept the news. The provider should use empathic disclosure techniques to deliver the news that the patient has died. The provider should use the word "dead" or "died" rather than euphemism such as "passed on." It is important to review terminology in advance with a hospital-based translator when the disclosure will be done in a language unfamiliar to the provider. The provider may start the disclosure with something like, "I am afraid I have bad news." After a pause, continue: "I am not sure if you know what happened today." Proceed to give a very short summary, in layman's terms, of the known events that occurred before the death. Then say something gentle but direct and simple, such as: "This may be difficult to hear, but Mr. X died." Stay with the family for a little while; expect emotional responses. Quiet presence and then an invitation to either leave the family alone for a while or to arrange for them to see the body is usually appropriate.

Special Issues

PATIENTS RECEIVING HOSPICE CARE

ED personnel may not always be familiar with hospice rules and protocols.[18] When hospice patients and families present to the ED, it may be because the patient and caregivers did not understand the dying process or because they were fearful that the patient had uncontrolled symptoms. Signs and symptoms of infection and changes in mental status are often difficult for patients and surrogates to negotiate, and short lengths of stay in hospice may make it difficult for hospice staff as well. The after-hours on-call nurse for the hospice may be unfamiliar with a particular issue but may have other important information, such as previously established resuscitation status and medications. Some patients and families may be in denial of the dying process and may be in search of additional opinions regarding treatment. These are all very difficult, often tense situations for the emergency provider. Emergency providers should treat the presenting symptoms but call the hospice before initiating invasive testing and detailed evaluations. Hospice care providers should take an active role in providing ED clinicians with as much information and support as possible when they are aware of a patient receiving hospice care who has presented to the emergency department.

LOSS OF SUPPORT DEVICES

Among patients with palliative care needs who present in the ED, the support devices most commonly lost include gastrostomy tubes and tracheal airways. Both losses can cause panic for patients and families. It is not uncommon for the device to be lost as a result of actions, by lay or even professional home care providers, such as moving the patient. Before acting, it is important for the provider to assess whether the patient or surrogate thinks that the device is still necessary. Presentation for care should not be assumed to mean that the patient or surrogate wants to continue using the device. A large amount of energy could be invested in the attempt to replace a device, only to learn that the patient or surrogate now wishes to discontinue its use. The patient or surrogate may view the occasion as an opportunity to explore the effectiveness of the device. The provider should give the patient or surrogate permission to discontinue using the support device if it is not meeting the patient's goals.

Enteral Feeding Devices

Numerous types of enteral feeding devices are available, and the percutaneous gastrostomy tube is the most commonly encountered. However, patients with head and neck cancer may have pharyngostomy or esophagostomy tubes, and patients with more complicated resections may have gastroenterostomy, duodenostomy, or jejunostomy tubes. The emergency palliative care clinician may not be able to tell what kind of enteral tube is in use by physical examination alone. The presence of a skin incision near the ostomy site suggests that the tube is not easily removable. Nonoperative tube replacements should be done only in patients who have well established and granulated tracts. Gastrostomy tubes come in different styles and materials, including rubber, silicone, and polyurethane. Many gastrostomy tubes are designed with a flange or a crossbar (bumper) to anchor them in the stomach and to prevent migration into the small bowel. Although a Foley catheter may be used as a replacement tube, it is more temporary and difficult to secure to the skin. The latex in the Foley balloon may be weakened by stomach acid over time. A Foley catheter can always be used temporarily in the ED (after which more definitive arrangements can be made) or permanently if life expectancy is limited (Figure 36-3).

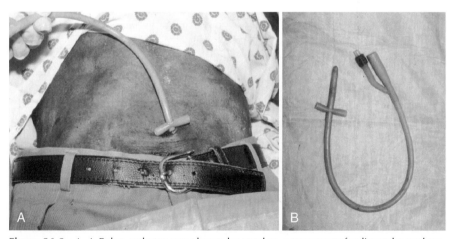

Figure 36-3. *A,* A Foley catheter can always be used as a temporary feeding tube replacement. The thin-walled Foley balloon usually only remains inflated for a month or so. A bolster can be made to prevent inward migration of the tube. *B,* In this case the previously removed Foley catheter was used to make the bolster for the new one. *(From Roberts JR, Hedges J, editors:* Clinical Procedures in Emergency Medicine, *ed 4, Philadelphia, 2004, Saunders.)*

If the tube is still present in the ostial lumen, contrast injection should be done to determine the final resting place of the tube and to determine patency. When radiographic services are not available, nonpatent tubes should be flushed gently with saline. When the device cannot be flushed and is more than 1 to 2 weeks old, a Foley catheter can be used to replace the feeding tube.

Airway/Tracheotomy Support Devices

Common complications of tracheostomies include tube dislodgement, occlusion, and fracture. These patients may present in acute respiratory distress, and this can be a very frightening experience for the patient, family, and care providers. A patient with a tracheostomy who is in respiratory distress should be considered to have a partially or fully obstructed device. Plugging of the trachea is usually the result of dried respiratory secretions, blood, or aspirated materials. Secretions may act as a ball valve that allows air in but restricts outward ventilation, thus causing the patient to appear in acute respiratory distress with agitation and fear. Granuloma formation just distal to the tube may also cause obstruction. Emergency management includes attempts to clear the trachea, high-flow oxygen, and immediate exchange of the tracheostomy (Figure 36-4). *Dislodgement or shifting* of the tracheostomy tube can

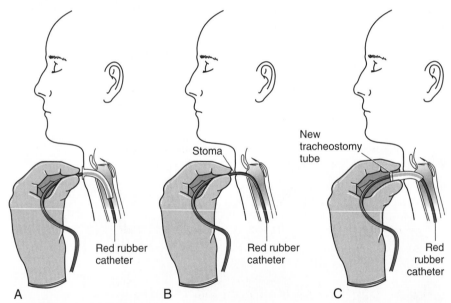

Figure 36-4. Changing a tracheostomy tube. *A,* Before the old tube is removed, a small red rubber catheter (or other guide catheter) is passed into the proximal trachea. *B,* The tracheostomy tube has been removed over the catheter, and only the catheter remains in the trachea. The catheter serves as a guide for easy and atraumatic insertion of a new tube. The neck should be slightly hyperextended. *C,* A new tracheostomy tube without the obturator is threaded over the guide catheter; once the tube is in place, the catheter is removed. Similarly, if the tracheostomy tube has already been removed, the catheter may be passed through the stoma before a new tube is advanced. An obturator or inner cannula is not used when changing a tube with this technique. *(From Roberts JR, Hedges J, editors:* Clinical Procedures in Emergency Medicine, *ed 4, Philadelphia, 2004, Saunders.)*

occur when the patient is intermittently ventilated and the tip of the tracheostomy is moved forward or when the head is flexed, causing the tube to be obstructed. Extension of the patient's head may solve the problem, or pulling back on the tracheostomy may help. *Bleeding* is a common complication; more than 20% of patients who present to the ED with tracheostomy difficulties have bleeding. Erosion of a major vessel from the cuff or tip of the tube is responsible for 10% of all tracheostomy hemorrhage and for most tracheostomy-related deaths. Minor bleeding is often postsurgical or the result of granuloma. Brisk bleeding from the tracheostomy, hemoptysis, or a history of either complaint should alert the clinician to the possibility of a life-threatening hemorrhage. Many patients experience "sentinel" bleeding hours or days before catastrophic bleeding. Some patients may report only a new cough or retrosternal pain. Any history or evidence of 10 mL or more of blood should be presumed to be arterial. Acute treatment in the ED includes an attempt to tamponade bleeding with a digit in the airway, a procedure that can cause significant discomfort to the patient. Topical thrombin-type agents may have a role. Consultation of surgical colleagues should rapidly ensue if the goals of care are consistent with airway stabilization.

PEARLS

- Time and information deficits are enemies. Anything that can be done to expedite information transfer and reduce delays is helpful.
- Emergency clinicians are typically willing and ready to provide comfort care when supported in appropriate guidelines or expertise.
- Functionally, emergency clinicians are trained to evaluate, treat, and decide disposition (admit, discharge or transfer). Palliative care consultants can help greatly in helping emergency clinicians with appropriate management and disposition.
- Emergency clinicians are procedurally competent and may be able to temporize difficult airway or enteral feeding issues until dealt with more permanently.

PITFALLS

- Failure to recognize the last hours of living can result in an inadvertent prolongation of life with therapies such as antibiotics, fluids, or mechanical ventilation, which may prolong active dying.
- Failure to contextualize the intercurrent illness within the global trajectory of terminal illness
- Discomfort with opioid dosing in opioid-tolerant patients
- Poor handling of death disclosure or family-witnessed resuscitation when protocols and training do not exist

Summary

Patients with palliative care needs who present in the emergency setting are a challenge because the practice setting emphasizes rapid disposition and because the patient and caregiver population tend to present in crisis. Practitioners in the emergency setting must be able to build trust rapidly and to deliver a global, "big picture" prognosis. A focus on sentinel ED presentations may more clearly identify the most appropriate treatment and disposition options for patients. Providers must be competent in death disclosure and must be familiar with the pros and cons of family-witnessed resuscitation. Skills in specific minor procedures are needed to care for the patient with support devices.

Resources

Education on Palliative and End-of-life Care—Emergency Medicine (EPEC-EM)
www.epec.net
Society for Academic Emergency Medicine Interest Group
www.comfort911.org

References

1. Kelly JJ, Njuki F, Lane PL, McKinley RK: Design of a questionnaire to measure trust in an emergency department, *Acad Emerg Med* 12:147–151, 2000.
2. Diem SJ, Lantos JD, Tulsky JA: Cardiopulmonary resuscitation on television: miracles and misinformation, *N Engl J Med* 334:1578–1582, 1996.
3. Jones GK, Brewer KL, Garrison HG: Public expectations of survival following cardiopulmonary resuscitation, *Acad Emerg Med* 7:48–53, 2000.
4. Takayesu JK, Hutson HR: Communicating life-threatening diagnoses to patients in the emergency department, *Ann Emerg Med* 43:749–755, 2004.
5. Ewer MS, Kish SH, Martin CG, et al: Characteristics of cardiac arrest in cancer patients as a predictor of survival after cardiopulmonary resuscitation, *Cancer* 92:1905–1912, 2001.
6. Marco CA, Bessman ES, Schoenfeld CN, et al: Ethical issues of cardiopulmonary resuscitation: Current practice among emergency physicians, *Acad Emerg Med* 4:898–904, 1997.
7. Yosefy C, Hay E, Ben-Barak A, et al: BiPAP ventilation as assistance for patients presenting with respiratory distress in the department of emergency medicine, *Am J Respir Med* 2:343–347, 2003.
8. Kelly AM, Georgakas C, Bau S, Rosengarten PL: Experience with the use of continuous positive airway pressure (CPAP) therapy in the emergency management of acute severe cardiogenic pulmonary oedema, *Aust N Z J Med* 27:319–322, 1997.
9. Poponick JM, Enston JP, Bennett RP, Emerman CL: Use of a ventilatory support system (BiPAP) for acute respiratory failure in the emergency department, *Chest* 116:166–171, 1999.
10. Bijur PE, Kenny MK, Gallagher EJ: Intravenous morphine at 0.1 mg/kg is not effective for controlling severe acute pain in the majority of patients, *Ann Emerg Med* 46:362–367, 2005.
11. Mercadante S, Portenoy RK: Opioid poorly-responsive cancer pain. Part 3: clinical strategies to improve opioid responsiveness, *J Pain Symptom Manage* 21:338–354, 2001.
12. Soares LG, Martins M, Uchoa R: Intravenous fentanyl for cancer pain: a "fast titration" protocol for the emergency room, *J Pain Symptom Manage* 26:876–881, 2003.
13. Tucker TL: Family presence during resuscitation, *Crit Care Nurs Clin North Am* 14:177–185, 2002.
14. Boudreaux ED, Francis JL, Loyacano T: Family presence during invasive procedures and resuscitations in the emergency department: a critical review and suggestions for future research, *Ann Emerg Med* 40:193–205, 2002.
15. Benenson RS, Pollack ML: Evaluation of emergency medicine resident death notification skills by direct observation, *Acad Emerg Med* 10:219–223, 2003.
16. Quest TE, Otsuki JA, Banja J, et al: The use of standardized patients within a procedural competency model to teach death disclosure, *Acad Emerg Med* 9:1326–1333, 2002.
17. Rutkowski A: Death notification in the emergency department, *Ann Emerg Med* 40:521–523, 2002.
18. Reeves K: Hospice care in the emergency department: important things to remember, *J Emerg Nurs* 26:477–478, 2000.

Further Reading

York NL: Implementing a family presence protocol option, *DCCN—Dimensions Crit Care Nurs* 23(2):84–88, 2004.

CHAPTER 37

Veterans, Veterans Administration Health Care, and Palliative Care

F. AMOS BAILEY and JOSHUA M. HAUSER

This chapter describes characteristics of the Veterans Administration Health System and then considers characteristics of veterans from different war eras. It describes two specific problems that veterans receiving palliative care may have faced in their history: posttraumatic stress disorder (PTSD) and military sexual trauma. Similar considerations may apply to the military from other countries, but for manageability this chapter focuses only on the U.S. military.

In the United States, the term *veteran* refers to men and women who have served in the armed services in the past and are now separated from the military. Veterans comprise up to 20% of the Americans who die in any given year.[1] This is in part because of the large number of men and women who served in the military during World War II and the Korean conflict who are now aging into their 70s, 80s, and 90s. Their illnesses, declines in health status, and, ultimately, deaths are usually not directly related to their military service. However, their military experiences during their years of service as young adults may have profound effects on how they cope with pain and suffering, interact with family and professional caregivers, and manifest emotional and spiritual distress. It is important for clinicians outside the Department of Veterans Affairs (VA) system to ask patients if they are a veteran as part of the social history, because many veterans receive their care outside the VA system. For many patients, it is important to explore the impact of their military service on

527

the current situation; from a practical point of view, many veterans are eligible for additional benefits that could help support both them and their family at the end of life. In collaboration with the National Hospice and Palliative Care Organization (NHPCO), the VA has established the We Honor Veterans campaign to help connect Veterans with existing hospice services.[2]

Military service has long been a defining experience for many Americans as they transitioned from youth to young adulthood. For the most part, military recruits are young, ages 18 to 21, just out of high school or with a General Equivalency Degree (GED). Veterans share the cultural diversity of our country; however, they also share a common bond of military service to their country.

The process of basic training, common to each branch of service, is an intense experience designed to transform distinct individuals into uniformed and uniform soldiers who are bound to each other as a group.[3] This is a remarkable experience that goes against much of the individualism and personal freedom that are valued in the larger American culture. Anthropologically and psychologically, this is an initiation into a select group; with this selection comes privileges, duty, and a connectedness that for many will continue for the rest of their lives, both in the military and after discharge as a veteran. The impact of military service has both positive and negative effects on the veteran and invariably impacts how the veteran will cope with the grief, loss, and suffering that are often experienced in the setting of serious illness.

Structure of the Department of Veterans Affairs

The Department of Veterans Affairs is a cabinet level department of the federal government tasked with provision of a wide range of benefits and services to veterans. The nascent formulation of the VA can be traced to President Lincoln's promise "to care for him who shall have borne the battle, and for his widow and his orphan," which greets visitors to the Department of Veterans Affairs offices in Washington, DC. The VA continues to grow and adapt to meet the changing needs of veterans and their families. The VA has three major programmatic charges—namely, to provide the following:

1. Pensions and benefits
2. Health care services
3. National military cemeteries and memorials

The VA health care (VAH) system is the most visible manifestation of the VA to the general public and to many veterans. VAH has 153 Veterans Administration Medical Centers (VAMCs) located throughout the United States that provide care for more than 5.5 million veterans annually.[4] These VAMCs provide acute hospital care, ambulatory primary and specialty care, long-term residential care, and home care programs. In addition, more than 800 Community Based Outpatient Care (CBOC) Clinics provide general primary and preventive care in local communities.[5] The CBOC structure is supported by linkages to VAMC for referral for specialty or inpatient care. Other affiliated organizations, such as the National Association of State Veterans Homes (NASVH),[6] are state, as opposed to federal, organizations.

Palliative care and hospice services are part of the required benefit package for veterans. The VAH recognizes that some of the veterans most in need have complex health and social problems, such as substance use disorder, homelessness, depression, and PTSD, that must be addressed to adequately and effectively provide health care services, including hospice and palliative care.

The VA has been a leader in hospice care in the United States. Some of the first and oldest inpatient hospice programs were started within the VA. In 2000, the VA began to evaluate the programmatic status of hospice and palliative care through the entire VAH system. This research revealed that there were a number of centers of excellence in hospice and palliative care but that variability was considerable.[7] Major deficiencies included linkage to home hospice programs in the communities where veterans live and fiscal support of home hospice care by purchase of contracted services. The result of these findings led to the development of Palliative Care Consult services, with interdisciplinary teams in every VAMC, and a corresponding rapid increase in the number of consults provided and veterans given these services.

In addition, it has become apparent that designated hospice and palliative care beds, staffed with trained providers, is a key to the provision of quality end-of-life care. The VA has embarked on an ambitious program to expand services, training and improve quality of care of veterans at end-of-life. The VA is striving to move palliative care upstream by integration of palliative care services with symptom management using an "open access" model that does not require veterans to choose between palliative care and disease-modifying treatment, but to individually combine services that best meet the needs and preferences of individual veterans.

At the same time that the VA has been working to increase institutional capacity to deliver palliative care, the VA has also been committed to increasing noninstitutional care in the home and community to honor veterans' preferences for type and location of care when appropriate. Although the VA has an extensive infrastructure to provide for residential, domiciliary, and nursing home care on VAMC campuses, many veterans would benefit from and prefer care in their own community. The types of home care assistance programs may include home-based primary care, home health aides and homemaker services, and attendant payments, support for durable medical supplies, and the purchase of contracted community-based care such as home hospice, home health, and nursing home care. These programs are allowing more veterans to be supported in their homes and community even when they have increasing debility near the end of life.

Impact of Veterans' Experiences on Response to Suffering at Life's End

Almost every society has a "warrior" class.[8] The warrior may choose this identity or have it thrust upon him or her by the circumstances of war and necessity. The first step to becoming a warrior is initiation, which is a process to "break down" individual citizens and reconstruct them as soldiers. The training is meant to prepare soldiers with the bravery to face hardship and danger and to win battles.

One of the major aspects of this training is the development of stoicism. Stoicism is the ability to tamp down the emotions and outwardly seem indifferent to hardship, pain, and grief. This is an important trait during military service, but this effective coping mechanism in a time of service or battle can have unanticipated and perhaps adverse, affects on how people deal with pain, grief, suffering, and even joy and pleasure at the end of life. Veterans as a group have been known to show incredible stoicism in the face of devastating injury and illness. This can lead some to underreport and minimize pain and other forms of physical suffering,[9] which can complicate pain and symptom control at the end of life. This attitude is sometimes articulated by veterans with phrases like "Big boys don't cry" or "No pain, no gain." Or it may be more subtly manifested by a veteran not reporting pain and other symptoms of suffering.

Although the majority (61%) of veterans were not in combat situations,[10] all veterans were prepared for the possibility of combat as part of their training. For those who were in combat situations, many were physically wounded and some left with lifelong physical disability. However, almost all veterans carry away some emotional, social, or existential suffering from the experience of battle. Those closest to the battle or in the fighting the longest are most likely to experience profound effects. Even those involved in support positions, such as nurses and physicians who cared for the wounded or those who maintained and repaired the equipment used in war are affected by the loss and suffering not only of comrades but also of the people in whose country the war took place. Some veterans have learned to cope well, whereas others have been unable to accommodate their profound responses. Wherever they fall on this spectrum, all veterans need to be cared for in a way that respects the life-changing experiences they had during their military service. These things must be taken into consideration to provide culturally competent hospice and palliative care to America's veterans.

Different Cohorts of Veterans

The time, location, branch of service, rank and mission during military service often lead to some common, shared health issues. This section discusses some of the unique issues related to service in particular war eras. It considers the experience of veterans who served during WWII, the Korean Conflict, Vietnam, Gulf War, and most recently, the wars in Afghanistan and Iraq (Operation Enduring Freedom/ Operation Iraqi Freedom—OEF/OIF).

WORLD WAR II

World War II began nearly 70 years ago. This aging cohort of veterans is rapidly decreasing in number. At this time, almost all World War II (WWII) veterans are more than 80 years old and many are in their 90s.

WWII veterans are almost uniformly proud of their military service and see their contribution to winning this war as an important part of their legacy at the end of life. However, although African Americans served, at that time the military was racially segregated.[11] This is still a painful memory for many African-American WWII veterans, who felt the sting of discrimination and rightly believed that their contributions were and still are underappreciated. This reality is sometimes neglected as the triumphs of some activities, such as the actions of the Tuskegee Airmen and the Navajo code writers,[12,13] are rightly celebrated. It is important to express gratitude and appreciation to all who served, but special effort should be made to recognize the contributions of African Americans, Native Americans, Hispanics, and other minorities that fought for our freedom as a country while their own freedom was not fully realized.

At the end of life, veterans of WWII may have complications related to injuries suffered during service. Combat injuries and environmental exposures such as cold injury, mustard gas exposure, and exposure to radiation due the use of atomic bombs in Japan at the end of WWII resulted in long-term consequences to veterans. The dangers of radiation exposure were not truly appreciated and exposure often occurred, such as during nuclear cleanup in Japan and during the early years of the Cold War caused by above-ground testing in remote islands in the Pacific. WWII veterans also may have had traumatic experiences that manifest themselves in nightmares or as part of delirium, which is a common occurrence at the very end of life. These can occur in the absence of a diagnosis of PTSD.

KOREAN CONFLICT

The Korean War is sometimes referred to as a "conflict" or a "police action" because there was never a formal declaration of war. Nearly half a million Americans served in Korea and more than 33,000 died there.[14] For veterans who served in Korea, there was no clear victory as there was with WWII. This often leaves Korean War veterans feeling that their service and the deaths of their comrades were not appreciated. The same source of pride that came from winning WWII may be missing for those veterans who served in Korea.

Korean War veterans often suffered from exposure to extremes of heat and cold. Often supplied with inadequate equipment to protect themselves from the elements, they struggled to survive the dual enemies of humans and the environment. Veterans certainly may re-live some of these experiences during times of stress or delirium. Uniquely, veterans may experience cold sensitivity that is associated with their experience of injury resulting from frostbite, including amputations. Some veterans feel painfully cold even when in a warm room. Special attention to extremities, using warm packs, careful range of motion, and positioning to reduce pain and prevent skin breakdown, should be incorporated into to overall hospice and palliative care for these veterans.

VIETNAM WAR

The Vietnam War has been and is a source of much angst for the United States. The Vietnam War was the first televised war, and the immediacy and violence of the fighting was a shock to the country.[15] Although war reporting goes back to Homer and Herodotus, television brought immediacy that stripped the war of the glamour it may have once had. Furthermore, because of the large number of personnel required and the existence of the draft for much of the war, a large percentage of the men entering the services possessed baccalaureate and higher degrees. At the conclusion of the war, many in the United States came to question the authority and veracity of some of the institutions of government.

The Vietnam War was the first U.S. guerilla war. For the personnel, the landscape, language, and culture were very different from the United States. In WWII and in Korea, the enemy had been in a defined uniform and the battle lines were clear. In Vietnam, it was often not possible to identify and separate combatants from civilians. As a result, soldiers could never let their guard down or feel safe. Soldiers did not generally feel any sense of gratitude from the Vietnamese, whom they were supposed to be there defending and helping. This new style of war, especially with its civilian casualties, made it hard for solders to have a sense of accomplishment.

For Vietnam veterans, the physical, emotional, and existential trauma was great. Improvements in medical and surgical trauma therapy, coupled with an enemy strategy to injure but not necessarily kill, meant that wounded soldiers were more likely to survive; but they survived with severe and disabling injuries that would make reintegration into society difficult. The emotional and existential trauma resulting from the war was significant.[16] During the war, alcohol and substance use was common among service personnel in Vietnam. For some, this would become substance addiction that they would bring home with them. The hypervigilance of guerrilla warfare still seems to have lead to a high prevalence of PTSD.

Vietnam veterans at the end of life often have struggled with mental health, addiction, or other social reintegration issues. Even for those who seem to have successfully transitioned to civilian life, there may be a resurgence of PTSD symptoms near the end of life, and especially during any episodes of delirium. Broken marriages and other relationships may also serve to reduce a veteran's social capital and make home care more difficult, increasing the need for institutional care.

Examples of physical issues that cause complications near the end of life include hepatitis C infection caused by intravenous drug use or complications related to Agent Orange exposure.[17] The physical manifestations of hepatitis C exposure include cirrhosis, liver failure, and hepatocellular cancer. Although the data regarding physical sequelae of Agent Orange exposure are controversial, they include soft tissue sarcomas, non-Hodgkin's lymphoma, chronic leukemia, multiple solid organ cancers, Parkinson's disease, and ischemic heart disease.[18] In addition, Agent Orange exposure may create a sense that the veteran was duped and suffered needlessly. It is important to discuss exposure with Vietnam veterans and refer and assist them and their families in making claims as appropriate. At the time of death, it is important to include Agent Orange exposure on the death certificate so as to aid families in obtaining important VA benefits.[19] Providing veterans with the peace of mind that can come from knowing they have access to all available benefits can be an important part of the psychosocial care plan at the end of life.

THE NEWEST VETERANS

Since the beginning of the Afghan and Iraq wars, approximately 1.64 million U.S. troops have been deployed for Operation Enduring Freedom (Afghanistan, OEF) and Operation Iraqi Freedom (Iraq, OIF).[20] There are some early data to suggest that the psychological morbidity and traumatic brain injury from these deployments may be higher than the other physical injuries of combat. Specifically, there is a high prevalence of PTSD and traumatic brain injury (TBI) among these veterans. There is also an increasing incidence of suicide and suicide attempts among returning veterans.[21]

Specific Issues with Veterans and Palliative Care

Two veteran-specific issues that may manifest in the palliative care setting are PTSD and military sexual trauma (MST). The discussion here introduces these topics and directs readers to sources for more in-depth discussion.

POSTTRAUMATIC STRESS DISORDER

Posttraumatic Stress Disorder is an anxiety disorder that can occur after an individual has experienced a traumatic event, such as the violence of war, military sexual trauma, or even the witnessing of these kinds of events. Although combat exposure is often the trauma that leads to PTSD in veterans, there are other types of trauma that veterans and nonveterans may experience, including sexual trauma and natural disasters. To meet the *Diagnosis and Statistical Manual of Mental Disorders,* revised fourth edition (DSM-IV-TR) criteria for PTSD,[22] the individual must have experienced, witnessed, or been confronted with an event involving actual or threatened death or serious injury, or a threat to the physical integrity of the individual or others. Additionally, the individual's response to the traumatic event must involve intense fear, helplessness, or horror. Diagnostic features of PTSD fall into three categories: intrusive recollections of the trauma, avoidant behaviors and numbing of general responsiveness, and hyperarousal.

War-related PTSD has been around for a long time, although it has been called by different names, such as "soldier's heart" in the Civil War era or "shell shock" in the World War I and II eras.[23] PTSD became recognized as distinct psychological syndrome after the Vietnam War. It was more fully characterized and was included in the third edition of the DSM in 1980[24]; it has since been included in subsequent editions of the DSM. As a consequence of this later formulation and inclusion in diagnostic categories, many veterans who may have had PTSD resulting from WWII and other conflicts have never been diagnosed. Older veterans, in particular WWII and Korean War veterans, tend to be quite stoic and humble about their wartime experiences. Many appear to have coped with their trauma by busying themselves in work and family life. For some, a reemergence of PTSD symptoms can be experienced on retirement when they have more time to reflect on the past.[25] PTSD symptoms can also reemerge or become more intense at the end of life.[26] Life review, either informal or as a specific part of psychosocial care, may lead some veterans and their families to better understand the impact that undiagnosed PTSD has had on the veteran's life and relationships. For other veterans, however, life review may serve as a trigger for their trauma and worsen their PTSD symptoms.

Facing death in and of itself may be a strong reminder of combat experiences, as may physical conditions, and these can also serve to activate symptoms of PTSD. Other feelings common at the end of life, such as loss of control or sensations related to dependence, can also activate PTSD. These can make the veteran with PTSD feel vulnerable, and that is a powerful reminder of trauma. There may also be a negative impact of coming into a hospital or hospice setting for a veteran with PTSD. It can be challenging for such people to be around others in a congregate living situation with frequent interruptions by strangers.

Many veterans with PTSD have anger toward authority (e.g., the government) and don't expect to be cared for properly. These feelings can be transferred to VA clinicians and community health care providers, especially in situations when the veteran feels he or she has no control over decision making. Although a veteran may begin the relationship with mistrust or even hostility, a caring and honest relationship with an emphasis on helping the veteran feel some control over his or her treatment can build trust over time and lessen hostility.

Flashbacks are disturbing events for patients, family, and health care providers caring for the patient. At end of life, the content of an episode of delirium may be combat related. However, true flashbacks may occur outside the context of delirium episodes. Flashbacks tend to be more short lived than episodes of delirium and have fewer disorders of orientation and fluctuating consciousness.

Screening questions exist that are designed to detect issues of hyperarousal, vigilance, and intrusive thoughts that characterize PTSD. One tool used in primary care settings can also be used in palliative care. It has four questions that begin with the common stem "In your life, have you ever had any experience that was so frightening, horrible, or upsetting that in the past month you …":[26,27]

1. "Have had nightmares about it or thought about it when you did not want to?"
2. "Tried hard not to think about it or went out of your way to avoid situations that reminded you of it?"
3. "Were constantly on guard, watchful, or easily startled?"
4. "Felt numb or detached from others, activities, or your surroundings?"

Management of PTSD includes pharmacologic management with selective serotonin reuptake inhibitors (SSRIs) and tricyclic antidepressants. Psychosocial management includes education of both staff and patients regarding the signs of PTSD and referral to mental health professionals with expertise in PTSD. As with depression, all patients with PTSD should be screened for suicidality, because it is a known risk factor for suicidality and suicidal ideation.[26,28] The VA maintains a comprehensive website of information and resources concerning PTSD that can be helpful for clinicians, patients, and families.[29]

MILITARY SEXUAL TRAUMA

Although military sexual trauma is not a DSM-IV-TR–defined diagnosis, it is a recognized condition by the Department of Veterans Affairs. MST is defined by U.S. Code Title 38, Section 1720D as "psychological trauma which in the judgment of a mental health professional employed by the Department, resulted from a physical assault of a sexual nature, battery of a sexual nature, or sexual harassment which occurred while the veteran was serving on active duty").[30]

MST is a common source of distress for veterans in the palliative care and end-of-life setting. The interdisciplinary palliative care team must be vigilant for a history of MST, be able to respond appropriately, be aware of the growing knowledge in this area, and reach out to those in the VA with expertise in this area as appropriate and needed for the veterans they serve.

As stated in the earlier definition, MST includes both sexual assault and sexual harassment. Sexual assault is any sort of sexual activity between at least two people in which someone is involved against his or her will—the person may be coerced into participation (e.g., with threats), not capable of consenting to participation (e.g., when intoxicated), or physically forced into participation. Although individuals of any sexual orientation may be targeted for sexual harassment, homosexuals or those perceived as homosexuals are often targeted for abuse and harassment and are often especially fearful of reporting perpetrators of abuse.

Sexual harassment is itself defined as "repeated, unsolicited verbal or physical contact of a sexual nature which is threatening in character." Any of these things occurring while a veteran was serving on active duty or training for active duty constitutes MST. In 2002, the Department of Defense conducted a large study of sexual victimization among active duty populations and found that 54% of women and 23% of men reported having experienced sexual harassment in the previous year. Rates of victimization by attempted or completed sexual assault were 3% for women and 1% for men.[31] The VHA now has universal screening of all veterans, and this is completed for 70% of veterans. This screening has revealed multiple physical and emotional sequelae of MST. The physical sequelae include reported associations with reproductive, gastrointestinal, cardiac, and pulmonary symptoms as well as chronic fatigue and chronic pain.[32] Emotional and psychological sequelae include depression, personality disorders, substance abuse, dissociative disorders, and PTSD. Of note, among the psychological disorders, PTSD and dissociative disorders have the largest odds ratios for both male and female victims of MST.[33]

Triggers for Manifestations of MST in Palliative Care Settings

Because of the nature of MST, medical, nursing, and personal care that involves touching, bathing, or toileting may be triggers that will bring memories of traumatic experiences to the present again. The issues of dependency and the power differential between the clinician and veteran create a complex dynamic in the palliative and end-of-life care settings that can make treatment difficult for both the veteran and the clinician.

Good practice on the part of the clinician includes the following:

- Explain all care and its purpose even if the veteran does not appear to be alert.
- Observe carefully for physical reactions to these potential triggers even when or if the veteran no longer appears to be alert.

Because of the nature of military sexual trauma, certain exams and treatments that involve the urinary and genital region, such as pelvic exams, bladder catheters, or simply bathing, cleaning, or changing pads or diapers, may be very traumatic. Additionally, distress related to sexual trauma could be triggered by things such as colonoscopy, the need for suppositories or enemas for constipation, oral care, and restraints of any sort, because the exact nature of the trauma may not be known.

When providing care for veterans who have experienced sexual trauma, it is important to give information and explain why and what needs to be done, always asking for permission to touch. Asking the veteran to assist the clinician with needed personal care and medical treatment can lessen the trauma associated with care.

PEARLS

- Ask all patients about whether they served in the military, even on non-VA settings: The majority of veterans receive care outside of the VA system.
- In patients with unexplained symptoms or psychological reactions near the end of life, consider the possibilities of PTSD.
- In veterans with a history of military sexual trauma, exercise special care when performing more intimate parts of the physical exam.
- Know hospice resources for veterans by consulting www.wehonorveterans.org

PITFALLS

- Assuming that veterans from all eras have had similar wartime experiences
- Forcing veterans to discuss their wartime experiences when they do not want to
- Assuming that all trauma leads to PTSD

Summary

Veterans will continue to turn to the VA for health care and, ultimately, palliative and end-of-life care. In this setting, health care professionals must provide the best care, which includes excellent symptom management as well as an understanding of the special needs of each individual and how military service and experiences as a veteran integrates into who the person is and what his or her needs are.

This purpose of this chapter is to introduce the basic aspects of military and veteran culture to foster cultural competency among all providers. In addition, this chapter reviews some aspects of the different war eras and how they can have health impacts that often are not appreciated but that profoundly affect end-of-life care. Finally, there are some unique health care issues, such as PTSD and military sexual trauma, that affect the health and experiences of many veterans near the end of life. The best teachers of veteran culture and needs are the veterans themselves, those whom we care for. It is important to routinely ask all patients if they are veterans and explore the nature of their military service, their experiences as veterans, and how these influence them when dealing with life-limiting illness.

References

1. NHPCO: Honoring our veterans includes caring for them at the end of life. Available at www.nhpco.org/i4a/pages/index.cfm?pageid=4390.
2. We Honor Veterans, www.wehonorveterans.org. Accessed November 29, 2010.
3. Huebner AJ: *The warrior image: soldiers in American culture from the Second World War to the Vietnam Era*, Chapel Hill, NC, 2008, University of North Carolina Press.
4. www1.va.gov/health/MedicalCenters.asp.
5. www2.va.gov/directory/guide/Allstate_flsh.asp?dnum=1.
6. National Association of State Veterans Homes main website: www.nasvh.org. Accessed November 23, 2010.
7. Office of Academic Affiliations, Geriatrics and Extended Care in the Office of Patient Care Services: Hospice and Palliative Care Services in the Department of Veterans: A Report of the TAPC Project Survey. Department of Veterans Affairs, February 2002.
8. Peters R: The new warrior class, *Parameters* (Summer):16–26, 1994.
9. Siddharthan K, Hodgson M, Rosenberg D, et al: Under-reporting of work-related musculoskeletal disorders in the Veterans Administration, *Int J Health Care Quality Assur* 19:463–476, 2006.
10. National Survey of Veterans: 2001. Chapter 4, pp. 4–9. Available at www1.va.gov/VETDATA/docs/SurveysAndStudies/MILITARY.pdf.
11. Modell J, Goulden M, Magnusson S: World War II in the lives of Black Americans: some findings and interpretation, *J Am Hist* 76:838–848, 1989.
12. Homan LM, Reilly T: *Black Knights: the story of the Tuskegee Airmen*, Gretna, La, 2001, Pelican Publishing.
13. Tuskegee Airmen, Inc: 2006. Available at www.tuskegeeairmen.org. Accessed August 17, 2009.
14. Chambers JW II, editor in chief: *The Oxford companion to American military history*, Oxford, UK, 1999, Oxford University Press.
15. Mandelbaum M: Vietnam: The television war, *Daedalus* 111(4):157–169, 1982.
16. Laufer RS, Gallops MS, Frey-Wouters E: War stress and trauma: the Vietnam veteran experience, *J Health Soc Work* 25:65–85, 1984.
17. Dominitz JA, Boyko EJ, Koepsell TD, et al: for the VA Cooperative Study Group 488: Elevated prevalence of hepatitis C infection in users of United States veterans medical centers, *Hepatology* 41(1):88–96, 2005.
18. Committee to Review the Health Effects in Vietnam Veterans of Exposure to Herbicides: Veterans and Agent Orange: Update 2008. Seventh Biennial Update, Institute of Medicine. Available at www.nap.edu/catalog/12662.html.
19. Department of Veterans Affairs, Office of Public Health and Environmental Hazards, Agent Orange Web-page. Available at: www.publichealth.va.gov/exposures/agentorange. Accessed November 23, 2010.

20. Invisible Wounds of War: Psychological and Cognitive Injuries, Their Consequences, and Services to Assist Recovery. Edited by Terri Tanielian and Lisa H. Jaycox. Available at: www.rand.org/pubs/monographs/MG720/. Accessed November 23, 2010.

21. CRS Report for Congress: Suicide Prevention Among Veterans, May 2008. Available at http://stanislaus.networkofcare.org/library/RL34471.pdf.

22. American Psychiatric Association: *Diagnostic and Statistical Manual of Mental Disorders: DSM-IV,* Washington, DC, 1994, American Psychiatric Association.

23. Hyams KC, Wignall FS, Roswell R: War syndromes and their evaluation: from the U.S. Civil War to the Persian Gulf War, *Ann Intern Med* 125(5):398–405, 1996.

24. American Psychiatric Association: *Diagnostic and Statistical Manual Of Mental Disorders: DSM-III,* Washington, DC, 1980, American Psychiatric Association.

25. Sherwood RJ, Shimel H, Stolz P, Sherwood D: The aging veteran: re-emergence of trauma issues, *J Gerontol Soc Work* 40(4):1540–4048, 73–86, 2004.

26. Feldman DB, Periyakoil VS: Posttraumatic stress disorder at the end of life, *J Palliat Med* 9:213–218, 2006.

27. Prins A, Ouimette P, Kimerling R, Cameron RP, Hugelshofer DS, Shaw HJ, Thraikill A, Gussman FD, Sheikh JI: The primary care PTSD (PC-PTSD) screen: development and operating characteristics, *Prim Care Psychiatry* 9:9–14, 2003.

28. Oquendo M, Brent DA, Birmaher B, et al: Posttraumatic stress disorder comorbid with major depression: Factors mediating the association with suicidal behavior, *Am J Psychiatry* 162:560–566, 2005.

29. National Center for PTSD: website: www.ncptsd.va.gov. Accessed April 16, 2010.

30. US Code Title 38, "Veterans' Benefits," Section 1720D, http://veterans.house.gov/documents/title38.pdf.

31. Street A, Stafford J: Military sexual trauma: issues in caring for veterans. Chapter 9 of Iraq War Clinician Guide, ed 2, June, 2004. Available at www.ptsd.va.gov/professional/pages/military-sexual-trauma.asp.

32. Frayne SM, Skinner KM, Sullivan LM, et al: Medical profile of women Veterans Administration outpatients who report a history of sexual assault occurring while in the military, *J Womens Health Gend Based Med* 8(6):835–845, 1999.

33. Kimerling R, Gima K, Smith MW, et al: The Veterans Health Administration and Military Sexual Trauma, *Am J Public Health* 97(12):2160–2216, 2007.

SECTION 3

Service Delivery

CHAPTER 38

The Interdisciplinary Team

JUDITH A. PAICE

The team approach is crucial to palliative care, but there has been little research on the optimal structure and function of an interdisciplinary team that is responsible for caring for those with a life-threatening illness. The interdisciplinary team approach to care is not unique to palliative care. Other disciplines that emphasize teamwork include rehabilitation, critical care, mental health, and geriatrics. Interdisciplinary teams include professionals from multiple disciplines (e.g., nurses, physicians, social workers) who work collaboratively and make group decisions about patient care. The primary difference between multidisciplinary and interdisciplinary care is the role of collaboration and consensus building that is present in interdisciplinary care. Regular meetings serve as the forum for this collaboration and consensus building, and each member contributes the knowledge and skills drawn from his or her own unique training and education.[1] This optimal approach to care, incorporating collaboration and interdependence, has been an historical cornerstone for hospice and palliative care and is the focus of this chapter.

Differences do exist regarding the definition of the interdisciplinary team, the criteria for an effective team, and methods for building and strengthening teams. A Medline search using the term "interdisciplinary" yields more than 17,000 citations; "multidisciplinary" generates more than 27,000 references. Nevertheless, significant overlap and confusion exist regarding the meaning and use of these and other related terms, such as transdisciplinary, interprofessional, and integrative teams. Multidisciplinary teams may consist of multiple disciplines, optimally working toward a common goal. Each individual team member performs his or her role within a formally defined scope of practice. The team members may function in parallel and, in less than ideal circumstances, with undefined or diverse goals. To add to the confusion, this term has also been used to describe teams that consist of multiple specialties

540

within the same discipline who work together to provide patient care. An example of this model is the multidisciplinary pain clinic that includes an anesthesiologist, a neurologist, and a psychiatrist, all of whom work to address the complex needs of individuals with chronic pain. Another example is a team of internists and gynecologists who work to provide the health care needs of women. These individuals are all of the same discipline (physicians), but they are trained in different subspecialties.

Other terms have been used which may result in confusion. *Interprofessional* is synonymous with interdisciplinary and has also been proposed as an alternative to avoid the confusion associated with teams that include collaboration among medical specialties. *Transdisciplinary* is used to denote a system in which one team member acts as the primary clinician and other members provide information and advice. The *integrative model* consists of an interdisciplinary team approach that incorporates conventional medicine with complementary and alternative health care. For purposes of this chapter, the term *interdisciplinary* is used to describe a team composed of members from multiple disciplines who work collaboratively to provide palliative care.

Despite the confusion regarding terminology, there is strong agreement that an interdisciplinary team approach is needed to address the complexities of today's health care system. The 1999 Institute of Medicine report, *To Err is Human: Building a Safer Health System,* identified "promoting effective team functioning" as one of several key principles necessary to create a safe health care environment. The Institute of Medicine's subsequent report, *Crossing the Quality Chasm: A New System for the 21st Century*, reiterated the critical need for collaboration to respond to the complex demands inherent in the current health care system and recommended that better opportunities be provided for interdisciplinary training. A recent appraisal of the progress made in this area acknowledged the slow pace of change and continued to endorse the need for team training as a means to improve patient outcomes. The Joint Commission (TJC) issued their 2006 National Patient Safety Goals, which include a critical objective to improve communication among caregivers. Additionally, this organization endorsed the need for interdisciplinary participation as teams and organizations develop a patient safety plan in the clinical setting.

Professional organizations support the role of interdisciplinary teams. The Society of Critical Care Medicine includes "integrated teams" and states that "Multiprofessional teams use knowledge, technology, and compassion to provide timely, safe, effective, and efficient patient-centered care" in their mission statement. The American Geriatrics Society also espouses the role of interdisciplinary care in their mission and goals statement. Although not explicitly stated in their mission statements, interdisciplinary care is clearly endorsed by the primary professional organizations devoted to palliative care. Such organizations include the American Academy of Hospice and Palliative Medicine, the Hospice and Palliative Nurses Association, the International Association for Hospice and Palliative Care, and the National Hospice and Palliative Care Organization.

Interdisciplinary Teams in Palliative Care

Interdisciplinary team membership is loosely defined in palliative care. Palliative care team members can comprise a variety of disciplines, including art therapists, chaplains, home health aids, nurses, nurse aides, nutritionists, pharmacists, physical and occupational therapists, physicians, psychiatrists, psychologists, social workers, and speech therapists.[2] The hospice core team members must include at least one physician, a nurse, and one other member from a psychosocial discipline.[3] Unique settings or populations may require specialized members.[4] These may include, for example, a neonatologist when providing palliative care in the special care nursery or an infectious disease specialist when addressing the needs of patients with human immunodeficiency virus infection.

Other members of the interdisciplinary team in palliative care can include volunteers and informal caregivers.[5] Even though both hospice and palliative care team members and patients and families find volunteers to be invaluable, few studies have evaluated the common or optimal role of these individuals within the team. In a survey of palliative care volunteers, investigators found the primary motivations for volunteering included the ability to ease the pain of those with a life-threatening illness. Other studies of palliative care teams reveal that volunteers were the least likely (37%) to consider leaving hospice work, compared with nurses (60% had considered leaving) and physicians (40%).

Informal caregivers include family members and friends of the patient who provide physical, emotional, and spiritual support. Numerous studies have documented the physical and psychological impact of providing care for loved ones who are dying. These include time constraints, physical tasks, financial costs, emotional burdens, and physical health risks. Rabow and colleagues suggested ways in which physicians can address the needs of informal caregivers, including good communication, encouraging appropriate advance care planning and decision making, supporting care within the home, demonstrating empathy, and attending to grief and bereavement needs.[6] Although directed to physicians, these recommendations apply to all interdisciplinary team members. Much research is needed to articulate fully the way informal caregivers optimally work together with the interdisciplinary team and how the team can best assist in meeting the caregivers' needs.

Although difficult to investigate, some evidence correlates improved outcomes with palliative care provided by interdisciplinary teams.[7] One controlled clinical trial of an outpatient palliative medicine consultation service revealed significant improvements in dyspnea, anxiety, sleep, and spiritual well-being when compared with patients who received standard care. Furthermore, patients who received palliative care from this interdisciplinary team experienced fewer visits to their primary care physician or at an urgent care setting. Other studies indicate improved relief of symptoms, improved use of advanced directives, more time at home, and reduced costs when care is delivered by interdisciplinary palliative care teams. A comprehensive review of the literature related to palliative care teams who care for dying patients in the intensive care unit (ICU) revealed high levels of family and staff satisfaction, as well as cost savings to the institution.

Criteria for Effective Team Functioning

As a result of limited research, few clear criteria are available to guide those attempting to build a strong and successful palliative care team. Experience suggests, however, that collaboration and communication are critical components to effective team functioning. Goals and roles must be clear and focused on the patient and family, and trust must be established. Leadership functions may be shared, and the strengths and contributions of all team members must be fully incorporated. The functioning and cohesiveness of the team should be viewed as more important than the individual identities of team members. Accepted signs of effective team function include strong rates of retention and satisfaction, trust among all members, participation by all members in leadership decisions, consistent attendance at meetings, successful attainment of quality indicators, and high satisfaction scores by patient and families.[8]

Threats to Team Functioning

There are inherent internal threats to the successful functioning of any group. Turnover of group members, along with role overload and conflict, can jeopardize team performance. This situation can be exacerbated by the stress of providing care to vulnerable patients and families with complicated needs, in a complex environment that may not provide sufficient fiscal and other support to allow effective team function.

INSTABILITY OF TEAM MEMBERSHIP

In the optimal situation, there is little staff turnover on an interdisciplinary team, but membership still changes at some point. Staff members may decide to leave for positive reasons (e.g., academic advancement or a partner who relocates out of town) or negative reasons (e.g., burnout). The program may decide that additional roles and positions are needed, and the resultant newcomers can produce temporary team instability. Furthermore, diverse settings present unique challenges to team solidarity. For example, when instituting palliative care in an ICU, some team members are based in the ICU, some visit the ICU, and some are consulted on a case-by-case basis.[9] This arrangement also occurs in dedicated palliative care units, where there may be a core interdisciplinary team based on the unit, personnel who visit the unit (e.g., the hospice chaplain whose patient is admitted for respite care), and members who are consulted for their expertise (e.g., psychiatry for assisting with a patient with complex mental health disorders). In each of these situations, the composition of the team changes in subtle ways, and team function may be altered.

In his classic studies of team function, Tuckman described four phases of team development: forming, storming, norming, and performing.[10] Forming describes the setting of goals and objectives as the team begins its task. Storming occurs when group members express discord in their approach to the task. Interpersonal conflicts may become apparent at this stage. Norming occurs when effective communication results in cooperation. Performing is achieved when the task is accomplished through collaboration and conflict resolution. Each time a new member is introduced to the team, some level of forming and storming takes place, and norming and performing follow these stages. Frequent staff turnover and repeated substitutions can be a significant burden and a threat to the stability of the team and its function.

ROLE CONFLICT

Disparities and conflict among clinical disciplines are common, but little research specific to palliative care has been conducted. Furthermore, most of the existing literature focuses on physician and nurse conflict and neglects potential sources of conflict among other members of the palliative care team. For example, in a survey of 90 physicians and 230 nurses who worked in the ICU setting, 73% of physicians rated collaboration and communication with nurses as high or very high. Conversely, only 33% of the nurses rated the quality of collaboration and communication with physicians at the same level. Specifically, the nurses in this study reported difficulties in speaking up to physicians, complained that conflict was often not resolved, and felt that their input was not valued.[10] The investigators concluded that some of this disparity in perceived effectiveness in collaboration and communication may be the result of differences in gender (most of the nurses were female and most physicians were male), status, authority, training, and responsibilities.

In a study of the role of various professionals working within a team, second-year postgraduate residents, advanced-practice nurses, and master-level social work students participated in the Geriatric Interdisciplinary Team Training. They were asked to respond to a survey regarding their beliefs about the roles of all team members.[11] Interprofessional differences appeared to be greatest for beliefs about the physician's role. For example, 73% of residents, but only 44% and 47% of social work and advanced practice nurse trainees, respectively, agreed that the team's primary purpose was to assist physicians in achieving treatment goals for patients. Compared with the advanced-practice nurses and social work students, twice as many residents believed that physicians had the right to overturn care plans developed by the team.[11] As in the previous study, differences in age, ethnicity, and gender among these groups may have correlated with the inconsistencies.

This theme of divergence and assumptions as a possible cause of impaired team functioning was echoed in another study of geriatric interdisciplinary team training.[12] The authors call the phenomenon "interdisciplinary split" and believe that attitudes and cultural traditions are important contributory factors. Physician trainees were the least enthusiastic about the interdisciplinary training. Specifically, physicians who were farther along in their training were more likely to perceive other team members as incompetent. The nature of the problem, according to the authors, was not incompetence but rather the clinical inexperience of some of the trainees. Thus, successful interdisciplinary training may need to consider the level of education and experience of the team members from different disciplines.

Other investigators have also identified cultural differences as threats to interdisciplinary care. The Council on Graduate Medical Education and the National Advisory Council on Nurse Education and Practice held a joint meeting to discuss collaborative education models to support patient safety. They defined culture as the language, ideas, beliefs, customs, codes, institutions, and tools used by physicians and nurses in their practices. The panel members concluded that existing professional cultural norms do not support the interdisciplinary team approach and believed that cultural change will be a critical factor in fostering interdisciplinary care.

Cultural differences exist among other disciplines as well. For instance, some disciplines are action oriented and focus on fixing a problem or performing a task. Medicine and nursing generally fall into this category. Other disciplines are more relationship oriented, processing interactions and interpreting their meaning. Social work and psychology provide examples of this approach. Similar divergent approaches may occur between members of one discipline. Teams may need to consider these cultural differences when analyzing specific instances of role conflict.

Role blurring refers to overlapping competencies and shared responsibilities.[13] This blurring can serve as a potential barrier to effective team function, particularly if resentment occurs because the skills of some team members are underutilized. Staff nurses, in particular, experience role blurring in interactions with advanced-practice nurses. Blurring also occurs when a physician's expectation of the nursing role differs

> **Box 38-1.** *Strategies to Address Role Confusion and Blurring*
>
> - Clarify role perceptions and expectations of each member.
> - Have each professional list his or her own competencies and the competencies of other team members, then compare these lists.
> - Discuss overlapping responsibilities and in what situations this overlap is most likely to arise.
> - Modify roles and expectations within the team based on these discussions.

from the nurse's expectation. Role blurring can be countered with clarification of the function of each team member. Williams and colleagues found that a clear definition of the roles and responsibilities of hospice chaplains was associated with less perceived stress.[14] Conflict resolution and unambiguous communication within a team can address this confusion regarding roles. Other strategies to address role blurring are listed in Box 38-1.

Aussman addressed the issue of role conflict and competition among health care professionals in an editorial, in which he charted the more recent history of medical care.[15] He described the demise of the era of solo practice in medicine, exemplified by the kindly family doctor (such as the television character Marcus Welby). A newer metaphor for the practice of the health care team is a symphony orchestra, with all musicians playing together with their own special instruments at the right time. The salient, and unanswered, question in palliative care teams is "Who should serve as the conductor?"

ROLE OVERLOAD AND BURNOUT

Although not well characterized, role overload (pressures related to the job) and burnout are potential barriers to the functioning of palliative care and other interdisciplinary teams.[16] Studies suggest that related components of role overload, including a lack of institutional support, a heavy workload, and a shortage of staff, contribute to reduced efficacy of palliative care team functioning. Conversely, a study of the effectiveness of an interdisciplinary team in long-term care found greater apparent resource availability (e.g., improved staffing) to be associated with increased perceived team effectiveness.[17]

Compassion fatigue occurs when health care professionals are constantly exposed to human suffering, and it is often evidenced by fatigue, anger, irritability, and emotional unavailability. Cumulative grief, related to and often a component of compassion fatigue, is a particular risk in palliative care and should be assessed.[18] If left unattended, compassion fatigue and grief can lead to burnout. Burnout has been described as a set of behaviors and responses to stressful environments and has been well characterized in oncology and ICU settings, among other places. Although burnout is common among all staff members, house staff members experience the greatest degree of burnout, according to a study of house staff, nurses, and medical oncologists who worked in a cancer hospital. Strategies used by the staff to counteract burnout included talking with friends and using humor. Nurses working in an ICU described experiencing burnout related to the stress of transitioning from cure to comfort care and particularly in providing what they perceived as "futile" care or

> **Box 38-2.** *Strategies for Addressing Burnout among Team Members*
>
> Get sufficient sleep.
> Take breaks throughout the day.
> Plan vacations.
> Engage in regular physical activity.
> Develop and cultivate hobbies.
> Seek balance between your professional and personal life.
> Learn time-management strategies.
> Create a personal space that allows reflection.
> Incorporate mindfulness exercises into daily life.
> Laugh.
> Keep a journal or other reflective writing exercises.
> Listen to music or view art.
> Talk with colleagues—seek mentors.
> Learn to grieve.
> Initiate grand rounds or other venues devoted to psychosocial issues (e.g., Schwartz Center rounds—see www.theschwartzcenter.org/ for specific information).
> Advocate for change when the system promotes factors that lead to burnout (e.g., unreasonable workload).
> Seek counseling to address unresolved concerns; do not self-medicate.

"torturing" the patient. These nurses also experienced distress when witnessing or becoming involved in the family discord surrounding a patient in the ICU. Strategies that assisted them in addressing this sense of burnout included feeling accepted as a professional member of the team and the use of cognitive, affective, and behavioral techniques to address this stress. Hospice nurses reported that the most important strategy for ameliorating the impact of witnessing unrelieved patient suffering was informal support from work colleagues. House officers rotating through hospice described their post as stressful, primarily as it related to staff conflict and caring for young patients. Almost one fourth of those surveyed had elevated scores on a test of psychological distress.

Of concern is the lack of self-awareness that can occur when burnout develops. A study of Scottish anesthesiologists found that many did not recognize the debilitating effects of stress and fatigue on their performance. This can lead to individual physical and mental health problems and can ultimately have a negative impact on team functioning. Strategies for managing burnout include lifestyle changes and self-care measures and are detailed in Box 38-2.[19]

Building and Strengthening Teams

Although much research is needed to guide the construction of effective interdisciplinary teams, experience has generated several recommendations. These include careful selection of team members, appropriate education and training of professionals regarding interdisciplinary approaches, and team building through effective communication. A creative exercise for the palliative care team may include reviewing literature, theater, or music, to compare situations within myth and the arts with the function of an interdisciplinary team.

CAREFUL SELECTION OF TEAM MEMBERS

In developing a palliative care interdisciplinary team, selection of team members is crucial. Team members must be skilled within their discipline and aware of their own limitations, as well as those of their specialty.[20] In a provocative article regarding network theory, computer modeling was used to determine the attributes of effective teams.[21] The most productive teams (broadly defined and drawing from business, science, and the arts) consist of individuals with the most skill who have experience in collaboration and are able to develop fresh ideas.[21] The model discourages including people with whom the team has worked before—"friends"—because this will eventually mar performance. Rather, the model encourages including the most qualified individuals.

INTERDISCIPLINARY EDUCATION

The literature supports the need for both early interdisciplinary training of all professionals and interdisciplinary teamwork education. Interdisciplinary education will ultimately instill respect for and understanding of the role and benefits of teams. Although these educational efforts are increasing, they remain relatively uncommon. In surveys of Canadian and US medical schools, fewer than 30% had formal training related to interdisciplinary teamwork, and most of these courses were elective. The lack of interdisciplinary education leads to diminished understanding of the roles of other team members and can result in isolation.[8]

One study of the outcomes of a day-long interdisciplinary palliative care course yielded high satisfaction rates. However, fewer medical students were involved when compared with other disciplines.[22,23] Early experience suggests that the timing of interdisciplinary educational efforts is critical and should occur within the first 2 years of education. Students must, however, have at least beginning competencies in their field to participate in and contribute to this education adequately.[23] Creative teaching strategies are necessary when providing palliative care education to interdisciplinary groups, including problem-based education, case studies, clinical experiences, and role playing, although some educators report that physicians are often reluctant to participate in these types of teaching methods.[24]

TEAM TRAINING

Along with providing interdisciplinary education during basic training, ongoing education is necessary to advance team function and growth.[1] Group interaction skills, communication techniques, and conflict resolution are all topics that teams must address.[8] Interestingly, much understanding of team training comes from other industries, particularly aviation. For example, a program called Crew Resource Management (CRM) was developed to ensure aircraft safety by fostering appropriate team attitudes among pilots and cockpit crews. This training has been successfully adapted to the health care setting. In a study of 489 physicians, nurses, technicians, and hospital administrators (most from the trauma unit and the emergency department) at Vanderbilt University Medical Center, in Nashville, Tennessee, who completed the Crew Resource Management training, most reported improvements in key areas such as addressing fatigue, creating and managing a team, recognizing adverse situations, cross-checking and communication techniques, decision making, and giving and receiving performance feedback.

In another example of successful interdisciplinary team building efforts, the Downstate Team-Building Initiative included students of medicine, nursing, physician assistants, physical therapy, occupational therapy, and diagnostic medical imaging. The students received training in group decision making, conflict mediation, and alliance building, along with multicultural skills. Team atmosphere improved 48%, group teamwork skills improved 44%, and interdisciplinary understanding improved 42% after the training.

Although focused on a single discipline, one study incorporated anesthetists who were asked to respond to simulated anesthesia scenarios to develop team skills. The program, Anaesthetists' Non-Technical Skills, included task management, team working, situation awareness, and decision making. Early trials established beginning validity and reliability of the simulated educational program. This is a creative program that may one day be adapted to enhance interdisciplinary team communication and to foster more efficient, productive interdisciplinary team meetings in palliative care.

Another example of team training that has demonstrated efficacy is TeamSTEPPS, promoted by the Agency for Healthcare Research and Quality and the Defense Department. Although this program is focused on safety and quality, many components could be adapted to team training in palliative care. The program focuses on increasing team awareness, clarifying roles and responsibilities, resolving conflicts, sharing information, and eliminating barriers to quality and safety. The program incorporates a training curriculum, along with vignettes, CDs, pocket guides, questionnaires, and other materials (for more information go to http://teamstepps.ahrq.gov/index.htm). This program and many others use the concept of a FLEXTRA Kit, a model for the development of resource materials to support inservice training and other educational efforts. The Kit includes a curricular guide and camera ready materials for handouts, slides, and videos, along with evaluation instruments.[25]

COMMUNICATION

An essential component of palliative care is communication, including conflict resolution. In studies of interdisciplinary teams in the ICU, clear and honest dialogue supported team functioning, in part by allowing team members to acknowledge differences regarding ethical issues. In other palliative care settings, communication training and the development of conflict management procedures have been found to support team building. A practical exercise that enhances communication and clarifies the work of the interdisciplinary team includes writing a mission and purpose statement and clarifying the roles of all team members. Conflict resolution should include respectful negotiation and avoidance of negative behaviors such as dominance, negativity, distraction, and avoiding blame.[20]

An interesting challenge to effective communication has been the introduction of electronic communication methods. Although intended to streamline communication, voice mail and e-mail can result in misunderstandings and, occasionally, hurt feelings. Strategies include projecting a courteous tone, reviewing content before sending a message, avoiding jargon, and being as brief as possible.[20]

An analysis of the structures, processes, and outcomes associated with effective palliative care team communication revealed several critical concepts.[26] Regarding structure, both internal and external concepts were essential. Internal concepts included the membership of the team, policies, procedures, and communication practices. These dictated the effectiveness of team communication. External structures that were crucial to team success included coordination with outside agencies and individuals. Team processes associated with effective communication included care planning, information exchange (how the team interacts with one another), teaching (both other team members as well as patients/families), decision making, negotiation, and leadership. These investigators found that several team outcomes were influenced by communication, including patient discharge planning, reintegration of the patient back into the community, effective disease management, patient and family satisfaction, and patient achievement of goals and objectives. These investigators recommend electronic methods to support the structure, process, and outcome of palliative care teams. Video or web conferencing and electronic patient records support internal and external structures associated with communication, as well as many of the processes so crucial to palliative care teams. These investigators caution that team agreement is needed about the type of communication channels to be used (e.g., telephone vs. email) and the frequency with which these channels will be monitored (e.g., hourly, daily).

INSTITUTIONAL SUPPORT

Institutional support is critical for effective interdisciplinary team function, yet recent trends in health care threaten this support. Time, the most valued resource, is needed to foster group process.[20] Adequate space, another precious commodity in today's environment, and physical proximity of team members, privacy, noise control, and comfortable seating are all necessary for interdisciplinary interaction.

In addition to physical attributes, the environment must support the work of the interdisciplinary team through unit level policies that support and value team.[4] The leadership structure within the institution should be interdisciplinary, and individual leaders must role model interdisciplinary communication.[4] Rewards offered for collaborative team work, rather than for individual achievements, will also serve to demonstrate the institutional support for this approach to care. The culture of the workplace must change to reduce unacceptable, intimidating behaviors, through improved dialogue, modeling of behaviors, and rewards for teamwork. Finally, the institution must foster and support an environment that allows the integration of interdisciplinary palliative care teams with existing services.

PEARLS

- The interdisciplinary team approach is crucial to palliative care. The Institute of Medicine, The Joint Commission, the Society of Critical Care Medicine, and others endorse the need for interdisciplinary care to address the complexities of today's health care system.
- Signs of effective team functioning include strong rates of retention and satisfaction, trust, attendance at meetings, attainment of quality indicators, and high satisfaction scores by patients and families.
- Careful selection of team members, interdisciplinary education, and institutional support are key to building successful teams.

PITFALLS

- Little research exists to define the criteria for an effective team, team structure, and methods for building and strengthening teams.
- Threats to effective team functioning include staff turnover, role conflict, role overload, and burnout.

Summary

Interdisciplinary teams are essential in the care of patients with life-threatening illnesses and their families. Interdisciplinary approaches to care also assist the professional in preventing stress and burnout. Obstacles to effective interdisciplinary team function include frequent change in team composition, as well as role conflict or blurring. Building or strengthening teams depends on careful selection of members, interdisciplinary education, and team training in communication techniques and conflict resolution, as well as appropriate institutional support. Cultural disparities among disciplines complicate effective communication and collaboration. Future research is needed to elucidate optimal interdisciplinary team functioning in palliative care.

Resources

Center to Advancer Palliative Care Center to Advancer Palliative Care
  www.capc.org/
This Web site provides practical information specific to interdisciplinary palliative care, including core and expert competencies for physicians, nurses, chaplains, social workers, and volunteers, as well as strategies for recruiting in interdisciplinary team.
Conflict Resolution Information Source
  http://v4.crinfo.org/
This Web site provides a wider variety of resources to learn about and how to address conflict.
Geriatric Interdisciplinary Team TrainingGeriatric Interdisciplinary Team Training
  www.gittprogram.org/
Sponsored by the John A. Hartford Foundation, Inc., this Web site provides information regarding interdisciplinary team training, videos, tools to assess team function, and many other resources.
National Consensus Project for Quality Palliative Care National Consensus Project for Quality Palliative Care
  www.nationalconsensusproject.org/
The Clinical Practice Guidelines for Quality Palliative Care are available on this Web site, highlighting the need for interdisciplinary teams and defining the core components of these teams.

References

1. Hall P, Weaver L: Interdisciplinary education and teamwork: a long and winding road, *Med Educ* 35:867–875, 2001.
2. Coyle N: Interdisciplinary collaboration in hospital palliative care: chimera or goal? *Palliat Med* 11:265–266, 1997.
3. Reese DJ, Sontag M: Successful interprofessional collaboration on the hospice team, *Health Soc Work* 26:167–175, 2001.
4. Baggs JG, Norton SA, Schmitt MH, Sellers CR: The dying patient in the ICU: role of the interdisciplinary team, *Crit Care Clin* 20:525–540, 2004.
5. Low J, Perry R, Wilkinson S: A qualitative evaluation of the impact of palliative care day services: the experiences of patients, informal carers, day unit managers and volunteer staff, *Palliat Med* 19:65–70, 2005.
6. Rabow MW, Dibble SL, Pantilat SZ, et al: The comprehensive care team: a controlled trial of outpatient palliative medicine consultation, *Arch Intern Med* 164:83, 2004.
7. Higginson IJ, Finlay IG, Goodwin DM, et al: Is there evidence that palliative care teams alter end-of-life experiences of patients and their caregivers? *J Pain Symptom Manage* 25:150–168, 2003.
8. Connor S, Egan K, Kwilosz D, et al: Interdisciplinary approaches to assisting with end-of-life care and decision making, *Am Behav Sci* 46:340–356, 2002.
9. Mularski RA, Bascom P, Osborne ML: Educational agendas for interdisciplinary end-of-life curricula, *Crit Care Med* 29:N16–N23, 2001.
10. Tuckman BW: Developmental sequence in small groups, *Psychological Bulletin* 63:384, 1965.
11. Leipzig RM, Hyer K, Ek K, et al: Attitudes toward working on interdisciplinary healthcare teams: a comparison by discipline, *J Am Geriatr Soc* 50:1141–1148, 2002.

12. Reuben DB, Levy–Storms L, Yee MN, et al: Disciplinary split: a threat to geriatrics interdisciplinary team training, *J Am Geriatr Soc* 52:1000–1006, 2004.
13. Mariano C: Inter-disciplinary collaboration: a practice imperative, *Healthcare Trends Transition* 3:10–12, 1992.
14. Williams ML, Wright M, Cobb M, et al: A prospective study of the roles, responsibilities and stresses of chaplains working within a hospice, *Palliat Med* 18:638, 2004.
15. Ausman JI: The kings and queens of medicine have died, *Surg Neurol* 63:290, 2005.
16. Vachon ML: Reflections on the history of occupational stress in hospice/palliative care, *Hosp J* 14:229–246, 1999.
17. Temkin-Greener H, Gross D, Kunitz SJ, Mukamel D: Measuring interdisciplinary team performance in a long-term care setting, *Med Care* 42:472–481, 2004.
18. Lyckholm L: Dealing with stress, burnout, and grief in the practice of oncology, *Lancet Oncol* 2:750–755, 2001.
19. Kearney MK, Weininger RB, Vachon MLS, Harrison RL, Mount BM: Self-care of physicians caring for patients at end of life, *JAMA* 301:1155–1164, 2009.
20. Lindeke L, Sieckert A: Nurse-physician workplace collaboration, *Online J Issues Nurs* 10:5, 2005.
21. Barabasi AL: Sociology. Network theory: the emergence of the creative enterprise, *Science* 308:639–641, 2005.
22. Latimer EJ, Deakin A, Ingram C, et al: An interdisciplinary approach to a day-long palliative care course for undergraduate students, *CMAJ* 161:729–731, 1999.
23. Latimer EJ, Kiehl K, Lennox S, Studd S: An interdisciplinary palliative care course for practicing health professionals: ten years' experience, *J Palliat Care* 14:27–33, 1998.
24. MacDonald N: Limits to multidisciplinary education, *J Palliat Care* 12:6, 1996.
25. Battles JB, Sheridan MM: The FLEXTRA Kit: a model for instructor support materials, *J Biocommunication* 6:1–13, 1989.
26. Kuziemsky CE, Borycki EM, Purkis ME, et al: Interprofessional Practices Team: an interdisciplinary team communication framework and its application to healthcare "e-teams" systems design, *BMC Medical Informatics and Decision Making* 9: article number 43, 2009.

Further Reading

Speck PW: *Teamwork in palliative care: fulfilling or frustrating?* New York, 2006, Oxford University Press.
Thomas EJ, Sexton JB, Helmreich RL: Discrepant attitudes about teamwork among critical care nurses and physicians, *Crit Care Med* 31:956–959, 2003.

CHAPTER 39

Palliative Care Nursing

JEANNE MARIE MARTINEZ

The (nursing) profession taught me so many lessons about the fragility of life, the importance of being mindful about the way you live, the need for appreciation of life's beauty and bounty while you are still healthy, and perhaps, most importantly, the worth of "unconditional positive regard," which is the way we were taught to approach our patients. Elizabeth Berg, RN.

The nursing specialty of palliative care has recently emerged. Its goals are to improve quality of life and symptom management, caring for the physical, emotional, and spiritual needs throughout the trajectory of illness. Nursing has provided leadership in the development of this specialty by defining the scope and standards of palliative nursing practice at both the generalist and advanced practice levels. The standards of palliative nursing practice can be applied to any care setting; they can be integrated into general patient care or used to guide specialist palliative care practice. Hospice programs currently provide the best example of structured, regulated palliative care. Future trends include the continued development and standardization of palliative care in inpatient and ambulatory care settings. These trends will likely drive the need for more advanced practice palliative care nurses (APNs) and improve palliative care for all.

Nursing Contributions

Dame Cicely Saunders, who started her career as a nurse, was the founder of the modern concept of hospice care; she opened St. Christopher's Hospice in Great Britain in 1967. She was instrumental in developing the core principles that provide the basis of all palliative care today. Her interest in care of the dying began when she was a volunteer nurse. Dame Cicely subsequently obtained a degree in social work and went on to become a physician before directing St. Christopher's Hospice. Florence Wald, a nurse, brought hospice care to the United States in 1974; she founded Connecticut Hospice in Branford, Connecticut, the first US hospice. A former Dean of the Yale University School of Nursing in New Haven, Connecticut, Florence Wald heard Dame Cicely lecture at Yale in 1963 and was so inspired by her work that she subsequently visited St. Christopher's to learn about hospice care. Connecticut Hospice was the first hospice to have a building designed specifically for hospice care, and it remains unique in other ways. It is licensed as a hospital and is identified primarily as an inpatient facility (as is St. Christopher's), although Connecticut Hospice is integrated with home care services that are provided throughout Connecticut. By contrast, most US hospices use a home care model and contract with inpatient facilities for services when patients cannot be cared for at home.

In 1984, the (then) Joint Commission on Accreditation of Hospitals developed its first standards for hospice programs.[1] Anne Rooney, RN, MS, MPH, was instrumental in defining these hospice accreditation standards, and was one of the first Joint Commission hospice surveyors. She is a former director of the Joint Commission's Home Care and Hospice Accreditation Program. In 1992, many of the original hospice standards were incorporated into the (renamed) Joint Commission on Accreditation of Healthcare Organizations (JCAHO) standards and applied to the care of dying patients in hospitals. Since that time, the (now named) Joint Commission has continued to incorporate palliative care standards into all patient care populations and settings. The best example of this is the Joint Commission standard asserting that pain management is a right for all patients.[2]

Madolon O'Rawe Amenta, PhD, RN, was another influential nurse in hospice development. She founded the Pennsylvania Hospice Network and was a founding member of the Hospice Nurses Association (HNA) in 1986. That same year, she co-authored one of the first nursing textbooks on end-of-life care, *Nursing Care of the Terminally Ill*, with Nancy Bohnet. Dr. Amenta served as the first HNA Executive Director from 1993 to 1997.[3] The HNA changed its name to the Hospice and Palliative Nurses Association (HPNA) in 1997.[4]

In May, 2004, the National Consensus Project for Quality Palliative Care (NCP), a collaboration of five major US palliative care organizations, published its comprehensive guidelines to promote consistent, high-quality palliative care by establishing a consensus on clinical practice guidelines. Five organizations participated in the development of these evidence-based palliative care guidelines: the HPNA, the American Academy of Hospice and Palliative Medicine, the Center to Advance Palliative Care, Last Acts/Partnership for Caring, and the National Hospice and Palliative Care Organization. The NCP provides this definition of palliative care: The goal of palliative care is to prevent and relieve suffering and to support the best possible quality of life for patients and their families, regardless of the stage of disease or the need for other therapies. Palliative care is both a philosophy of care and an organized, highly structured system for delivering care. Palliative care expands traditional disease-model medical treatments to include the goals of quality of life for patient and family, optimizing function, helping with decision-making and providing opportunities for personal growth. As such it can be delivered concurrently with life-prolonging care or as the main focus of care.

More than a dozen nursing organizations have endorsed the NCP guidelines, as well as the American Alliance of Cancer Pain Initiatives and the Society of Critical Medicine. The second edition was published in 2007.[5]

Defining a Specialty

According to the NCP, "Specialist Palliative Care providers are professionals whose work is largely or entirely involved with palliative care and who have received appropriate training and credentialing in the field." The American Board of Nursing Specialties (ABNS), the only accrediting body dedicated specifically to nursing certification, accredits specialty nursing certification programs if the organization has demonstrated compliance with rigorous standards for certification. The ABNS considers "specialty nursing certification THE standard by which the public recognizes quality nursing care." Of the eighteen ABNS accreditation standards, the first ABNS Standard 1 requires a definition and written scope, describing the nursing specialty, along with evidence of a distinct body of scientific knowledge that is unique and distinct from that of basic nursing. Hospice and Palliative Nursing has been approved by ABNS as a distinct nursing specialty.[6]

In 2000, the HPNA published their statement on the scope, standards of care, and standards of practice of the specialty of hospice and palliative nursing.[4]

SCOPE

The defined scope of the specialty of hospice and palliative nursing includes the following:

- Pain and symptom management
- End-stage disease process care
- Psychosocial and spiritual care of patient and family
- Culture-sensitive care of patient and family
- Interdisciplinary collaborative practice
- Loss and grief care
- Patient education and advocacy
- Bereavement care
- Ethical and legal considerations
- Communication skills
- Awareness of community resources

STANDARDS

The Standards of Hospice and Palliative Nursing Practice are authoritative statements that describe the responsibilities for which practitioners are accountable. They are divided into the Standards of Professional Performance and the Standards of Care.

The Standards of Professional Performance, which reflect the consistency of language and structure recommended by the American Nurses Association 1998 Standards of Clinical Practice[7] are as follows:

Standard I: Quality of Care. The hospice and palliative nurse systematically evaluates the quality and effectiveness of nursing practice.

Standard II: Performance Appraisal. The hospice and palliative nurse evaluates own nursing practice in relation to professional practice standards and relevant standards and regulations.

Standard III: Education. The hospice and palliative nurse acquires and maintains current knowledge and competency in hospice and palliative nursing practice.

Standard IV: Collegiality. The hospice and palliative nurse contributes to the professional development of peers and other health care professionals as colleagues.

Standard V: Ethics. The hospice and palliative nurse's decisions and actions on behalf of patient and family are determined in an ethical manner.

Standard VI: Collaboration. This use of interdisciplinary team and other resources includes collaborating with patients and family in developing the care plan and supporting team decisions.

Standard VII: Research. The hospice and palliative nurse uses research findings in practice, identifies research issues, and supports research studies.

Standard VIII: Resource utilization. The hospice and palliative nurse considers factors related to safety, effectiveness and cost in planning and delivering patient and family care.

Types of Care Activity

Beyond the standards of professional performance, the Standards of Care describe palliative nursing care activities for all patients and their families. The processes encompass all significant actions taken by nurses when providing care, and they form the foundation for clinical decision making.[4] They are described below.

Standard I: Assessment—The Hospice and Palliative Nurse Collects Patient and Family Health Data

Whether assessing a newly admitted hospital patient with severe pain, caring for someone who is actively dying, performing intake at home for hospice services, or responding to a palliative care consultation, a nursing assessment is often the initial act of care in the nursing specialty of palliative care. In every circumstance, the patient's evaluation needs to be holistic and should identify current problems that encompass the physical, emotional, social, and spiritual care realms. It is essential that patient and family care goals be identified and communicated to the health care team. Problems need to be responded to according to the patient's identified priorities (or the family's priorities if the patient is unable to communicate). When palliative care is provided by a specialist in a consultative role, it is critical for the palliative care nurse to communicate with the patient's current care team, respond to the initial consultation, elicit their concerns, and provide a model of excellent team work.

Caring for patients with end-stage disease and for those who are actively dying entails the challenge of ensuring that the assessment itself does not pose a burden on patients or significant others. Because a thorough physical assessment may sometimes exacerbate symptoms, determining the cause of a symptom may not be realistically possible. Empirical symptom management, titrated to patient relief, may be the best option, along with intense intervention for immediate physical, emotional, and spiritual needs and immediate needs of the family. For actively dying patients, family support needs related to grieving must be assessed and should particularly identify those at risk for complicated grieving or those with a history of poor coping skills.

Standard II: Diagnosis—The Hospice and Palliative Nurse Analyzes the Assessment Data in Determining Diagnosis

Diagnoses are derived by the analysis of multidimensional assessment data and the identification of problems that may be resolved, diminished, or prevented. Whenever possible, diagnoses are validated with the patient, family, and other interdisciplinary team members and health care providers, and they should be consistently communicated to other team members.

Standard III: Outcome Identification—The Hospice and Palliative Nurse Develops Expected Outcomes

Realistic, derived outcomes are mutually formulated with the patient, family, and (as appropriate) other members of the interdisciplinary team. Expected outcomes should be attainable, given the prognosis of the patient; they can provide direction for continuity of care across all care settings and from the time of admission through bereavement. When possible, expected outcomes are documented as measurable goals.

Standard IV: Planning—The Hospice and Palliative Nurse Develops a Plan of Care that Prescribes Interventions to Attain Expected Outcomes

Care is planned in collaboration with the patient, family, and other interdisciplinary team members within the context of patient and family goals of care. It is individualized to the spiritual, emotional, physical, social, psychological, and cultural needs of the patient and family. The plan of care is dynamic and should be updated regularly as the status, goals, and priorities of the patient and family change. If goals of care are not clarified, the plan of care may go in the wrong direction.

Standard V: Implementation—The Hospice and Palliative Nurse Implements the Interventions Identified in the Plan of Care

All interventions need to be weighed by a benefit versus burden calculus that is, ideally, determined by or negotiated with the patient or surrogate decision maker. Although a palliative care approach generally focuses on symptom management, the nature of a particular symptom may lead a clinician to consider aggressive treatment to eradicate the cause, similar to an acute care approach. However, consideration must be given to the impact on the patient's quality of life, the patient's desire for intervention, and the potential for the intervention to cause further suffering. In patients with end-stage disease, the timeliness of the effect of an intervention must also be weighed against the amount of time an individual may have. Another important aspect of nursing intervention is timely referral to other health care disciplines and services and coordination of care to facilitate the interdisciplinary team expertise that is often required to meet the needs of the patient and family.

Many routine nursing interventions other than treatment can also be burdensome to patients with end-stage disease, particularly in inpatient settings. These include such routine tasks as daily weights, blood pressures, blood draws for laboratory studies, and even bathing and feeding. Inpatient facility routines, often designed for efficient diagnosis and disease management procedures, can also be burdensome to frail patients or those with end-stage disease. Care needs to be individualized and designed to optimize symptom management, to allow patients to maintain as much control as possible, and to enhance quality of life.

Standard VI: Evaluation—The Hospice and Palliative Nurse Evaluates the Patient and Family's Progress toward Attainment of Outcomes

The effectiveness of the plan is evaluated in relation to achievement of the intended or acceptable outcomes. Palliative care interventions must consider the response of the patient and family to care as one of the most critical measures of effectiveness. The plan of care should be reviewed and revised according to the effectiveness of interventions at the time and according to the patient's current priorities.

Patient Education

Throughout the nursing process, a critical role of the nurse is to guide the patient and family through all the information that is needed to understand care options. The emotional context of coping with illness, of grieving the many losses, and of anticipating death can make education and learning a challenge. Nurses in palliative care and hospice roles often need to tell people information that they may not want to hear. They also need to provide or reinforce a great deal of information in a short amount of time. The need for frequent repetition of information to patients and families should be expected, and the use of written educational materials to reinforce information can be helpful. Common education needs for patients and families include information related to the following:

- Disease, expectations for disease progression, and prognosis
- Treatment options, including realistic, expected outcomes of treatment
- Advanced care planning information and tools
- Patients' rights, especially as related to decision making and pain management
- Care options, including hospice services and experimental treatments
- How to provide physical caregiving (for family caregivers)
- Signs of impending death
- Community regulations related to dying at home
- The grieving experience
- Resources for grief counseling and bereavement services

The HPNA provides patient teaching sheets that address many of the foregoing needs. These can be accessed at www.hpna.org.

Effective Communication

Because the emotional aspects of care can often be intense, it is critical that the care team be clear, consistent, and empathetic communicators throughout assessment, care, and evaluation. Nurses need to anticipate the difficult and common themes that accompany serious illness and end-of-life care. These themes include the meaning of illness, the desire to know when death will occur, truth telling among family members, and fears about suffering at the time of death. Other common fears are fear of pain and other physical symptoms, loss of control, and fear of the unknown. Palliative care practitioners need to anticipate these issues, feel comfortable discussing them, and develop competency in using clear and comforting verbal and body language.

To attain patient goals and to ensure continuity of care, effective communication must also extend to colleagues. All involved members of the interdisciplinary team need to be able to provide input in care planning, and be cognizant of patients' goals of care. Another critical part of the communication process is for every team member to give a consistent message to patients and families, who are often struggling with difficult and emotional care decisions. Receiving mixed messages from members of the health care team can create anxiety and add to distress for all involved.

Spiritual Dimensions

A spiritual assessment, which includes cultural aspects of beliefs and values, is the first step in addressing spiritual needs. Nurses need to elicit important spiritual beliefs and needs, which can vary greatly among patients and their family members. It is important for nurses to understand some of the common beliefs, values, and rituals of cultural backgrounds of patients and families that may differ from their own. However, rather than making assumptions based on the culture of the patient and family, beliefs must be assessed individually. Some common spiritual needs include exploring the meaning of suffering, the existential issues of patients and families, and resolving unfinished issues or life tasks. Spiritual distress may exacerbate physical suffering, and it can greatly affect quality of life. Helping patients and families work through spiritual issues can also have a positive impact on the family's grieving after the patient's death.

Spiritual distress may be a concern for many patients and their family members, but nurses also need to be open to cues and opportunities for spiritual growth. For example, patients can be empowered to guide their family's communication by being open about feelings, take the opportunity to resolve problem relationships, and explore religious beliefs.

Although some experienced nurses may be able to address spiritual issues and guide patients and families through spiritual tasks adequately, nurses also need to ensure that patients and families have access to the appropriate providers who can address spiritual needs. Ideally, this is a chaplain, community clergy member, spiritual guide, or other counselor who is also competent in addressing suffering for persons with serious and end-stage illness.

Nurses need to be aware of their own beliefs and values and ensure that they do not impose them on patients and families. It is important to be open to diverse ways of coping, grieving, and dying, rather than holding preconceived notions of how others should feel or behave.

Presence and Support

In providing care, there are many instances when physical presence is the most effective supportive nursing intervention. It may be a silent presence that allows the patient and family to express emotion, or it may be companionship during times of anxiety, loneliness, despair, dying, and intense grieving. The value of presence is to be in the moment and to model the importance of "being" rather than "doing" for families, friends, and other caregivers.

Ethical Issues

PROFESSIONAL BOUNDARIES

Providing hospice and palliative care can be an intense, intimate experience, and boundaries between the patient and nurse can become blurred. Violating professional boundaries may be a greater risk for home care and hospice clinicians who are unaccompanied during visits in the patient's home environment. Highly functioning interdisciplinary teams help to provide the support and perspective necessary to prevent individual clinicians from crossing boundaries. Professional caregivers who have had their own losses or suffer from unresolved grief may also find themselves at risk of over-identifying with patients and families, or unintentionally seeking to have their own needs met. Nurses should be aware of signs of their own or a colleague's over-involvement. These include the following, as set forth by the National Council of State Boards of Nursing[7]:

- Excessive self-disclosure: The nurse discusses personal problems, feelings, or aspects of his or her intimate life with the patient or family.
- "Super nurse" behavior: The nurse believes that only he or she understands and can meet the patient's needs. Other members of the team are not utilized in the usual way.
- Secretive behavior: The nurse keeps secrets with the patient or becomes defensive when someone questions his or her interactions with patients or family.
- Selective communication: The nurse reports only some aspects of patient care or patient behavior.
- Flirtations: The nurse communicates in a flirtatious manner, perhaps employing sexual innuendo or off-color jokes.

Nurses may need help from a supervisor or other team member to set limits with some patients and families and to explore the reasons for their behavior. Crossing boundaries can be harmful to patients and families and, ultimately, can be a source of burnout for the nurse.

WITHHOLDING/WITHDRAWING THERAPY

The withholding and withdrawing of life-prolonging or life-sustaining therapy or treatment are governed by the ethical principle of *autonomy,* which is an individual's right to refuse or accept treatment. However, the emotional component of deciding not to initiate treatment and of withdrawing treatment can feel very different in the clinical setting. Nurses need to be clear that withholding therapy and withdrawing therapy are legal and ethical equivalents. However, the knowledge of this equivalency may not make the decision to withdraw therapy easier for family members or, at times, professional members of the health care team. This issue should, therefore, be a consideration when recommending trials of life-sustaining or life-prolonging treatments that are unlikely to be effective or may need to be withdrawn in the future. When treatment trials are proposed, it is helpful to establish success or failure markers and a time frame for achieving success in advance of the trial so the groundwork is laid for withdrawal.

The difficulty in many of these decisions depends on who is making the decision and what therapy is being withheld or withdrawn. The decision is usually easier when a person is able to communicate clearly his or her wishes about refusing treatment. There is particular emotionality associated with withholding or withdrawing artificial food and fluids.[8] The very public 2005 case of Terri Schiavo, a 41-year-old woman who had been in a persistent vegetative state for more than 15 years, provides an extreme example of the volatility of such decisions. Ms. Schiavo's parents fought with her husband (the legal surrogate decision maker) for many years to prevent removal of her feeding tube. This situation presented the combination of a young person who could not speak for herself and the decision to withhold artificial nutrition and hydration.[9]

PALLIATIVE SEDATION

Palliative sedation (formerly called terminal sedation) refers to the intentional use of pharmacological agents to induce sleep for relief of distressing symptoms that cannot be controlled by other means. Sedation is used in home and inpatient palliative care settings for relief of refractory symptoms, both physical and existential. The most common reasons for palliative sedation include pain, vomiting, terminal delirium, dyspnea, and psychological distress. This intervention should be reserved as a last resort at end of life. The pharmacological agents used in palliative sedation vary but may include opioid analgesics, benzodiazepines, anticholinergics, and neuroleptic medication classes. Indications for palliative sedation are rare, and it should be used only within the context of specialty palliative care to ensure that optimal, current symptom management has been provided, including nonpharmacological interventions such as assessment of spiritual distress, psychosocial support, and environmental alterations. Although governed by the ethical principle of *double effect*, palliative sedation practice varies and is rare enough that not every health care team member will feel comfortable with every intervention.[8] Professional team members may have different opinions about whether palliative sedation is indicated, particularly when it is used for psychological distress. Some team members may feel that continual sedation is too similar to euthanasia, eliminates patient control, and does not allow the patient to continue to consent. Nurses should become involved in developing and revising protocols for defining the practice of, and indications for, palliative sedation in their practice settings, and also ensure that palliative care specialists are available to guide the intervention. Policies and protocols need to allow for "conscientious objection" by individual team members, but still ensure that palliative sedation is an available option, when needed.[10]

INDIVIDUAL COMPETENCY

For nurses to improve palliative care, they need to take responsibility for their individual practice, including self-assessment of knowledge and skills, to identify areas where competency needs to be attained or improved. Although most nurses practice within a nursing specialty, palliative care needs are present in all care settings and most nursing practice. Areas of competency may include updating knowledge of symptom management, improving communication skills, assessing spiritual needs, and learning better methods of teaching patients and families. Another method for self-assessment is evaluating one's own practice outcomes. This can occur through quality improvement studies, medical record reviews, case studies, and clinical supervision.

Self-Care

The emotional nature of working with patients and families who are living with, and dying of, chronic and end-stage illness can be stressful for many practitioners. Nurses need to acknowledge that they and other professional caregivers will also experience feelings of loss and helplessness during the course of providing palliative and end-stage care. Individual nurses need to expect these feelings, to acknowledge them, and to find healthy strategies for coping with their feelings. A nurse's stress can affect his or her quality of life, as well as the ability to give optimal patient care. Some strategies that have been shown to be effective include: relaxation, using a variety of techniques such as guided imagery, meditation, and passive relaxation; self-reflection; teaching or mentoring others; exercise; yoga; and journaling. Each nurse needs to monitor his or her own stress level and to find the most effective, individual coping strategies.

Every member of the palliative care team should be sensitive to any coping difficulties experienced by colleagues. Some hospice and palliative care programs offer formal support mechanisms for professionals, such as support groups or debriefing sessions for the team. Many organizations also provide individual, confidential counseling services through employee assistance programs that employees can access at any time. Many team members find it helpful to seek out individual colleagues who understand their work and with whom they can debrief and explore feelings when needed.

Nurses Integrating Care

Nurses have the opportunity to affect the organizations where they practice by integrating palliative care into all care settings. Initiatives can come from a variety of mechanisms. Organizational quality improvement measures, such as improving utilization of advanced directives, are often a good way to integrate palliative care because these indicators already have organizational support and are often recognized as both important and needing improvement. Another helpful mechanism for improving palliative care in organizations is to seek out and join others in the organization with interests in improving specific aspects of palliative care. These may include departments or groups such as pharmacy, pastoral care, ethics committees, and pain consultation teams. In addition, other nurses (including advance practice nurses who function in specific roles in pain management), educational and quality care departments, and specialties such as geriatrics, oncology, care of acquired immunodeficiency syndrome, pediatrics, and critical care often welcome support in improving patient comfort, decision making, and symptom management.

For all patient care, the benefits and applicability of integrating palliative care concepts into nursing practice apply to diverse care settings, including ambulatory care, intensive care, pediatrics, and emergency departments and cover areas such as pain and symptom management, advance care planning, bereavement care, and optimizing care at the time of death. In 1997, the American Association of Nursing Colleges identified 15 nursing competencies necessary for the care of patients during the transition at the end of life (Box 39-1). Enhancing the care environment is another way to affect organizational improvement in palliative care. Some examples are furniture designed for family comfort, a designated space for family cell phone use, lighting that can be softened and controlled by patients, and calming colors and art work in patients' rooms.

> **Box 39-1.** *Competencies Necessary for Nurses to Provide High-Quality Care to Patients and Families During the Transition at the End of Life*
>
> Recognize dynamic changes in population demographics, health care economics, and service delivery that necessitate improved professional preparation for end-of-life care.
>
> Promote the provision of comfort care to the dying as an active, desirable, and important skill, and an integral component of nursing care.
>
> Communicate effectively and compassionately with the patient, family, and health care team members about end-of-life issues.
>
> Recognize one's own attitudes, feelings, values, and expectations about death and the individual, cultural, and spiritual diversity existing in these beliefs and customs.
>
> Demonstrate respect for the patient's views and wishes during end-of-life care.
>
> Collaborate with interdisciplinary team members while implementing the nursing role in end-of-life care.
>
> Use scientifically based standardized tools to assess symptoms (e.g., pain, dyspnea [breathlessness] constipation, anxiety, fatigue, nausea/vomiting, and altered cognition) experienced by patients at the end-of-life.
>
> Use data from symptom assessment to plan and intervene in symptom management using state-of-the-art traditional and complementary approaches.
>
> Evaluate the impact of traditional, complementary, and technological therapies on patient-centered outcomes.
>
> Assess and treat multiple dimensions, including physical, psychological, social, and spiritual needs, to improve quality at the end of life.
>
> Assist the patient, family, colleagues, and one's self to cope with suffering, grief, loss, and bereavement in end-of-life care.
>
> Apply legal and ethical principles in the analysis of complex issues in end-of-life care, recognizing the influence of personal values, professional codes, and patient preferences.
>
> Identify barriers and facilitators to patients' and caregivers' effective use of resources.
>
> Demonstrate skill at implementing a plan for improved end-of-life care within a dynamic and complex health care delivery system.
>
> Apply knowledge gained from palliative care research to end-of-life education and care.

From American Association of Nursing Colleges: *A Peaceful Death*, Washington, DC, 1997, American Association of Nursing Colleges.

The Approach

In some organizations, palliative care has been integrated so nurses in general care units or ambulatory settings routinely assess patients from a holistic perspective and identify palliative care needs, thus establishing an optimal, individualized care plan. In other organizations, palliative care (including the transition from acute care to comfort care at the end of life) often does not occur without a specialty palliative care consultation. The ideal nursing care model incorporates both: palliative care standards integrated into all patient care *and* the availability of specialty palliative care consultations for complex patients. Complex patients can include those with intractable symptoms, difficult symptoms of dying such as terminal delirium, suffering related to psychosocial or spiritual needs, and ethical concerns, such as requests for euthanasia from the patient or family. A nurse who is competent in providing palliative care will be able to do so in any role and for any patient population. Some general guidelines that illustrate a palliative care approach are listed in the following subsections. The nurse will always assess or establish these elements from the assessment of other team members when beginning care with a patient.

ESTABLISH WHAT THEY KNOW

The nurse begins each patient assessment by ascertaining what the patient and family members understand about the patient's disease status and prognosis. Not only does this provide insight into the patient's and family's knowledge base, but also it often provides clues about how each person is coping emotionally.

DETERMINE THE LEGAL PROXY

The nurse needs to determine whether the patient has the capacity to make decisions and who the surrogate decision maker will be should the patient be unable to make decisions. Even a weak or dying patient who has capacity has the right to make decisions for himself or herself. Patients may delegate decision making to another, but they need to be aware of the laws that guide medical decision making if they wish to delegate to someone who is not the legal next of kin, unless previous legal arrangements have been made. The health care team needs to be aware of and to document these arrangements to honor them when the patient can no longer participate in decisions. Patients with capacity who verbally delegate medical decisions or information flow to another person should still be asked by members of the health care team, periodically and in private, whether they wish to continue to delegate in this way. When patients have a language barrier with their caregivers, medical translators who are not friends or family need to be provided when critical information is communicated and when decisions are needed. When patients lack capacity, the nurse needs to determine the legal decision maker and to provide the name and contact information to other members of the health care team so communication and decisions are directed to the correct person.

DETERMINE THE PATIENT'S PROGNOSIS

Information from the patient's primary care provider and other health care consultants, and the patient's current status, will provide information about the likely prognosis. If it is probable that the patient is imminently dying, assessments and individualized interventions must be accelerated to facilitate a peaceful, comfortable death that honors the values of the patient and family. Counselor members of the team such as social workers, chaplains, and the patient's community clergy, if applicable, should be alerted to the patient's imminent dying, to assist in planning care and support at the time of dying.

IDENTIFY GOALS OF CARE AND PATIENT PRIORITIES

In the context of the patient's prognosis, reasonable goals of care need to be determined. Patients and family members should be encouraged to express their current concerns, unaddressed issues, and priorities. The nurse addresses any immediate needs identified by the patient and family and discusses the reason for the referral, if it resulted from a hospice or palliative care consultation. The nurse communicates or clarifies goals of care to other members of the health care team.

ASSESS PAIN AND OTHER SYMPTOMS

The nurse assesses the level of distress and meaning of symptoms to the patient and formulates a care plan based on the patient's priority for symptom management on an ongoing basis. Pain and symptoms need to be assessed using standardized assessment tools that are tailored to the patient's cognitive abilities, developmental stage, and preference. For example, a patient with mild dementia may not be able to use a 10-point visual analog pain scale but may be able to describe pain as mild, moderate, or severe. It is essential to communicate with the health care team about which assessment tools are best suited to the individual patient to ensure consistency in the use of tools among all team members.

A palliative care approach includes anticipation of symptoms related to disease progression and the dying process so these symptoms can be prevented or minimized. For example, a dying patient may lose the ability to swallow. Nurses need to collaborate with the medical team about which medications could be discontinued and for alternate administration routes for medications needed to manage symptoms. Nurses also need to continually assess for burdensome interventions that may cause discomfort or negatively affect the patient's quality of life, such routine vital signs, laboratory studies, and other diagnostic tests when they cease to provide information that will influence the patient's care.

ASSESS EMOTIONAL ISSUES

The nurse needs to be competent at discussing difficult topics related to prognosis and questions or fears about dying that patients and family members need to process. The nurse should review previously identified preferences related to advanced care planning and listen for values and beliefs expressed by the patient and family members. The competent nurse will be emotionally prepared and comfortable discussing psychosocial and spiritual concerns, and will be able to anticipate many of the questions patients and families may ask. This often means listening to expressions of sadness and grief in situations where there are no real answers and understanding the value of empathetic presence and support.

MAKE REFERRALS

After assessment of the patient's status, the nurse collaborates in a timely manner with the primary health care provider and other professional team members to communicate the need for orders and referrals to address the patient's needs. The team reviews the patient's and family's goals of care and determines what other goals need to be discussed or clarified. The team then determines who will document goals and plans in the medical record, who will communicate what to the patient and family, and, if necessary, who will communicate with any other professional caregivers.

FACILITATE GRIEVING

The nurse should be prepared to provide spiritual support and grief resources before and at the time of the patient's death, in addition to the support provided by the patient's own clergy, counselor, or the counseling members of the health care team. The nurse ensures that written information about normal grief reactions and sources for grief support and counseling are also provided.

FOSTER QUALITY OF LIFE

A goal of the art of palliative nursing is to assist patients in the identification and accomplishment of remaining life goals. This may mean helping patients move to the place where they wish to die, helping to complete a task, or communicating important information to loved ones. Some patients wish to plan or have input in their funeral arrangements and may look to members of the health care team for help with this task. Enhancing the patient's immediate environment impacts quality of life, especially for the bed-bound person. For inpatient facilities, this may mean moving furniture to accommodate better window views and providing a quiet environment with dimmed lighting, music of the patient's preference, and items from home. Whether at home or in an inpatient setting, the nurse should collaborate with family and caregivers to create or enhance ways to help the patient have some control over his or her own environment and daily routine.

FACILITATE A "GOOD DEATH"

At the time of dying, the nurse facilitates privacy for the patient and family and any other changes to the patient's immediate environment that may enhance the comfort of the patient or family. At the time of dying, it is critical for inpatient routines to be altered and tailored to the needs of the patient and family. Space to rest and sleep in the patient's room, areas outside the room for consultation, family respite, and telephone calls are helpful to visiting family members. Nurses need to provide a balance between support and privacy and should check frequently to ensure that the patient and family feel cared for and supported, not abandoned. An increase in the frequency of professional visits may be necessary for patients who are dying at home. Family members should be assured of a timely, knowledgeable, and sensitive response from the health care team, including the on-call team members.

Nurses and other members of the health care team should encourage family expressions of grief, even when their loved one can no longer communicate. Family members will need information about the dying process, what to expect at the time of death, and information on local laws regarding funerals and burial. Nurses need to assess for cultural and religious practices and rituals that may be important to families and should act as facilitators. Nurses should be a role model of compassionate, respectful patient care. One way to assist the family's grieving is to ensure that the patient's death "went well" from their perspective.

Professional Associations

Membership in local, regional, and national nursing and other professional organizations provides opportunities for nurse networking, peer support, and education. Nurses who become involved in professional organizations at the committee or board level can directly affect specialty nursing practice through policy development, professional presentations, and committee work. Professional organizations depend largely on the volunteer expertise of professional nurses. The rewards to the individual nurse are enormous in enhancing their individual, professional development.

The HPNA has grown to represent more palliative nurses than any other organization in the world. The HPNA provides special interest groups in the areas of pediatrics, advanced practice geriatrics, administration, and research. Technical assistance is available to regional HPNA groups to give hospice and palliative care nurses local networking opportunities, as are resources and expertise from the national organization. HPNA has provided a variety of educational opportunities for nurses through their journal (the *Journal of Hospice and Palliative Nursing*), an annual clinical conference, teleconferences, and many educational publications. In addition, the HPNA hosts train-the-trainer conferences throughout the year, the End-of-life Nursing Education Consortium, and the HPNA Clinical Review to provide curricula and teaching strategies that allow professional nurses to teach their colleagues.

Specialty Certification for the Nursing Team

In 1994, the first specialty certification examination in hospice nursing was offered by the (then) National Board for Certification of Hospice Nurses. In 1996, a role delineation study conducted by this organization demonstrated a common core of practice for hospice and palliative nurses. This provided the validation for broadening the specialty beyond those who practice in hospice programs to include palliative care nurse specialists in non-hospice settings. Subsequently, The National Board for Certification of Hospice Nurses and the HNA changed the names of their organizations by adding "palliative," to reflect the expanded scope of the specialty.

The NBCHPN has expanded specialty certification for other members of the hospice and palliative nursing team. Specialty certification for nursing assistants began in 2002 and in September 2004 for Licensed Practical and Vocational Nurses. The NBCHPN collaborated with the American Nurses' Credentialing Center in 2003 to create the first Advanced Practice Palliative Care Certification. In 2005, the NBCHPN became sole proprietor of the certification for APNs. Successful candidates who attain specialty certification earn the credentials identifying their specialty. Credentials for Hospice and Palliative Certified Members of the Nursing Team are:

Advanced Practice Nurse (APN): ACHPN
Registered Nurse (RN): CRNH
Licensed Practical Nurse of Licensed Vocational Nurse (LPN/VN): CHPLN
Nursing Assistant (CNA, HHA): CHPNA

Future Trends

PALLIATIVE CARE SPECIALISTS

The need for palliative care specialists is anticipated to continue to increase as the population ages and more people are living with chronic, serious illnesses. The success of treatments that allow people to live longer also creates an increased need for symptom management for diseases that can be managed but not cured. Because palliative care services are not currently regulated, there is an inconsistency in the ability to meet the needs of patients and families comprehensively and holistically. Palliative care programs need to standardize care by adhering to the recommended standards developed by the NCP, regardless of the palliative service practice model.[5]

ADVANCED PRACTICE PALLIATIVE NURSES

APNs are increasing in number and are poised to assume a variety of necessary roles in palliative care. In 2003, the first certification examination for APNs was offered through a collaborative effort between the American Nurses Credentialing Center and the NBCHPN. APNs are prepared at the master's degree level or beyond and are either nurse practitioners or nurse clinicians. APNs are prepared for leadership roles in clinical care, education, consultation, and research.[11]

PALLIATIVE EDUCATION

Palliative care practice will improve on a large scale only when undergraduate nursing programs incorporate palliative care education into their curricula and more graduate level programs in palliative care become available. The End-of-life Nursing Education Consortium project originally designed its curriculum to allow undergraduate programs to adapt and learn from it. Madonna University in Michigan offers interdisciplinary hospice education programs. The Breen School of Nursing at Ursuline College in Ohio was the first program to prepare advanced practice nurses in palliative care.[12] More graduate and postgraduate programs will be needed to fill future needs.

NURSING RESEARCH

In addition to the common barriers in nursing research (e.g., lack of research funds and a limited number of nursing researchers), research in end-of-life nursing care faces a set of unique issues. Some of these research challenges include study accrual issues related to rapidly declining subjects and late referrals to hospice and palliative care programs. In addition, there are the ethical considerations (e.g., the ability of subjects to provide consent) and the challenge of conducting research on emotionally and physically vulnerable patient and family populations. Research tools need to be designed that balance scientific rigor and potential burden to the subject, and must be sensitive to the fact that, for these subjects, time, especially quality time, is a limited commodity.[12] Conversely, many seriously ill patients and their families respond positively to requests for participation in research studies. Some patients see this as a way to contribute to science and the well-being of others, providing some sense of purpose and allowing them to feel that they are giving as well as being cared for.

The National Institute of Nursing Research (NINR) developed an end-of-life research agenda after the publication of the Institute of Medicine report on the scientific knowledge gaps about end-of-life care. In August 2000, the NINR was joined by the National Cancer Institute, the National Center for Complementary and Alternative Medicine, the National Institute of Allergy and Infectious Diseases, the National Institute of Dental and Craniofacial Research, and the National Institute on Aging to collaborate on the theme of "Quality of Life for Individuals at the End of Life." The NINR has since funded more than 22 research projects and 7 training and career development awards related to end-of-life care.[13]

PEARLS

- Careful listening is a key skill for every palliative care practitioner.
- At the end of life, patients may have capacity for decision making at some times, but not others. Patients should always be assessed for capacity and should be allowed to make decisions when they are able.
- Conflicting goals among the patient, family members, and health care team require respectful negotiation and clear communication.
- Nurses should appreciate the value of therapeutic presence, even when traditional nursing interventions are no longer effective or needed.
- The nurse should anticipate what family members need to know, because most will not know what to ask or be able to articulate all their needs.
- The dying experience can be improved in *any* care setting.

PITFALLS

- All members of the health care team should communicate with the designated decision maker, rather than the most convenient family member or caregiver.

- Do not avoid discussion of imminent dying with family members who do not appear "ready" to hear the information. They still need to be informed, supported, and coached through their grieving.

- Decreasing medications and burdensome interventions should not be equated with decreasing care. Nurses need to ensure that patients are frequently monitored for comfort needs, and families are well supported by the entire health care team.

- The nurse needs to rely on the entire team to meet the needs of the patient and family and should not assume that he or she is the only one with the expertise or relationship that is needed.

Summary

Nursing has been instrumental in the evolution of modern palliative care by developing and defining this nursing specialty to meet the needs of a society where people are living longer with chronic, serious illnesses and wish to die on their own terms. In many ways, palliative care is an ideal nursing practice because it combines the art and science of nursing within the context of interprofessional collaborative practice, thus positively affecting patients, families, and society.

Resources

Educational resources can be found at http://www.supportivecarecoalition.org/EducationalOpportunities/elnec.htm.

Two respected curricula on palliative care for nursing are provided by TNEEL and ELNEC which can be found, respectively, at http://www.tneel.uic.edu/tneel.asp and http://www.aacn.nche.edu/elnec/curriculum.htm.

Two associations that provide educational materials and other resources are: The Hospice and Palliative Nurses Association and The National Board for Certification of Hospice and Palliative Nurses.

References

1. Joint Commission on Accreditation of Hospitals: *Accreditation manual for hospice*, Chicago, 1986, Joint Commission on Accreditation of Hospitals.
2. Joint Commission: *Comprehensive accreditation manual for hospitals. Standard I: rights, ethics and responsibilities*, Oakbrook Terrace, Ill, 2009–2010, The Joint Commission, RI-3.
3. Association news, *J Hosp Palliat Nurs* 7:2, 2005.
4. Sheldon JE, Dahlin C, Zeri K: *Statement on the scope and standards of hospice and palliative nursing practice: the hospice and palliative nurses association*, Dubuque, IA, 2000, Kendall/Hunt Publishing.
5. National Consensus Project for Quality Palliative Care Clinical Practice Guidelines for Quality Palliative Care: 2009. Available at www.nationalconsensusproject.org.
6. American Board of Nursing Specialties Accreditation Standards. Available at www.nursingcertfication.org/pdf/ac_standards_short/pdf.
7. National Council of State Boards of Nursing Professional Boundaries: a Nurse's Guide to the Importance of Appropriate Professional Boundaries. Available at www.ncsbn.org.
8. Schwarz KA: Ethical aspects of palliative care. In Matzo ML, Sherman DW, editors: *Palliative care nursing: quality care to the end of life*, New York, 2001, Springer Publishing, pp 493–504.
9. Grady D: The hard facts behind a heartbreaking case, *New York Times* 493–504, June 19, 2005.

10. Quill TE, Lo B, Brock DW, et al: Last resort options for palliative sedation, *Ann Intern Med* 151(6):423, 2009.
11. Phillips SJ: A comprehensive look at the legislative issues affecting advanced nursing practice, *Nurse Pract* 30:14–47, 2005.
12. Ferrell BR: Research. In Ferrell BR, Coyle N, editors: *Textbook of palliative nursing*, Oxford, 2001, Oxford University Press, p 702.
13. National Institute of Nursing Research: Available at www.ninr.nihgov/ninr/research/diversity/mission.html.

CHAPTER 40

Social Work Practice in Palliative Care: An Evolving Science of Caring

MATTHEW J. LOSCALZO

Definition of Social Work	Prospective Identification of Barriers to Quality of Life through Biopsychosocial Screening
Psychosocial Context of Palliative Care	
Credentialing	Physical Quality of Life: Education, Advocacy, and Skills
Social Work Values in Palliative Care	Practical Quality of Life
Social Work Competencies in Palliative Care	Psychological Quality of Life
Emerging Role of Palliative Care Social Work	Social Quality of Life
	Spiritual Quality of Life
Social Work in Action: Maximizing Quality of Life	Pearls
	Pitfalls
	Summary

Social work is a younger profession than either medicine or nursing. Although some form of social work has been present wherever social systems have been in place, social work as a health care profession has its roots in the early 20th century. Social work in health care has always been closely aligned with underserved populations; it focuses on the interplay between individuals and society. Serving the underserved has been both part of its core calling and a liability for the social work profession. The liability comes from being aligned with those (the underserved) who are not privileged in society.

In some ways, social work's unconditional acceptance that all humans have value both to the individual and to society and the opposition of behaviors that are harmful to self or others has been influenced by the fact that social work evolved from a feminine perspective. Although it is difficult to make generalizations about gender, feminine culture places value on fairness, justice, allocation of resources, interpersonal relationships, and the personal internal experience of the individual, especially as it relates to the *processes* of communication and interaction. The importance of the female perspective in the evolution of professional social work is discussed elsewhere.[1] Social work, with its perspective, has the potential to challenge the value

570

systems of society generally and medicine specifically.[2] Mainstream medicine has traditionally tended to be *outcome* focused, whereas social workers value *process*. Palliative care has the potential to integrate the very best that diversity and technology offer while putting the spirit of sharing and healing back into the uniquely human experience of making prolonged efforts that are often needed to protect people from suffering.

Definition of Social Work

Numerous formal definitions of social work have been proposed. One of these, from the International Federation of Social Workers, follows:

> *The social work profession promotes social change, problem solving in human relationships and the empowerment and liberation of people to enhance well-being. Utilizing theories of human behavior and social systems, social work intervenes at the points where people interact with their environments. Principles of human rights and social justice are fundamental to social work.*[3]

However, at present, there is no established definition of palliative care social work. A patient's experience of serious life-threatening or debilitating illness is influenced by at least three domains that are a target for professional social work: personality and coping, family system patterns, and practical resources. The palliative care social worker needs to be expert at assessing and implementing approaches within a systems perspective to maximize the well-being and functioning of the patient/client and the family in all these domains. In addition to providing patient care, social workers discover new knowledge through research, develop educational programs, and advocate for social change that furthers skilled and respectful care for all members of a diverse society. The social worker may take on varied roles, as noted in Table 40-1.

Table 40-1. Social Work Roles

Advocate	Group leader
Change agent	Information giver
Clinician	Program developer
Colleague	Problem solver
Consultant	Researcher
Communicator	Role model
Counselor	Systems expert
Educator	Teacher
Ethicist	Team builder and catalyst

From LP Gwyther, T Altilio, S Backer, et al: Social work competencies in palliative and end-of-life care, *J Soc Work Palliat Care* 1:87–120, 2005.

Psychosocial Context of Palliative Care

Social workers meet the needs of patients and their informal caregivers by supporting efforts to maximize their well-being, independence, and problem-solving abilities. Attachment, commitment, challenge, loss, grief, death, reintegration, resolution, and growth characterize the continuum of the human experience throughout life. It is within the psychosocial context, not the disease, that people live their lives. In a study that reviewed the patient's perspective at the end of life, patients with chronic obstructive pulmonary disease, cancer, or acquired immunodeficiency syndrome were asked what their physicians could do to improve the quality of care they provided. For all three diseases, the importance of emotional support, communication, accessibility, and continuity was emphasized.[4] These are all essential elements of the psychosocial domain. A number of studies across chronic diseases have recently demonstrated the effectiveness of self-management involving education, problem-solving, and social support.[5] People need to feel participatory and to feel that they have been heard. Social work stresses the importance of assessing the person-in-context and establishing a therapeutic alliance.

Palliative care needs differ by socioeconomic group. Most individuals (70%–80%) in industrialized nations will die in their later years from a known chronic, degenerative disease that may last for years.[6] In the Unites States, especially for the rural and urban poor, coping with loss and bereavement may be disproportionately experienced as a consequence of violence. Sudden, violent loss requires specialized support and management, and the psychosocial interventions, where and when they exist, are highly condensed. Other clearly definable disenfranchised segments of society, including the elderly, must also bear the unequal and added burden of having to understand and navigate a patchwork health care system that is poorly organized, reactive, inefficient, and sometimes unable to meet their needs.[7] Social workers help provide services independent of socioeconomic group. They are often engaged in the tasks of helping people access the system who are having difficulty doing so. This is true in palliative care no less than other aspects of medicine. Some of the many settings in which social workers practice are set out in Table 40-2.

Table 40-2. The Many Settings of Social Workers

Adoption agencies	Mental health centers
Adult protective services	Military centers
Assisted living	Morgues
Child welfare	Places of worship
Community centers	Poverty relief organizations
Disease-specific advocacy groups	Prisons
Financial counseling services	Private counseling practices
Funeral homes	Schools
Health care settings (e.g., home health care, nursing homes, hospices)	Social supportive agencies
Homeless shelters	Substance abuse clinics
Immigration offices	Rehabilitation programs
Legal and court systems	Relief organizations responding to natural disasters and terrorism
Mediation centers	Research foundations

Social workers do not see their patients/clients as separate and distinct from the social milieu in which they exist. Social workers help people to solve problems and to make hard decisions, often in the face of great uncertainty. Social workers serve as the connective tissue of the health care and social systems by supporting, advocating, informing, educating, sensitizing, counseling, and synergizing all available resources and inherent strengths to the benefit of the patient, family, and society. Social workers have an ethical duty to go beyond direct services to patients and families, a responsibility that always includes awareness of the greater good to society. Social workers need to see challenges and opportunities from a systems perspective because the focus of the intervention may just as easily be on the individual, the institution, or both simultaneously.

People with chronic life-threatening illness and their committed family members are generally not in a position to find the time, focus, energy, or resources to fight for structural systems change. So, although many of the barriers to living a meaningful life are not caused by the individual, the individual must ultimately manage the problem within existing systems. Social workers aim to promote self-reliance and independence while ensuring that a realistic assessment of the situation is made and clearly communicated. Social workers, regardless of the practice setting, value and actively work to promote social justice. Palliative care highly values and maximizes the benefits of the supportive social milieu of the patient and family in a way that modern medicine has long forsaken. It is not by accident that palliative care services are often provided in the home. The home is the territory of the patient and the family. Palliative care provides an opportunity to change not only how health care is practiced but also how society as a whole treats its ill members.

People receiving palliative care are usually facing and must learn to live with increasing levels of loss—loss of function, dreams, relationships, and more. The degree of physical deterioration, the number of internal resources, and social support factors are key interacting variables in how people manage challenge and live meaningful lives. Within the context of palliative care, social workers are attuned to the potential meanings ascribed to the inherent sense of loss related to chronic debilitating illness and how it is manifested at all developmental stages. For example, social workers are aware that Medicare recipients with life-threatening illness are more likely to access higher-quality medical centers and to spend less time in the hospital if they are married (compared with Medicare recipients who are widowed).[8] People who are married are less likely than unmarried people to spend the end of their lives in a nursing home.[9] Because men often die at least 5 years earlier than women, at the end of life women are at risk of being unmarried and alone. People are particularly vulnerable at the end of life, given the myriad complex demands related to the need to understand medical information, important decisions that must be made, and the implications of these decisions for the person and the family. Although managing the demands of chronic illness is a challenge to all patients and families, certain factors significantly increase vulnerability. Being financially disadvantaged is one of the most important risk factors for inadequate medical care and premature death.

Losing control over matters that are most important to people, such as an emotional connection to the person they knew, may be exacerbated by the presence of unmanaged psychiatric symptoms. According to the Institute of Medicine's report of 2001, "A major problem in palliative care is the under recognition, under diagnosis, and thus under treatment of … significant distress … ranging from existential anguish to anxiety and depression".[10] Psychiatric symptoms of depression, anxiety, and delirium in the chronically ill and in the final stages of life are frequently overlooked, and problems in the spiritual, psychosocial, and existential suffering domains are virtually ignored. Psychosocial concerns of the dying patient include not prolonging death; maintaining a sense of control; minimizing family caregiving burdens; and strengthening ties.[11] When patients' priorities are not followed, emotional distress will also be experienced by the family caregivers.

Family caregivers experience many mini-losses on multiple levels and for extended periods in the face of serious debilitating illness. The accumulation of assaults on their integrity can undermine the ability to respond in an adaptive manner. The family caregivers of people with advanced disease can also be affected by the caregiver's own disabling psychiatric problems, although fewer than half these caregivers ever access mental health services.[12] Social workers are trained to identify psychiatric and social problems and they usually have more communication with the families than the rest of the health care team. In cancer settings, social workers are estimated to provide approximately 75% of the mental health services overall.[13] Because families know the patient best, they are able to see changes that a busy physician may not perceive. Patients and family members are also more likely to share information about emotional and family problems with the social worker because they perceive this to be a social work function and also because they do not want to "bother" the doctor with their personal problems. Patients and families perceive the delineation of duties in their own minds and act accordingly. These perceptions are reinforced by the environment and by the attitudes of health care professionals. Social workers may also have the time, interest, and training to talk about emotions, family problems, and psychosocial concerns that some physicians and nurses do not. Ultimately, managing the sense of loss and sadness inherent in having a serious chronic illness or intractable noxious symptoms comes down to trying to put a life into an overall context and staying connected to loved ones even as the reality of separation and loss becomes evident. Within this context, loss is an ongoing process of not being able to control those things that are most valued.

Social work focuses on the strengths of individuals, families, and systems to find resources to manage challenges of loss. By analogy with the traditional pathology and physiology models that focus on the origin of disease and care, the psychosocial model is interested in the genesis of processes that maximize the inherent strengths of people and their systems.[14] Seeing people as part of a social system generates many opportunities for assistance, support, and problem solving. Social workers are best known for their practical problem-solving skills and their ability to identify, link, and actively engage supportive resources.

Credentialing

Medicine has recently made significant progress in credentialing in palliative care. At present, there is no formal process to credential, board certify, or license social workers specifically in palliative care, but this may be changing. As with other professions, there is an increasing consensus that credentialing in palliative care is necessary. Social work organizations and other interprofessional organizations are invested in ensuring the quality of services provided by psychosocial professionals within palliative care. In addition, educational material in the form of comprehensive books and journals focusing on social work competencies in palliative care are now available. The National Association of Social Workers (NASW) in the United States now has online courses on care at the end of life available to its membership of more than 160,000. There are now many conference-based opportunities for social workers to gain knowledge and skills in palliative care.

Most social workers have a 2-year master's degree from an accredited school of social work. Bachelor's degrees in social work (BSW) are also awarded and are especially helpful in underserved areas where masters in social work (MSW)–educated social workers are not available. Increasingly, the doctorate in social work will be favored, especially in academic medical institutions. Because social work is present in so many settings, schools of social work are hard pressed to prepare social workers for all the specialty areas. However, palliative care has gained momentum in universities in recent years, and training for social workers in this area has improved significantly.

Social workers differ from other professions in that so many social workers come to the field in the middle of their careers or in midlife. Some of these social workers have experienced significant loses in their own lives and know how to support people as they manage the emotional and practical aspects of healing. The wisdom, maturity, and experience that social workers bring to palliative care offer a great resource for them and for the people they serve.

Social Work Values in Palliative Care

In 1993, the NASW produced the "Client Self-Determination in End-of-Life Decisions," a policy statement that delineated the needed role of social workers in ensuring that the client's rights are respected, that clients are fully informed, and that quality of life be valued as an end in itself.[15] In 2003 the NASW reinforced in further policy statements the natural synergies and values between palliative care and social work.[16]

In their 1999 position paper on euthanasia, the Association of Oncology Social Work supported a person's right to make informed choices, including through open discussion, information gathering, and advocating for best services available, while at the same time clearly limiting the level of social work participation. AOSW does not support assisting in hastening death. Inherent in these statements is the acknowledgment that to begin to address the needs of the chronically ill and the dying, social workers are frequently put in emotionally laden situations of great ambiguity, without adequate training, and within a health care system in dire need of reform. In 1999, a survey supported by the Project on Death in America documented the lack of training opportunities in palliative care for social workers, including education, clinical care, and research.[17]

Social Work Competencies in Palliative Care

A consensus statement of the Social Work Leadership Summit on End-of-Life and Palliative Care 2002[18] outlined the need for standards of practice. Knowledge competencies, skills competencies, and practice values and attitudes were used as the three organizing concepts for social work competencies across practice settings. The summit conference developed a core statement that guides the functions of all social workers regardless of the setting. Complementing this work is that by leaders in social work who have identified areas the social worker should have awareness of and management skills in. Competency areas are noted in Box 40-1. The clarification of

Box 40-1. *Knowledge Competencies*

- Patient and family as the focus of care
- Biological, psychological, social, emotional, spiritual, practical, informational, and financial variables
- Care and setting options
- Common biopsychosocial disease and treatment-related symptoms throughout the illness experience
- Cognitive behavioral, psychodynamic, crisis, and environmental interventions that manage distress
- Signs and symptoms of imminent death
- Clinical and culturally aware information about death and related expectations of particular patients and families
- Religious, spiritual, and cultural values and rituals and beliefs
- Ethical and legal principles
- Experience of grief, loss, and bereavement
- Equity in access to care
- Insurance, entitlements, and financial processes and challenges
- Community resources
- Standards of care established by professional and legislative organizations

SKILLS COMPETENCIES
- Assessment as the foundation of social work practice
- Consideration of physical, functional, financial, social, emotional, spiritual, and psychological factors
- Strengths and coping resources maximized
- Family functioning
- Cultural expectations in communication and decision making
- Spiritual and religious beliefs
- Emotional issues
- Body integrity and functioning and level of dependences
- Barriers to maximizing health and quality of life
- Legal and ethical principles used to make health care decisions
- Safety issues, abuse or neglect, suicide, requests to hasten death

TREATMENT PLANNING AND INTERVENTIONS
- Treatment plans revised according to ongoing needs and tailored according to race, age, culture, religions socioeconomic, educational, and lifestyle
- Education, information, communication enhancement, supportive counseling, Gestalt techniques, brief therapies, life review, stress management, problem solving, family counseling and therapy, cognitive behavioral therapy, spiritual support, crisis intervention, conflict resolution, advocacy, case management, expressive therapies
- Varied modalities, including groups, families, couples, and individuals
- Teamwork by fostering communication, suggesting enhancements, documenting information and suggestions, sharing patient and family concerns, role modeling the management of team conflict, supporting self-awareness and self-care
- Program planning to include research, education, and clinical care
- Community outreach and education
- System change to enhance functioning and services at all levels
- Psychosocial research to identify and meet community needs
- Advocacy for human and dignified care for all populations, especially the most vulnerable

> **Box 40-1.** *Knowledge Competencies—cont'd*
>
> **PRACTICE VALUES AND ATTITUDES**
> - Client-centered care that is compassionate, sensitive, respectful with an openness to diversity at all levels
> - Recognition of personal attributes and attitudes as opportunities and challenges
> - Demonstrated respect for values and desires of patients and family
> - Active support to work with others on team and in the community
> - Support for an environment of support and hope
> - Commitment of personal growth and to advance new knowledge in the field through research

roles and duties will be helpful in developing clinical, educational, and research programs. In addition to these areas, attention is needed on the area of screening for psychosocial needs—something to which social workers are well-suited.[19]

Emerging Role of Palliative Care Social Work

Both palliative care and social work seek to build on personal strengths and encourage people to maximize their abilities to live a meaningful life that benefits society. Both fields share the view of the human being as having inherent worth, regardless of the situation, and share a focus that looks beyond and above disease diagnosis, while actively nurturing those qualities that have meaning for a particular individual. The very aspects of the human experience that create complexity and ambiguity also create the greatest opportunities to forge new relationships, to deepen existing ones, to review a life lived, and to decide how to live and be in the moment.

The United States Medicare Hospice Benefit, enacted in 1982, recognized the importance of psychosocial factors at the end of life and mandated coverage for social work in the care of the dying. In 1999, the Social Work Section of the National Hospice and Palliative Care Organization conducted the National Hospice Social Work Survey. Their findings can be summarized as follows[20]:

1. Social work services supported desired hospice outcomes.
2. Social workers were an important part of the intake and assessment process.
3. Frequent contacts by social workers were highly supportive of the hospice mission.
4. Social workers were instrumental in preventing crises.
5. Experienced social workers with a master's degree had better client outcomes.
6. Social workers who were supervised by a social worker also had better outcomes.
7. Increased social work involvement led to decreased hospitalizations, fewer home health aide visits, and higher patient satisfaction scores.
8. Greater social work involvement resulted in lower hospice costs.

Social workers value and enhance teamwork. Further, they enhance the values of autonomy and self-determination because these can be realized only when they are based on a sound foundation of honesty and open communication, and social workers are very strong in both these areas. Although people are resilient, they require accurate and honest information to make rational decisions and to begin integrating the emotional realities of their lives. There are serious long-term costs to ignoring reality, borne mostly by the patient and family. The patient and family lose invaluable time, trust in the health care system is eroded, and futile procedures are performed. Social workers also foster trust. For example, if research is perceived to be an important part of an institution's mission, there may be an inherent actual or perceived conflict in timely referrals to palliative care services. Patients and family members frequently need assurances that their trust in the health care team is well placed and that appropriate referrals will be made, especially when levels of stress and vulnerability are high. Generally, the ongoing demonstration of the quality of *both* the medical services and psychosocial support are needed for a relationship of trust. For example, in the Simultaneous Care Study (funded by the National Cancer Institute), a physician–nurse–social worker team teaches problem solving to enable cancer patients, family members, and health care professionals who are participating in clinical trials to make key transitional decisions together.[21]

Social Work in Action: Maximizing Quality of Life

Patients who are receiving palliative care tend to have many complex medical and psychosocial problems. Five to 10 years after the initial diagnosis of cancer, patients who are in remission or cured are often sicker and have more symptoms than a general population.[22] This finding is important because so many of the struggles of the chronically ill are invisible to a harried health care system strongly leveraged to reactive, intense, and episodic interventions focused on cure. Social workers can bridge between disease-directed treatment and the inherent human capabilities and strengths to maximize well-being in the presence of serious debilitating disease.

Prospective Identification of Barriers to Quality of Life through Biopsychosocial Screening

One effective way to identify barriers to quality of life is through prospective universal biopsychosocial screening of patients and families. Screening has been shown to be an efficient way to identify problems in a manner that does not stigmatize patients. It allows for triage to the appropriate person or resource and communicates that the health care team cares for and about the patient.[23]

Many of the problems manifested by people with serious illness are overshadowed by the focus on cure. The psychosocial aspects of care, though central to the patient and family, may be seen by health care professionals as time-consuming, potentially disruptive, and too emotionally charged to acknowledge within the busy clinical setting. There may also be the perception that if psychosocial problems were actually identified there would not be the professional services or resources to manage these concerns. This "don't ask don't tell" attitude is quite common even in large health systems. Patients and families are reluctant to discuss psychosocial and spiritual concerns because of fear of distracting the physician from focusing on the medical conversation and because they may not perceive the medical encounter as friendly to their personal problems. Finally, the influence of stigma around sharing highly personal vulnerabilities (e.g., mental illness, substance abuse, lack of financial resources) is underestimated by health care professionals and is reinforced by the lack of a systematic approach to discussing these potential barriers to family functioning and to maximizing the benefits of medical care and support. The National Comprehensive Cancer Network in 2005, and more recently the Institute of Medicine Report in 2007 (Cancer Care for the Whole Patient: Meeting Psychosocial Health Needs), recommended systematic biopsychosocial screening as the standard of clinical care for patients with serious illness.[24,25]

In the early 1990s two social workers introduced the first prospective program of biopsychosocial screening at a National Cancer Institute (NCI)–designated comprehensive cancer center in the United Sates.[26] This program established the feasibility of biopsychosocial screening in the busy clinical setting with good acceptance of cancer outpatients. Building on this experience in another NCI-designated comprehensive cancer center, a highly evolved screening instrument and program was introduced using touch-screen technology.[27,28] The Institute of Medicine recognized this program as a model for the country.[23] More recently, the City of Hope developed a touch-screen program called *SupportScreen* that identifies problems with an electronic interface that facilitates patient, physician, and multispecialist communication and automates personalized referrals in real time. The program identifies the patient's physical, social, emotional, spiritual, financial, psychosocial, and psychiatric problems at the time of diagnosis and at set times throughout the illness experience. It also creates a Summary Report that is provided to the designated health care team, so that communication is maximized and the team knows which member of the team is managing which problem.

PHYSICAL QUALITY OF LIFE: EDUCATION, ADVOCACY, AND SKILLS

Social workers play a crucial role by educating patients about the importance of easing the impact of physical symptoms and clarifying their expectations for effective management. This can be achieved by the following:

- Encouraging patients to share perceptions about what is happening to their bodies and why
- Communicating physical symptoms and side effects with the rest of the health care team
- Teaching those who lack the verbal skills or cognitive abilities to communicate effectively

Social workers also remind the team to address symptoms. When assistance is not readily available in the immediate setting, the social worker's advocacy efforts expand. The social worker may identify symptom management experts in the community when skill or motivation is lacking in the present setting. As with all health care professionals, the primary commitment is first to the patient and then to the institution. When this is not the case, the patient and family should be fully informed.

The social worker's role is to increase the sense of entitlement as it relates to management of physical discomfort and to advocate for what is possible. Given the concerns that patients, family members, and health care professionals commonly share about the use of narcotics and fear of addiction, the social worker has a role in clarifying the issues. Underserved groups and minorities are at particular risk for undertreatment of pain, so it is essential that social workers be thoroughly informed about the issues and skills in advocating for these groups.

Finally, social workers should be skilled in at least some interventions that directly reduce physical distress and tension, such as supportive counseling, distraction, relaxation, meditation, hypnosis, Lamaze breathing, and guided imagery.[29] For most patients, these skills can be readily taught and reinforced by involving family members or by audiotaping the exercises and skills.

PRACTICAL QUALITY OF LIFE

The importance of the practical needs of people can be invisible to the health care system until it interferes with care or follow-up. Housing, transportation, finances, health insurance, food, and comorbidities in the family are all powerful influences on the ability to access health care and the ability to live a meaningful life free from unnecessary suffering. Social workers are able to work within the system to make adjustments to maximize the benefit of medical and psychosocial care.

PSYCHOLOGICAL QUALITY OF LIFE

Fear, anxiety, depression, confusion, psychological numbing, lack of a sense of control and predictability, vulnerability, and feelings of being lost and adrift are examples of common experiences among patients in palliative care. Information, skills training, supportive counseling, advocacy, and referrals are used by socials workers to help patients and family members maintain a sense of direction, hope, and focus on function, comfort, and meaning.

SOCIAL QUALITY OF LIFE

Debilitating or life-threatening illness creates an intense sense of isolation, exposure, and vulnerability. The social milieu of the patient and family is the reference point for their lives, *not the hospital or the health care team.* Family, close friends, work relationships, and other support systems are where and how people function. Family members are often more distressed than the patient. In most situations, by actively supporting the family and social structure, the health care team can significantly help the patient and family to create an environment of empowerment and meaning that will continue after the death of the patient.

SPIRITUAL QUALITY OF LIFE

Most or all people have some sense of spiritual or existential yearnings and a connection that extends beyond the boundaries of their lives. Although most people also have an identified religious or spiritual belief system, some do not, and they also face the end of life. The ability to find a place in the universe where one's existence can have meaning is a powerful balm and a respite from the many challenges experienced by people with debilitating or life-threatening illness. Understanding how the individual uses his or her religious or spiritual belief system is essential in being able to help maximize a sense of well-being and connection to others.

The role of the social worker is to support existing adaptive belief systems that enable people to stay positively connected to something bigger than they are. This is usually best accomplished by encouraging people to communicate their beliefs openly, to stay connected to support systems, and to strive to make a legacy connection to those around them. Giving personally, materially, or otherwise to valued others is always a healing experience, especially when time is limited and life is emotionally condensed.

PEARLS

- Frail voices may belie the clarity of the condensed wisdom of a lifetime that offers great potential benefit to all society's children.
- The value system of palliative care has the potential to effect changes in the health care system and in societal norms.
- It is within the psychosocial context, *not the disease,* that people truly live their lives.
- Resources and resiliency should be explored early in the relationship to allow the health care provider, the patient, and the family to see beyond the illness and suffering.
- From the first encounter, stress the importance of psychosocial variables and family integrity as an essential element of medical care.
- Social work focuses on the strengths of individuals, families, and systems to find the resources necessary to manage the challenges of daily living.

PITFALLS

- The emotional impact of psychosocial concerns of patients on health care professionals can be underestimated.
- One may fail to recognize that the connection between mental health and social injustice is amplified in vulnerable persons.
- The social milieu of the patient and family is their reference point for their lives, *not the hospital or the health care team.*

Summary

Social workers in palliative care provide for the biopsychosocial needs of individuals with life-threatening or debilitating illness and their families, based on a value system that recognizes the worth of people regardless of the setting or individual situation. Social workers understand that it takes responsibility, knowledge, and courage to speak for those whose voices are too frail to be heard. Social workers also realize that if they do not actively speak for the vulnerable, without apology, the silence will eventually deafen and deaden the better parts of all of us. Frail voices may belie the clarity of the condensed wisdom of a lifetime that offers great potential benefit for all society's children.

Because of the incredibly broad range of settings in which social work services are provided, it is not possible to delineate the true scope of practice in a manner that would be truly reflective of even most social workers. However, this discussion of palliative care social work does provide an initial and evolving paradigm that can serve to stimulate a higher level of discussion that identifies the common values of social work and palliative care and the contributions social work will make in the future. Social work has played a key role in the evolution of palliative care and has clearly defined the contributions and relevance of the psychosocial perspective as practiced by highly trained social work clinicians and administrators. It is now essential that social work research and educational programs also be developed that clearly define a research agenda that fosters an environment where interprofessional programs can discover new knowledge that leads to a deeper sense of caring and respect for all individuals with life-threatening or debilitating illness, their families, and society overall. It is only when there is a true *science of caring* that whole patient–centered care will become our long sought after reality.

Resources

American Academy of Hospice and Palliative Medicine. This organization is dedicated to the advancement of palliative medicine through prevention and relief of patient and family suffering by providing education and clinical practice standards, fostering research, facilitating personal and professional development, and by public policy advocacy.
www.aahpm.org

American Psychosocial Oncology Society. This group includes all health care professionals who seek to advance the science and practice of psychosocial care for people with cancer.
http://apos-society.org

Association for Death Education and Counseling. This interprofessional group is dedicated to promoting excellence in death education, care of the dying, and bereavement counseling.
www.adec.org

Association of Oncology Social Work. Social work services are designed to assist individuals, families, groups, and communities through counseling, stress and symptom management, care planning, case management, system navigation, education, and advocacy.
www.aosw.org

NASW Standards for Social Work Practice in Palliative and End of Life Care. This is the most comprehensive overview of social work role in palliative care.
www.socialworkers.org/practice/bereavement/standards/default.asp

National Family Caregivers Association. This group supports, empowers, educates, and speaks up for the more than 50 million U.S. residents who care for a chronically ill, aged, or disabled loved one.
www.nfcacares.org

People Living With Cancer. This patient information Web site of the American Society of Clinical Oncology provides oncologist-approved information on more than 50 types of cancer and their treatments, clinical trials, coping, and side effects.
www.plwc.org

Cancer Support Community (formerly the Wellness Community and Gild's Club). This national nonprofit organization is dedicated to providing free emotional support, education, and hope for people with cancer and their loved ones.
www.cancersupportcommunity.org

References

1. Freedberg A: The feminine ethic of care and the professionalization of social work, *Social Work* 38:535–541, 1993.
2. Emmanuel L: Feminist perspectives in medical ethics, *N Engl J Med* 328:361, 1993.
3. International Federation of Social Workers: 2000 Definition Social Work. Available at www.ifsw.org/Publications/4.6e.pub.html.
4. Curtis JR, Wenrich MD, Carline JD, et al: Patients' perspectives on physician skill in end-of-life care: Differences between patients with COPD, cancer and AIDS, *Chest* 124:771–772, 2003.
5. VonKorff M, Gruman J, Schaefer J, et al: Collaborative management of chronic illness, *Ann Intern Med* 12:1097–1102, 1997.
6. Battin P: *The death debate: ethical issues in suicide*, Prentice-Hall, 1997, Upper Saddle River, NJ, pp 176–203.
7. Reinhardt UE: Does the aging of the population really drive the demand for healthcare? *Health Affairs* 22:27–38, 2003.
8. Iwashyna TJ, Christakis NA: Marriage, widowhood, and health-care use, *Soc Sci Med* 57:2137–2147, 2003.
9. Freedman VA: Family structure and risk of nursing home admission, *J Gerontol B Psychol Sci Soc Sci* 51:S61–S69, 1996.
10. Foley KM, Gelband H, editors: *Improving palliative care for cancer: institute of medicine and national research council*, Washington, DC, 2001, National Academy Press, p 208.
11. Singer PA, Martin DK, Kelner M: Quality and end of life care patients' perspectives, *JAMA* 281:163–168, 1999.

12. Vanderwerker LC, Laff RE, Kadan-Lottick NS, et al: Psychiatric disorders and mental health service use among caregivers of advanced cancer, *J Clin Oncol* 23:6899–6907, 2005.

13. Coluzzi PH, Grant M, Doroshow JH, et al: Survey of the provision of supportive care services at the National Cancer Institute–designated cancer centers, *J Clin Oncol* 13:756–764, 1995.

14. Loscalzo MJ, Zabora JR: Identifying and addressing distress and common problems in cancer patients and committed caregivers through skill development. In Spitzer W, editor: *The strengths based perspective on social work practice in healthcare. National society for social work leadership in healthcare,* Petersburg, Va, 2005, Dietz Press, pp 33–55.

15. National Association of Social Workers: Client self-determination in end of life decisions. In *Social Work Speaks: National Association of Social Workers Policy Statements*, ed 6, Washington, DC, 2003–2006, NASW Press, pp 46–49.

16. National Association of Social Workers: Client self-determination in end of life decisions. In *Social Work Speaks: NASW Policy Statements*, ed 3, Washington, DC, 2003, National Association of Social Workers, pp 58–61.

17. Christ G, Sormanti M: The social work role in end-of-life care: a survey of practitioners and academicians, *Soc Work Healthcare* 30:81–99, 1999.

18. Gwyther LP, Altilio T, Blacker S, et al: Social work competencies in palliative and end-of-life care, *J Soc Work End-of-Life Palliat Care* 1:87–120, 2005.

19. Zabora J, Brintzenhofeszoc K, Curbow B, et al: The prevalence of psychological distress by cancer site, *Psychooncology* 10:19–28, 2001.

20. National Hospice Foundation: 1999 National Hospice Foundation Survey. Available at www.nhpco.org.

21. Ferrell BR: Late referrals to palliative care, *J Clin Oncol* 23:1–2, 2005.

22. Yabroff KR, Lawrence WF, Clauser S, et al: Burden of illness in cancer survivors: finding from a population-based national sample, *J Natl Cancer Inst* 96:1322–1330, 2004.

23. Institutes of Medicine: *Cancer care for the whole patient: meeting psychosocial health needs,* Washington, DC, 2007, IOM, pp 222–223.

24. Holland JC, Andersen B, Breitbart WS, et al: Distress management: clinical practice guidelines in oncology, *J Natl Compr Canc Netw* 8:448–485, 2010.

25. Institutes of Medicine: *Cancer care for the whole patient: meeting psychosocial health needs,* Washington, DC, 2007, IOM.

26. Zabora JR, Loscalzo MJ, Weber J: Managing complications in cancer: identifying and responding to the patient's perspective, *Semin Oncol Nurs* 19:1–9, 2003.

27. Clark KL, Bardwell WA, Arsenault T, et al: Implementing touch screen technology to enhance recognition of distress, *Psycho-Oncol* 18(8): 822–830, 2009.

28. Loscalzo M, Clark K, Dillehunt J, et al: SupportScreen: a model for improving patient outcomes at your fingertips, *J Natl Compr Canc Netw* 8:496–504, 2010.

29. Loscalzo M, Jacobsen PB: Practical behavioral approaches to the effective management to pain and distress, *J Psychosoc Oncol* 8:139–169, 1990.

CHAPTER 41

Spiritual Care

MELISSA J. HART

At some point, people who are diagnosed with a life-limiting condition or illness generally realize that they are in transition to something unknown, either to the process of living differently with the condition or perhaps to the process of dying with it. Their time during this transition is precious. It may be a last opportunity to live as fully as one can, to be authentically oneself, to communicate meaningfully with loved ones, or to experience life in a different way.

The spiritual questions and concerns of people in this kind of life transition are often universal in scope. It appears to be inherent to the human condition to ask, "What has my life been about? What will it be about now?" Understanding our beliefs and finding a purpose can help to strengthen, calm, and root us when we are feeling knocked about by life or victimized by circumstance. This is true for patients as well as for those involved in their care, including loved ones, hired caregivers, and medical professionals.

Until they breathe their last breath, people often are still growing, appreciating, seeing things from a new perspective, and making meaning. They are engaged in the last developmental stage of life as we know it, and being with people at this stage in their development can be an amazing, invigorating experience.

As Confucius observed thousands of years ago, "everything has its beauty, but not everyone sees it." Our society in the United States focuses on death and dying as a tremendously negative and painful experience. We dismiss our last phase of life as a terrible series of losses that is devoid of value. It does not have to be so.

584

The physical, emotional, and spiritual challenges that people face at this stage can be met with respect, compassion, and guidance. A closely knit palliative care team that is devoted to the dignity and comfort of both patients and families can facilitate a positive, meaningful experience of illness, dying, death, and bereavement. By valuing and being present at the last developmental stage of life, we open ourselves to the wonder and opportunity that lies therein. Part of that opportunity is to find a sense of comfort, contentment, and completeness by the time death occurs.

How do we help people get there? How do we make our way toward a greater sense of wholeness as we move toward the end of life?

Clinicians who specialize in palliative care are trained to combine highly effective medications with complementary therapies to address physical concerns. So, too, effective tools and guides are available to help lead a person toward a place of emotional and spiritual comfort at this critical time in his or her life.

Common Fears

Change is usually stressful for human beings—not just unwanted change, but even changes that we desire. People may deem as positive a new job, marriage, or children. Changes we may judge as negative include the diagnosis of a life-limiting illness, going through treatment, or losing a loved one. Why are both kinds of change taxing? Change represents loss. After integrating the change, we will not be the same person and are thus called on to form a new identity. Such an invitation may be perceived as both a curse and a blessing, and moving toward this unknown can be extremely frightening.

Why does fear of death seem larger than fear of other unknowns? First, the other unknowns, such as marriage, childbirth, and the diagnosis and treatment of a life-limiting illness, have usually been survived by and reported by others. Because dying is the only unknown that has no survivors who can report the experience, it is harder to comfort those who may be moving closer to death. Witness the human fascination with near-death experiences—we are looking for reassurance from those who have gone before us.

In addition, if change inherently brings loss, then death is the ultimate change: the loss of everything as we know it and the integration of a new understanding of ourselves and the greater world. Some people think of it as the ultimate leap of faith; others describe it as the greatest letting go they will ever experience.

Individuals express fears around illness and dying in three principal ways: physical concerns, emotional concerns, and spiritual concerns. People often wonder about the actual, physiologic process of becoming sicker and dying: Will it hurt? Will it be awful? People may form a graphic picture in their mind of specific, uncontrolled symptoms overtaking their bodies. For some individuals, the only image of dying they have comes from the sensationalism of movies and television. Others may have watched an elderly loved one experience illness or death without symptom relief years ago.

Individuals often describe their emotional concerns in terms of worry—worry about burdening loved ones and, later, about the possibility of leaving loved ones behind. People with life-limiting illness sometimes wonder what they will be missing and how loved ones will function without them.

In terms of spiritual concerns, a person with a serious illness tends to reflect on some combination of the following questions:

What is happening to my body? Will I die?

Why have I been afflicted?

Do I believe in an organizing intelligence or connectedness in the universe? Do I believe in God? What *kind* of greater world do I believe in?

What has my experience of the foregoing been thus far? Does my experience match what I say I believe?

What has my life meant?

What gives my life meaning right now?

What will give my life meaning in the future?

How have I treated people and the world at large?

Do I live true to my values? Do I live true to my beliefs?

In general, at critical life junctures in which spiritual counsel is offered, it seems to be inherent to the human condition to ask the following:

Where have I been?

Where am I standing right now?

Where am I going?

Purpose of Spiritual Care

Illness is a highly personal experience that no one else can have for us; no one can adjust to the limitations and losses incurred from illness but the person himself or herself. In the words of the Buddha, "Peace comes from within. Do not seek it without." Life-limiting illness can be an extremely lonely experience.

Thus, spiritual care has two aims: to address the deep sense of isolation that accompanies serious illness and to help patients and loved ones find their own internal sense of comfort, strength, and balance. When these goals are achieved, the person may unearth a broader or deeper understanding of his or her relationship with the larger world. Patients and caregivers often describe this discovery process with words of wonder and relief, finding a quiet, inexplicable gift hidden within the illness.

Definitions

There are countless ways to describe spirituality and religion, and admirably rigorous works that examine the issues have been well set out elsewhere.[1] Simply put, spirituality is about a relationship between ourselves and the greater world, whereas religion is an expression of this relationship by a particular group. Spiritual care addresses both the universal and the particular—the interior awareness of our connection to the world at large and the specific form that relationship takes. Both may influence some or even all aspects of a person's daily life, thus presenting a person with abundant resources in which to find solace.

Methods of Spiritual Care: The Role of the Chaplain

Reviews of the role of clinicians in providing spiritual care are excellently provided elsewhere.[2] Deeper spiritual work usually is provided by a chaplain. There are three primary roles for a spiritual care professional in palliative care. One is simply to be with the patient in the experience of transition and hope to alleviate some of the patient's isolation. Another is to connect the patient with clergy from a particular tradition, if that is what the patient desires. A third role is to be present for the patient's exploration of spiritual concerns and questions.

PRESENCE

First, it is of utmost importance to offer a humane, compassionate presence. Although we cannot take away the deep sense of isolation that patients and caregivers tell us they experience, we do aim to lessen it to the extent possible. How do we do this? Simply by being present with people as they struggle through their challenges. They may not have any interest in discussing religious, spiritual, or emotional matters and may, in fact, describe themselves as "areligious," "nonbelievers," or "not spiritual." This should not be a deterrent to the spiritual care professional in palliative medicine. We are there to provide a quiet, supportive presence for those who desire to be accompanied, to meet people on a path they may never have walked before, and to hold their hand, figuratively or literally. If watching a baseball game with a patient brings comfort to him or to her, that is how the relationship begins to be built.

Even if a patient is comatose, spiritual care professionals visit the bedside to talk, or meditate, or sing, or hold a hand. We hope that with the sound of the human voice or the touch of the human hand, such a patient may feel a bit less alone.

TRADITION AND COMMUNITY

The second role for the spiritual care professional is to facilitate connection between patients (or caregivers) and their religious tradition. We do this by offering to contact clergy and congregations from each individual's particular faith tradition. Even when an individual or family tells us of a lapsed or nonexistent relationship with the institutional part of religious tradition, we offer to arrange for clergy or congregants of the faith tradition to visit. Such a visit may allow individuals or families to take part in religious observance through ritual, prayer, holiday celebration, story telling, or conversation. Although a person's interest in religious observance may have lapsed during adulthood, he or she will often find a significant, new relevance in participating, much to the surprise of loved ones.

If the prospect of a visit seems too much to bear or feels too invasive and the person still desires some form of connection with his or her own faith tradition, we also offer the opportunity to be included on a prayer list of a particular religious community. In either case, experiencing the link to the heritage and rituals and community of one's own faith tradition brings some people a sense of belonging and relief, relief at remembering one's connection to a larger community of faith.

REFLECTION

The third role for the spiritual care professional is to invite individuals and families to bring their spiritual joys and concerns to light. Spiritual counselors are trained to facilitate the exploration of one's inner experiences of meaning and faith, as well as one's understanding of being as it relates to the greater world. Such exploration may uncover both spiritual strengths and stressors, areas of vigor and unease. By helping an individual to hold the fullness of these, the person's interior experience is received in total with respect and compassion. The person may begin to feel less isolated by his or her circumstances and may begin to move toward a greater sense of wholeness and integration.

Paths to Meaning

Traditional forms of spiritual care include prayer, the holy scriptures of one's faith tradition, and spiritual reflection. Sitting in silent companionship may also provide a supportive presence that feels comforting to some people. Sometimes people with a life-limiting illness may not wish to (or be able to) expend precious energy on speaking. Even facial reactions require a certain amount of vigor that may not be available to the very sick.

There are other, very simple ways to provide care for the human spirit when a person is seriously ill. The list is limitless, really, but several ideas follow that may start the reader thinking. They show how each of us is touched in different ways, some visual, some auditory, some kinesthetic.

LOCATION, LOCATION, LOCATION

First, a bed-bound person may find the bedroom setting too isolated from the rest of the household. Consider moving the bed to a more central location, such as the living room, where the person may become integral to the natural flow of household activity, rather than being set apart. Physical proximity to the daily bustle of life may increase the bed-bound person's sense of participation and connection and can often result in a boost in spirit.

NATURE: THE FIVE SENSES

Next, many people experience an increased sense of well-being when they are in the presence of nature. Some relate that they feel most connected to the universe or God, most peaceful and whole, when they are outdoors in the natural world.

Moving a bed close to a window with a view of the natural world can work wonders for the spirits of such individuals. One attentive family I met even installed a special bird feeder in the window that attracted birds within the patient's view, and the patient delighted in the variety of lively, petite birds that visited her window each morning.

When this is not possible, a video or audio recording of the natural world can bring the sights and sounds of nature to the bedside. Watching sapphire blue waves lapping at a sandy beach bathed in the glow of an orange sunset or listening to the chirping of tiny, soft birds atop tall, green trees swaying in the wind can be very calming and soothing to the human spirit.

Aroma can also help people feel connected to the larger world. The fragrances of incense and spice are part of some religious traditions, and favorite scents of flowers and foods can delight the hearts of those who love them. One daughter I met told me of peeling the thick skin of a fresh orange beneath her mother's nose, because the bright fragrance released by the natural oils in the orange peel had been one of her mother's daily joys in life when she was well. Another person described her happiness and memory of wholeness simply at having the taste of coffee put on her tongue.

The pleasure of touch can also revive the spirit. For those who are seriously ill, touch is often a neglected sense, yet it is one that can return people to an early memory of wholeness, caring, and value. The warmth of a gentle, furry animal or even the soft squishiness of a velvety stuffed animal can help people to remember their connection to love, security, and comfort. Light massage can help people regain a memory of wholeness and contentment, as well, and can remind people that they are still fully human and part of the larger world.

ART

Some people feel intimately connected with the greater world through art. Consider Kim. Kim had her bed moved to the living room, beside her favorite window view, and then asked that her favorite painting be hung close to her new location. She had fond memories of complete absorption in that painting and knew that she needed its familiar comfort with her now. For other individuals, creating art or watching art be made at the bedside may feel nourishing to the spirit.

MUSIC

Similarly, some individuals experience a deep sense of connectedness to the larger world through music. Hearing live music played at the bedside, singing, or listening to recorded music can help to enhance a person's sense of inner strength and balance. Consider Tim, a gentleman with lifelong medical problems of increasing acuity, who felt fortified and at ease after regular visits from the music therapist. The therapist nurtured Tim's love and knowledge of classical music with discussion, live performance, and recordings specific to Tim's musical interests.

CREATING A SPIRITUAL LEGACY

Some people wish to record what they have experienced, what they have learned in life, and their wishes for the future. Those who are inclined to write may put their thoughts down on paper, in a form of their choosing, such as journal entries, poetry, short stories, a biography, a letter, or an ethical will. Others may dictate their thoughts aloud to someone who will write for them. Some may wish to relay the meaning they have found in life by speaking directly to loved ones or making a recording. Still others may desire assistance in making a scrapbook or photograph album that captures something of their life that they would like to have remembered in years to come.

Ethical Wills: Staying Connected after Death

What is an ethical will? Basically, all wills are sets of instructions. A will of inheritance directs distribution of one's material property at death and is a set of financial instructions. A living will directs which treatments a person wishes to accept and refuse near death and is a set of medical instructions. An ethical will encapsulates the wisdom a person has gleaned in life and is a set of spiritual instructions for those they leave behind.

An ethical will summarizes a person's journey in life, their values, and their closing wishes. It can be general or specific, short or long. There are no rules for developing an ethical will, but there are simple guidelines. Although ethical wills are classically thought of as written documents meant to be shared with loved ones, the wisdom they hold may also be disseminated verbally (as in the Bible). In today's world, this often takes the form of audio and video recordings, without being formally named as such. In any form, creating an ethical will gathers and names the wisdom acquired over a lifetime. Leaving this spiritual legacy for heirs, friends, or caregivers can have a positive impact on all involved. Both patients and loved ones may benefit from decreased feelings of loss and isolation, as well as an increased sense of meaning, connection, and well-being.

Ancient Roots of Ethical Wills. For many people, the concept of an ethical will is appealing, even when it is not named as such. Leaving behind closing wishes, values, and spiritual instructions for heirs is an ancient practice, and early examples are described in the Bible. For those who would like to learn more about these roots, several Biblical references follow.

In *Genesis: 48–49*, Jacob offers parting words about what he sees for the life ahead of each of his sons, as well as burial instructions for himself. In *Deuteronomy: 33*, Moses speaks to the tribes of Israel. Moses discusses the journey of the people, with God accompanying them, and he blesses each of the tribes individually. In *I Kings 2: 2–4*, King David speaks to his son Solomon and gives him instructions for spiritual and moral fortitude. Today, ethical wills are used for these same purposes—to pass on wishes, guidance, values, and life lessons—to bless those that follow.

Sample Questions for Ethical Wills. Following are some suggestions for questions to answer when writing an ethical will.

- What have you learned from life?
- What values, wisdom, or life lessons would you like to pass on?
- What is important to you?
- What would you want your loved ones to remember about you? About life? About themselves?
- What do you want your grandchildren and great-grandchildren to know about your life?
- What are your hopes and dreams?

ENERGY WORK

Some people experience their spiritual connection to the greater world in a physical way, through their body. Many who meditate and pray or practice physical disciplines, such as running, yoga, knitting, or tai chi, report a feeling of calm, clarity, and wholeness permeating their body both during and after the activity. For those who no longer have the capacity to engage in these forms of spiritual connection but who still desire a way to be filled with the sense of balance and strength they bring, there is energy work, experienced through the laying on of hands.

As far back as the Bible, there are myriad examples of the healing power of touch, or the laying on of hands. Today's medical world offers treatments based on this real phenomenon. Continuing education programs in nursing teach healing touch and many health professionals, including physicians and chaplains, study the art of Reiki. (Although other types of energy work abound, only two are named here.) Practitioners are trained to place hands either very lightly on the patient or even slightly above the patient. During and after treatments, patients often report an internal sense of wholeness and balance returning. Other benefits patients express include feelings of soothing, calm, and well-being.

When does energy work seem appropriate for spiritual care? Consider Susie, a woman in her 40s who has cancer. Susie was raised in a religious home and attended private religious schools, but she never related to the beliefs and practices she was taught. As an adult, she did not find herself drawn to any faith traditions. Now very sick and home-bound, conserving energy by limiting her movement and speaking, Susie longed for a way out of her spiritual isolation. When she described the sense of wholeness she used to experience when exercising outdoors, and how she wished desperately to return to that feeling, I asked Susie whether she would like to sample energy work. Anxious to try anything that would not drain her resources (as she found that talking did) and wanting physically to feel the comfort she described as "prayer flowing through her body," Susie readily agreed. A Reiki practitioner (who was also a registered nurse) was dispatched to her home to work with a laying on of hands, both directly on and slightly above the body. Susie felt spiritually connected and calmed during the first treatment and asked the nurse to return for regular treatments. During the second and third visits, Susie began to describe her fears about the stage she had been so surprised to reach with her illness—one of watching her body fragment and disintegrate. The practitioner continued the treatments and witnessed Susie's return to wholeness in spirit.

Susie was someone who connected to her spirituality kinesthetically, had extremely limited energy for talking, and did not relate to traditional religion. This made her an excellent candidate for at least a trial with energy work. Although individuals differ in *how* they experience their spiritual connection to something larger, the longing for that connection is virtually universal. Chaplains creatively seek to access and provide resources that facilitate meaningful connection to that which is greater, for everyone.

Spiritual Assessment and Cases

Spiritual assessment can be thought of as analogous to physical assessment in palliative care—that is, "Where/when/how does the patient hurt? Where/when/how is the patient at ease?" The health care practitioner assesses these basics, through history taking and physical examination, to create a care plan best suited to the unique person before him or her. The clinician can also screen for spiritual distress so that a specialist may be called in if need be. To do so, he or she may use questions from one of the published screening instruments designed for the purpose.[3–4]

In the same way that a clinician takes a thorough history pertaining to physical aspects of an illness, the spiritual care practitioner takes a thorough history of an individual's spiritual strengths, vulnerabilities, and proclivities. The goal of the assessment is to begin building a spiritual care plan that is tailored to be most helpful to a particular individual. When a person's spirit is tended to, walking through the unfamiliar territory of life-limiting illness may feel just a bit less lonely or less impossible.

In palliative medicine, the chaplain attends to the spiritual life not only of the patient, but also of the entire system involved in the patient's circle of care. This may include hired caregivers, beloved friends, and family members, each of whom may be deeply challenged by the patient's illness. All are equally important in the eyes of the visiting palliative care team, and whoever desires spiritual care may receive it.

As with physical assessment, spiritual assessment is usually done by a specialist (in this case by a chaplain) and elucidates one of the following three circumstances: well-being, distress, or camouflage for psychological or emotional struggles. In addition, spiritual assessment may note a person's lack of apparent connection to spirituality or meaning, which also guides a chaplain in building an appropriate care plan.

Although an initial assessment (physical or spiritual) may point to the overall direction for a care plan, assessment is ongoing. As the relationship between practitioner and patient develops, additional information may present itself, either spoken by the patient or hinted at in the patient's body language or demeanor.

Many people have fears and anxieties about the actual process of living and dying with a life-limiting illness that they may or may not verbalize. Physically, what will it be like? Will it be painful or scary? Spiritually, what will the process of dying be like? Will it be painful or scary? If I am not in control, who or what is?

If the team senses unacknowledged concerns in persons they are serving, they may attempt to assess further to discern the underlying nature of the perceived disquiet. In the examples of the unease just described, the appropriate team member (in this case, the physician or the chaplain, respectively) may then begin to address the individual concerns directly. This can prove immensely reassuring and comforting to patients, who may have been suffering silently with their wonderings.

SPIRITUAL WELL-BEING

Virginia was a traditional and deeply religious woman in her middle 50s who suffered with cancer pain. Until the palliative team was able to control her pain, the chaplain focused on prayer, hand holding, and quiet companionship. Day by day, Virginia's physical comfort improved.

Virginia was very sure of her religious beliefs and her prayer life, and this certainty gave her a spiritual comfort that she began to discuss. Still, even without saying so, she appeared to be quite frightened about the actual process of dying. Sensing this, the chaplain asked Virginia whether she would like to hear about his experience of sitting with individuals as they are dying. Eagerly and with surprise in her eyes, Virginia nodded her head. The chaplain described what he most often beheld: a peaceful, quiet, beautiful, and sacred experience. A great sense of peace and relief came over Virginia's face and her body relaxed into her bed.

Bess was a strong woman in her 90s with old-fashioned values of home and hearth, and she described herself as having a private, personal spirituality. She did not discuss her beliefs. She did not want to see a clergyperson, nor did she relate to institutional religion, and her family was of a similar mind. Chaplaincy visits to Bess and her family were intended to build and maintain a supportive relationship. When Bess's pain suddenly became uncontrolled while she waited for new medications to take effect, her nephew Brian tried to cheer her up with vibrant, joyous, reggae music, which Bess used to enjoy. It now made her shriek. The palliative team educated Brian about using silence or gentle, calming music to help lower Bess's rising level of internal stimulation (from the pain). Opportunities to help Bess and the family cope better presented themselves week after week, and because a supportive relationship had been built, the chaplain was able to make a difference in the comfort level of both the patient and the family.

In the foregoing situations, both Virginia and Bess came to their illness with a foundation of spiritual well-being. Proper assessment allowed the chaplain to build a care plan around this strength and to be of increasing assistance as needs arose. Sensitivity, respect, and a genuine desire to learn what would be most supportive for each individual patient facilitated the assessment process.

SPIRITUAL DISTRESS

Catherine was a pillar of her religious community. She had dedicated herself to years of committed service, by leading task forces for worthy causes while raising a large, participative family. After describing her deep religious involvement to the hospice chaplain, Catherine asked to see a clergyperson from her faith tradition, but not one from her own places of worship. Rather, she liked the idea of finding clergy from a local university, where they were "smarter about discussing the tough questions."

After Catherine met with university clergy, she confessed to the hospice chaplain what she had intended to discuss with the clergyperson, but found herself unable to disclose. "What if, all this time, I've been kidding myself? What if I die and there's really no heaven, no God waiting for me with open arms, nothing else for me?" The hospice chaplain talked and prayed with Catherine, acknowledging the paradox of belief amidst nonbelief as part of the human condition, citing many scriptural examples. Catherine found relief from her distress in her honest expression of doubt alongside faith.

The initial spiritual assessment for Catherine may have pointed to spiritual well-being, but it also may have begun to hint at spiritual distress when Catherine wanted to meet with university clergy, rather than her own. By being sensitive to Catherine's request and staying close to the evolving assessment process, the chaplain was able to support Catherine in her distress in a way that was meaningful to Catherine.

RELIGIOUS CAMOUFLAGE FOR PSYCHOLOGICAL STRUGGLES

Debra was extremely anxious about dying. A woman in her 70s, she had lived a very active life within the stability of a long, loving marriage. Debra described herself as a religious person who relied on the tools of her faith tradition to help her with life's challenges, but she did not seem to be using them in this situation. Although Debra did not have clergy or a religious community, she agreed to meet with clergy from her tradition to talk about her concerns and to receive partnership for working with the tradition's prayers and meditations. The chaplain on the palliative care team arranged and attended the first meeting with the clergy and Debra. After the meeting, Debra stated that she did not want to work any further with the specifics of her religious tradition. When asked, she told the palliative team's chaplain of her underlying emotional and psychological concerns.

Debra acknowledged that she derived her self-esteem only from her competence in the external world and that she had little awareness of the internal world (her own heart and mind) that needed her attention and care as well. The chaplain worked with Debra in two primary ways: broadening Debra's concept of compassion to include compassion for herself as well as for others and awakening Debra's awareness to the fact that, although she may have learned how to give during her life thus far, she perhaps did not yet know how to receive. Debra had spent a lifetime in compassionate action for others, but she seemed to fight the possible opportunity provided by her illness to receive love, gentleness, and honor, from others and from herself. The chaplain was then able to create prayer and meditations with Debra that were specific to Debra's unique world view, lifelong fears, and persistent psychological struggles. Debra finally found peace and rest as her enormous tensions dissolved into meditations created specifically for her.

The initial spiritual assessment for Debra indicated emotional distress. When the chaplain attempted to draw on Debra's stated religious foundation to alleviate some of her emotional distress, the foundation seemed metaphorically to fall away, leaving nothing to support Debra. Ongoing assessment, as well as consultation with the team's social worker, allowed the chaplain to discern where Debra was in her own emotional and spiritual development. This process of ongoing assessment and consultation was critical in designing an appropriate care plan for Debra, one that supported her as she finally found her way to the balance, comfort, and strength waiting inside her.

LACK OF APPARENT CONNECTION TO SPIRITUALITY OR MEANING

Joseph was a gentleman in his late 90s who relayed that, although he was born to a particular religion, he had lived his life without it. Like so many others, he had been working, and working hard. He had neither the time nor the patience for religion, and he did not have anything to discuss. Did he believe in God? Maybe, maybe not, but there was no need to talk about it. Nothing was going to change his circumstances.

Joseph had a very off-putting manner in describing his lack of need for chaplaincy and social work visits, yet both the chaplain and the social worker agreed that there was something inexplicable in his manner that kept them wanting to try again. After all, he was all alone in the world—as with so many others his age, he had outlived friends and relatives, and Joseph had never raised any children.

At first, Joseph used his abrupt manner to try to get rid of these friendly faces, but gradually, seeing them return again and again, he began to tolerate their gentle, nondemanding presence. Over time, Joseph quietly began to come out of his shell and started talking about different phases of his life. He slowly developed relationships with the entire palliative team and allowed them glimpses into his mind and heart while his body gradually deteriorated. The care team threw Joseph birthday parties, helped him to hire caregivers, and brought him his favorite foods.

One day, Joseph told the story of his involvement with his religious tradition as a youth, and what prompted him to leave and never return. Joseph began telling the story over and over to the team, across many weeks, as though he were attempting to integrate a long-lost part of himself. Joseph wept at the loss. The chaplain invited him to restart his religious studies and prayer life, and Joseph spent the next months and years enjoying his "return to God." At his senior residence, he came to be known as a person of strong character who quietly lived a life of gentleness and kindness toward all. Staff and residents alike spoke to the visiting palliative team about how they admired the genuine and inspiring way in which Joseph conducted himself. He became a role model for the other seniors with whom he lived. Joseph seemed to die a happy, religious man.

In this instance, the team followed their instincts at initial assessment and attempted to provide a nondemanding presence in Joseph's life. Because this was well tolerated, ongoing assessment guided the team to stay in step with Joseph and try to provide him with a sense of family. Joseph seemed to feel so safe and cared for in his relationship with the team that he eventually brought to the team's attention a painful part of his spiritual life that he had jettisoned, but dearly missed. With the team's support, he reclaimed his religious heritage and his relationship with God.

ATTENDING TO CURRENT AND FORMER RELIGIOUS NEEDS

Although some adults may adopt a religious practice that differs from the tradition into which they were born, in palliative care we find that the person is often holding the full circle of their life experience, remembering all the phases of their life. Thus, the chaplain may consider offering to bring in clergy from a person's current faith practice as well as their initial faith. Depending on circumstance, comfort or healing may be found in the rituals and prayers of one's childhood.

Similarly, if a seriously ill person has lived his or her adult life without interest in religion or spirituality, family members may decline chaplaincy visits for that person. It is probably best for the chaplain to offer to visit anyway and explain to the family that the purpose of the visit is not to press spiritual matters, but simply to assess.

The family is often not aware of how the ill person was raised as a small child, and they may not realize that comforting rituals and prayers, music, and language from a very young age are still lodged in an older person's mind. Even if someone is non-responsive or lives with dementia, the earliest parts of memory can often be engaged, producing visible pleasure for the ill person and sometimes enormous surprise for family members.

POSSIBLE PROBLEMS

In all assessments, it is vital that practitioners engage the person before them with the awareness that they do not know fully that person's story and that they desire to learn more. Entering the life of a patient with respect and sensitivity for the complete person is of paramount importance. A genuine posture of humility and openness on the part of the practitioner is necessary to be able truly to serve the person before him or her.

When assessment is approached from this premise, practitioners may then have the highest likelihood for designing a care plan that is uniquely supportive and meaningful to that individual. In that vein, team members and consultants should not be allowed to bring a preconceived spiritual care agenda to the palliative patient. The resultant assessment and care plan could then become skewed toward a particular end in spiritual care, regardless of whether that end is experienced as meaningful, helpful, or even relevant by the individual patient. At worst, the patient may experience the interaction as disrespectful, destructive, or even traumatizing. When patients are already at their most vulnerable as they try to live with serious illness, there is no room for risking harm.

WHO PROVIDES SPIRITUAL ASSESSMENT AND CARE?

Chaplains, pastoral counselors, spiritual counselors—these are all terms that may be used interchangeably for the person on the palliative team who facilitates spiritual care. Pastoral counseling began as an effort to help persons who had experienced a crisis and were trying to make sense of it within the context of their religious beliefs and their experience of God. Persons who are braving a life crisis or major personal change often find themselves in startling and unfamiliar territory. Sometimes this leads to a crisis of meaning or faith, perhaps because the new realities can seem to challenge an unexamined or basic assumption. Pastoral counselors are guides who help navigate these dark and rocky waters.

There are several ways to become a chaplain, two of which are described here. Both combine theology and psychology, spirituality and counseling. One path consists of attending seminary in one's own religious tradition, becoming ordained clergy, and then taking additional training in counseling (which may not be emphasized in seminary). However, one need not be clerical to receive the proper training to provide spiritual care. Another path is a graduate degree in pastoral counseling, a program that integrates counseling with issues of meaning and faith. Professional associations for chaplains oversee requirements, equivalencies, and credentialing to maintain high standards of spiritual care.

HOW THE TEAM CAN HELP

Any member of the palliative team should be able to refer individuals to the chaplain for spiritual assessment and care. The entire team visits patients and families, and any team member may notice opportunities where spiritual care could be helpful. For example, a physician making early rounds or a nurses' aide bathing and dressing patients each morning may be the first to hear a patient describe vivid dreams from the night before—with distress, joy, or, contentment.

Why may dreams be noteworthy for the team? Dreams can provide rich spiritual imagery for individuals throughout life, perhaps taking on even greater significance as people move toward meaningful milestones, such as the end of life. For a person rooted in scripture, dream connections to present life circumstances may be of even deeper, religious interest, because the Bible, for example, is replete with examples of the spiritual content of dreams. In any case, a team member who hears from a patient about a particularly distressing or strengthening dream is encouraged to contact the chaplain for a possible spiritual care referral. Similarly, when a physician hears a patient, loved one, or hired caregiver discussing concerns about purpose, meaning, or faith and the team is unaware, it is a good time to give the chaplain a call.

Even though a trained chaplain will have attempted a thorough, initial spiritual assessment at, or soon after, every palliative care admission, some individuals may decline spiritual support at the start of their care, by citing lack of concern, interest, or need. As serious illness progresses, however, patients, caregivers, or loved ones may find themselves flooded with unexpected experiences, thoughts, and feelings for which they have no context. When this window of opportunity opens, however slightly, the team should be ready to reintroduce the idea of spiritual support and should alert the chaplain to a possible point of reentry.

The team is also fortified when each professional is in close touch with his or her own spiritual strengths and vulnerabilities. Consider how your personal spiritual beliefs affect you in your work. Do they help to increase your sense of balance, comfort, and strength with the struggles you face in caring for patients? Do they help to decrease your own sense of isolation with the challenges you encounter in medicine?

Consider, too, how will you respond when a patient asks you to pray with him or her? There is no right answer here; the question just requires some thought on your part before the situation arises. Whatever your response, deliver it with integrity and kindness, honoring both your own beliefs and those of your patient. And call the chaplain.

PEARLS

- Remember that people may still be developing spiritually, even as they decline physically and mentally.
- Accompany people through life-limiting illness. This may reduce a deep sense of isolation and help people to find their own internal sense of comfort, balance, and strength.
- Realize that people tend to find meaning in relating to a greater world beyond themselves; this appears to be a virtually universal human need.
- Alert the chaplain to possible spiritual developments discovered during routine care.
- Stay in close touch internally with your own spirituality, and note where it strengthens you and renders you vulnerable in your life and in your work.
- Practice from a genuine posture of humility and openness. Desire to learn what will provide the most meaningful support to the person before you.

PITFALLS

- Do not discount or dismiss the last stages of life as devoid of value.
- See beyond brokenness of body and mind to the wholeness of the person.
- Consider that someone who is not religious may be helped by spiritual care.
- Know that a person's initial decline of spiritual care need not be static throughout the progression of an illness.
- Be quietly aware of one's own spiritual beliefs.
- Do not bring a preconceived spiritual care agenda to the person for whom you are caring.

Summary

How does spiritual care help people who are facing life-limiting illness to find courage and equanimity? How does it help people find balance, comfort, and strength?

The added dimension that spiritual care brings to palliative medicine has enormous capacity to improve the quality of life for patients, for families, and for physicians. Attending to the needs of the spirit can bring great comfort to the palliative care patient and to his or her entire circle of care. If spiritual care is offered with respect, sensitivity, and a supportive disposition, and if it is not agenda driven, it should rarely present any disadvantage.

By being present with people and attending to them in a way that is meaningful to them, the palliative team shows patients that they are valued as fully human—that the team *sees* the whole of them, no matter how broken the physical body. When patients seemingly no longer have control over their circumstances, the palliative team gives them control wherever possible by respecting their needs and wishes. The care team functions with the understanding that all of us want to know we are loved, we belong, and we are not alone.

This is the condition of being fully human. Spiritual care helps people to remember this.

Resources

American Art Therapy Association
www.arttherapy.org
American Music Therapy Association
www.musictherapy.org
Association of Professional Chaplains
www.professionalchaplains.org
Ethical Wills
www.ethicalwill.com
Healing Touch
www.healingtouch.net
International Center for Reiki Training
www.reiki.org
National Association of Catholic Chaplains
www.nacc.org
National Association of Jewish Chaplains
www.najc.org

References

1. Puchalski C: Spirituality. In Berger AM, Shuster JL, Von Roenn JH, editors: *Principles and practice of supportive oncology and palliative care*, ed 3, Philadelphia, 2007, Lippincott Williams & Wilkins, pp 633–644.
2. Chochinov HM, Cann BJ: Interventions to enhance the spiritual aspects of dying, *J Palliat Med* 8(Suppl 1): S103–S115, 2005.
3. Lo B, Ruston D, Kates LW, et al: Discussing religious and spiritual issues at the end of life. A practical guide for physicians, *JAMA* 287:749–754, 2002.
4. Puchalski CM, Romer AL: Taking a spiritual history allows clinicians to understand patients more fully, *J Palliat Med* 3:129–137, 2003.

CHAPTER 42

Palliative Care in Long-Term Care Settings

JENNIFER M. KAPO and SEEMA MODI

The world's population is aging. Worldwide, 1 in every 10 persons is more than 60 years old. By year 2050, the number is expected to increase to 1 in every 5 persons. Palliative care clinicians will increasingly be confronted with providing end-of-life care for frail, older persons who are dying with multiple chronic illnesses. Palliative care clinicians must therefore develop expertise in the evaluation and treatment of geriatric patients.

This chapter provides an overview of three fundamental issues in the care of chronically ill, older patients: long-term care options and the option of including hospice or palliative care within the long-term care setting; the challenges of prognostication in chronically ill older adults; and the indications for and alternatives to artificial nutrition and hydration.

Long-Term Care

Clinicians who care for chronically ill, older patients who are near the end of life need to be aware of the community resources and sites of long-term care that are available for those who can no longer live independently. This section describes long-term care options, including home care, assisted living, nursing home care, day care programs such as Programs for the All-Inclusive Care of the Elderly, and integrated programs such as the Edmonton Regional Palliative Care Program. Although this information may not be universally applicable, the aim is to provide examples of the diverse options that may be available in different communities.

HOME HEALTH CARE

Many chronically ill patients wish to remain in their own homes as long as possible. Home health care aims to provide health and social services for older adults in their own homes to improve and maintain their function and to prevent institutionalization. Services may include skilled nursing and psychiatric nursing, physical and occupational therapy, home health aide assistance, and social work support.

Although more research is needed to define the most effective strategies for providing palliative care in a patient's home, numerous benefits of home palliative care are described in the international literature and in this textbook (Chapter 43) and include increased satisfaction of the family caregivers with the care provided, decreased time spent in the hospital at the end of life,[1] and improved primary care physician management of symptoms. Another study has shown that incorporating a palliative care program into an existing home care program results in improved family satisfaction with care, fewer emergency room visits, and decreased costs.

DAYCARE AND OTHER PROGRAMS FOR ELDERS

Adult daycare programs are designed to provide daytime care for patients who have minimal personal care needs and have family caregivers who are able to provide care only at night. Adult daycare offers a range of supportive and social services in the United States, the United Kingdom, Canada, Italy, and other countries. Most centers provide recreation, socialization, meals, some social services, personal care, and transportation. The medical care provided varies from site to site, however. Some centers offer specialized services such as dementia programs and incontinence programs. Although some may offer pain management, they rarely offer comprehensive end-of-life care.

One notable daycare program is found in the United States, the Program for the All-Inclusive Care for the Elderly (PACE).[2] PACE is a community-based, comprehensive care program funded by Medicare and Medicaid dollars. PACE programs enroll older persons who would otherwise be eligible for nursing home placement and provide them with comprehensive medical, rehabilitative, social, and personal services delivered by an interdisciplinary team. In the evening, the members return home to be cared for by families and friends. Care is provided in a daycare environment and in the participant's home, tailored to the participant's needs and social resources. PACE programs commit to caring for patients until the end of life, and these patients are no longer eligible for the Medicare hospice benefit while they are enrolled in PACE.[2]

There are no published national standards for the provision of palliative care by PACE, and research suggests wide variation among programs. However, PACE may help clinicians, patients, and families to address important palliative care goals. Specifically, patients enrolled in PACE are more likely to die at home, to avoid the use of invasive medical technology in the last months of life, and to have documented advance planning conversations, compared with Medicare recipients who are not enrolled in PACE. In addition, because the same interdisciplinary team follows patients from primary care to hospitalization to long-term care, the errors and distress that accompany transitions of care may be minimized under PACE. To improve the quality of palliative care provided, many programs have developed educational programs. However, research is needed to determine the specific needs of this group and how best to meet those needs.[2,3]

Another model of care that integrates a home palliative care program is the Edmonton Regional Palliative Care Program in Alberta, Canada. This program was created with the goal of increasing the access to palliative care services, decreasing the number of cancer-related deaths that occur in acute care facilities, and increasing the participation of primary care physicians in the end-of-life care of their patients. In the pilot program, four interdisciplinary teams provided consultative services for patients enrolled in a palliative care system that integrated several sites of care, including hospital-based services, inpatient palliative care units and hospices, and continuing care facilities, as well as a regional home care program. During the study period from 1992 to 1997, there was a decrease in the number of patients who died in the acute care facility and a significant decrease in the average length of stay in the acute care facility and the cancer center. It is likely that these outcomes not only met the goals of patients and families for a "good death" but also resulted in significant cost savings. Further research is needed to define both these benefits of home palliative care programs.

ASSISTED LIVING

Individuals who are less ill and more functionally intact may choose to reside in an assisted living facility. Typically, these facilities provide a combination of housing, personalized support services, and health services. Personal care homes, board and care homes, supportive care homes, residential care homes, and domiciliary care are all examples of assisted living housing. In the United States, as well as other countries, assisted living facilities are quite heterogeneous, reflecting divergent regulations and variable institutional practices and levels of care offered.[4]

Staffing and payment sources vary considerably among facilities. The most complete description of this can be found in literature from the United States. Although they are not required to do so by law, some assisted living facilities provide on-site physician visits and 24-hour nursing care. However, a national study of assisted living facilities in the United States reported that only 30% to 40% were staffed with a full-time registered nurse (40 hours/week).[5] In addition, only 15 of 50 states have minimum staffing laws, 22 of 50 states allow unlicensed staff members to distribute medications, and only 11 of 50 states require training for the nurse's aides.

Palliative care delivery in assisted living facilities may be hindered by a variety of factors, including lack of 24-hour coverage by a nurse, lack of an interdisciplinary care team, difficulty dispensing opioids because of limited nursing care or a lack of secure storage, insufficient numbers of physician visits, and minimal staff education about end-of-life issues. However, some assisted living facilities are piloting programs to improve care at the end of life in an attempt to provide adequate care for dying individuals.[4] One study compared the dying experience in assisted living facilities with that in nursing homes. In the last month of life, the assisted living residents were more likely to report untreated pain (14.8% vs. 1.8%; $P = .013$) and inadequately treated shortness of breath (12.5% vs. 0%; $P = .004$) compared with nursing home residents. Despite these inadequacies in symptom management, however, family and staff members reported greater satisfaction with end-of-life care in assisted living facilities compared with nursing homes.[6] Although this study reported high satisfaction with care by both the families and the staff, this study also found substantial unmet palliative care needs. More research is needed to understand potential care interventions for assisted living residents. With the aging of the population, it is likely that the number of persons who will receive care in an assisted living facility will grow substantially.

NURSING HOME CARE

Nursing home care is available to patients who develop significant functional and physical impairments during the course of their illness and can no longer live at home or in an assisted living facility. Broadly defined, nursing homes are long-term care institutions that provide inpatient, 24-hour nursing care, as well as medical, social, and personal services to persons in need of short-term nursing and rehabilitation or long-term maintenance.

Increasingly, nursing homes have become the site of death for frail, older persons. It is projected that by the year 2020 approximately 40% of Americans will die in a nursing home. Given this trend, nursing home clinicians will likely assume an increasingly important role in the provision of end-of-life care.

Palliative care in nursing homes is frequently suboptimal. Research has highlighted important concerns with the quality of care in nursing homes from untreated pain,[7] family dissatisfaction with the quality of care, and care that is not consistent with the disease trajectory or patient preferences.[8] Research indicates that 33% to 84% of residents have ongoing pain that impairs ambulation, reduces quality of life, and increases the incidence of depression.[7] In one study, 29% of nursing home residents with cancer reported daily pain, and only 26% of those with daily pain were treated with daily analgesics.

In another study, pain was reported by 69% of nursing home residents who were able to communicate. In 34% of these cases, however, the attending physician failed to recognize and treat the resident's pain. In a large study of 15,745 nursing homes, the staff reported that 3.4% of the residents had experienced daily excruciating pain during the previous week.[7] Many dying nursing home residents with daily pain are either not receiving adequate pain management treatments or are receiving treatments that are inconsistent with pain management guidelines.[9] Experts have identified barriers to the provision of excellent palliative care, including frequent staffing turnover, lack of palliative training and knowledge among the staff, and tension between goals of restorative care and those of palliative care.

Nursing home staffing issues may create a barrier to palliative care delivery. Staffing and services can vary substantially among nursing homes. Physician visits may be infrequent. A large portion of direct patient care is provided by nursing assistants, who usually have no formal training in geriatrics or palliative care.

The level and types of palliative care services provided vary among nursing homes. For example, some nursing homes have separate palliative care units or beds and specialized dementia care units. Some may be able to administer intravenous medications and complete frequent pain assessments, but others may not. Nursing home residents at one institution may have immediate access to clinicians such as physicians, social workers, and chaplains, whereas others may have infrequently available contacts.

The quality of care also depends on staff turnover. Higher staff-to-patient ratios are associated with higher quality of care, and longer relationships with staff result in greater satisfaction with care. However, many facilities experience frequent staff turnover. High turnover of nurse aides has been associated with inadequate staffing and stressful working conditions. Organization-wide efforts to improve quality of end-of-life care are difficult to sustain without a stable staff. Lack of continuity of care has the potential to affect the quality of pain assessments and other end-of-life care adversely.[10] Therefore, efforts to retain staff are particularly important. Additional education and training may be one strategy to decrease staff turnover.

Data describing educational and quality improvement programs that target physicians, nurses, and other nursing home staff members show an increase in family satisfaction with end-of-life care, increases in patient comfort (i.e., decreased pain intensity), and increases in job satisfaction among the nursing home workers.[11,12] Thus, staff education may lead to improved care because of an augmented knowledge base, as well as a more stable staff.

Another challenge to the provision of palliative care in nursing homes may be related to regulatory environments. In the United States, experts in both long-term care and palliative medicine note that regulations and reimbursement systems may be at odds with the use of hospice and palliative care in nursing homes.[10,12,13] In the United States, the 1987 Omnibus Budget Reconciliation Act (OBRA) stated that a major goal for nursing homes is to maintain or improve physical functioning (OBRA 1987) and mandated comprehensive assessments of all residents using the Minimum Data Set (MDS). The MDS, which includes 400 items that assess health and functional status, is used for clinical assessment and quality improvement. The information is also used to determine levels of reimbursement. Therefore, nursing homes with negative findings on their residents' MDSs are at risk for financial losses, as well as deficiency citations from state surveyors and possible decertification.

The desire to optimize the measures included in the MDS may be at odds with high-quality end-of-life care that is consistent with patient preferences. For example, weight loss secondary to dysphagia is a common terminal event in persons with dementia. Nursing home staff may believe that they will be cited or perform poorly on quality indicators if they respect a patient's wish not to have a feeding tube. It is important that these concerns be addressed with the nursing staff that cares for actively dying persons and that appropriate documentation outlining goals of care be noted in the medical record. Current reimbursement policies and the professional culture of many nursing homes focus on restorative care and the use of life-sustaining treatment such as artificial nutrition and hydration. Such financial incentives are one of the reasons cited for the underuse of and late referral of nursing home residents to hospice services or a focus on palliation in the nursing home setting. Palliative care clinicians need to be aware of these tensions to understand the decision-making process at the institution where they practice.

In Canada, limited funding for nursing home patients and similar staffing issues may also interfere with appropriate provision of quality end-of-life care. Research in Canada over the past decade has shown that the quality of care in for-profit nursing homes is lower than that in not-for-profit nursing homes in many areas, including staffing levels and turnover; increased use of restraints, catheters, and tube feeding; and more unwanted outcomes such as pressure ulcers, infections, and hospitalizations.

One way to improve end-of-life care in nursing homes is to increase access to palliative care or hospice involvement for appropriate nursing home residents. Nursing home residents who died with hospice care in place had improved pain assessment and management, a greater likelihood of receiving an opioid for pain, and lower rates of hospitalization, restraint use, and artificial nutrition and hydration. Furthermore, in nursing homes with a larger proportion of residents enrolled in hospice, the non-hospice residents, as well as the hospice residents, experienced lower rates of hospitalization, higher frequency of pain assessment, and higher rates of opioid use for control of pain or dyspnea, when compared with decedents from nursing homes with limited or no hospice presence.

Nonrandomized, case-controlled studies have shown that families rated symptom management as significantly improved after the addition of hospice services to U.S. nursing home care, and overall family satisfaction with end-of-life care was higher. Hospice or palliative care teams can teach family members and other caregivers to care for the dying patient and can offer emotional, psychological, and spiritual support to the patient and family, as well as bereavement care and counseling to family and friends before and after the patient's death.

A major factor cited for the low rate of hospice involvement in nursing homes is the difficulty in prognostication, especially in residents with a non-cancer diagnosis because they have a less predictable illness trajectory.[14] Other barriers to hospice referral include poor recognition of terminal illness, lack of knowledge within the facility about hospice, and the presence of artificial nutrition or expensive palliative care treatments.[10]

Given that hospice involvement can improve the quality of end-of-life care, many residents will benefit from efforts to increase enrollment in hospice programs. One study found that a quality improvement intervention involving the development of palliative care leadership teams who taught a structured curriculum to all nursing home staff in selected nursing homes led to increases in hospice enrollment, pain assessments, nonpharmacologic pain treatment, and discussions about end-of-life care from baseline.[12] A randomized controlled trial of 205 residents demonstrated that those residents who received a "case-finding" intervention (including "jump-starting" conversations about hospice) were more likely to enroll in hospice within 30 days, had fewer acute care admissions, spent fewer days in an acute care setting, and had families who rated care more highly than the families of those who received the usual care.[15]

Proactive discussion may minimize any conflict that may arise if the nursing home staff members believe that the hospice team members do not respect and value their opinions and care, or if nursing home staff members see the hospice as duplicating or interfering with their work or as another source of criticism and oversight. Nursing homes should focus more on care of the dying as part of their mission. Regulators need to recognize that caring for the dying is part of the nursing facility's mission, and that these populations require different services and measures of quality of care than those who are receiving custodial care. Nursing facility staff and regulators need training in appropriate means of caring for the dying.

Artificial Nutrition and Hydration

Malnutrition and dehydration are serious and common problems among older people in nursing and residential care homes, especially among those at the end of life. Malnutrition is highly prevalent in the elderly populations in long-term care facilities, with estimates ranging from 30% to 85%. In addition to resident factors, specific barriers in long-term care staffing may contribute to poor nutrition, such as a lack of training, responsibility for the care of too many residents, poor food quality, and a lack of teamwork between nurse and nursing assistant. More than half of nursing home residents need feeding assistance. In addition, 40% to 60% of nursing home residents may have some degree of dysphagia. Higher staff levels have been associated with a reduced risk of malnutrition.

The prevalence of artificial nutrition and hydration for nursing home residents with dementia is higher in the United States than in many other countries. In one cross-sectional cohort study, approximately 6.6% of older nursing home residents in the United States received long-term artificial nutrition by feeding tubes, compared with 6.4% in Ontario, Canada. Of the two, the U.S. cohort was almost three times as likely to have a diagnosis of dementia.[16] In a 1999 study of all U.S. Medicare- and Medicaid-certified nursing homes, more than one third of severely cognitively impaired residents had feeding tubes. The prevalence of artificial nutrition and hydration was associated with the residents' clinical features and the nursing home's demographic, financial, and organizational features. Palliative care clinicians may be asked to assist patients and families in making decisions about artificial nutrition and hydration.

EVIDENCE SUMMARY: RISKS AND BENEFITS

Most literature about artificial nutrition and hydration in the long-term care setting focuses on patients with advanced cognitive impairment. Although there are no randomized, controlled studies that compare tube feeding with hand feeding, little evidence indicates that artificial nutrition and hydration prolong life, improve nutritional status, prevent aspiration, decrease development or promote healing of pressure ulcers, or improve a patient's comfort.[17] A large retrospective study showed that nursing home residents with dysphagia and advanced dementia did not have any survival benefit from receiving artificial nutrition and hydration, even after correcting for medical comorbidities. Another study reported that the median survival among elderly patients after percutaneous gastrostomy tube placement was 5.7 months, with 1-month mortality of 24% and 1-year mortality of 63%.[18]

A prospective cohort study of relatively younger residents (mostly without dementia) and observational studies of nursing home residents with advanced dementia found that artificial nutrition did not provide consistent improvement in weight or serum albumin. There is no evidence from existing studies that artificial nutrition and hydration via gastrostomy tube prevents aspiration.[17] Cohort studies have failed to demonstrate any benefit of artificial nutrition and hydration on prevention or healing of pressure ulcers.

In addition to this lack of evidence of improved outcome, artificial nutrition and hydration have adverse effects at the end of life. There are complications related to the placement of a gastrostomy or jejunostomy tube, such as local infection, perforation, and aspiration secondary to sedation. Long-term complications can include tube dislodgement or clogging, diarrhea, aspiration pneumonia, *Clostridium difficile* colitis, and the use of restraints to prevent removal of the tube.

COSTS OF TUBE FEEDING

A small prospective cohort study examined U.S. health care costs associated with gastrostomy tube feeding over 1 year. The average daily cost of tube feeding was $87.21 (median, $33.50). The estimated cost of providing 1 year of feeding via gastrostomy is $31,832 (median, $12,227). The main components of this cost include the initial tube placement (29.4%), enteral formula (24.9%), and hospital charges for rare but costly major complications (33.4%).

Another small study examined the cost of caring for 11 severely demented U.S. nursing home patients with artificial nutrition and hydration versus another 11 patients without artificial nutrition and hydration. Items assessed included nursing time, physician assessments, food, hospitalizations, emergency room visits, diagnostic tests, treatment with antibiotics and parenteral hydration, and feeding tube insertion. Costs of nursing home care were higher for the residents who were not receiving artificial nutrition and hydration (i.e., receiving hand feeding) than for those receiving artificial nutrition and hydration ($4219 ± $1546 vs. $2379 ± $1032, $P = .006$).

ETHICAL ISSUES REGARDING ARTIFICIAL NUTRITION AND HYDRATION

Ethical issues surrounding artificial nutrition and hydration often involve decision-making conflicts between the health care provider and patient's surrogates about the decision to initiate and the eventual decision to withdraw artificial nutrition and hydration. When a resident's wishes about artificial nutrition and hydration are known, it is reasonable to respect them, unless doing so will bring about obvious harm, such as increased respiratory distress or pain. Unfortunately, a resident's advance directive regarding wishes for artificial nutrition and hydration is often not available. When a patient's preferences are unknown, the surrogate or substitute decision maker should make a decision based on substituted judgment or knowledge of the patient's probable wishes. When the patient's probable wishes are not known, the surrogate must consider how a reasonable person would make a decision under the same circumstances. When artificial nutrition is being considered, clinicians should prepare patients and surrogates to consider a trial of therapy, with eventual withdrawal if it does not achieve the desired effects.

Education of a resident's surrogate decision makers can greatly aid the process of decision making, but this education is often limited or nonexistent. Routine education at the time of nursing home admission may be helpful. Proactive education of decision makers about the lack of known benefits for tube feeding in advanced dementia may lead to more informed decisions, to greater satisfaction with decisions, and possibly to decreased tube placement in patients with advanced dementia.[19,20]

Education should focus first on general goals of care instead of technical options and should involve listening to the patient's or surrogate's perspective and addressing any disagreements with a mutual exchange of information. Disagreements are more likely to arise when patients or surrogates have unrealistic goals, if they have received mixed messages or mistrust the medical establishment, if they are in denial about the poor prognosis, or if the surrogate feels guilt about his or her own involvement in the patient's care. Language barriers and sociocultural differences can exacerbate the challenges of communication.

A critical question for discussion is whether the particular treatment or intervention will restore or enhance the quality of life for the patient. For example, artificial nutrition and hydration may meet goals of care in some long-term care populations, such as patients in the acute phase of a stroke or head injury, those receiving short-term critical care, or those with certain bowel conditions, but artificial nutrition and hydration in other populations, such as patients with advanced dementia, may not achieve any of the mutually determined goals of care.

The value systems of patients and surrogates should play a role in decisions. Although most available evidence suggests that artificial nutrition does not improve survival or quality of life in many situations and, in fact, may worsen outcomes, this evidence conflicts with beliefs that many people have that all nutrition is basic care and must be provided, just as patients must receive shelter and basic personal care. This view may be linked to cultural or religious beliefs or a belief that forgoing artificial nutrition results in suffering and "starvation." In this sense, artificial nutrition sometimes represents more to patients and families than simply another medical treatment.

Specifically, cultural differences in perceptions of feeding may account for discrepant care. In Japan, physicians sometimes institute tube feeding in older patients with dysphagia out of consideration for strong family emotions, religion, public opinion, and social customs. Japanese physicians may agree to use feeding tubes out of fear that they will be accused of refusing such treatment for economic reasons. However, 90% of family members caring for tube-fed patients would not want to receive a feeding tube themselves in a similar situation. U.S. data suggest that African-American patients with advanced dementia receive feeding tubes at higher rates than do white patients. Regional differences also exist in the United States, with higher rates of use in urban settings and lower rates of use in rural settings. Physicians must acknowledge these cultural differences and accept that sometimes a well-informed surrogate will choose tube feeding for a nursing home resident with advanced dementia or other end-stage disease. To provide artificial nutrition in such cases can provide relief of psychological, spiritual, or social distress in the dying process for the patient and family. Conversely, adequate education of risks, benefits, and alternatives to tube feeding may allow patients legitimately to refuse a feeding tube if they do not want tube feeding but feel societal pressure to accept it. National standardization of practice through the use of guidelines that are based on evidence from trials may be one method of eventually changing societal norms.

In developing countries, cost may be a major additional consideration. Decision making may also be influenced by health care settings and clinical circumstances; for example, decisions about artificial nutrition and hydration are more likely to occur in a nursing home than in an acute care hospital. Standardized methods of capturing patient preferences may assist facilities in documentation.

If artificial nutrition and hydration are already in place, then ongoing discussion of the goals of care should occur. The same ethical principles apply to withdrawal of artificial nutrition and hydration as to its initiation. Artificial nutrition can be withdrawn if it is no longer consistent with mutually determined goals of care. Patients who forego or request the withdrawal of artificial nutrition and hydration should receive high-quality palliative care.

ALTERNATIVES TO ARTIFICIAL NUTRITION AND HYDRATION

Extrapolation from other situations of impaired eating at the end of life suggests that discomfort from not eating is rare and, when it occurs, can be improved by measures other than artificial nutrition and hydration.[21] It is important to reassure patients and families that decreased food and fluid intake at the end of life is normal and is an expected part of the dying process and that, in fact, it usually leads to a more comfortable death by minimizing secretions, urine output, and edema. This information will minimize guilt that families may feel and will decrease the assumption that a needed treatment, nutrition, is not being given.

Family members who attend meals and who bring in favorite foods from a restaurant or from home can help to restore pleasure in eating. At visits, the family can offer snacks in a non-pressuring manner. Other practical interventions include creating an atmosphere that promotes mealtime as a pleasurable social activity; providing smaller portions more frequently; offering lactose-free nutritional supplements between meals as well as with medication passes; encouraging favorite foods; and avoiding diabetic, low-salt, low-fat, and low-cholesterol diets. In residents with dysphagia, a change in food texture and thickened liquids or changes in body positioning can improve swallowing. However, patients may dislike the modified food because the food can be less tasteful and thus makes eating less enjoyable, and this could inadvertently lead to further weight loss. For patients who do not take adequate fluids and who appear to have dry mouth, good oral care can improve comfort, and moistening the mouth can decrease the sensation of thirst.

In addition, residents should be assessed for unrecognized and inadequately treated medical conditions that can contribute to decreased appetite, including certain medications; dental caries or infection; poorly fitting dentures; dry mouth; pain; constipation or fecal impaction; urinary retention; and burden of symptoms, such as nausea, vomiting, sedation, agitation, and dyspnea. The benefits and burdens of a comprehensive workup must be determined by taking into account the patient's condition, family expectations and desires, and any health care directives.

Patients should be assessed and treated for anxiety, insomnia, and depression, and the use of antidepressants with appetite-stimulating effects, such as mirtazapine, should be considered. If improved appetite meets mutually determined goals of care, the clinician should consider the use of other appetite-stimulating medications, such as dexamethasone, 1 to 2 mg twice daily, prednisone, 10 to 20 mg twice daily, or megestrol, 80 to 400 mg twice daily (for a typical trial of 6–8 weeks). The efficacy of dronabinol, nabilone, and oxandrolone as appetite stimulants is controversial.

PEARLS

- Understand local long-term care options, including home care, assisted living, nursing home care, daycare programs such as Programs for the All-Inclusive Care of the Elderly (PACE), and any integrated programs such as the Edmonton Regional Palliative Care Program.

- Use home health care services to improve and maintain function and to prevent institutionalization.

- Use home palliative care to increase caregiver satisfaction, decrease hospital and emergency department visits, and decrease costs.

- Use adult daycare programs for patients with minimal personal care needs whose caregivers are able to provide care only at night.

- Use assisted living facilities to provide a combination of housing, personalized support services, and health services.

- Provide decision makers with alternatives to tube feeding, such as good palliative care.

PITFALLS

- Providers may fail to incorporate hospice or palliative care into the care plan of nursing home residents.
- Providers may not recognize the limitations of providing palliative care in different sites of care such as assisted living programs and nursing homes.
- Providers may not understand the lack of evidence for use of artificial nutrition in patients with advanced dementia.
- Providers may not recognize the ethical issues surrounding artificial nutrition and hydration, especially conflicts in decision making between health care providers and patients' surrogates.
- Providers may fail to respect a resident's known wishes about artificial nutrition and hydration.
- Providers may not acknowledge cultural differences in attitudes toward artificial nutrition and hydration.
- Providers may not accept that a well-informed surrogate may choose tube feeding for a nursing home resident with advanced dementia or other end-stage disease.

Summary

In summary, there is a dearth of evidence supporting the use of tube feeding in nursing home residents at the end of life. There should be advance care planning on every admission to the nursing home to determine the resident's or surrogate's wishes regarding this issue, with clear discussion of the lack of evidence of benefit in most situations, especially in advanced dementia. Despite this lack of evidence, many decisions about tube feeding are based on a patient's values, which often vary based on cultural and religious backgrounds. In this light, any well-informed decision regarding tube feeding should be respected. Good palliative care provides many alternatives to tube feeding.

As the population ages, there will be a greater need for palliative care physicians who are expert in determining the level of care an older, functionally impaired individual will require to be comfortable and safe near the end of life. In addition, families and patients will need advocates and guides to help them make difficult decisions regarding goals of care and treatments, particularly regarding the use of artificial hydration and nutrition.

Resources

European Association for Palliative Care
  www.eapcnet.org/index.html
International Association for Hospice & Palliative Care
  www.hospicecare.com
International Observatory on End of Life Care
  www.eolc-observatory.net

References

1. Grande GE, Todd CJ, Barclay SI, Farquhar MC: Does hospital at home for palliative care facilitate death at home? Randomised controlled trial, *Br Med J* 319:1472–1475, 1999.

2. Eng C: Future consideration for improving end-of-life care for older persons: Program of All-inclusive Care for the Elderly (PACE), *J Palliat Med* 5:305–310, 2002.
3. Covinsky KE, Eng C, Lui LY, et al: The last 2 years of life: functional trajectories of frail older people, *J Am Geriatr Soc* 51:492–498, 2003.
4. Mitty EL: Assisted living: aging in place and palliative care, *Geriatr Nurs* 25:149–156, 163, 2004.
5. Hawes C, Phillips CD, Rose M, et al: A national survey of assisted living facilities, *Gerontologist* 43:875–882, 2003.
6. Sloane PD, Zimmerman S, Hanson L, et al: End-of-life care in assisted living and related residential care settings: comparison with nursing homes, *J Am Geriatr Soc* 51:1587–1594, 2003.
7. Teno JM, Kabumoto G, Wetle T, et al: Daily pain that was excruciating at some time in the previous week: prevalence, characteristics, and outcomes in nursing home residents, *J Am Geriatr Soc* 52:762–767, 2004.
8. Teno JM, Clarridge BR, Casey V, et al: Family perspectives on end-of-life care at the last place of care, *JAMA* 291:88–93, 2004.
9. Miller SC, Mor V, Wu N, et al: Does receipt of hospice care in nursing homes improve the management of pain at the end of life? *J Am Geriatr Soc* 50:507–515, 2002.
10. Miller SC, Teno JM, Mor V: Hospice and palliative care in nursing homes, *Clin Geriatr Med* 20:717–734, 2004.
11. Steel K, Ribbe M, Ahronheim J, et al: Incorporating education on palliative care into the long-term care setting: National Consensus Conference on Medical Education for Care Near the End of Life, *J Am Geriatr Soc* 47:904–907, 1999.
12. Hanson LC, Reynolds KS, Henderson M, Pickard CG: A quality improvement intervention to increase palliative care in nursing homes, *J Palliat Med* 8:576–584, 2005.
13. Teno JM, Claridge B, Casey V, et al: Validation of toolkit after-death bereaved family member interview, *J Pain Symptom Manage* 22:752–758, 2001.
14. Fox E, Landrum-McNiff K, Zhong Z, et al: Evaluation of prognostic criteria for determining hospice eligibility in patients with advanced lung, heart, or liver disease: SUPPORT Investigators. Study to Understand Prognoses and Preferences for Outcomes and Risks of Treatments, *JAMA* 282:1638–1645, 1999.
15. Casarett D, Karlawish J, Morales K, et al: Improving the use of hospice services in nursing homes: a randomized controlled trial, *JAMA* 294:211–217, 2005.
16. Mitchell SL, Berkowitz RE, Lawson FM, Lipsitz LA: A cross-national survey of tube-feeding decisions in cognitively impaired older persons, *J Am Geriatr Soc* 48:391–397, 2000.
17. Finucane TE, Bynum JPW: Use of tube feeding to prevent aspiration pneumonia, *Lancet* 348:1421–1424, 1996.
18. Rabeneck L, Wray NP, Petersen NJ: Long-term outcomes of patients receiving percutaneous endoscopic gastrostomy tubes, *J Gen Intern Med* 11:287–293, 1996.
19. Monteleoni C, Clark E: Using rapid-cycle quality improvement methodology to reduce feeding tubes in patients with advanced dementia: before and after study, *Br Med J* 329:491–494, 2004.
20. Mitchell SL, Tetroe J, O'Connor AM: A decision aid for long-term tube feeding in cognitively impaired older persons, *J Am Geriatr Soc* 49:313–316, 2001.
21. McCann RM, Hall WJ, Groth-Juncker A: Comfort care for terminally ill patients: the appropriate use of nutrition and hydration, *JAMA* 272:1263–1266, 1994.

CHAPTER 43

Home Palliative Care

RUSSELL GOLDMAN

Clinician Competencies	System Capacities
Thinking Ahead	24/7 Access
Managing with Limited Access to Diagnostic Interventions	Access to Physicians
	Access to Patient Information
Delegating Medical and Nursing Tasks to Family Members	Supplies, Medication, and Equipment
The Interdisciplinary Team in the Home	**Predictors of a Home Death**
Clinicians Taking Care of Themselves on the Streets	**Home Palliative Care Is Not for Everyone**
	Pearls
Respecting the Patient's "Bad" Decision	**Pitfalls**
	Summary

Survey results of different populations vary considerably with regard to preference for home as the location of death. A 2000 systematic review of studies found that, overall, the majority of the general population as well as patients and caregivers would prefer to die at home, but the findings varied considerably by study, with the percentage of people preferring to die at home ranging from 25% to 100%.[1] There can be profound shifts in patient and caregiver preference for location of death as the illness progresses. Hinton found that the preference for a home death changed from 90% initially to 50% as death approached.[2]

Regardless of the ultimate preference for location of death, it is generally agreed that most people would prefer to stay at home as long as possible. Data from the U.S. National Hospice and Palliative Care Organization reveal that in 2008, 95.9% of hospice patient care days were spent at home.[3] A primary goal of home palliative care providers should be to provide pain and symptom management that is comparable to the care received on an inpatient unit while striving to maintain the patient at home as long as possible if that is the patient's wish.

Clinician Competencies

With most clinicians receiving little exposure to home visits in their training and even fewer receiving exposure to home palliative care visits, a number of skills and competencies for those providing care at home must be highlighted.

611

THINKING AHEAD

A critical element in keeping end-of-life patients at home and out of the emergency room is the capacity to anticipate what crises a given patient may encounter, especially over the next 24 to 48 hours. In an inpatient facility, staff, supplies, and medication are available and readily accessible. For patients at home, it may take hours for a nurse or physician to attend to the patient and even longer to arrange for special supplies and medications. This may be particularly problematic at night or on the weekend. A basic task of the clinician providing care at home is to inform the patient and caregivers about what might occur in the near term of the next few days. For many people, "forewarned is forearmed." With appropriate education, caregivers will be able to implement appropriate interventions if they have been adequately prepared. The home care clinician is responsible for ensuring that the necessary medications and supplies are in the home. The items that it is possible to have on hand are fewer than in the in-patient setting. However, hospice palliative care providers in many areas have developed emergency medication and supply kits.[4] These kits typically contain the supplies necessary to deal with the common palliative care emergencies. The kit may be placed in the home either at the time of first visit or when the team feels it is appropriate. In the event of a crisis, caregivers can be instructed to open the box and access the necessary medications. Other providers have taken a more focused approach and will order medications and supplies to have on hand that are specific to a given patient's needs. An extreme example of this is the patient at risk for sudden airway obstruction who wishes to stay at home to die. The family and patient should be fully informed as to what to expect if the patient develops signs of airway obstruction. A common approach in this situation would be to insert a subcutaneous line to allow for parenteral access and have preloaded syringes of an opioid and sedative on hand. Caregivers can be taught how to administer a "stat" dose of the appropriate medication while telephoning for further direction or awaiting a member of the home hospice palliative care team.

MANAGING WITH LIMITED ACCESS TO DIAGNOSTIC INTERVENTIONS

A hallmark of modern medicine is easy access to laboratory tests and diagnostic imaging. The clinician providing home hospice/palliative care must learn to cope with limited access to these modalities. Bloodwork at home may be available, but it may only be on a delayed basis. Mobile radiography and ultrasound may not be available or practicable at all in many jurisdictions. Given the frail state of most patients at this stage of their illness, careful consideration must be given before deciding to transport someone for tests. As a result, the home hospice/palliative care clinician must be comfortable with a certain degree of diagnostic uncertainty when confronted with an acute or unexpected situation. In these situations, one should be reminded of the dictums from training; *history, history, history* and *common things are common*. In some situations, *time will tell the tale*. Initially, it may be hard to determine on the basis of a history and physical alone if the house-bound ovarian cancer patient with abdominal pain and no bowel movement for 5 days is constipated or obstructed. The clinician would not want to give laxatives to a patient who is obstructed. Similarly one could worsen the condition of the constipated patient by implementing a treatment algorithm for bowel obstruction. Symptom progression over time may help one sort out this diagnostic dilemma without having to transport the patient for an x-ray examination. Clinicians should openly discuss the issue of diagnostic uncertainty with the patient and family as part of the consent for your recommendations. There will be patients who are prepared to accept a certain amount of uncertainty if it means they do not have to make a trip for tests. Others may push themselves in an extreme fashion to have a specific test performed to know "exactly what is going on." Regardless of their inclination, patients and their families will generally be very understanding of the limitations imposed by the circumstances and will appreciate your careful consideration of their situation.

DELEGATING MEDICAL AND NURSING TASKS TO FAMILY MEMBERS

Patients and their families are frequently called upon these days to provide complex medical care in the home. It is amazing, at times, to see the care that laypeople with appropriate instruction are able to provide to their loved ones. Family members are routinely taught by hospice providers to accomplish rather advanced skills such as changing wound dressings, changing intravenous bags or even managing central lines, or administering artificial nutrition whether through the intravenous route or through a percutaneous endogastric tube. For patients at the end of life, family members can be enlisted to assess and manage symptoms, administer opioids, and utilize pain pumps. However, it is important that the clinician never assume that all caregivers and family members are up to the task at hand. Although many people are willing and able, a significant number are unwilling or unable to assist with care in this way. It is easy for family members to feel "guilted" into assisting with care that they are uncomfortable providing. Furthermore, once a caregiver has agreed to provide a certain type of care, the hospice palliative care providers must ensure that people are well trained and well educated about the task. For example, family members who are providing opioids when needed for pain at the end of life must be advised of the possibility that they may give a dose of medication and see their love one stop breathing a short while later. Given the common myths about opioids, it is easy to envision this person believing that their action of administering medication had a direct impact on the timing of their loved one's death. Appropriate counseling about the possibility of there being a "coincidence" in the timing of a dose of medication and the person's death must be provided before a family member administers a PRN (as needed) or even an RTC (round-the-clock) opioid dose at this point in the illness. Active, hands-on caregiving can be an enormously satisfying experience for some family members, whereas for others it can be extremely stressful and embarrassing. Clinicians providing home palliative care must take the time to assess a given family member's capacity and willingness to perform various tasks.

THE INTERDISCIPLINARY TEAM IN THE HOME

The interdisciplinary team is the cornerstone of palliative care. The role and function of the interdisciplinary team is covered in elsewhere in this textbook. However, a few issues regarding the interdisciplinary team in the home setting should be highlighted.

There may be a need for greater fluidity in roles in the home care setting than there is in an inpatient facility. As a result, members of the various disciplines may have to stretch their "comfort zones" and perform tasks that may not be typically part of their discipline. In an institutional setting, the social worker who walks in the room to find a patient in a pain crisis can go out into the hall to find a nurse to assist. In the home setting, the social worker, as part of the interdisciplinary team, would be expected to be able to assess the situation, assist the patient to take some break-through medication, and call the nurse or physician to report in and request follow up. Similarly, a physician performing a home visit to follow up on medication changes from last week may need to counsel the patient's children when one is enraged that the other is not "pulling their weight." In this situation, the physician would need to perform some initial family counseling and arrange for follow up with the social worker.

It should be noted that not all home palliative care patients have access to the full range of professionals who, ideally, should make up an interdisciplinary team. Depending on where one lives and how home palliative care services are funded, the interdisciplinary team may be composed of a nurse and a physician. In some instances, the nurse is the only one seeing the patient, with the physician providing orders and medication from afar at the nurse's recommendation. Under these circumstances, clinicians may really find themselves stretching to fulfill the various roles. For some, this can be extremely rewarding and refreshing as it forces one to "get out of the box" and learn new skills. However, it can also lead to burnout. Clinicians must be mindful of their limits and should create systems of supports both for themselves and their patients. Often, this entails actively recruiting others, such as the patient's spiritual leader, if they have one, to be a "member" of that patient's care team. Teams can come together around a given patient and disband at the time of death. Over time, these individuals working in the community may come to know each other and be able to function at an increasingly high level. For their own mental health, the clinician may need to identify a few peers with whom they can discuss cases and vent when neces-sary. Although most palliative care providers find their work highly rewarding, working in an environment where one is the "lone ranger" may not be conducive to a lengthy career in the field.

CLINICIANS TAKING CARE OF THEMSELVES ON THE STREETS

Clinicians need to be cognizant of personal safety when providing home palliative care. Good clinical records on a patient before the initial visit may include sufficient information on the home situation. Working in the community involves a type of risk beyond that experienced by most health care providers who work in facilities. In addition to the angry and occasionally violent patients and families one has to deal with in health care facilities, the home health care worker may have to contend with areas of high crime, aggressive panhandlers, gangs, prostitution, poor driving conditions, and unsafe parking areas as they travel between patients.[5] Exact statistics are hard to come by. A study done in Saskatchewan, Canada, in 1995 showed that nurses working in urban settings experienced twice as many assaults and five times as many threatening situations as their rural counterparts.[6] Become knowledgeable about your organization's safety policies and procedures and undertake appropriate safety education. Risk minimization strategies should be identified and implemented when relevant. Having two members of the team do a joint visit can be a very effec-tive care intervention while providing a degree of peace of mind for the providers. It is essential that once a risky situation has been identified, a system exists to dis-seminate this information to the other team members and home health providers who may be involved in providing on-call and after-hours coverage. Some home care services provide escorts for clinicians in some settings. However, one should question whether a given patient is a candidate for home palliative care if an escort is truly required.

RESPECTING THE PATIENT'S "BAD" DECISION

Health care providers have all, at some point in training or practice, had a patient who has made a decision that is hard to agree with. For instance, we may be deeply troubled by a decision to insist on staying at home to die. Clinicians are often troubled by the 82-year-old widow with congestive heart failure who has no children and no family, lives in a squalid apartment, and insists that she will only leave her home "feet first," or the 66-year-old bed-bound man with advanced cancer who is being abused and neglected by his alcoholic wife and similarly won't leave his home to be cared for at an inpatient unit.[7] Patients are well within their legal and ethical right to refuse offers of care, and we must respect their rights to make these decisions as long as they are competent. Caring for patients under these circumstances can exact an emotional toll on the clinician. Case conferences and team meetings should be used to discuss these challenging situations and allow providers an opportunity to share their feelings and frustrations.

System Capacities

In addition to personal skills and competencies, a number of system capacities are necessary for the provision of quality home palliative care.

24/7 ACCESS

Patients can only be maintained at home if they have access to advice and assistance 24/7. Where there is no formal home palliative care program, individual clinicians have been successful at coming together as a call group to provide the necessary coverage. It is difficult to expect that families can care for someone at home if assistance and support are only available from 9 to 5 or from 7 am until 11 pm. Many eventualities can be anticipated and planned for, but there will always be the 3 am phone call from a patient or the family when an unexpected or unforeseen event occurs. Efforts should be made to ensure that the after-hours call system is simple and easily accessed with a timely response. It would be challenging for someone in a crisis to have to handle multiple options on an automated answering service and then have to wait 2 hours for a reply. Creating an easily accessible after-hours network can be extremely difficult, and if it seems unrealistic, home hospice may not be right for that person's setting.

ACCESS TO PHYSICIANS

Physician involvement in home palliative care varies significantly from country to country and within countries as well. Anecdotally, the degree of physician involvement seems to be influenced by how home palliative care is organized, by reimbursement schemes, and by the local medical culture. In certain areas it is the norm for physicians to provide home visits, whereas in other nearby areas it may be exceedingly rare. Access to a physician has been shown to have a significant impact on end-of-life quality of care. Burge and colleagues, using administrative data from Nova Scotia, Canada, demonstrated an association between a family practice continuity of care index and emergency department visits. Patients experiencing low continuity made 3.9 (rate ratio 3.93; 95% CI = 3.57–4.34) times more emergency department visits than those experiencing high continuity.[8] Barbera and colleagues, using administrative data sets from Ontario, Canada, showed that a physician house call or a palliative care assessment were associated with decreased odds of emergency department visits, intensive care unit admissions, and chemotherapy in the last 2 weeks of life. These indicators were selected by the study's authors as measures of poor end-of-life care.[9]

The challenge in many jurisdictions has been how to involve and maintain the involvement of the primary care physician for the patient who requires home palliative care. Barriers to primary care physician involvement have been explored in several studies. Lack of clinical expertise, the challenge of scheduling home visits, poor remuneration, the emotional toll of caring for dying patients, and the lack of resources within the health care system have all been identified as impediments to the provision of home palliative care by primary care physicians.[10,11]

ACCESS TO PATIENT INFORMATION

Ideally, there should be timely flow of patient information between providers from different organizations and between providers within the same organization. This is particularly problematic for patients being discharged for home palliative care follow-up. For all patients, there are significant deficits in information flow. A 2007 U.S. study found that direct person-to-person communication between hospital physicians and primary care physicians was infrequent (3%–20%). Furthermore, the availability of the discharge summary at the first post-discharge visit was poor (12%–34%), with only modest improvement by 4 weeks (51%–77%). When the discharge summary was available, it was frequently found to be missing key information such as course in hospital, discharge medications, and follow-up plans.[12] The study authors felt that computer-generated summaries with standardized formats might remedy some of the identified deficits.

Sharing information among the home palliative care providers may be even more of a challenge. Patients generally have a chart in the home that can be utilized when the clinician is in the home. However, not infrequently, patient contacts may occur by phone. This information will at best then only be updated in the home chart at the next visit. Furthermore, the chart in the home is of no help to the on-call clinician who gets called after hours for a patient that the clinician may not be personally following. Many palliative care programs have implemented electronic medical records to address these gaps in information sharing. Systems now allow remote access such that a provider can log on to the network and access a given patient's chart at all hours. Recently, a patient with amyotrophic lateral sclerosis suffered a choking episode and was taken to the emergency department unconscious after the panicked caregiver called 911. The patient's power of attorney had yet to arrive. The emergency physician contacted the palliative care program as a decision was required about intubation. The on-call clinician was able to log into the patient's chart and advise the emergency physician that the patient did not want to be intubated. Comfort measures were instituted and the patient was returned home based on her previously stated wish to die at home. Her family was able to be with her at home when she died 24 hours later.

Electronic medical records are very costly and there are significant challenges associated with their implementation. However, they can be exceedingly valuable from a patient care perspective as long as the appropriate information is being entered into the system in a timely fashion.

SUPPLIES, MEDICATION, AND EQUIPMENT

Access to supplies, medication, and equipment also varies from location to location, depending on care organization and funding. It is a necessary system capacity feature that patients being cared for at home have timely access to the necessary medications, equipment, and supplies to ensure that they can be adequately cared for at home.

Predictors of a Home Death

A number of factors are predictive of a patient staying at home to die. Highly significant are the patient's stated preference to die at home and the presence of a caregiver.[13–16] These two factors were significant in studies from a number of different countries. In an effort to better understand variation in place of death in the United States, Gruneir and colleagues conducted a systematic review and multilevel analysis in which they linked death certificates with county and state data. Their findings indicate that Americans who are white have greater access to resources and social support, and Americans who have cancer are more likely to die at home. The multilevel analysis revealed that minority status and lower educational attainment increase the probability of death in hospital. Nursing home deaths were associated with a higher density of nursing home beds and a higher state Medicaid payment rate.[17] As can be seen, both individual level characteristics and health care system characteristics impact the rate of home deaths.

Home Palliative Care Is Not for Everyone

Although a home death is an extremely rewarding and enriching experience that lessens the pain of loss for many families, for others it can be a highly stressful and negative experience.[18] Home palliative care clinicians may sometimes need to help families relieve themselves of the burden of a promise to their loved one to care for them at home by encouraging the patient to consider other options. Perhaps the most challenging scenario is when the patient is no longer able to make decisions for himself, but he did indicate his prior wish to be cared for at home, and the family is not coping. In this situation, the substitute decision maker has to decide whether to respect the patient's wishes to stay at home or acknowledge that the family is unable to manage and authorize an admission to an inpatient unit. The home palliative care team must help the decision maker consider immediate needs against the prospect of guilt from a broken promise down the road. There is little in the literature that provides guidance on this question. For some, the prospect of long-term regret is such a concern that they may elect to tough it out for a few more days or weeks. For others, the immediate stress will overcome a hypothetical concern of regret in the future.

Clinicians must be aware of their own biases and beliefs and be careful not to inject them into the decision-making process. Injecting our own biases and beliefs can be extremely damaging, as is illustrated in this quote of an interview of a health care provider from a Canadian ethnographic study examining the social context of home-based palliative caregiving.

> I remember one family I worked with, and they wanted their loved one admitted [to the hospital]. They asked me, "What would you do if it was your father?" And I said, "Well, I'll tell you what I did when it was my mother. I took a leave of

absence and I just stayed with her." And they just looked one to the other and said, "Oh, we can't afford to do that." And I said, "I couldn't afford not to."[18]

Home palliative care is not for all clinicians either. Most palliative care clinicians find their work to be extremely rewarding and professionally fulfilling.[19] However, for some, providing frequent palliative care can exact an emotional toll. Providers must be conscious of their own personal tolerance to being exposed to significant suffering on a daily basis. Working with supportive and caring colleagues is a key element to a long career in the field.

PEARLS

- Do think ahead and prepare patients and their families for anticipatable events.
- Be cautious of your own safety.
- Accept and manage the challenge of diagnostic uncertainty in the home.
- Advocate for system changes when needed.

PITFALLS

- Failing to acknowledge and recognize when the work is taking an emotional toll on you.
- Injecting your own biases and beliefs about the importance of a home death into a decision-making discussion with a patient and their family.

Summary

There are many unique challenges to providing home palliative care. A home palliative care clinician must be aware of the unique competencies required of the individual as well as the vagaries of the health care system he or she is practicing in. In many countries, there is still much work to be done to achieve the necessary system capacities. Although a home death may not be the wish of all palliative care patients and their families, care at home will compose a significant portion of most hospice patients. For those who do wish to die at home, high quality care with appropriate resources to support the patient and family should be the objective of the palliative care team and the health care system.

References

1. Higginson IJ, Sen-Gupta G: Place of care in advanced cancer: a qualitative systematic literature review of patient preferences, *J Palliat Med* 3:287–300, 2000.
2. Hinton J: Which patients with terminal cancer are admitted from home care, *Palliat Med* 8:197–210, 1994.
3. National Hospice and Palliative Care Organization: *NHPCO facts and figures: Hospice care in America*, Alexandria, VA, 2009, NHPCO.
4. Wowchuk SM, Wilson EA, Embleton L, et al: The palliative medication kit: an effective way of extending care in the home for patients nearing death, *J Palliat Med* 12(9):797–803, 2009.
5. Anderson NR: Safe in the city, *Home Healthc Nurse* 26:534–540, 2008.
6. Steinberg A: Safety and home care nurses: a study, *Saskatch Regi Nurses Assoc* 24:24–26, 1995.
7. LoFaso V: The doctor-patient relationship in the home, *Clin Geriatr Med* 16, 2000.
8. Burge F, Lawson B, Johnston G: Family physician continuity of care and emergency department use in end-of-life cancer care, *Med Care* 41:992–1001, 2003.

9. Barbera L, Paszat L, Chartier C: Indicators of poor quality end-of-life care in Ontario, *J Palliat Care* 22:12–17, 2006.
10. Aubin M, Vezina L, Allard P, et al: Palliative care: profile of medical practice in the Quebec City Region, *Can Fam Physician* 47:1999–2005, 2001.
11. Burge F, Lawson B, Johnston G, Cummings I: Primary care continuity and location of death for those with cancer, *J Palliat Med* 6:911–918, 2003.
12. Kripalani S, LeFevre F, Phillips CO, et al: Deficits in communication and information transfer between hospital-based and primary care physicians: implications for patient safety and continuity of care, *JAMA* 297:831–841, 2007.
13. Gyllenhammar E, Thoren-Todoulos E, Strang P, et al: Predictive factors for home deaths among cancer patients in Swedish palliative home care, *Support Care Cancer* 11:560–567, 2003.
14. Klinkenberg M, Visser G, Broese van Groenou MI, et al: The last 3 months of life: care, transitions and the place of death of older people, *Health Soc Care Community* 13:420–430, 2005.
15. Bruera E: Place of death and its predictors for local patients registered at a comprehensive cancer center, *J Clin Oncol* 20:2127, 2002.
16. Brazil K, Bedard M, Willison K: Factors associated with home death for individuals who receive home support services: a retrospective cohort study, *BMC Palliat Care* 1:2, 2002.
17. Gruneir A, Mor V, Weitzen S, et al: Where people die: a multilevel approach to understanding influences on site of death in America, *Med Care Res Rev* 64:351–378, 2007.
18. Stajduhar K: Examining the perspectives of family members involved in the delivery of palliative care at home, *J Palliat Care* 19:27, 2003.
19. Brown JB, Sangster M, Swift J: Factors influencing palliative care, *Can Fam Physician* 44:1028–1034, 1998.

CHAPTER 44

Integrating Palliative Care Guidelines into Clinical Practice

RICHARD H. BERNSTEIN and CHRISTOPHER DELLA SANTINA

This chapter provides an overview of guidelines, their purpose, characteristics, and steps to successfully disseminate and implement them in everyday practice. The goal of this chapter is to encourage the adoption of evidence-based palliative care practices. This challenge requires not only guidelines but also approaches to behavioral change among clinicians, patients, and caregivers, as well as changes in social settings, professional organizations, educational institutions, and regulatory agencies. Specific examples of palliative care guidelines are noted in the text or cited in the Resources section of this chapter.

620

About Guidelines

Several terms are used to describe consensus statements about clinical practices.

Practice policies are recommendations intended to be applied to populations of patients with a particular condition within a specified medical context. Eddy describes three types of practice policies: standards, options, and guidelines.[1] **Standards** are considered best practices backed by well-documented research and experience. Failure to follow standards might be a basis for a malpractice claim. **Options** represent interventions for which outcomes are unknown or for which outcomes are known but patient preferences vary. **Guidelines** are more flexible than standards and are intended to aid or guide clinical decision making.

The Institute of Medicine defines clinical practice guidelines as "systematically developed statements to assist practitioner and patient decisions about appropriate health care for specific clinical circumstances".[2] Guidelines are intended as aids, and deviations are common and in many cases appropriate. The quality of the underlying evidence varies,[3] and systems for rating the strength of evidence have been codified by the Canadian Taskforce on the Periodic Health Examination and the U.S. Preventive Services Taskforce. Well-formulated guidelines have an explicit description and evaluation of the evidence used, the potential benefits and harms, and the resulting grade of recommendations made. Additional terms, such as *clinical practice guidelines, protocols, clinical pathways, critical pathways, care maps, clinical algorithms,* and similar terms are generally used synonymously. The balance of this chapter employs *clinical guidelines,* or *guidelines,* for short.

Guidelines have multiple applications, depending on the user (e.g., clinicians, educators, quality-of-care evaluators, patients, policy makers, payers, and others) and on how they are designed. Clinical guidelines may introduce recent innovations into clinical practice, suggest recommendations for education programs, outline methods for evaluating practices, and provide a basis for pay-for-performance initiatives. They may also aid patients and consumer groups to better understand medical decision making, inform policy makers to help set research agendas, and identify best practices for payers and regulators to reduce unnecessary and cost-inefficient practices. Over the past 2 decades, the number of clinical practice guidelines in general and those for palliative care in particular have proliferated exponentially. They are usually available via the internet in comprehensive databases (see Resources section at the end of this chapter).

Ideal guidelines should be user friendly, evidence based, and identify key decision points along with the possible benefits and burdens of options at those decision points.

Barriers to Guideline Use

The quality, applicability, and utility of individual guidelines vary considerably. Furthermore, it can be daunting for practicing community clinicians to sort through the literature to assess the quality of evidence and the strength of recommendations to guide decision making in individual clinical circumstances.

Another challenge facing guideline writers and other stakeholders (clinicians, patients, families, administrators, payers, etc.) with an interest in improving the quality of palliative care is the difficulty of getting guidelines adopted within a particular care delivery system. Clinicians, patients, and families may be resistant to recommendations, and the community context of the practice may also influence treatment decisions.[4] Thus, the ease with which recommendations can be integrated into the existing clinical care settings and the likelihood of their acceptance by both physicians and the communities they serve directly affects the probability that the intended beneficial outcomes of the guideline will be realized.

Finally, the relative dearth of hospital-based palliative care specialists, particularly in smaller community hospitals or rural settings, is another limiting factor to improving access to quality palliative care.

Status of Guidelines in Palliative Care

PROFESSIONAL CONSENSUS ABOUT THE IMPORTANCE OF QUALITY PALLIATIVE AND END-OF-LIFE CARE

Over the past decade, palliative care has gained wide acceptance as a quality standard for all care settings in which serious, life-threatening conditions are treated. Fourteen national specialty societies and the Joint Commission (formerly the Joint Commission on the Accreditation of Healthcare Organizations) have adopted recommendations and policies that embrace the core principles of palliative care. Palliative care is now a recognized subspecialty with a well-defined set of practice standards.

In 2005, the American College of Surgeons (ACS) Committee on Ethics developed and approved its principles of palliative care, which includes patients at all stages of disease, in a "Statement on Principles of Palliative Care" (available at www.facs. org/fellows_info/statements/st-50.html). The Accreditation Council for Graduate Medical Education (ACGME) began certifying fellowship training programs in palliative medicine in 2007, and in 2008 the American Board of Medical Specialties (ABMS) began offering subspecialty certification in hospice and palliative medicine.

Related efforts are underway to ensure that palliative care is provided in intensive care units,[5] where 22% of all deaths in the United States occur during or after admission.

One of the largest representative efforts to codify practice guidelines for palliative care was the National Consensus Project for Quality Palliative Care (see Resources section in this chapter). Its guidelines were developed and agreed upon by five major palliative care organizations in the United States: the American Academy of Hospice and Palliative Medicine, the Center to Advance Palliative Care, the Hospice and Palliative Nurses Association, Last Acts Partnership, and the National Hospice and Palliative Care Organization. It referred to prior efforts of the Institute of Medicine reports (*Approaching Death*, *When Children Die*, and *Crossing the Quality Chasm*), the American Association of Colleges of Nursing report *Peaceful Death*, the National Hospice Work Group and the Hastings Center in association with the National Hospice and Palliative Care Organization monograph, *Access to Hospice Care: Expanding Boundaries, Overcoming Barriers*. It was noted that all these reports call for substantive changes to improve access to palliative care across the life span, in all health care settings, during all stages of debilitating chronic or life-threatening illness or injury. These changes include enhancements in the quality of care, restructuring of health care system regulations on service, education of health care professionals and research to support evidence-based palliative care practice.

Translating the corpus of these principles into user-friendly tools that allow practicing community physicians or institutionally based practices to easily translate them into culturally sensitive practice guidelines remains a challenge. Great Britain's National Health Service has made major progress in meeting this challenge. An initiative, called the Gold Standards Framework (GSF), was started by a single general practitioner and is designed to educate community-based primary care physicians on palliative care standards. GSF provides a toolkit for assessing prognosis and counseling individuals with a limited prognosis (see www.goldstandardsframework.nhs.uk). It has now been now adopted by 4500 practices covering half the English population.

A set of useful resources is available to clinicians to facilitate developing these skills (see www.hospicecare.com/resources/treatment.htm, in addition to the Resources section in this chapter).

Besides broad agreement about the principles and practice of palliative care, there is also general recognition that changes in the health care system need to occur. These include the following:

- Broader access to palliative care in all stages of life-limiting conditions
- A focus on the quality of end-of-life care
- More professional education in palliative care
- More research to enhance the scientific basis for palliative care practice and guidelines

Although clinical guidelines can be expected to make a contribution to several of these goals, they are not sufficient to achieve all these aspirations. Moreover, guidelines are not likely to be effective in changing traditional practice patterns unless they are disseminated to more physicians, and unless physicians are motivated to adopt such guidelines and be held accountable for performance consistent with the guidelines. Steps to facilitate these critical behavioral changes will be more fully addressed in the next section.

Beyond Guidelines: Steps to Effect Behavioral Changes among Professionals, Patients, and Their Caregivers

IMPROVING THE PALLIATIVE CARE CONTENT WITHIN GENERAL AND SPECIALTY CLINICAL GUIDELINES

Ideally, palliative care standards should be integrated into the care pathways of all clinical management guidelines that focus on life-limiting conditions. Studies indicate that this is not the case. Mast and co-workers surveyed 91 guidelines representing nine significant life-limiting conditions for palliative care guidance and found that only 10% had significant palliative care content, and 64% had minimal content.[6] The absence of palliative care references in such guidelines may undermine the importance of palliative care in the eyes of generalists and specialists who manage such diseases.

As described previously, experts in palliative care have developed guidelines for specialists in their own field. Nonetheless, there is a critical need for palliative care principles to be disseminated more broadly, especially to non–palliative care physicians who use disease management guidelines in their clinical practices. The American Hospice Foundation Guidelines Committee recognized the lack of end-of-life issues in most chronic disease management guidelines. In 2004, this group developed a template that recommended how other medical specialty guidelines could integrate palliative care principles into the initial assessment, diagnosis, treatment, and concluding phases of managing life-limiting diseases.[7]

STRATEGIES TO INCORPORATE GUIDELINES INTO CLINICAL PRACTICE

The gap between existing evidence-based recommendations and actual clinical practice is well documented. A variety of interventions to close this gap (such as medical record audits and feedback, academic detailing, chart-based reminders, computer decision support, and benchmarking) have been studied and tried, although no one intervention has been shown to consistently change behavior among health care professionals across all settings. It is clear that passive dissemination alone, such as traditional continuing medical educational (CME) efforts, is one of the least effective techniques; however, a recent study demonstrated that CME utilizing a more interactive format with multimedia and live demonstration can improve knowledge, practice behavior, and clinical practice outcomes.[8]

THE CHALLENGE OF CHANGING PATIENT AND CAREGIVER BEHAVIOR

Effective implementation strategies to ensure that guidelines are broadly disseminated must also involve patients and caregivers in medical decision making and self-management. Fortunately, public versions of guidelines are available and formatted in ways that are understandable to the layperson and caregivers. Such material is available in multiple formats (e.g., brochures, videos, audiotapes, websites).[9] Examples can be found on various websites, including Get Palliative Care (www.getpalliativecare.org), Palliative Care, The Relief You Need When You're Experiencing the Symptoms of Serious Illness (www.ninr.nih.gov/NR/rdonlyres/01CC45F1-048B-468A-BD9F-3AB727A381D2/0/NINR_PalliativeCare_Brochure_508C.pdf), and Aging With Dignity (www.agingwithdignity.org/5wishes.html); books on advanced care planning, such as Molloy's *Let Me Decide* (see http://www.planningwhatiwant.com.au/Documents/c%20let%20me%20decide.pdf); and booklets and videos in several languages used in Canadian studies on the implementation of health care choices for life-threatening illness, cardiac arrest, and nutritional support.

An innovative video series of relatively short patient interviews has been designed to improve patient decision making on difficult end-of-life care issues. Volandes has tested these in a variety of populations in the United States and abroad. This approach enabled patients to better visualize what "comfort care," "limited care," and "life-prolonging care" would mean to them. Seeing the videos had a measurable influence on their decisions compared with those who received only more traditional one-on-one counseling about such decisions (see http://news.harvard.edu/gazette/story/2009/06/video-can-help-patients-make-end-of-life-decisions/).

Diffusion of Information and Training: Applying Lessons to the Adoption of Palliative Care

Diffusion studies is a field that analyzes the processes that contribute to or inhibit the dissemination of an innovation. Effectively applying its insights can help make quality palliative care more available.

Palliative is a form of innovation—that is:

> An idea, practice, or object that is perceived as new by an individual or another unit of adoption.... Diffusion is the process by which an innovation is communicated through certain channels over time among the members of a social system...The four main elements are the innovation, communication channels, time, and the social system. These elements are identifiable in every diffusion research study, and in every diffusion campaign or program.[10]

Innovation, including the adoption of comprehensive, quality palliative care in clinical practice, embodies a set of valuable principles that should be readily embraced by all physicians. Nonetheless, lack of familiarity with advances in palliative care generates indifference or resistance or may raise questions about its value to patients, compared with how generalists or specialists usually deal with end-of-life issues.

Potential adopters of an innovation may also be influenced by their perceptions of the acceptability of palliative care guidelines by their patients and colleagues in their particular practice setting. Also important is adopters' perceptions about the feasibility of implementing guideline recommendations given the available resources (e.g., time, technical skills, facilities) in their practice setting.

Innovation-oriented physicians may be early adopters and appreciate the relative advantage of palliative care over the standard medical model. Others focus on its comprehensiveness and multidimensional nature and become discouraged. For example, the previously cited National Consensus Project for Quality Palliative Care takes more than 25 pages to describe 8 separate domains of care and 19 guidelines with 120 criteria that should be addressed. As shown with the Gold Standards Framework, much work can be done to simplify such guidelines.

Communication channels to educate physicians about palliative care exist in many venues and are important tools for the dissemination of information about a field's general ideas. Some examples include the Education in Palliative and End-of-Life Care (EPEC) Project, whose mission is to educate all health care professionals on the essential clinical competencies in palliative care (www.epec.net); End of Life/Palliative Education Resource Center at the Medical College of Wisconsin (EPERC; www.eperc.mcw.edu; and End-of-Life Nursing Education Consortium (ELNEC; www.aacn.nche.edu/ELNEC/index.htm). In addition, the Liaison Committee for Medical Education (LCME), which establishes undergraduate medical education requirements, and the Accreditation Council on Graduate Medical Education, which defines requirements for residency and fellowships programs in the United States, have both recognized training in end-of-life care issues in their review criteria.

Despite these efforts, deficiencies continue to be prevalent. In a 2003 survey that evaluated the experiences of medical students, residents, and faculty, Sullivan and coworkers found that fewer than 18% of students and residents received formal end-of-life education, 39% of students reported being unprepared to address patients' thoughts and fears about dying, and nearly half felt unprepared to manage their own feelings about patients' deaths or to help bereaved families.[11] In addition, palliative care has not been adequately represented in medical textbooks.[12]

Physicians have also relied on other continuing medical education resources to maintain and improve their skills and knowledge. Traditional formats, such as attending lectures and reading textbooks, journals, and published clinical guidelines, are supplemented by newer methods that are more learner-centered and self-directed. The latter include computer-based interactive technologies. Conclusions about which educational methods are most effective in influencing clinical practice and improving outcomes may be determined by factors unique to the individual targeted, such as review of actual records. This becomes more practical with the installation of electronic health records.

Despite the ease and availability of the internet and the variety of traditional continuing medical education venues, innovation studies suggest that the most effective way of influencing behavioral changes, especially those involving new patterns of practice, are interpersonal experiences, especially those that include face-to-face contact. This allows a clear exchange about the key elements of the innovation, an opportunity to positively influence the initiate's attitude toward the innovation, and, ultimately, to persuade physicians to try implementing these changes in their practice.

Diffusion investigations show that most individuals do not evaluate an innovation on the basis of scientific studies of its consequences, although such objective evaluations may be especially relevant to the very first individuals who adopt them. Instead, most depend primarily on a subjective evaluation of an innovation that is conveyed to them from other individuals like themselves. The dependence on the experience of near peers suggests that the heart of the diffusion process consists of the modeling and imitation by potential adopters of their network partners who have previously adopted the innovation. Thus, diffusion is a very social process.

The availability of mini-residencies for community physicians or invitations to attend palliative care units and palliative care rounds as CME-creditable activities may be important complements to courses, conferences, journal articles, books, and guidelines in palliative care.

The pace or rapidity with which those exposed to the concepts of palliative care actually adopt it will vary. Innovation studies consistently describe four groups: early adopters, an early majority, a late majority, and laggards.

The social system in which innovative ideas occur affects the likelihood of innovations being adopted and how quickly they are adopted. The presence of opinion leaders who are respected members of a peer group and a nexus of relationships that reinforce the acceptability and desirability of new changes has a strong influence on the rate of adoption of innovation.

The challenge here is threefold. First, the presence of fellowship-trained palliative care physicians in more institutions is a critical step to improving access to expert consultations and care and to influencing the attitudes and practices of non–palliative care physicians elsewhere in the hospital and related institutions. At present, there are fifty hospice and palliative care medicine fellowship programs in the United States, and these programs are expected to graduate more than 100 fellows each year. This number falls far short of the need, and therefore all medical residents and fellows need to be trained in basic palliative care skills. This is part of the curriculum stipulated by the Accreditation Council on Graduate Medical Education, although the details of this aspect of the curriculum and the qualifications of the teachers of palliative care are not specified.

Second, many physicians in practice may not define their core responsibilities as including palliative care or early palliative care referral. It is therefore important to further encourage specialty societies to include palliative care principles in their clinical guidelines, board exams, recertification exams, and residency program accreditation requirements; to include courses in palliative care principles in major meetings; to encourage palliative care–oriented journal articles in specialty journals; and to have specialty society leadership explicitly stress the inclusion of palliative care responsibilities within the professional expectations of each specialty.

Third, there is a need to reach relatively isolated physicians in rural practices or those without active hospital privileges and to find practical ways to invite such individuals into model palliative care centers so that such physicians will learn to better manage their patients and make appropriate referrals.

TECHNOLOGY AS A TOOL FOR DIFFUSING INNOVATION

Technology also has an important role in the dissemination of palliative care. As previously mentioned, the comprehensiveness of palliative care generates hundreds of potential interventions in multiple domains of care. When viewed from the standpoint of paper-based guidelines and paper-based medical records, the translation of these guidelines into practice is indeed daunting. Digitizing health information is crucial for many reasons, not least of which is that electronic health records (EHRs) allow programming of prompts or reminders to clinicians about needed care for individual patients. These rules-driven reminder systems incorporate evidence-based guidelines and help busy physicians adhere to even complex sets of recommendations.

The initiative of the U.S. and British governments, as well as managed care and pharmaceutical firms, to subsidize the purchase of EHRs and the development of computerized networks will make such prompting systems more prevalent. The ease with which guidelines can be downloaded to handheld personal digital assistants (PDAs and tablet PCs) should also facilitate the diffusion of the important principles of palliative care into everyday practice, in both hospital and office settings.

Given the slow rate of adoption of EHRs, a low-technology approach, such as the Gold Standards Framework, may allow a more rapid diffusion of high quality palliative care, if it is supported by professional organizations, pay-for-performance initiatives, and private and public quality rating organizations.

Linking Palliative Care Guidelines to Quality of Care: Major Challenges

The implementation of palliative care guidelines is fundamentally a means to improve quality of care in large systems. Because end-of-life and palliative care must be individualized and take into account patient preferences and values, clinical judgment is more complex. As a result, palliative care guidelines must allow for broad flexibility in provider decision making. This complicates the ability to measure "guideline adherence," which characterizes most assessments of quality. Similarly, setting performance benchmarks or metrics may not be feasible in a population of individuals with terminal illness. There are multiple potential sources of bias in evaluating outcomes and even satisfaction: the variation in patient values and goals of care, the difficulty establishing prognosis, the definition of the dominant diagnosis in the presence of multiple comorbidities, the variation in the quality of caregiver support, the changing level of cognitive function, and the variable response to medication for relief of symptoms, all of which impact on the effectiveness of palliative care interventions.

The Gold Standards Framework used an "audit questionnaire" completed by health care providers to gauge effectiveness of the program. The majority of practices reported that quality of palliative care improved, despite the lack of financial incentives built around this.[13] Although encouraging, the self-report is open to selection and other biases that complicate research focused on palliative care outcomes.

THE PROBLEM OF PAY-FOR-PERFORMANCE INCENTIVES IN PALLIATIVE AND END-OF-LIFE CARE

National attention to improving quality of care and patient safety has prompted the development of pay-for-performance (P4P) or pay-for-improvement (P4I) initiatives by large health plans and the Centers for Medicare and Medicaid Services (CMS). Quality of care is measured, and financial incentives for physicians and hospitals are linked to performance measures. There are now well-established metrics in these pay-for-performance models that can be used to assess quality based on preventive care and longitudinal care for a variety of chronic diseases. The primary focus of these incentive programs is to motivate physician compliance with evidence-based clinical guidelines.

Although these programs hold much promise for improving quality of care in a variety of areas, performance payment models for palliative care delivery are problematic and, to our knowledge, have not been implemented. Challenges in the design and implementation of such incentives include the development of standardized, validated measures, adjusting payments based on case mix and severity, and building in financial incentives that are significant enough to encourage providers to focus on quality. Ethical considerations must be addressed to ensure that financial incentives would not encourage inappropriate care.

THE ROLE OF HOSPITAL EVALUATION, ACCREDITING ORGANIZATIONS, AND LEGISLATION TO PROMOTE PALLIATIVE CARE AND QUALITY MEASUREMENT

The Joint Commission is a national accrediting body that can foster practice changes in hospitals. The audits by this organization are based on practice standards. Current standards recognize the patient's right to refuse care, the patient's wishes relating to end-of-life decisions, and the patient's right to pain management, along with comfort and dignity, during end-of-life care. The Joint Commission has not incorporated other elements of palliative care principles in its audits, although the Center to Advance Palliative Care has developed a "Crosswalk" of the Joint Commission's Standards and a broad spectrum of palliative care policies, procedures, and support tools (www.capc.org/jcaho-crosswalk).

The Leapfrog Group (www.leapfroggroup.org) is a well-recognized employer-driven organization that is using evidence-based standards in the areas of safety, quality, and affordability of health care. Its goal is to inform health care consumers and to provide recognition for excellence in hospital performance. It has developed incentive programs to encourage hospitals to adopt its standards. These initiatives are supported in part by the Agency for Healthcare Research and Quality (AHRQ). The Leapfrog Group could influence the rate of availability of palliative care within hospitals if it were to accept certain structural standards, such as the importance of staffing hospitals with palliative care teams to improve access to quality end-of-life care.

The National Quality Forum (www.qualityforum.org) has hospital standards for palliative care programs in its report "National Framework and Preferred Practices for Palliative and Hospice Care Quality" (see www.qualityforum.org/Projects/n-r/Palliative_and_Hospice_Care_Framework/Palliative__Hospice_Care__Framework_and_Practices.aspx).

The Center to Advance Palliative Care (www.capc.org) offers materials based on preferred hospital palliative care practices developed by the National Quality Forum (www.capc.org/support-from-capc/capc_publications/nqf-crosswalk.pdf).

The National Committee for Quality Assurance (www.NCQA.org) is the most widely accepted accrediting organization for managed care organizations. Because of their emphasis on coordinated and comprehensive care, managed care organizations potentially offer an ideal delivery model to promote palliative care guidelines. Nonetheless, NCQA has not adopted standards for quality palliative care. This suggests an opportunity for palliative care leadership to further their goals by influencing the priorities of this accrediting organization.

Unfortunately, the few palliative care standards within the corpus of the Joint Commission and the lack of any NCQA standards convey to those being audited that either there are no evidence-based guidelines upon which to base audits or that palliative care is not a priority for assessing quality of care. Political considerations may be another factor affecting some organizations, given the critical reaction to health care reform efforts that tried to incorporate palliative care counseling. Nevertheless, many managed care organizations have adopted palliative care guidelines or developed novel programs to better manage end-of-life patients.[14]

THE ROLE OF GOVERNMENT IN PROMOTING ACCESS TO PALLIATIVE CARE

The Center to Advance Palliative Care and the National Palliative Care Research Center recently completed a state-by-state survey of access to palliative care in our nation's hospitals (www.capc.org/reportcard) in America's Care of Serious Illness. Overall, the country received a "C" grade, meaning 41% to 60% of hospitals had a palliative care program.

The report's recommendations included involvement of the government in several areas including legislation that would require access of all hospitalized patients to palliative care as a condition for Medicaid and Medicare reimbursement. Palliative care quality indicators for Medicaid recipients and the provision of funding for palliative care training are other ways the government could promote the diffusion of palliative care and greatly reduce the unneeded suffering of its citizens with life-limiting diseases.

PEARLS

- Clinical practice guidelines have the potential to crystallize large bodies of scientific evidence into actionable recommendations to improve the quality of clinical outcomes, reduce unnecessary and harmful care, and reduce the cost of care.

- Ideally, guidelines are evidence based and include objective evaluation of risk-stratified outcomes, incorporate patient preferences, and allow weighing of benefits and burdens of various treatment options.

- Most guidelines do not fulfill the ideal characteristics, and this is true of many elements within palliative care guidelines. This limitation of palliative care guidelines is understandable, given the multifaceted nature of palliative care's scope (as opposed to a single disease focus) and the difficulty of doing scientific research with a frail and vulnerable population that may be unwilling or unable to cooperate with strict research protocols.

- Despite these limitations, there is a broad consensus about what quality palliative care entails.

- It is critical that the curricula for medical students, residents, and postgraduate students incorporate palliative care more extensively. This should be reinforced through accreditation bodies and certification examinations.

- Templates can help specialty societies and other organizations enrich their guidelines that deal with life-limiting conditions so that they incorporate key principles of quality palliative care.

- Diffusion studies suggest a variety of strategies for reaching those slow to adopt innovations. For palliative care this might include a user-friendly toolkit, such as the one developed by the Gold Standards Framework; interactions with one-on-one near peer role models in mini-residencies or rounds; technology such as electronic prompting systems within EHRs; pay-for-performance incentives that reinforce palliative care best practices; and the Joint Commission, Leapfrog, and NCQA standards that stress palliative care.

PITFALLS

- Guidelines that employ informal or formal consensus among subject matter are more subject to bias, especially if the scientific evidence upon which opinions are based is not well documented.

- Guidelines that do not take into account expected patient outcomes for various subgroups are problematic, because they make it difficult for both physicians and patients to confidently apply the recommendations.

- Despite its difficulty, the effect of patient preferences should also be incorporated into guidelines, especially those that involve palliative care.

- These ideal attributes are rarely characteristic of clinical practice guidelines and contribute to the lack of widespread adoption of clinical practice guidelines.

- Changing clinical practice patterns and widely diffusing innovations such as high-quality palliative care must involve changes in many dimensions of medicine as a social system. As a result, we cannot expect to see the goals of palliative care fully realized in the near term.

Summary

Clinical guidelines have the potential to improve the quality of care and patient outcomes, decrease the variation in clinical practice, and reduce the cost of care. They can help educate clinicians at all levels about evidence-based recommendations on state-of-the art practices.

There has been general acceptance about the attributes of ideal guidelines and the process for creating effective guidelines. In addition, there is a general consensus among palliative care organizations about what constitutes high-quality palliative care. The guidelines that derive from this consensus are not ideal, nor are they easy to implement, especially for the busy practicing physician. Nonetheless, with a more user-friendly format and simplification to make it a practical tool for community-based clinical practices, it could form a foundation to make palliative care more accessible.

There is a need to expose physicians to more palliative care training. Medical schools, residency programs, and board exams should reinforce this. In addition, templates have been formulated to help incorporate palliative care into guidelines developed by specialty societies and interdisciplinary groups that address the care of life-limiting conditions. Dissemination of guidelines alone cannot be expected to change practice patterns, especially among the majority of physicians who had little or no exposure to palliative care during their training.

Diffusion studies suggest several changes that will be needed to ensure that recommendations about quality palliative care are more broadly instituted by those physicians who treat the many patients who could benefit from such guidelines. These include the influence of one-on-one near peer teaching, reinforcement of the importance of palliative care by opinion leaders, and the use of technology to facilitate the translation of comprehensive guideline recommendations into electronic prompting systems in hospital and office settings. Pay-for-performance incentives and the incorporation of palliative care standards into the Joint Commission, Leapfrog, the National Quality Forum, and NCQA would also help those who are slower at integrating palliative care into their practice patterns. Finally, support from government, including legislation to promote the diffusion of palliative care, can also help reduce the suffering of its citizens with life-threatening illnesses.

Resources

National Guideline Clearinghouse, Agency for Healthcare Research and Quality (U.S.). A general guideline database.
   www.guideline.gov
At present, there are four general categories of palliative care guidelines. Following are four resources for current lists of these guidelines: The National Consensus Project for Quality Palliative Care. General palliative care policy guidelines that deal with palliative care from a comprehensive perspective.
   www.nationalconsensusproject.org/Guidelines_Download.asp
Integrating Principles of Palliative Care into Disease Management Guideline Development.
   Emanuel LL, Alexander C, Arnold R, et al: Integrating palliative care into disease management guidelines, *J Palliat Med* 7:774–783, 2004.
TIME: A Toolkit of Instruments to Measure End-of-life Care. Guidelines specifically intended for health care practitioners who provide palliative care.
   www.chcr.brown.edu/pcoc/choosing.htm
National Comprehensive Cancer Network (NCCN) Clinical Practice Guidelines in Oncology. Disease management–based guidelines for life-limiting conditions that include aspects of end of life care (requires registration).
   www.nccn.org/professionals/physician_gls/f_guidelines.asp

References

1. Eddy DM: Designing a practice policy: standards, guidelines, and options, *JAMA* 263:3077–3084, 1990.
2. Field MJ, Lohr KN, editors: *Clinical practice guidelines: directions for a new program*, Washington, DC, 1990, National Academy Press.
3. Wilson MC, Hayward RSA, Tunis SR, et al: Users' guides to the medical literature. VIII. How to use clinical practice guidelines B. What are the recommendations and will they help you in caring for your patients? *JAMA* 274:1630–1632, 1995.
4. Greer AL, Goodwin JS, Freeman JL, et al: Bringing the patient back in. Guidelines, practice variations, and the social context of medical practice, *Int J Technol Assess Health Care* 18:747–761, 2002.
5. Bradley CT, Brasel KJ: Developing guidelines that identify patients who would benefit from palliative care services in the surgical intensive care unit, *Crit Care Med* 37:946-950, 2009.
6. Mast KR, Salama M, Silverman GK, et al: End-of-life content in treatment guidelines for life-limiting diseases, *J Palliat Med* 7:754–773, 2004.
7. Emanuel LL, Alexander C, Arnold R, et al: Integrating palliative care into disease management guidelines, *J Palliat Med* 7:774–783, 2004.
8. Marinopoulos SS, Dorman T, Ratanawongsa N, et al: Effectiveness of continuing medical education, *Evid Rep Technol Assess* 14:1–69, 2007.
9. Michie S, Lester K: Words matter: increasing the implementation of guidelines, *Qual Saf Health Care* 14:367–370, 2005.
10. Rogers EM: *Diffusion of innovations*, New York, 1995, The Free Press.
11. Sullivan A, Lakoma M, Block S: The status of medical education in end-of-life care: a national report, *J Gen Intern Med* 18:685–695, 2003.
12. Rabow MW, Hardie GE, Fair JM, et al: End-of-life content in 50 textbooks from multiple specialties, *JAMA* 283:771–778, 2000.
13. Dale J, Petrova M, Munday D, et al: A national facilitation project to improve primary palliative care: impact of the Gold Standards Framework on process and self ratings of quality, *Qual Saf Health Care* 18:174–180, 2009.
14. Brumley RD: Future of end-of-life care: the managed care organization perspective, *J Palliat Med* 5:263–270, 2002.

CHAPTER 45

Palliative Care Services and Programs

ALEXIE CINTRON and DIANE E. MEIER

In this chapter, we discuss the types of palliative care services that are available in the United States and Canada. Palliative care services are most often provided in one of two settings: the hospital and the patient's home. Hospital-based palliative care programs include palliative care consult teams, palliative care units, and ambulatory palliative care services. Non–hospital-based programs include hospice care, home care, and bridge programs. A major criticism of hospice programs and some bridge programs is that enrollment is restricted to those individuals with a terminal prognosis. Provision of palliative care services should be based on need, not on prognosis. Conflating palliative care with end-of-life care can lead to late referrals to palliative care services.

Although primary palliative care can be provided by all health care professionals and is part of the basic competency of individual practitioners, secondary and tertiary palliative care encompasses a set of specialist services that exceed the skills of primary care providers and are therefore provided by providers with specialty training in palliative care. Palliative care providers should have skills and training in complex medical evaluation, pain and symptom management, professional-to-patient communication, addressing difficult decisions regarding goals of care, sophisticated discharge planning, and providing bereavement support while adhering as closely as possible to clinical practice guidelines such as those put forth by the National Consensus Project for Quality Palliative Care. Certification for hospice and palliative

633

care nursing is granted by the National Board for Certification of Hospice and Palliative Nurses (NBCHPN), and certification of physicians is granted by the American Board of Medical Specialties (ABMS).

Palliative care can be provided to patients with advanced serious illness by a variety of services in numerous settings. This chapter discusses the types of palliative care services that are available. The types and availability of palliative care services are discussed within the context of Medicare, the major payment system for palliative care in the United States. We then end with an overview of training core skills necessary to provide palliative care, as well as training requirements for obtaining certification in hospice and palliative care.

Levels of Palliative Care Delivery

As with general medical care, palliative care can be delivered at three levels: primary, secondary, and tertiary. Primary palliative care can be provided by all health care professionals in any setting where patients receive care and should be part of the basic competency of individual practitioners.[1] Moreover, primary palliative care is an expected part of primary care service models, and primary care physicians can acquire the knowledge, attitudes, and skills needed to provide palliative care to their patients. Local and national policy initiatives can ensure that providers demonstrate palliative care competencies. For example, an initiative of the Joint Commission (formerly the Joint Commission on Accreditation of Healthcare Organizations) on pain aims to ensure that pain control is part of the primary care of all patients in its accredited institutions.[1] Accreditation of health care institutions in Canada by the Canadian Council on Health Services Accreditation now includes a specific section on palliative and end-of-life care.

Secondary palliative care is a set of specialist services that exceeds the skills of primary care providers.[1,2] These services are provided through specialized consultation teams. Although the recommendations made by palliative care consultation services may overlap with care that every physician should be able to provide, providers with special interest and training in palliative care possess attitudes, knowledge, and skills not yet acquired by most physicians. Palliative care specialists are equipped to handle the very time-consuming and complex interventions required by some patients with serious illness. Examples of secondary palliative care are hospices, palliative care teams and specialists, home palliative care services, and palliative care units. Pain specialists are not considered secondary palliative care providers because their practice patterns and target populations are generally different from those of palliative care specialists.[1] Standards for specialist palliative care training have been developed and are discussed later in this chapter.

Tertiary palliative care exceeds the ability of secondary palliative care and is provided by referral centers with expertise in difficult problems.[1,2] Providers of tertiary palliative care are responsible for educating and conducting research in palliative care.

Hospital-Based Programs

Hospital-based palliative care teams have evolved from the modern palliative care movement as a result of national initiatives in the United States and Canada that called for improved pain and symptom management and for psychosocial, social, and spiritual support for patients and families living with serious illness.[3,4] These programs aim to improve hospital care for patients living with serious illness, care that is often characterized by untreated physical symptoms, poor communication between providers and patients, and treatment decisions in conflict with prior stated preferences. Patients with serious illness spend at least some time in a hospital during the course of their illness. These patients need expert symptom management, communication and decision-making support, and care coordination. Consequently, the number of hospital-based palliative care programs has grown rapidly in recent years.[5–7] Various secondary and tertiary palliative care models have developed in hospital settings, including palliative care consultation teams, palliative care units, and ambulatory palliative care services.

PALLIATIVE CARE CONSULTATION TEAM

The palliative care consultation team is the predominant hospital-based, specialist-level palliative care delivery model.[2,6] The goal of such a service is to assess the physical, psychological, social, spiritual, and cultural needs of patients with advanced, serious illness. The consultation team then advises the consulting provider on how to address these needs, thus providing support and supplementing the care of other physicians for their most complex and seriously ill patients, as well as providing direct care collaboratively with the referring care team. Effective palliative care teams understand that the referring team is also a client and that, although the work of the palliative care consultation team directly benefits the patient, the team should demonstrate a benefit to these clinicians. The team roles include educating clinicians about the components of care and the benefits of palliative care, generating visibility and awareness of the program and the need for better quality end-of-life care, and building clinical partnerships and support for its services. Evidence exists that palliative care consult services improve outcomes.[8]

The design of a successful palliative care program should fully reflect the unique mission, needs, and constraints of the hospital it serves, as well as nationally accepted standards. It also adjusts to accommodate shifts in hospital priorities and patients' needs.[9] Ideally, palliative care consultation services should consist of an interdisciplinary team that includes a physician, an advanced nurse practitioner, and a social worker. Other team members may include chaplains, volunteers, rehabilitation professionals, psychologists, and psychiatrists. Many programs have adopted a solo practitioner model that consists of a physician or an advanced nurse practitioner. The choice between starting a program with a solo practitioner or a full team often depends on the availability of trained palliative care staff. However, as more trained staff becomes available, the model can transition from a solo practice to a full team model.[8,9]

Everyone on the team is responsible for assessing and following patients referred by an attending physician and contributing to the care plan. The team then provides advice to the referring team based on the assessment, care plan, and follow-up. On occasion, the team may assume all or part of the care of the patient, including writing the patient's orders. Other functions of the consultation team are to participate in conferences about patient and family needs, to refer the patient to needed services, to discharge the patient to appropriate care settings, and to communicate the plan of care with all the patient's providers.[8]

Palliative care consultations are ordered by the most responsible physician. In some institutions, nurses, social workers, and even family members may initiate a consultation request if approved by the responsible physician. Once the consultation is ordered, the first task of the palliative care consultation team is to elicit the specific reasons for consultation from the primary service. Reasons for palliative care consultation include relief of pain and other symptoms, assistance with communication about goals of care and support for complex medical decision-making, provision of psychosocial and bereavement support, and assistance with care coordination and continuity.[10]

The approach to the patient and the family begins with a comprehensive assessment of any physical and psychological symptoms and other social, spiritual, and cultural aspects of care, using validated assessment instruments whenever possible. Any active symptoms should be treated first because a discussion of realistic goals and overall goals of care cannot be held until the patient is comfortable enough to do so. The team can then elicit from the patient and the family their understanding of the disease and its treatment and the patient's opinion about what constitutes an acceptable quality of life. The consultation team can coordinate a family meeting to discuss goals of care and to address advance care planning. The formulation of an appropriate plan of care and a discharge plan should take into account the family's support system and financial resources and should be consistent with the established goals of care. Throughout this process, the consultation team maintains a close working relationship with the referring team. The consultation team should encourage participation from the referring service at family meetings; should encourage participation from nursing and support staff in the formulation of the patient's care plan; and should educate the medical, nursing, and support staff in particular aspects of the patient's management and care plan. The team should also provide staff with support regarding difficult patient situations and treatment decisions.[8]

This consultation process is time consuming. Because an initial evaluation can take more than 2 hours, the process often requires several visits over several days. Most of this time is spent communicating information and providing counseling.[8]

PALLIATIVE CARE UNIT

Palliative care consultation services advise the primary providers on how best to provide palliative care to patients with serious illness. In contrast, palliative care units become the primary providers for these patients. Palliative care units provide expert clinical management to patients who have severe symptoms that have been difficult to control, to patients who are imminently dying, and to patients with advanced serious illness that cannot be managed in any other setting. When staff members in other settings are untrained, uncertain, uncomfortable, or unable to formulate and implement a suitable palliative care plan for a patient with serious illness, it is appropriate to admit this patient to a dedicated palliative care unit where expert and trained staff and consistent-quality care plans can be ensured. The palliative care unit can also be a place where interdisciplinary training in palliative care practice can take place and a venue for conducting research projects that require careful monitoring of patients with serious illness.[1]

Palliative care units often have a physical environment that is much different from that of other parts of the hospital. The staff is more experienced in providing palliative care and is more attentive to palliative care issues compared with the rest of the hospital staff. Patients and families can find a more cheerful, comfortable, and "homelike" environment that affords privacy, peace, and quiet. Ideally, palliative care units provide a room for family meetings and educational resources, such as computer access and printed literature. Finally, dedicated palliative care units allow for expanded or unrestricted visiting hours so family, children, and even pets can spend quality time with their loved ones.[1]

Palliative care units have been organized in a variety of ways to meet the particular needs of distinct hospitals and surrounding communities. These units have consisted of scattered hospital beds, dedicated palliative care beds on another inpatient unit, and dedicated inpatient palliative care units. Table 45-1 describes various palliative care unit models available.[1]

Table 45-1. Palliative Care Unit Models

Unit Model	Model Characteristics
Acute palliative care beds or units	Operated under hospital license
	Rules that govern the operation of the unit are the same as the rules that apply to other in-hospital units
	Available in both academic and community hospitals
	Third-party payer covers if patient meets criteria for being in an acute care hospital
Subacute units	Provide postacute care where the focus is on providing treatment for problems identified during acute hospitalization
	Focus on short-term rehabilitation and discharge
	Beds not exclusively used for palliative care; possible conflicts in overall goals of care under the reimbursement rules or the unit's philosophy
Hospice units	Beds may be scattered in the institution, located in a dedicated unit, or located within a limited area of the hospital, such as an oncology unit
	May operate under the hospital's or hospice's license
	If patient has opted for Medicare Hospice Benefit, then hospice is responsible for overall plan of care and is reimbursed under Medicare hospice inpatient fee schedule; in turn, hospice reimburses the hospital under negotiated contract
	Usually for short-term care

AMBULATORY PALLIATIVE CARE

Ambulatory services are an important aspect of the continuum of palliative care. Ambulatory palliative care programs are available on a consultation basis to ambulatory patient with serious, complex, or life-threatening illness. These practices can offer a range of services from ongoing symptom management to follow-up for patients discharged from inpatient services. They can also address the various needs of patients and families through a multilevel, interdisciplinary practice. In general, patients seen in such clinics are seen earlier in the course of their illness, and they may be receiving palliative care in conjunction with active, disease-modifying therapy.[1]

Ambulatory palliative care may be provided as a stand-alone service, or it may be incorporated into another clinic such as oncology, infectious disease, geriatrics, or general internal medicine. Programs are staffed by physicians and nurses with specialized skills in palliative care. Therefore, this model allows for assessment and management of symptom control problems; provision of psychosocial support, information, counseling, and bereavement services; continuity of care and contact with the medical system; triage of patients to other specialty services offered by the institution or community; and 24-hour access to care providers on call via telephone. When appropriate, patients seen by the ambulatory palliative care practice can be admitted directly to an inpatient palliative care unit if hospitalization is required to manage intractable symptoms or complex medical situations.[1]

Non–Hospital-Based Programs

Throughout history, most people spent their last days at home surrounded by their loved ones. As hospitals increasingly became places of care in Western countries, more people were dying in these institutions rather than at home. Renewed interest in helping dying persons spend their last days at home, rather than in the hospital, gave rise to the field of home palliative care.

HOSPICE CARE IN THE UNITED STATES

Hospice care is specialized care designed to relieve the suffering of people facing life-limiting illness. Through an interdisciplinary approach, hospice aims to alleviate physical, psychological, emotional, and spiritual distress and provides support that specifically addresses the needs and wishes of the patient and his or her loved ones. The focus of hospice care is to improve the patient's quality of life rather than pursuing curative therapy for the life-limiting illness. Most hospice care, approximately 90%, is provided at home, but hospice is available wherever the person lives, including hospitals, nursing homes, and assisted living facilities.[11]

How does hospice care work? In general, the care of the patient is primarily managed by a family member, and this family member also helps make decisions on behalf of the patient. Members of the hospice staff make regular visits to the patient's home to assess and treat the patient's symptoms and to provide support and other services. A member of the hospice staff is available to patients and family 24 hours a day, 7 days a week, by phone or pager. The hospice staff usually consists of the patient's primary physician, a hospice physician or medical director, nurses, home health aides, social workers, clergy or other spiritual counselors, trained volunteers, and speech, physical, and occupational therapists.[12]

What services does hospice provide? The following is a list of services provided by hospice staff[12]:

- Assess and manage the patient's pain and other symptoms
- Provide support to the patient and family for emotional, psychosocial, and spiritual concerns
- Provide medications, medical supplies, and durable medical equipment
- Coach the family on how to care for the patient
- Deliver speech, physical, and occupational therapy when needed
- Make short-term inpatient care available when pain or other symptoms become too severe or too difficult to manage at home or when the patient's primary caregiver needs respite
- Provide counseling and bereavement support to surviving loved ones

Besides the patient's home, hospice care can be provided by a nursing home hospice unit, a freestanding hospice unit, or a residential hospice.[1] Hospice programs in nursing homes may provide routine home care or continuous home care services to residents because the nursing facility is considered to be the resident's home. However, because nursing home legislation has focused on promoting maintenance of function and prevention of premature death, residents who elect hospice care must be cared for by a certified hospice program that has a contract with the nursing facility.[1] Moreover, the Medicare Hospice Benefit does not cover the cost of room and board. Consequently, a nursing home resident who receives partial or full room and board coverage under Medicare Part A (usually during the first 120 days of the nursing home stay) is suddenly responsible for all the room and board expenses should he or she choose to enroll in the hospice program while continuing to live in the nursing home.

Freestanding hospice units provide inpatient care, respite care, and residential care. Individual units provide one, two, or all three levels of care. A hospice unit must be Medicare certified so patients can use the Medicare Hospice Benefit in this program. Freestanding hospice programs have made arrangements with hospitals to provide patients with certain services, such as radiation therapy for spinal cord compression resulting from metastatic cancer, that are not available in the freestanding unit.[1]

COMMUNITY VOLUNTEER HOSPICES IN CANADA

The term *hospice* in Canada has most often referred to community volunteer hospices that provide a range of volunteer services for patients and families that complement formal professional palliative care programs. These services include trained volunteers to provide part of the care team at home, grief programs, complementary therapy, spiritual counseling, and other services.[13] Some services labeled hospices actually have full interdisciplinary teams that usually concentrate on care in the home.

RESIDENTIAL HOSPICES

Some hospice programs provide care in a residential setting where patients go to live the last days, weeks, or months of their lives.[1] Residential hospices are still scarce in the United States and Canada, yet they embody the image that many people have of hospice. For residents of these hospice units, the costs of room and board are generally covered by Medicaid programs, managed care or other commercial insurance, private pay, philanthropy, or, in Canada, even by some government funding. If patients require a more intense level of care to treat symptoms, the residential hospice can intensify staffing or can transfer the patient to a hospital or palliative care unit.

HOME PALLIATIVE CARE PROGRAMS IN CANADA

Depending on the province and its organization of palliative care and home care, home palliative care programs may provide comprehensive palliative care on a local or regional basis. These are usually interdisciplinary and consist of physicians, advance practice nurses, primary palliative nurses, and others. These programs often are attached to organizations that provide institutional palliative care and collaborate extensively with community volunteer hospices. These home palliative care services provide around-the-clock care. Funding comes from a combination of hospital and government funding and donations.[13]

HOME CARE AGENCIES

Home care agencies provide a wide range of assistance to patients who wish to receive care at home for their acute, chronic, or advanced illness. Home care agencies can provide skilled nursing care, home health aide and personal support worker services, and physical, occupational, or speech therapy to supplement the caregiving of the family. They can also provide practical guidance on planning for the illness as well as counseling to the patient and the family. Finally, home care services can be available to the patient and the family 24 hours a day, 7 days a week, to provide rehabilitative, maintenance, or palliative care at the home.[1]

In the United States, Medicare reimburses the home care agency under a prospective payment system that is related to severity of illness and medical need. Coverage for these services can also be provided by Medicaid and commercial insurance, although these benefits vary widely. Medicare covers physicians' services at home. As more of these agencies have developed palliative care programs for patients with serious illness, home care programs have become an alternative for patients who are unable to access hospice services, who do not qualify for hospice, or who are not yet willing to forgo life-prolonging treatment for the terminal illness.[1]

In Canada, home care is a benefit under provincial health care schemes, but the provinces vary with respect to services covered, copayments, and drug coverage. There has been a recent provincial and federal accord to increase home care services to dying patients.[13]

BRIDGE PROGRAMS IN THE UNITED STATES

Home care programs in the United States, however, are often limited because they restrict eligibility to those patients who are home bound, those who need skilled nursing services, and those whose needs are episodic, with a potential for restoration of function.[14] As mentioned earlier, hospice is limited by the requirement that a physician certify that the patient has 6 months or less to live and that the patient forego curative treatment for the illness in favor of symptomatic treatment for the illness. Because of the regulatory limitations of both hospice and home care services, an alternative mode of providing palliative care has emerged: prehospice or bridge programs. Ideally, these programs provide a smooth transition, or bridge, to hospice.[14,15]

Bridge programs provide some of the services provided by hospice without requiring a 6-month prognosis or that patients forego life-prolonging treatment. These programs provide interdisciplinary supportive care to patients with advanced serious illness and their families concurrent with potentially curative or life-prolonging therapy. They are also able to provide advanced palliative care treatments that may be too expensive for hospices to cover under the current per diem reimbursement scheme. Unlike the usual home health programs, whose staff may not have much experience caring for patients near the end of life, bridge programs provide access to hospice-trained nurses. An interdisciplinary team provides treatment of pain and other physical symptoms; care management and coordination services; support with advanced care planning; and other psychosocial, spiritual, and bereavement support.[14,15]

Services from bridge programs are covered by Medicare Part B or Medicare Advantage (formerly Medicare + Choice) managed care plans, which are private health plans for Medicare beneficiaries and include both coordinated care plans and private fee-for-service plans at costs that are usually lower for the beneficiary.[16] Although the scientific literature does not currently provide much evidence of their effectiveness, bridge programs provide an opportunity to extend the benefits of hospice care to a wider population and spare patients the difficult choice between curative or life-prolonging treatment and high-quality palliative care.

Training and Certification

Ideally, palliative care should be provided by an interdisciplinary team that consists of at least a physician, a nurse, and a social worker with appropriate training and education in palliative care. Other team members may include chaplains, rehabilitation professionals, psychologists, and psychiatrists. The team should have skills and training in complex medical evaluation, pain and symptom management, psychosocial care, professional-to-patient communication, addressing difficult decisions about the goals of care, sophisticated discharge planning, and providing bereavement support. The team should provide coordinated assessment and services adhering as closely as possible to accepted guidelines of care and accepted practice standards. In the United States, the National Consensus Project for Quality Palliative Care has identified eight domains as the framework for its clinical practice guidelines.[17] These domains are as follows:

- Structure and processes of care
- Physical aspects of care
- Psychological and psychiatric aspects of care
- Social support
- Spiritual, religious, and existential aspects of care
- Cultural considerations
- Care of the imminently dying patient
- Ethics and the law

The Canadian Hospice and Palliative Care Association's Norms of Practice form the basis for both institutional and professional practice in the area of palliative care. The components of care are summarized by the "square of care" depicted in Figure 45-1.[13]

Proper adherence to guidelines and standards requires that members of the team have special training or work experience in palliative medicine, hospice, or nursing home settings, as well as familiarity with the demands and standards of the acute

Square of Care

COMMON ISSUES	Assessment	Information Sharing	Decision-making	Care Planning	Care Delivery	Confirmation
	History of issues, opportunities, associated expectations, needs, hopes, fears Examination—assessment scales, physical exam, laboratory, radiology, procedures	Confidentiality limits Desire and readiness for information Process for sharing information Translation Reactions to information Understanding Desire for additional information	Capacity. Goals of care Requests for withholding/potential for benefit, hastened death Issue prioritization Therapeutic priorities, options Treatment choices, consent Surrogate decision-making Advance directives Conflict resolution	Setting of care Process to negotiate/develop plan of care–address issues/ opportunities, delivery chosen therapies, dependents, backup coverage, respite, bereavement care, discharge planning, emergencies	Careteam composition, leadership, education, support Consultation Setting of care Essential services Patient, family support Therapy delivery Errors	Understanding Satisfaction Complexity Stress Concerns, issues, questions

PROCESS OF PROVIDING CARE

Patient/Family

Left-column common issues:

- **Disease Management**: Primary diagnosis, prognosis, evidence; Secondary diagnoses—dementia, delirium, psychoses; Co-morbidities—delirium, seizures; Adverse events—side effects, toxicity; Allergies
- **Physical**: Pain, other symptoms; Cognition, level of consciousness; Function, safety, aids; Fluids, nutrition; Wounds; Habits—alcohol, smoking
- **Psychological**: Personality, behavior; Depression, anxiety; Emotions, fears; Control, dignity, independence; Conflict, guilt, stress, coping responses; Self image, self esteem
- **Social**: Cultural values, beliefs, practices; Relationships, roles; Isolation, abandonment, reconciliation; Safe, comforting environment; Privacy, intimacy; Routines, rituals, recreation, vocation; Financial, legal; Family caregiver protection; Guardianship, custody issues
- **Spiritual**: Meaning, value; Existential, transcendental; Values, beliefs, practices, affiliations; Spiritual advisors, rites, rituals; Symbols, icons
- **Practical**: Activities of daily living; Dependents, pets; Telephone access, transportation
- **End of Life/ Death Management**: Life closure, gift giving, legacy creation; Preparation for expected death; Management of physiological changes in last hours of living; Rites, rituals; Death pronouncement, certification; Perideath care of family, handling of body; Funerals, memorial services, celebrations
- **Loss, Grief**: Loss; Grief—acute, chronic, anticipatory; Bereavement planning, mourning

Figure 45-1. The square of care. *(From Ferris FD, Balfour HM, Bowen K, et al: A model to guide hospice palliative care. Ottawa, Canada, Canadian Hospice Palliative Care Association, 2002, with permission from the U.S. Cancer Pain Committee.)*

hospital culture. Equally important is the team's ability to work well and communicate effectively with each other and with other health professionals.[1]

How do health care providers develop these core skills? The Education on Palliative and End-of-Life Care (EPEC) project educates professionals by combining didactic sessions, videotape presentations, interactive discussions, and practical exercises.[18] The curriculum is geared to an interdisciplinary audience and teaches fundamental palliative care skills such as comprehensive assessment, symptom management, communication, and ethical decision making, thus preparing professionals in the provision of primary palliative care. The complete EPEC curriculum is available as online learning for continuing medical education credit. The American Academy of Hospice and Palliative Medicine provides courses[1,2] in the United States. In Canada, education of primary care providers is available through a variety of government- and organization-sponsored comprehensive courses, as well as presentations at appropriate conferences. Preceptorships, involving primary care providers who work with expert palliative care providers, are also available.

The End-of-Life Nursing Education Consortium (ELNEC) provides a comprehensive education program to improve end-of-life care by nurses in the United States. The ELNEC core curriculum was developed to prepare educators to disseminate the information to nursing schools and health care agencies.[18]

Nursing staff members who wish to seek certification in hospice and palliative care nursing can do so at one of four levels: hospice and palliative advanced practice nurse, hospice and palliative care nurse, hospice and palliative licensed practical/vocational nurse, and hospice and palliative nursing assistant. The NBCHPN is responsible for determining eligibility, administering the examination, and awarding certification credentials. The purpose of the examination is to "test the ability to apply the nursing process in helping patients and their families toward the goal of maintaining optimal functioning and quality of life within the limits of the disease process, while considering factors such as fear, communication barriers, economic issues and cultural issues".[19] Table 45-2 summarizes the eligibility requirements and the examination content for each of the four levels of nursing certification.[19] In Canada, the Canadian Nurses Association now offers a certification examination for registered nurses in palliative care.

In the United States, physicians who seek subspecialty training in hospice and palliative medicine generally do so through one of two avenues: experiential practice for at least 2 years after residency or fellowship training or completion of an accredited fellowship in palliative medicine. The ABMS is the body responsible for credentialing physicians in the practice of hospice and palliative medicine. The Hospice and Palliative Medicine Certification Program is developed by the American Board of Internal Medicine (ABIM), the American Board of Anesthesiology (ABA), the American Board of Emergency Medicine (ABEM), the American Board of Family Medicine (ABFM), the American Board of Obstetrics and Gynecology (ABOG), the American Board of Pediatrics (ABP), the American Board of Physical Medicine and Rehabilitation (ABPMR), the American Board of Psychiatry and Neurology (ABPN), the American Board of Radiology (ABR), and the American Board of Surgery (ABS). The examination is administered to candidates from all boards at the same time in the same testing centers. The American Board of Internal Medicine is responsible for administering the examination; however, candidates from cosponsoring boards must register for the certification exam through the primary board by which they are certified.[20]

Table 45-2. Summary of Eligibility Requirements and Examination Content for Each of Four Levels of Nursing Certification

Level of Nursing Certification	Eligibility Requirements	Examination Content
Hospice and Palliative Advanced Practice Nurse	1. Hold currently active registered nurse license 2. Graduated from accredited institution having didactic and clinical component leading to graduate-level academic credit 3. Hold one of: master's or higher degree from an advanced practice palliative care program; post-master's certificate with supervised clinical practice in palliative care; master's, post-master's, or higher degree from advance practice program as palliative care clinical nurse specialist or nurse practitioner	Nine domains of practice tested: clinical judgment, advocacy and ethics, professionalism, collaboration, systems thinking, cultural and spiritual competence, facilitation of learning, communication, and research
Hospice and Palliative Care Nurse	1. Hold current license as registered nurse 2. Have at least 2 years experience in hospice and palliative nursing practice (recommended)	Seven domains of practice tested: end-stage disease process in adult patients, pain management, symptom management, care of patient and family (including resource management; psychosocial, spiritual, and cultural aspects; and grief and loss), education and advocacy, interdisciplinary practice, and professional issues
Hospice and Palliative Licensed Practical/ Vocational Nurse	1. Hold current license as practical/vocational nurse 2. Have at least 2 years experience in hospice and palliative licensed practical/vocational nurse practice (recommended)	Eight domains of practice tested: end-stage disease process in adult patients; pain and comfort management; symptom management; treatments and procedures; care of patient, family, and other caregivers (including resource management; psychosocial, spiritual, and cultural aspects; and grief and loss); education and advocacy; interdisciplinary practice; and practice issues

Table 45-2. Summary of Eligibility Requirements and Examination Content for Each of Four Levels of Nursing Certification (Continued)

Level of Nursing Certification	Eligibility Requirements	Examination Content
Hospice and Palliative Nursing Assistant	1. Documentation of at least 2000 practice hours under supervision of registered nurse in past 2 years 2. Have at least 2 years experience in hospice and palliative nursing assistant practice (recommended)	Four domains of practice tested: patient and family care; psychosocial and spiritual care of patient and family; interdisciplinary collaboration; and ethics, roles, and responsibilities

Eligible candidates for board certification must hold a current unrestricted medical license in the United States (or equivalent in other countries) and must be certified by an ABMS-approved board, an osteopathic medicine equivalent, or the equivalent in other countries.[20] Those who choose to apply for board eligibility through the experiential track must have been in the clinical practice of medicine for at least 2 years after residency or fellowship, must have directly participated in the active care of at least 50 terminally ill patients (the requirement for pediatricians is 25 terminally ill and 25 severely chronically ill pediatric patients) in the preceding 3 years for whom palliative medicine was the predominant goal of care, and must have worked as a physician member of an interdisciplinary team for at least 2 years. The 2012 certification examination will be the last one accepting applicants from the experiential track. Beginning with the examination in 2014, all candidates must apply through the postfellowship track. Those who apply through the postfellowship track must have successfully completed an accredited fellowship in hospice and palliative medicine.[20] The examination covers the following nine content areas: hospice and palliative approach to care, psychosocial and spiritual issues, impending death, grief and bereavement, pain management, non–pain symptom management, communication and teamwork, ethical and legal decision making, and prognostication. ABIM certification is valid for 10 years.[20]

In Canada, a 1-year residency program in palliative medicine is offered at most medical schools. This is a joint program between the College of Family Physicians of Canada and the Royal College of Physicians and Surgeons of Canada.[13] Fellowships and preceptorships are also routes to achieving advanced knowledge. There is no certification examination. The Canadian Society of Palliative Care Physicians provides opportunities for advanced learning for palliative medicine physicians.

PEARL

• Provision of palliative care services should be based on need and not on prognosis.

PITFALL

• Conflating palliative care with end-of-life care can lead to late referrals to palliative care services.

Summary

Whereas primary palliative care can be provided by all health care professionals and is part of the basic competency of individual practitioners, secondary and tertiary palliative care encompasses a set of specialist services that exceed the skills of primary care providers and are therefore provided by providers with specialty training in palliative care.

Hospital-based palliative care programs include palliative care consult teams, palliative care units, and ambulatory palliative care services; non–hospital-based programs include hospice care, home care, and bridge programs.

Palliative care providers should have skills and training in complex medical evaluation, pain and symptom management, professional-to-patient communication, addressing difficult decisions regarding goals of care, sophisticated discharge planning, and providing bereavement support while adhering as closely as possible to clinical practice guidelines such as those put forth by the National Consensus Project for Quality Palliative Care.

In the United States, certification for hospice and palliative care nursing is granted by the NBCHPN, and certification of physicians is granted by the ABMS. In Canada, there is no certification examination.

Resources

American Academy of Hospice and Palliative Medicine
  www.aahpm.org
Canadian Hospice Palliative Care Association
  www.chpca.net
Center to Advance Palliative Care
  www.capc.org
Centers for Medicare and Medicaid Services
  www.cms.hhs.gov
National Consensus Project for Quality Palliative Care
  www.nationalconsensusproject.org

References

1. Von Gunten CF, Ferris FD, Portenoy RK, Glajchen M, editors: *CAPC Manual: how to establish a palliative care program*, New York, 2001, Center to Advance Palliative Care.
2. Von Gunten CF: Secondary and tertiary palliative care in US hospitals, *JAMA* 287:875–881, 2002.
3. Fischberg D, Meier DE: Palliative care in hospitals, *Clin Geriatr Med* 20:735–751, 2004.
4. Standing Senate Committee on Social Affairs, Science and Technology: The health of Canadians: the federal role. Recommendations for reform (Kirby Report). In The Final Report on the State of the Health Care System in Canada, vol. 6, October 25, 2002. Available at www.parl.gc.ca.
5. Billings J, Pantilat S: Survey of palliative care programs in United States teaching hospitals, *J Palliat Med* 4:309–314, 2001.
6. Pan CX, Morrison RS, Meier DE, et al: How prevalent are hospital-based palliative care programs? Status report and future directions, *J Palliat Med* 4:315–324, 2001.
7. Morrison RS, Maroney-Galin C, Kralovec PD, Meier DE: The growth of palliative care programs in the United States, *J Palliat Med* 8:1127–1134, 2005.
8. Manfredi P, Morrison RS, Morris J, Goldhirsch SL: Palliative care consultations. How do they impact the care of hospitalized patients? *J Pain Symptom Manage* 20(3):166–173, 2000.
9. Center to Advance Palliative Care: *A guide to building a hospital-based palliative care program*, New York, 2004, CAPC. Available at www.capc.org.
10. Morrison RS, Meier DE: Clinical practice: palliative care, *N Engl J Med* 350:2582–2590, 2004.
11. Mayo Foundation for Medical Education and Research: Hospice Care: When Comfort, Not Cure, Is the Focus. Available at www.mayoclinic.com/invoke.cfm?id=HQ00860.
12. National Hospice and Palliative Care Organization: What is Hospice and Palliative Care? Available at www.nhpco.org/i4a/pages/index.cfm?pageid=3281.

13. Canadian Hospice Palliative Care Association: A Model to Guide Hospice Palliative Care: Based on National Principles and Norms of Practice, March 2002. Available at www.chpca.net/publications/norms/A-Model-to-Guide-Hospice-Palliative-Care-2002.pdf.
14. Stuart B, D'Onofrio CN, Boatman S, Feigelman G: CHOICES: promoting early access to end-of-life care through home-based transition management, *J Palliat Med* 6:671–680, 2003.
15. Casarett D, Abrahm JL: Patients with cancer referred to hospice versus a bridge program: patient characteristics, needs for care, and survival, *J Clin Oncol* 19:2057–2063, 2001.
16. Centers for Medicare and Medicaid Services: Choices for Medicare Advantage. Available at www.cms.hhs.gov/healthplans/rates.
17. National Consensus Project for Quality Palliative Care 2004 Clinical Practice Guidelines for Quality Palliative Care. Brooklyn, NY. Available at www.nationalconsensusproject.org.
18. Center to Advance Palliative Care: Training and Education. Available at www.capc.org/palliative-care-professional-development/Training.
19. National Board for Certification of Hospice and Palliative Nurses: Candidate Handbook. Available at www.nbchpn.org/CandidateHandbook.asp.
20. American Board of Internal Medicine: Hospice and Palliative Medicine Certification. Available at www.abim.org/specialty/hospice.aspx.

CHAPTER 46

The Role of the Physician in Palliative and End-of-Life Care

DENISE MARSHALL

In ancient cultures, physicians did not have central roles in caring for the dying. Physician skills were focused on caring for those for whom a cure was possible. From medieval times on through to the Reformation, religious organizations were important providers of care for the dying.[1] The role of the physician remained peripheral. Much of the care of the dying through many centuries, including the ancient hospice movement, involved family and community members and those with nursing/religious training as the central figures in care.

In a world that now has embraced scientific medicine, the role of the physician as a skilled clinician has accelerated and the role of the physician as a care provider with capacities to relieve suffering in the seriously ill and dying has emerged.

Prominence of the role of the physician in care of the dying was heightened in the second half of the 19th century with the creation of sanatoriums and the realization that tuberculosis was an infectious disease. The result was institutionalization and medicalization of seriously ill and dying patients. The circle of care shifted to involve the physician as a central figure, often in a position of gatekeeping the role that family and community could or should play in care for these patients.

The role of the physician in palliative and end-of-life care is rooted in the genesis of the modern hospice movement. In the late 19th century, Christian-based residential care of the dying became prominent. With the development of the modern hospice movement some 30 years ago and the increasing focus on pain and symptom management, the role of the physician as a key skilled clinician in care of the dying has rapidly developed.[1]

648

According to Lewis,[2] sociologists describe three prevalent death typologies: traditional, modern, and late modern. "Traditional" is described as deaths from infectious diseases or trauma, where these rather sudden deaths evoke robust death rituals and the need to connect the dead person to the collective group from which they came. "Modern" is described as the cancer death, one that is managed by physicians and involves death in institutions. "Late modern" is described as death from chronic illnesses or degenerative diseases and a new focus on ways to search for meaning and quality of life during a long trajectory. Indeed, advances in life-prolonging medical knowledge over the last century, combined with the rise in illnesses with a longer period of morbidity before death such as cancer and heart disease, have resulted in a dying trajectory that can most appropriately be described as a phase of life. Comorbid conditions, complex syndromes, and medication regimens, as well as an aging population, have necessitated the development of physicians with adequate knowledge, attitudes, and skills to meet the demands of increasingly complex dying patients.[3]

Thus, the role of the physician in palliative/end-of-life care very much mirrors the development of the modern death typology, the rise in scientific medicine, and the genesis of the modern hospice movement.

The Role of the Family Physician in Palliative Care

The essence of the physician–patient relationship makes family physicians ideally suited to provide palliative/end-of-life care. Cassell has said that this relationship is the very means to help relieve suffering. An in-depth understanding of suffering of those who are seriously ill, and responding to it, is a fundamental role of family medicine.[4] When asked, patients consistently speak to the desire for continuity of care both in terms of the physician's expertise and also in terms of maintaining the physician–patient relationship, as essential to their sense of nonabandonment at the end of life.[5,6] They also describe the need for closure with the physician, with whom they have had an ongoing relationship.[5] The family physician's role allows him or her to be able to attend to the patient holistically, in the context of the patient's family and friends, by virtue of his or her longstanding relationship with the patient. Family physicians have the capacity to stay available and involved in care in a way that is reassuring to patients and alleviates patient suffering. Patients repeatedly emphasize the importance of the role of a family physician with whom they have had close ties over the years, and for this role to continue through the palliative stages of life.[7] The family physician is also well positioned to address the concerns of the patient's loved ones and assist in coping with grief, as these persons are often patients in the physicians' practice.[8,9]

The Role of the Specialist Physician in Palliative Care

Although family physicians are ideally suited to roles in palliative/end-of-life care by virtue of their training and vocational calling—in essence, the "core business" of being a family physician—palliative/end-of-life care is not the exclusive focus of their practice. They need to be excellent providers of basic palliative care but not necessarily expert providers of palliative medicine.[3,10] Expert providers of palliative medicine are needed as opinion leaders and experts in end-of-life care who have the breadth of skills to inform knowledge generation, acquisition, and translation.[3,10] Thus, there is a need for physicians engaged in this pursuit full time and for physician experts who do so in relationship with academic medicine.

Palliative medicine meets the criteria of a specialty within the discipline of medicine.[11] The area of practice for palliative medicine specialists encompasses practicing with knowledge of many different disease states and the ability to assess and manage a wide range of symptoms in physical, psychological, spiritual, and social realms. The physician specialist must be adept at dealing with ethical dilemmas, advanced care planning, decision making, family conflict, and issues regarding physician-assisted suicide and euthanasia.[11]

The role of the expert palliative care physician can also be described in terms of a physician subspecialist.[10] Palliative medicine is a subspecialty in the United States, Australia, New Zealand, the United Kingdom, Ireland, and multiple other European countries.[10] Subspecialty status in medicine requires that an in-depth body of knowledge exists, that the area has identifiable competencies, that there is evidence of need for this status, and that there is adequate infrastructure, including professional organization and recognition, to sustain the specialty/subspecialty.[10] Palliative medicine meets the criteria for subspecialty in Canada, and much like Australia, the United States, and the United Kingdom, this subspecialty designation can meet the standard for entry and eligibility from both family medicine and specialty colleges and boards.

The Role of the Physician and Models of Care

Family physicians express the wish to remain active in the care of their dying patients[9] but find it challenging to address the complexity of physical and psychosocial issues at end of life. This is described as primarily the result of time and funding pressures, lack of education and experience, and lack of familiarity with the modern and postmodern dying trajectories.[12,13] They also may experience difficulty in accessing interprofessional specialist resources to support them in providing comprehensive palliative home care.[14,15] Sustainable models of palliative care that support optimal care and death at home can be achieved when family physicians work in collaborative, integrated ways with interprofessional specialist palliative medicine physicians and teams.[8,12,16,17] Throughout the United Kingdom, the United States, Australia, Canada, and other countries, models of care that support family physicians through facilitated practice with specialists and enhanced care coordination through nurse case managers demonstrated improvement in all parameters of community-based care.[8,16-19]

Specific Skills and Competencies

The field of palliative medicine is concerned with quality of life, value of life, and meaning of life.[20] Healing requires competency in scientific diagnosis and treatment but also compassion as demonstrated through solidarity with the patient.[2] Physicians who make an open-ended, long-term caring commitment to joint problem solving demonstrate the concept of nonabandonment in care. This is seen as the very essence of medical practice. Morrison and Meier articulate five broad areas of skills that form the core of palliative medicine: physician–patient communication; assessment and

Table 46-1. Physician Roles in Palliative Care

Physician Skills (Morrison & Meier, 2004)	Physician Roles (American Board of Hospice and Palliative Medicine [ABHPM])
Patient–Physician Communication • Goals of care • Communicating bad news • Discussing treatment and cessation of treatment	**Care for Patients** • Guidance, assessment, support, diagnosis, intervention • Presence, advocacy, collaboration • Teaching and research
Assessment and Treatment of Pain and Other Symptoms	**Care for Family Members** • Information, decision making • Teach patient care techniques • Education and emotional support
Psychosocial, Spiritual, and Bereavement Support • Assessment and interventions • Family support	**Care for Self** • Professional competency • Peer support • Self-care
Coordination of Care • Social and medical services • Financial, program planning, and support	**Care for the Team** • Participate in meetings • Ask for and give help and advise • Attend to team members needs and emotional status
	Care for the Organization • Stewardship of resources • CQI, administration • Human resource management

treatment of symptoms; psychosocial, spiritual, and bereavement care; and coordination of care.[21] This involves defining practice standards, responsibility for educational development and implementation, research in partnership with the academy, and program and systems needs. The American Board of Hospice and Palliative Medicine describes roles for palliative medicine physicians that correspond well to Morrison's and Meier's categories. A compilation of these can be found in Table 46-1.

Education

The literature repeatedly suggests that physicians do not currently receive adequate palliative care education during their residency training.[13,15,22,23] Given the recent shift to competency-based frameworks in medical education,[24,25] with increasing emphasis on patient care outcomes, training physicians for their roles in palliative/end-of-life care has received some focus. National organizations such as the College of Family Physicians of Canada, Educating Future Physicians in Palliative and End-of-Life Care (EFPPEC), and the American College of Graduate Medical Education have identified palliative and end-of-life care core competencies for residents.[26,27] The CanMeds competencies framework for medical residency education contains most of these same competencies.[25] Despite these initiatives, there is no consensus as to the most effective methods by which to educate future physicians about palliative care. It has even been questioned as to whether these skills can be taught, or whether they need to be inherent to the clinician.[20]

A systematic review of postgraduate training programs in palliative care[28] stresses that a multifaceted approach with some intentional focus on individual competencies will be necessary to meet all the educational requirements of postgraduate physician learners in end-of-life care. Communication skills in palliative care can be effectively taught with the use of simulated patients in a short 2-hour to full-day workshops. The use of faculty-observed patient interviews appears feasible and acceptable but still needs to be better evaluated using a reliable tool to assess observable behaviors. Educational modules can produce improvements in focused areas of knowledge such as appropriate use of opioids and criteria for hospice care, with the former showing sustainability at 6 months. Moderate- or high-intensity interventions with longer seminar series or a clinical component appear to be necessary to more broadly improve knowledge base in end-of-life care. It is possible that the intensity of the intervention may have a significant impact on sustainability of knowledge, confidence, or attitude; however, this has not been well measured. An ideal teaching program for attaining the skills and competencies required for physicians likely requires simulated patients and role play to address communication skills, along with highly relevant clinical exposure supplemented with academic sessions, resource material, or educational modules to address knowledge and other clinical skills. This approach is supported by the literature from continuing professional development. A recent systematic review of educational interventions to increase primary care physicians' knowledge and skills in palliative care suggested that a multifaceted approach may be most effective.[29] There are a multitude of educational resources now available for practicing physicians to enhance their palliative/end-of-life care knowledge and skills through both formal and informal means. A partial listing of these can be found in Appendix 2 (available online at www.expertconsult.com).

Physician Well-Being

Physicians working in end-of-life care have to respond to overwhelming human suffering and often must do so in the absence of adequate system supports or resources.[30,31] This can contribute to both physician compassion fatigue and burnout. Compassion fatigue evolves specifically from the relationship between the physician and patient and has been seen as the cost of caring for others in emotional pain. It is also known as vicarious or secondary traumatization and has been compared to posttraumatic stress disorder.[30] Compassion fatigue may lead to burnout.

Burnout is described in the literature as a form of mental distress that arises from the clinician's interaction with the work environment and includes feelings of emotional exhaustion, cynicism, and depersonalization and a low sense of personal accomplishment.[30,32] Physician burnout, and its associated feelings, can affect the quality of medical care and has been associated with suboptimal patient care and medical errors.[31,33] It appears to be more prevalent in younger and less experienced care providers, and particularly those professionals who are highly motivated personalities with intense involvement in their work life. There has been much research looking at burnout in palliative care.[30,31] Practitioners identify various factors that they feel are stressors to them: constant exposure to death; inadequate time with dying patients; large caseloads; emotional responses and poor coping strategies when a patient dies; the need to simply carry on when a patient has died; difficult communication issues; attachment to patient and family; and distress when unable to provide the kind of "good death" that they hoped for.[30] Constant reminders of death, and caring for dying patients, forces physicians to confront, at some level, their own mortality and affect many aspects of the physician's life.[34,35]

Several factors have been found to mitigate burnout and compassion fatigue. Support from palliative care team members and sharing leadership responsibilities seem to be important. Personal hardiness (i.e., a sense of commitment, control, and challenge) has been found to help alleviate burnout.[30] Resilience in physicians[36] helps shift the focus from what might be pathologic stress to successful adaptation. Compassion satisfaction, identified as the pleasure derived from the work of helping others, may be a factor that counterbalances the risks of compassion fatigue and contributes to resiliency.[37] The concept of "exquisite empathy" has been put forward as a protective practice that enhances caregivers satisfaction and can help to prevent or mitigate compassion fatigue. This is described as "highly present, sensitively attuned, well boundaried, heartfelt empathic engagement," the practice of which serves to invigorate rather than deplete professional connection.[30] Palliative care physicians must adopt a self-awareness–based approach to self-care to stay healthily engaged in the practice of palliative medicine. Kearney describes this as a combination of self-knowledge with the development of dual awareness, "a stance that permits the clinician to simultaneously attend to and monitor the needs of the patient, the work environment, and his or her own subjective experience".[30] A number of measures that help prevent physician burnout are outlined in Box 46-1. In particular, mindfulness meditation and reflective writing have shown effectiveness in randomized trials. These practices enable physicians engaged in end-of-life care to care for their patients "with a greater compassion, sensitivity, effectiveness and empathy".[30]

Box 46-1. *Measures that May Help Prevent Burnout*

Mindful meditation
Reflective writing
Adequate supervision and mentoring
Sustainable workload
Promotion of feelings of choice and control
Appropriate recognition and reward
Supportive work community
Promotion of fairness and justice in the workplace
Training in communication skills
Development of self-awareness skills
Practice of self-care activities
Participation in research
Mindfulness-based stress reduction for team
Meaning-centered intervention for team

From Kearney MK, Weininger RB, Vachon ML, et al: Self care of physicians caring for patients at end of life, *JAMA* 301(11):1155–1164, 2009. Used with permission.

PEARLS

- Expected competencies for the role, knowledge, skills, and attitudes of the physician in palliative/end-of-life care are now well articulated.
- A plethora of well-developed training materials and programs exist to help physicians attain these competencies and feel adept in their roles.
- Dying is a "postmodern" phase of life that requires the engagement of a range of physicians and interactions, from the occasional practitioner through to the leading expert.

PITFALLS

- The very definition of the "palliative patient" is a moving target. Physicians' roles and skills need to adapt to this evolving reality.
- Compassion fatigue and burnout are ongoing occupational hazards for the physician practicing palliative/end-of-life care. Self-care must be part of the therapeutic mandate.

Summary

Palliative medicine is now a field of medicine and encompasses both the primary care practitioner and the expert clinician. Given the modern trajectory of dying, it seems that the role of the physician as a member of the collaborative interprofessional "team" of care will remain essential for quality patient care and good outcomes at the end of life. There is a robust understanding of the core competencies and skills needed for physicians to succeed at their roles in palliative/end-of-life care. Well-researched models of care exist to support the role of the physician, and training programs are increasingly based on specific palliative care competencies that can effectively position the physician for his or her work.

Resources

End of Life/Palliative Educational Resource Centre (EPERC)
　　www.eperc.mcw.edu/
Education on Palliative/End of Life Care (EPEC)
　　www.epec.net
American Association of Hospice and Palliative Medicine (AAHPM)
　　www.aahpm.org
Canadian Virtual Hospice
　　www.virtualhospice.ca
Palliative.Info
　　www.palliative.info
The Pallium Project
　　www.pallium.ca
Canadian Society of Palliative Care Physicians
　　www.cspcp.ca
Centre to Advance Palliative Care
　　www.capc.org
University of Massachusetts Centre for Mindfulness in Medicine, Healthcare, and Society
　　www.umassmed.edu/cfm/mbsr/
Pain Management
　　www.Paincare.ca

Educating Future Physicians on Palliative/End of Life Care
www.afmc.ca/efppec
Medications for Palliative Care
www.palliativedrugs/com
World Health Organization—Palliative Care
www.who.int/cancer/pallliative/en/

References

1. Saunders M: Foreword. In Doyle D, Hanks G, Cherny N, et al, editors: *Oxford textbook of palliative medicine*, ed 3, Oxford University Press, 2005, New York, pp xviii.
2. Lewis MJ: *medicine and care of the dying: a modern history*, Oxford, UK, 2006, Oxford University Press, pp 3–5.
3. Librach SL: Role of family physicians in end-of-life-care, *Can Fam Physician* 47:1941–1943, 2001.
4. Daneault S, Dion D: Suffering of gravely ill patients, *Can Fam Physician* 50:1343–1345, 2004.
5. Back AL, Young JP, McCown E, et al: Abandonment at the end of life from patient, caregiver, nurse and physician perspectives, *Arch Intern Med* 169(5):474–479, 2009.
6. Heyland DK, Dodek P, Rocker G, et al: What matters most in end-of-life care: perceptions of seriously ill patients and their family members, *Can Med Assoc J* 174(5):627–633, 2006.
7. Daneault S, Lussier V, Mongeau S, et al: *Primum non-nocere*: could the health care system contribute to suffering? *Can Fam Physician* 52(12):1574e1–1574e5, 2006.
8. Mitchell J: How well do general practitioners deliver palliative care? A systematic review, *Palliat Med* 16:457–464, 2002.
9. Lehman F, Daneault S: Palliative care: first and foremost the domain of family physicians, *Can Fam Physician* 52:417–418, 2006.
10. Shadd J: Should palliative care be a specialty? *Can Fam Physician* 54(6):840–842, 2008.
11. Librach SL: The specialty of palliative medicine. In Walsh DT, et al, editor: *Palliative medicine*, Philadelphia, 2009, Saunders Elsevier.
12. Higginson I: Palliative care services in the community: what do family doctors want? *J Palliat Care* 15:21–25, 1999.
13. Grande GE, Barclay SI, Todd CJ: Difficulty of symptom control and general practitioners' knowledge of patients' symptoms, *Palliat Med* 11:399–406, 1997.
14. MacDonald N, Findlay HP, Bruera E, et al: A Canadian survey of issues in cancer pain management, *J Pain Sympt Manage* 14:332–342, 1997.
15. Oneschuck D, Bruera E: Access to palliative medicine training for Canadian family medicine residents, *Palliat Med* 12:23–27, 1998.
16. Phillips JL, Davidson PM, Jackson D, et al: Enhancing palliative care delivery in a regional community in Australia, *Austral Health Rev* 30(3):370–379, 2006.
17. Marshall D, Howell D, Brazil K, et al: Enhancing family physician capacity to deliver quality palliative home care: an end-of-life, shared-care model, *Can Fam Physician* 54(12):1703–1703, e7, 2008.
18. Finlay IG, Higginson IJ, Goodwin DM, et al: Palliative care in hospital, hospice, at home: results from a systematic review, *Ann Oncol* 13(4):257–264, 2002.
19. National Gold Standards Framework Centre: Gold Standards Framework, 2010. Available at www.goldstandardsframework.nhs.uk.
20. Doyle D, Hanks G, Cherny N, et al: Introduction. In Doyle D, Hanks G, Cherny N, et al, editors: *Oxford textbook of palliative medicine*, ed 3, New York, 2005, Oxford University Press, p 4.
21. Morrison RS, Meier DE: Clinical practice: Palliative care, *N Engl J Med* 350(25):2582–2590, 2004.
22. Bugge E, Higginson I: Palliative care and the need for education: do we know what makes a difference? A limited systematic review, *Health Ed* 65:101–125, 2006.
23. Mullan PB, Weissman DE, Ambuel B, et al: End-of-life care education in internal medicine residency programs: an interinstitutional study, *J Palliat Med* 5:487–496, 2002.
24. Carraccio C, Wolfsthal SD, Englander R, et al: Shifting paradigms: from Flexner to competencies, *Acad Med* 77:361–367, 2002.
25. Frank JR, editor: *The CanMEDS 2005 physician competency framework. Better standards. Better physicians. Better care*, Ottawa, 2005, The Royal College of Physicians and Surgeons of Canada.
26. Association of Faculties of Medicine of Canada: Educating Future Physicians for Palliative and End of Life Care: Postgraduate Family Medicine Common Competencies/Learning Outcomes. Accessed December 18, 2009. Available at www.afmc.ca/efppec/docs/pdf_2006_june_postgraduate_fam_med_common_competencies.pdf.

27. Weissman DE, Block SD: ACGME requirements for end-of-life training in selected residency and fellowship programs: a status report, *Acad Med* 77:299–304, 2002.
28. Shaw EA, Marshall D, Howard M, et al: Systematic review of post graduate palliative care curricula, *J Palliat Med*, accepted for publication.
29. Alvarez MP, Agra Y: Systematic review of educational interventions in palliative care for primary care physicians, *Palliat Med* 20:673–683, 2006.
30. Kearney MK, Weininger RD, Vachon ML, et al: Self-care of physicians caring for patients at the end of life, *JAMA* 301(11):1155–1164, 2009.
31. Meier DE, Back AL, Morrison RS: The inner life of physicians and care of the seriously ill, *JAMA* 286(23):3007–3014, 2001.
32. Swetz KM, Harrington SE, Matsuyama RK, et al: Strategies for avoiding burnout in hospice and palliative medicine: peer advice for physicians on achieving longevity and fulfillment, *J Palliat Med* 12(9):773–777, 2009.
33. West CP, Huschka MM, Novotny PJ, et al: Association of perceived medical errors with resident distress and empathy: a prospective longitudinal study, *JAMA* 296(9):1071–1078, 2006.
34. Kutner JS, Kilbourn KM: Bereavement: Addressing challenges faced by advanced cancer patients, their caregivers, and their physicians, *Prim Care Clin Office Pract* 36:825–844, 2009.
35. Solomon S: Personal correspondence, February, 2010.
36. Jensen PM, Trollope-Kumar K, Waters H, et al: Building physician resilience, *Can Fam Physician* 54(5):722–729, 2008.
37. Stamm BH: Measuring compassion satisfaction as well as fatigue: developmental history of the compassion satisfaction and fatigue test. In Figley CF, editor: *Treating compassion fatigue*, New York, 2002, Brunner-Routledge, pp 107–119.

SECTION 4

The Social Context

CHAPTER 47

The Economic Burden of End-of-Life Illness

ALEXANDER A. BONI-SAENZ, KENNETH E. COVINSKY, and
SANDRA Y. MOODY

The economic domain is not often a priority topic for clinicians; however, economic issues permeate the health care experience of clinicians, patients, and their families and caregivers. For example, reimbursement policies can affect the choice of treatment options available to patients, and caregiver employment status can affect the types of informal support that are available to patients. Prescription drug compliance can be related to insurance coverage, and the social care supports available to the caregiver can determine levels of strain that, in turn, affect caregiving quality and productivity at work. These issues are especially important to patients at the end of life and to those families on the lower end of the socioeconomic spectrum, but the lessons learned in providing high-quality care and support are applicable to all patient populations.

Palliative care is a movement and a philosophy dedicated to holistic patient care. In contrast to the biomedical model of medicine, this type of care has as its "trademark" a comprehensive assessment of the different domains of illness-related human experience, including the physical, psychological, social, and spiritual.[1] Illness-related suffering can have its origins in any of these domains and can threaten the identity and humanity of the patient, as well as the caregiver.[2] Another important feature of palliative care is that caregivers and family members are considered part of the unit of care. This perspective recognizes the support networks the patient may have, as well as the knowledge that life continues for other individuals after a patient dies. Support for caregivers and family members is important both for the patient and as good preventive care for these other individuals.

This chapter focuses on how economic burdens may contribute to the suffering of the patient and relevant third parties and how these burdens are expressed in various domains of the human experience. Through adequate assessment and treatment of the problems in economic domains, the interdisciplinary team in palliative care can help to alleviate the associated effects of economic burden. We first examine what constitutes the economic domain with respect to end-of-life illness and care. Following that, we review the empirical evidence about the economic impact of illness, with special attention given to dementia and cancer. Finally, we provide brief, practical guidance for dealing with the economic issues that may arise in treatment of patients.

Understanding the Economic Domain

The economics of end-of-life and palliative care need to consider the variety of costs borne by the patient and the caregiver, as well as the possibilities that palliative care interventions can provide economic benefits.[3] Costs and benefits can be categorized first in terms of whether they affect the patient or the family, including nonfamily informal caregivers. When dealing with resources such as family savings that may pertain or belong to the patient as well as the family, this line may become blurred. However, a change in the health status of a caregiver has a clear effect on the family.

The second distinction is between medical and nonmedical costs and benefits.[3] Medical costs and benefits are those that affect the cost of health care or health status for the patient or family. These costs can be monetary, coming in the form of insurance premiums or out-of-pocket costs for medical care. However, health status is also included here because economists often use measurements of quality of life or health utility to calculate the cost effectiveness of interventions through a quality-adjusted life year (QALY) type of analysis. This is a reminder that even abstract health effects can have economic implications. Nonmedical costs and benefits are those that affect areas such as workplace productivity or school absenteeism. These are measured in terms of job wages or time or opportunity lost while taking care of a sick relative.

Economics of End-of-Life Illness

Anecdotal evidence suggests that end-of-life illness can have substantial burdens on patients and their families. However, because most cost-of-illness studies focus on the cost to health systems and insurers, surprisingly little is known about the costs of terminal illness to patients and families. Over the past decade, several studies have begun to fill the gap by providing clear empirical evidence that the economic burdens of end-of-life illness are substantial. To illustrate this point, we summarize evidence from several sources: the Study to Understand Prognoses and Preferences for Outcomes and Risks of Treatment (SUPPORT), the Commonwealth-Cummings Study of the burdens of terminal illness, and studies of labor market and economic burdens of dementia and cancer, and studies of medical bankruptcy.

IMPACT OF SERIOUS ILLNESS ON PATIENTS' FAMILIES: FINDINGS OF THE SUPPORT PROJECT

The SUPPORT project was a landmark study of prognoses, preferences, and decision making in patients with one of nine serious life-threatening illnesses.[4] One of the goals of the SUPPORT project was to develop a better understanding of the impact of serious illness on the families of patients. Surrogate and patient interviews about the impact of illness on the family were obtained for 2129 patients who survived an index hospitalization. The interviews were obtained between 2 and 6 months after the hospitalization. Patients represented a wide age range (15% < 45 years; 45% > 65 years).

Table 47-1 describes the frequency of burdens described by SUPPORT subjects. Families noted several severe burdens. For example, 20% reported that a caregiver made a major life change to care for the patient, and this often included quitting or taking time off from work. In 31% of cases, most of the family savings was lost, whereas in 29% of cases, a major source of family income was lost. Seventeen percent reported a major change in family plans, such as moving to a less expensive home, delaying medical care for another family member, or altering educational plans for another family member. At least one major burden was reported by more than half (55%) of families.

Although rates of burdens were high for all patient subgroups, several characteristics defined families most likely to suffer adverse financial impacts. For example, loss of most of the family savings was more common in families of patients with severe functional dependence than in those without severe functional dependence (37% vs. 29%) and in families with incomes higher than $25,000 a year than in those with lower incomes (35% vs. 22%). Young patient age was, however, the strongest predictor of loss of family savings. Loss of savings was reported for 43% of families

Table 47-1. Burdens of Serious Illness on Families

Burdens Described by SUPPORT Families	Burden Percentage (%)
A family member made a major life change to care for the patient	20
Quit or took time off from work	11
Other major life change	9
Others in the family became ill or unable to function normally because of the stress of the illness	12
Most of the family savings was lost	31
A major source of family income was lost	29
A major change in family plans was made because of the cost of the illness	17
Moved to a less expensive home	6
Delayed medical care for another family member	6
Altered educational plans for another family member	4
Other change	4
Suffered any of the above adverse impacts	55

SUPPORT, Study to Understand Prognoses and Preferences for Outcomes and Risks of Treatment.

of patients younger than 45 years compared with 25% for patients older than 75 years. There are probably several reasons families of younger patients were at higher risk than families of older patients. Because most older patients receive Social Security, their income is less likely to be threatened by severe illness. In contrast, it is more likely that younger patients and their caregivers will need to give up work as the result of severe illness. Moreover, older patients are more often eligible for social and other support services than younger patients, and it is possible that some of these services offer some measure of protection.

The SUPPORT study did not identify the mechanisms of these burdens. However, because 96% of patients in SUPPORT had health insurance, it is likely that many of these burdens were the result of expenses not covered by insurance. Undoubtedly, a major source of financial burden is the loss of employment income for patients and caregivers. Many illness-related costs associated with terminal illness are not covered by most health insurers. This includes the costs of home health aides and assistance with basic activities of daily living (ADLs), home modifications, and long-term care costs. Although some of these costs are covered by hospice, many terminally ill patients are never enrolled in hospice, and those who are enrolled usually enter hospice for the last few weeks of their illness.

COMMONWEALTH-CUMMINGS STUDY

The Commonwealth-Cummings Project shed some more light on the mechanisms of burden that the SUPPORT project did not identify.[5] Within 6 selected regions, 988 terminally patients (identified by their physicians as having a life expectancy of less than 6 months) and 893 of their caregivers were chosen for interviews. Fifty-nine percent of the subjects were more than 65 years old. Overall, 35% of patients had at least moderate need for nursing home care, homemaking, or personal care. Eighteen percent had unmet needs for nursing care, and 23% had unmet homemaking needs. Greater functional burdens, older age, and low income were associated with greater care needs. Substantial care needs, female gender, and African-American ethnicity were associated with unmet care needs.

The study strongly suggested that substantial care needs were a key contributor to economic and other burdens. For example, significant depressive symptoms were reported by 31% of caregivers of patients with high care needs, compared with 25% of caregivers of patients with few needs. Similarly, caregivers of patients with high care needs were more likely to report that caregiving interfered with their personal needs (36% vs. 24%). Interestingly, having an empathic physician seemed to buffer these burdens. Among caregivers of patients with high caregiving needs, those who reported that the needs and opinions of the caregiver were addressed by the physician were less likely to be depressed (28% vs. 42%) and less likely to feel that caregiving interfered with their personal life (32% vs. 48%).

The results of this study suggest an explanatory model for the burdens critical illness places on caregivers. In this model, factors such as poor performance status, older age, incontinence, and low income lead to high caregiving needs. These high caregiving needs lead to both economic burdens and health burdens such as depression.

ECONOMIC IMPACT OF DEMENTIA

Dementia differs from other end-of-life conditions because the later stages of the disease are often protracted, and the prognosis is unpredictable. Dementia also imposes special challenges on a patient's family because patients often require extensive caregiving assistance. This caregiving assistance is generally required because of a combination of memory impairments, behavioral disturbances, and impairments in physical functioning. Although dementia is the leading cause of nursing home placement, most patients with dementia are cared for at home by family members. However, although it seems probable that dementia care would impose high costs on families, only a limited number of studies have addressed the economic costs of dementia care.

One of the most important economic costs of dementia caregiving may be on the ability of caregivers to work. Because many caregivers need to provide continuous supervision, the ability to be employed is often compromised. In a study of patients newly enrolled in the Program of All-Inclusive Care for the Elderly (a new capitated benefit authorized by the Balanced Budget Act of 1997 that features a comprehensive service delivery system and integrated Medicare and Medicaid financing), 25% of patients with dementia had at least one caregiver who either quit working or reduced the number of hours worked to care for the patient.[6] Loss of employment was considerably more common in patients of African-American and Hispanic ethnicity, as was the case in the Commonwealth-Cummings Study of terminally ill patients, a finding suggesting that this economic burden of caregiving may be disproportionately endured by minority communities. Loss of employment was also more common when the caregiver was a woman.

One method of estimating the value of the time family members spend caring for patients with dementia is to estimate the opportunity cost of caregiving. *Opportunity costs* of caregiving generally represent the estimate of how a caregiver's time would be valued if they could provide their services within the labor market. Using this approach, Langa and colleagues used the Asset and Health Dynamics (AHEAD) study, a nationally representative sample of community-dwelling elderly persons, to conduct a study of the cost of informal caregiving for elders with dementia.[7] The market value of caregiving was estimated using the average wage of a home health aide. In 2001, Langa and colleagues determined that patients with mild, moderate, or severe dementia required an additional 8.5, 17.4, and 41.5 hours, respectively, of caregiving per week compared with elders without cognitive impairment. The yearly opportunity cost of this caregiving was $3600, $7420, and $17,700, respectively, in these three groups. This represented a national annual opportunity cost of more than $18 billion. This estimate is striking because the total national expenditure for all paid home services (for all conditions) was $29 billion in 1998. Because the $18 billion cost estimate considers only one condition, it seems almost certain that the economic cost of family caregiving (generally unpaid) exceeds the current economic cost of paid home care.

Caregiving also has substantial personal costs. Although these costs are incurred in many end-of-life illnesses, they are best documented for caregivers of patients with dementia. In particular, caregivers of patients with dementia have repeatedly been found to be at higher risk for depression. In a study of more than 5000 patients with advanced dementia, for example, 32% of caregivers were classified as depressed based on a high number of depressive symptoms.[8] Rates of depression varied depending on patient and caregiver characteristics. Patient characteristics associated with higher rates of caregiver depression included younger age, white or Hispanic ethnicity (compared with black), low education, dependence on the caregiver for activities of daily living, and behavioral disturbances. Caregiver characteristics associated with high rates of depression included low income, female gender, more hours spent caregiving, and poor functional status. Thus, caregiver depression appears to be a complex process that is influenced by ethnicity, as well as by patient and caregiver characteristics. Depression is also associated with labor productivity losses. In one study, workers with depression had 5.6 hours per week of lost productive time compared with an expected 1.5 hours per week. Most productivity costs were explained by reduced performance while at work.[9]

Some evidence suggests that caregiving for a frail elder is sometimes associated with more global health effects. For example, Schulz and colleagues demonstrated that caregivers who reported emotional strain while caring for disabled spouses had a 63% higher risk of death than nonspousal caregivers.[10] Because spousal caregivers who did not have strain were not at higher risk for death, this study illustrated the importance of identifying caregivers who are experiencing adverse emotional outcomes from caregiving. There is also evidence suggesting that dying a "good death" by receiving palliative care services in the form of hospice may also have positive effects for spouses. Christakis and Iwashyna retrospectively matched 30,838 couples, in which the decedent in one group used hospice while the matched decedent in the other group did not.[11] After 18 months, bereaved wives whose husbands had used hospice showed a significantly lower mortality than those wives whose husbands did not use hospice. This finding suggests that high-quality palliative care has the potential to soften the blow of widowhood.

ECONOMIC IMPACT OF CANCER

Cancer is a leading cause of death, particularly among elderly persons. Although cancer affects all ages, the studies on the economic costs of cancer to patients and their families have focused on the elderly. Although initial studies used small convenience samples to examine the out-of-pocket costs related to cancer, more recent studies have exploited the data available from the 1995 AHEAD study. A study by Langa and colleagues examined the relative out-of-pocket medical expenditures of community-dwelling elderly persons who were more than 70 years old and who had cancer.[12] In this sample of 6370 respondents, 84% reported no cancer or history of cancer, and 13% reported a history of cancer but no current treatment regimen, whereas 3% reported a history of cancer and current treatment. Adjusted mean annual out-of-pocket expenditures were significantly different at $1220, $1450, and $1880 for each of the groups, respectively. The major sources of costs were prescription medications and home care services. Low-income individuals undergoing cancer treatment spent 27% of their yearly income on out-of-pocket expenses, a demonstration of the staggering effect that cancer can have on low-income individuals and their families.

Pain is a frequent and feared symptom of patients with cancer. Optimizing pain management remains an important clinical goal. However, considering pain as a mere physical symptom ignores the social and economic effects it can have on the patient and the family. In a study of 373 outpatients with cancer, investigators estimated the direct and indirect costs of cancer pain.[13] Sixty-nine percent of patients had a direct medical cost associated with cancer pain, be it an emergency room visit or cost of analgesic medication. These costs are absorbed by insurance after copayments and deductibles; however, patients without insurance shoulder the whole cost, which was, on average, $825 per month, or almost $10,000 per year. Excluding productivity losses, 57% reported at least one indirect cost associated with cancer pain.

These expenses are borne almost entirely by the patient and family and totaled $61 per month, or more than $700 per year. The most frequently cited expense was transportation, followed by the costs of purchasing over-the-counter medication. The largest predictors of both types of costs were pain intensity, pain interference, and breakthrough pain. This finding indicates that high-quality pain management in palliative care not only frees the patient from physical ailments but also aids in the reduction of economic costs.

Although the previous study excluded labor costs, further analysis of the first wave (1993) of AHEAD data using similar methods to calculate the costs of dementia caregiving provides estimates of these numbers.[14] Even though the informal caregiving costs for elderly patients with cancer are less than those with dementia, they are still significant at $1200 a year per patient, for a total of nearly $1 billion annually.

ILLNESS AND BANKRUPTCY

Filing for bankruptcy involves petitioning a federal court for protection from creditors under bankruptcy laws. It is not a step to be taken lightly, as it has negative consequences for access to credit, reputation, and employment prospects.[15] Himmelstein and colleagues have shown the strong and increasingly powerful link between illness and bankruptcy.[16] In their most recent study, they surveyed a random national sample of 2,314 bankruptcy filers from 2007, finding that 62.1% of bankruptcies were medical in nature. This is a nearly 50% increase in medical bankruptcy since 2001. The primary medical contributors to bankruptcy included unpaid medical bills and income loss as a result of illness. Most bankruptcy filers were middle-class, well-educated, privately-insured, and homeowners, revealing that even those who are financially well-off can be subject to the negative economic effects of illness.

How Clinicians Can Handle the Economic Dimension of Care

As the empirical evidence has demonstrated, economic issues permeate many different dimensions of illness and care. Clinicians should recognize that economic distress can be one of the consequences of end-of-life illnesses. Economic costs can be paired with physical symptoms such as pain, or they can be associated with psychological ailments suffered by caregivers, such as depression. Economic costs can come in the form of transportation expenses, deductibles for insurance, or loss of income as a result of work absenteeism. These effects are not limited to the patient; they affect caregivers, spouses, and children as well. There are steps the clinician can take to help alleviate these economic burdens. We suggest several steps that a clinician can employ.

ECONOMIC ASSESSMENTS

Comprehensive assessment should involve a simple screening question about the financial burden of end-of-life illness. End-of-life screening tools such as the Needs at the End-of-Life Screening Tool contain a question about the financial burden ("How much of a financial hardship is your illness for you or your family?") that can help to guide this process.[17] Those performing the assessment should be aware of the cultural differences with respect to money and health status that may exist with the patient or the family members, including variability about when financial hardship is identified and articulated. Clinicians should avoid implying that the patient is a burden to the family or that the family is unwilling to support the patient financially. Assessments can be conducted in informal conversations with the family or in planned formal family meetings. Assessment of the economic situation of the patient and caregiver or family should be a continuous process because it may be common to have economic situations "flare up" at different points during the course of the illness.

MAKING USE OF THE INTERDISCIPLINARY TEAM

One of the benefits of palliative care is the emphasis on care by the interdisciplinary team, which is associated with increased quality of care and satisfaction of the patient and family, though further randomized controlled trials are required to quantify the effects.[18] If the patient demonstrates a significant financial burden, it may be appropriate to make a referral to a social worker who may be adept at providing financial guidance and finding sources of support for the patient and family. There are often sources of support, from the government, nonprofit organizations, or religious community organizations that the clinician can help mobilize to help the family to cope with caregiving stresses or economic burdens.

Other members of the interdisciplinary team may be useful in preventing economic burdens. For instance, a chaplain may help family members to deal with the existential issues surrounding death, which could have the impact of increasing work productivity and adjustment to loss after the patient dies. If the patient is still able to work and has the desire to do so, an occupational therapist may be able to alter the work environment of the patient and may help to navigate issues of accommodations with employers. Many economic stressors also have a legal dimension, because they may involve access to public benefits and health insurance or bankruptcy and foreclosure. The integration of attorneys into the interdisciplinary team could assist with addressing these issues as well.[19]

REIMBURSEMENT

All clinicians should have some rudimentary knowledge of the different funding streams for palliative care. Although the main type of palliative care funding comes in the form of the Medicare Hospice Benefit, this benefit does not necessarily provide coverage for elements of palliative care provided in hospitals and nursing homes. In these settings, palliative care services may be limited by the internal budgets of the organization or by the priorities that have been set for care. However, early referral to hospice may be beneficial to patients and their families because it gives families access to some benefits, such as health aides and pain medications, which may not be available otherwise. Medicaid, through specialized state waiver programs, may provide services that can enable the patient to stay at home. This may reduce the costs of institutionalization. In addition, for those younger clients who lack Medicare, clinicians should inquire and work with the patient and family to ensure that the medical services provided to the patient that are not justified by the benefit do not cause financial harm to the family because they are not reimbursable under the patient's private insurance.

EMPATHY AND COMMUNICATION

As demonstrated in the Commonwealth-Cummings study, simple interventions such as clinician empathy can buffer the burdens of caregiver stress. As a result, simply asking about economic burdens can help to stem depressive symptoms of informal caregivers. The trajectory of bereavement is highly influenced by the type of care that was provided before the death of the patient.[20]

INEQUITIES IN ACCESS TO PALLIATIVE SERVICES

Despite the successful growth of hospice programs in the United States, there has been limited success in providing equal access to palliative care services in vulnerable populations, including patients with low income and members of minority groups. As indicated in a review by Brenner,[21] hospice programs have been most successful "in addressing the needs of middle class, white, elderly persons with cancer who have family members able to care for them at home." It has been a challenge for hospice programs to serve low-income, nonwhite, non–English-speaking individuals without health insurance. Additionally, some of the initial admission criteria to hospice may continue to have an impact. Some of the following examples highlight this fact:

1. To be admitted, patients must have supportive families with a primary caregiver.
2. Patients must agree to a do-not-resuscitate order (this is not a legal requirement).
3. Patients must discontinue certain therapies before admission to the program.
4. Patients must live in a safe enough neighborhood that the hospice is willing to visit.

Since 1995, many of these criteria have been changed substantially to reduce barriers to hospice and palliative care.[22] Nevertheless, access to hospice and palliative care remains an issue, and recent studies have shown that several of the foregoing criteria are the very reasons that certain minority groups do not enter hospice programs. The issue of access, however, is not simple. It is not simply economics, and yet many of the barriers that prevent individuals from different racial and ethnic minority backgrounds from accessing good end-of-life care are intricately linked to economics.

Studies of access have been predominantly of white populations. Therefore, little is known about the use of hospice care by individuals of different racial and ethnic groups. However, in a secondary analysis of the 1993 National Mortality Followback Survey, Greiner and colleagues[23] examined hospice use by minorities in the last year of life and found that African Americans were 34% less likely to use hospice than white Americans, even after controlling for socioeconomic status. Greiner and colleagues concluded that "economic, educational, and access-to-care differentials between African Americans and white [Americans] are not the primary explanation for the variations in hospice use between these groups".[23] Indeed, many studies of seriously ill hospitalized patients have indicated that African-American individuals have fewer do-not-resuscitate orders, receive cardiopulmonary resuscitation more frequently, tend to have written advance directives less often, and prefer more aggressive care for terminal illness. Other studies have shown that individuals of Latino descent also use hospice less often than white individuals.[6] Smith and colleagues concluded that effective use of interpreters, sensitivity to family dynamics and cultural factors, and universal strategies of clear health communication would help in providing culturally congruent care to Latinos and their families at the end of life.[24] Although it is still not entirely clear why differences in treatment preferences exist, they continue to influence access to hospice care for African Americans and Latinos, and they lead to higher systemic costs at the end of life for these groups as well.[25]

Table 47-2. Barriers to Hospice Use among Minorities

Barrier	Impact
Medicare Hospice Benefit requirement for a full-time (≥19 hours/day) personal caregiver to care for the patient	Low-income patients and minority patients have working family members, which may lead to reduced work hours or job loss.
Physicians are primary sources of referral to hospice	Physicians may be less likely to refer Asian Americans to hospice because of assumptions about cultural preferences.
Linguistic barriers	Language barriers preclude adequate communication between patients and physicians.
To be eligible for hospice services, informed consent is required, which requires knowledge and acceptance of a terminal diagnosis and prognosis	In contrast with the principles of patient autonomy and informed consent, many Asian American and Pacific Islanders may value filial piety, indirectness in communicating bad news, and family-centered model of decision making (studies have shown that African American and Mexican American patients also favor a less individualistic and more family-centered model of decision making).

In 2003, Ngo-Metzger and colleagues[26] performed a study using the Surveillance, Epidemiology, and End Results program data to examine hospice use by patients of Asian and Pacific Islander descent compared with white patients and to assess whether hospice use differs by birthplace (United States vs. abroad). These investigators found that Asian-American and Pacific Islander patients used hospice 33% less often than did white Americans, and that those who were foreign-born were especially less likely to enroll in hospice. The authors highlighted several important possible reasons why Asian Americans and other racial and ethnic minorities use hospice less often, including sociocultural factors (Table 47-2).[26]

In summary, access to hospice and palliative care among racial and ethnic minority patients is a complex issue and requires consideration not only of economic factors but also of the relationships among economic, social, and cultural factors. Overcoming inequities to hospice use will require major efforts from physicians, researchers, policy makers, and hospice and palliative care organizations.

PEARLS

- Make sure the comprehensive assessment includes a screening question about economic burdens of end-of-life illness.
- Know about the insurance status and coverage of patients, including details of reimbursement.
- Maintain awareness of the informal supports available to the patient.
- Make use of interdisciplinary team members, including interpreters, social workers, attorneys, and chaplains, to help the patient and family members deal with complex financial, social, and spiritual matters.

PITFALLS

- Do not present the ill patient as a burden on the family or other caregivers.
- Do not avoid or ignore cultural differences in discussing and dealing with money and end-of-life illness.
- Do not forget to perform a continuing assessment of economic status (it may have changed because of loss of employment or other "shocks").
- Do not assume the economic status or preferences of the patient or family members.
- Do not miss the signs of caregiver stress and its associated health effects.

Summary

Advanced illness is often costly to patients and families. The economic costs to families are frequently different from those measured in traditional analyses of health care costs because they often include expenses not reimbursed by insurance (e.g., informal home supports), the patient's lost income, and the opportunity cost of foregone employment on the part of the caregiver. It is important that clinicians and policy makers recognize that economic costs can be an important component of the burden experienced by patients and families facing end-of-life illness.

Resources

Agency for Healthcare Research and Quality: Evidence Report/Technology Assessment, no. 110: End-of-Life Care and Outcomes. Publication no. 05-E004-2, 2004.
   www.ahrq.gov
Americans for Better Care of the Dying
   www.abcd-caring.com/mainpagemain.htm
Good Endings
   www.goodendings.net
Promoting Excellence in End-of-Life Care
   www.promotingexcellence.org/i4a/pages/index.cfm?pageid=1
Department of Pain Medicine and Palliative Care: StopPain.org
   www.stoppain.org/for_professionals

References

1. Saunders C: *Care of the dying*, London, 1959, Macmillan.
2. Cassell E: The nature of suffering and the goals of medicine, *N Engl J Med* 306:639–645, 1982.
3. Boni-Saenz AA, Dranove D, Emanuel LL, et al: The price of palliative care: toward a complete accounting of costs and benefits, *Clin Geriatr Med* 21:147–163, 2005.
4. Covinsky KE, Goldman L, Cook EF, et al: The impact of serious illness on patients' families: SUPPORT Investigators. Study to Understand Prognoses and Preferences for Outcomes and Risks of Treatment, *JAMA* 272:1839–1844, 1994.
5. Emanuel EJ, Fairclough DL, Slutsman J, Emanuel LL: Understanding economic and other burdens of terminal illness: the experience of patients and their caregivers, *Ann Intern Med* 132:451–459, 2000.
6. Covinsky KE, Eng C, Lui LY, et al: Reduced employment in caregivers of frail elders: impact of ethnicity, patient clinical characteristics, and caregiver characteristics, *J Gerontol A Biol Sci Med Sci* 56:M707–M713, 2001.
7. Langa KM, Chernew ME, Kabeto MU, et al: National estimates of the quantity and cost of informal caregiving for the elderly with dementia, *J Gen Intern Med* 16:770–778, 2001.
8. Covinsky KE, Newcomer R, Fox P, et al: Patient and caregiver characteristics associated with depression in caregivers of patients with dementia, *J Gen Intern Med* 18:1006–1014, 2003.
9. Stewart WF, Ricci JA, Chee E, et al: Cost of lost productive work time among US workers with depression, *JAMA* 289:3135–3144, 2003.

10. Schulz R, Beach SR: Caregiving as a risk factor for mortality: the Caregiver Health Effects Study, *JAMA* 282:2215–2219, 1999.
11. Christakis N, Iwashyna T: The health impact of health care on families: a matched cohort study of hospice use by decedents and mortality outcomes in surviving, widowed spouses, *Soc Sci Med* 57:465–475, 2003.
12. Langa KM, Fendrick MA, Chernew ME, et al: Out-of-pocket health-care expenditures among older Americans with cancer, *Value Health* 7:186–194, 2004.
13. Fortner BV, Demarco G, Irving G, et al: Description and predictors of direct and indirect costs of pain reported by cancer patients, *J Pain Symptom Manage* 25:9–18, 2003.
14. Hayman JA, Langa KM, Kabeto MU, et al: Estimating the cost of informal caregiving for elderly patients with cancer, *J Clin Oncol* 19:3219–3225, 2001.
15. Himmelstein DU, Warren E, Thorne D, et al: Illness and injury as contributors to bankruptcy, *Health Aff* [Web Exclusive] 2005. Available at: http://content.healthaffairs.org/cgi/content/full/hlthaff.w5.63/DC1. Accessed May 18, 2010.
16. Himmelstein DU, Thorne D, Warren E, et al: Medical bankruptcy in the United States, 2007: results of a national study, *Am J Med* 122:741–746, 2009.
17. Emanuel LL, Alpert HR, Emanuel EE: Concise screening questions for clinical assessments of terminal care: the Needs near the End-of-life Screening Tool, *J Palliat Med* 4:465–474, 2001.
18. Zimmerman C, Riechelman R, Krzyzanowska M, et al: Effectiveness of specialized palliative care: a systematic review, *JAMA* 299:1698–1709, 2008.
19. Zuckerman B, Sandel M, Lawton E, et al: Medical-legal partnerships: transforming health care, *Lancet* 372:1615–1617, 2008.
20. Bass DM, Bowman K, Noelker LS: The influence of caregiving and bereavement support on adjusting to an older relative's death, *Gerontologist* 31:32–42, 1991.
21. Brenner PR: Issues of access in a diverse society, *Hosp J* 12:9–16, 1997.
22. Storey P, Knight CF: *UNIPAC One: the hospice/palliative medicine approach to end-of-life care. The American Academy of Hospice and Palliative Medicine UNIPAC Series: Hospice/Palliative Care Training for Physicians: A Self-Study Program*, ed 2, New York, 2003, Mary Ann Liebert.
23. Greiner KA, Perara S, Ahluwalia JS: Hospice usage by minorities in the last year of life: results from the National Mortality Followback Survey, *J Am Geriatr Soc* 51:970–978, 2003.
24. Smith AK, Sudore RL, Pérez-Stable EJ: Palliative care for Latino patients and their families: whenever we prayed, she wept, *JAMA* 301:1047–1057, 2009.
25. Hanchate A, Kronman AC, Young-Xu Y, et al: Racial and ethnic differences in end-of-life costs: why do minorities cost more than whites? *Arch Intern Med* 169:493–501, 2009.
26. Ngo-Metzger Q, EP McCarthy, Burns RB, et al: Older Asian Americans and Pacific Islanders dying of cancer use hospice less frequently than older white patients, *Am J Med* 115:47–53, 2003.

CHAPTER 48

Addressing the Social Suffering Associated with Illness: A Focus on Household Economic Resilience

LINDA L. EMANUEL*, TAPAS KUNDU**, EVA B. REITSCHULER-CROSS, KAREN GLASSER SCANDRETT, MELISSA SIMON*, and S. LAWRENCE LIBRACH

Economic devastation is a fairly common consequence of illness. As described in the previous chapter, in the United States, even among employed, higher socioeconomic groups with financial reserves and health insurance, terminal illness results in lost assets for the household that can take more than 6 years to recover and can result in bankruptcy. Regions with stronger social safety net policies may have lower rates of economic damage to households, and resource-challenged countries with weaker social safety net policies appear to have higher rates of illness-related economic devastation. However, even in Canada, with its national health scheme and perhaps better social safety net, patients and families bear some significant costs as a result of terminal illnesses, mostly in family caregivers' time.[1]

Much of the economic impact of illness is usually related to the lost work income of the patient if the patient is a bread-winner and to the lost work income of the

*Also contributing for the Kellogg-Feinberg Economics and Illness Study Group listed at the chapter's end.
**While carrying out this research, Tapas Kundu has been associated with the Centre of Equality, Social Organization, and Performance (ESOP) at the Department of Economics, University of Oslo. ESOP is supported by the Research Council of Norway.

family caregiver if full or partial exit from the workplace is required to take care of the patient. However, some of the economic impact is caused by the direct costs of care services. This component of economic impact should be considered a side effect of treatment and the usual informed consent procedures should be taken; that is, steps should be taken to ensure that the patient is aware of the side effects and still wants the intervention, and to minimize the side effect's impact.[2]

A serious commitment to medical professional values demands attention to the mechanisms of illness-related economic distress and sources of its amelioration. This is particularly true in palliative care, in which field the care of social dimensions of illness is a distinguishing feature. The capacity to minimize impact and maximize recovery can be summarized in one term: *resilience.* Enhancing economic resilience of households coping with serious and terminal illness is an essential part of palliative care.

Since the beginning of modern hospice and palliative care several decades ago, programs have offered more support to the household than many other types of medical care. In so doing, in economic terms, palliative care programs variously infused monetary and human capital into the household by (1) maximizing the patient's ability to stay in the workplace by optimizing symptom management; (2) training the family caregiver to care for the patient (a form of skills training); (3) supporting bereavement and thereby optimizing family caregiver resumption of life in the workplace; and (4) offering return-to-work assistance.

Providers of palliative care need to understand and optimize this aspect of care and leverage its impact for households toward the goal of achieving household economic resilience as part of palliative care. Toward the goal of continued growth in understanding and intervention in this area, improvements in household economic resilience should be a quality outcome measure for palliative care services in the future.

The Mechanism of Illness-Poverty Cycles

It is nearly axiomatic in public health that poverty increases both the risk of getting sick and the difficulty of fighting illness. Through many mechanisms, including poor living conditions, limited access to primary and preventive health care, and accepting whatever employment can be found even if it entails social, mental, or physical risk (such as prostitution, mining, etc.), poverty can lead to declining health in the individual and more prevalent disease in the community. The cycle comes full circle, as disease can directly lead to or deepen poverty, because of the incurrence of doctors' fees, paying for diagnostic and therapeutic interventions, transportation costs, and so on. Disease also frequently decreases a patient's work productivity, further worsening the financial burden through significant wage losses.

THRESHOLDS FOR AN ILLNESS–POVERTY TRAP

The financial burden caused by illness has long-term implications. Poor households can be trapped in poverty for generations when illness affects occupational choices of the household. Studies show that children in disease-affected families are less likely to remain in school. They may be needed at home to take care of the patient when families cannot bear the costs of professional nursing or families may be unable to afford school fees.[3] Lack of education adversely affects future occupational choices and further results in low future income for households. In this fashion, disease can trap households into an illness–poverty trap over generations.[4] Economic studies on health and development demonstrate this apparent illness–poverty trap in various resource-constrained countries.[5,6] The severity of this trap multiplies in countries without adequate social welfare programs, where low income is highly correlated with lack of healthy living conditions and a greater risk for disease.

Households with income below certain critical thresholds are vulnerable to the illness–poverty trap. With income being almost insufficient to meet current consumption need, these households rationally respond to the additional financial burden caused by illness by altering its members' current and potentially future occupational choices. It is therefore important for clinicians to estimate when the financial impact of illness becomes detrimental to health, either for the patient or for the patient's household members. Efforts can then be made to prevent that level of hardship and to assist recovery from it.

However, research has offered relatively sparse guidance on this topic. One researcher estimated that 10% loss in income in developing countries could be catastrophic.[7] Importantly, the threshold level at which financial impact becomes detrimental depends on factors internal to the household and external to it. So calculation of impact in a way that meaningfully relates to this threshold can be problematic.

One common-sense rule of thumb that clinicians can use is that if a household is unable to sustain the patient's medical care without significant jeopardy to any of its members' food intake, substantive medical care, workplace involvement, or education, then the household may be at or near economic devastation, and intervention may be imperative and health care service choices must be appropriate if an illness–poverty trap is to be prevented.

Why Is Health Care Spending High Near the End of Life?

The issues of economics and health care reach their greatest proportions when the illness is life threatening. Across an average person's lifetime, a large majority of health care spending occurs in the last months of life.[8] Further, the indirect costs are very large and probably track the time course of direct costs, or even rise further during home hospice care when care relies heavily on family support.[9] For this reason, palliative care clinicians see patients at a time and in a circumstance in their lives when their vulnerability to the economic impact of illness is probably at a lifetime high for them.

CHANGING PROGNOSIS, CHANGING VALUES, AND THE RULE OF RESCUE

For many years, awareness that costs of health care were highest at a time when prognosis was worst lead to a general assumption that something irrational or involuntary was driving decisions to intervene inappropriately with medical care. Why, so the logic went, would anyone want to spend exorbitantly on something destined to fail when one could be having low-technology quality of life with one's loved ones? However, the reverse analysis that the spending is appropriate is also persuasive for two reasons. First, the less it looks like a person has time to live, the more that person may value what does remain. Second, the less time one has to spend whatever resources are available, the more inclined a person might be to spend it—after all, as the logic goes, "the dying can't take money with them." The motivation to preserve resources for the next generation may be challenged by the desperation to live, and for many people, illness-related suffering does not engender altruism.

EXISTENTIAL EQUANIMITY AT A PERSONAL, FAMILY, AND SOCIETAL LEVEL

Individuals who seek to make use of palliative care services and eschew further curatively intended intervention have often reached a psychological point that accepts the inevitability of death. For some, this is because they have tried every available curative intervention and their illness and suffering is increasing despite every effort; often they are simply exhausted from all the suffering. For others, it is because they value quality of remaining life over the suffering associated with curative interventions.

But for many, reaching such a point is very difficult. The presence of palliative care programs that do not require refusal of further life-sustaining interventions appears to allow many more people to access palliative care and also seems to result in reduced direct costs of care.[10]

Quite likely, peoples' decisions are driven by their level of resolution and acceptance of mortality, a state of mind that might be called *existential equanimity* or *maturity*.[11] It is not easy to assess this state of mind formally or directly in the present state of palliative care's development as a field because measures do not exist for it. However, the clinician can probably gain a pretty good sense of the patient's disposition by engaging in discussion about his or her hopes for the future.

In terms of planning care interventions, the clinician can and should stay in frequent touch with the patient (or family as relevant) about any changes in the primary goals of care. Clinicians can also tailor the schedule of medical interventions and make sure the patient has the option for care settings (especially home) that allow for intergenerational visits and care by a social worker, psychologist, or pastor who may, without rushing things, facilitate life narratives or other stage of life–appropriate legacy-making, baton-passing activities that may foster some settledness and acceptance in the patient.

What Is Economic Resilience?

The definition of economic resilience of other social structures, usually countries, can be adopted for use in describing household economic resilience in the face of illness. We adjust one such definition from economists[12] here:

> *Economic resilience of the household in the face of illness is the "nurtured" ability of the household's economic state to recover from or adjust to the effects of illness.*

Components of economic resilience of the household in the face of illness are, however, less readily adopted from national economics. A practical way to think of the situation for clinicians is to focus on the nurtured components of economic resilience. These can be considered as twofold—those that (1) help prevent households from falling into poverty even in the face of illness and (2) help households get out of the illness–poverty cycles.

The Capacity of Palliative Care to Engender Economic Resilience

STAYING AWAY FROM THE ILLNESS–POVERTY TRAP

Optimizing Use of Goals of Care and Advance Care Planning

Hospice and palliative care have evolved as disciplines focused on the goals of symptom management, quality of life, acceptance of natural death, and care of the family as well as the patient. Even as its scope broadens to include patients seeking to extend life, still palliative care focuses on the patient's goals for what remains of his or her life and on the corresponding medical care goals. Attentive matching of the patient's goals to care provided ensures that at least the care provided for is desired care.

Advance care planning discussions can also be helpful so that goals of care are clear for the event that the patient cannot communicate them. However, it is also known that goals for care change with the experience of serious illness. It is appropriate to let patients know this when they are making their advance care plans and ask the patient's wishes about how to take this phenomenon into account for him or her. Some patients will ask to have current wishes honored; others will allow for the substituted decision maker or proxy to determine what the patient would have wanted had he or she been able to return momentarily to a condition in which a wish and its communication were possible. Many patients, desiring to minimize family burden, want the decision maker to also consider what is best for the family. Completion of advance care planning in the presence of the surrogate decision maker allows the decision maker to become familiar with the patient's values for their own quality of life, including the threshold beyond which the patient would no longer want to have invasive treatment, as well as the degree of flexibility they want the decision maker to have. This knowledge may help with decisions in unpredictable situations, relieving the stress experienced by the decision maker, decreasing feelings of guilt or conflict during bereavement, and consequently lessening the risk of complicated grief. Overall, since many will ask to have current, supportive care goals honored, the population's cost of care will likely decline with such an approach.

Patients who enjoy equanimity about their mortality appear to have a higher quality of life than those who have unresolved concerns or are fearful of death. Patients also respond overwhelmingly positively to engagement in activities such as Dignity Therapy (see Chapter 41). Clinicians can invite patients and their families to participate in these life review, intergenerational role-passing type of activities. It is not known whether such activities foster equanimity and perhaps less inclination to spend resources exhaustively near the end of life, but it seems possible. Because that kind of care has independent worth, and as long as it is not felt by any party to be promoting premature closure, clinicians should be trained, or should provide professionals who are trained, to offer it.

Optimizing Symptom Management and Family Caregiver Support

Palliative care has another capacity to minimize the economic impact of illness on the household. This capacity derives (1) from the improved symptom management for the patient that allows longer duration in the workplace and less dependence on the family caregiver, and (2) from the support offered to the family caregiver,

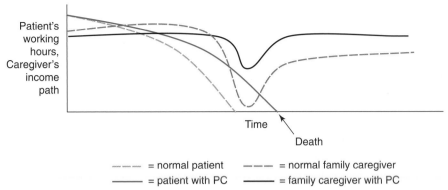

Patient's working hours, Caregiver's income path

Time

Death

----- = normal patient   ----- = normal family caregiver
——— = patient with PC   ——— = family caregiver with PC

Figure 48-1. Describes a theoretical case of a bread-winning parent (the patient) becoming terminally ill. It assumes that the spouse (the caregiver) has less earning capacity at the outset. In the normal scenario, health falls at an increasing rate and finally becomes zero at the time of death. With palliative care, the patient's health depreciates at a relatively low rate because of good symptom control under palliative care. The patient can stay in the workforce longer with palliative care. The orange lines describe the parent participating in the workforce in two different scenarios. In the normal scenario, the spouse leaves the workforce to care for the patient as she or he gets sick and has difficulty returning to full economic capacity caused by debts and psychosocial burden after that. The spouse's situation is improved by palliative care because of support received and because the patient is less symptomatic and more independent. The income path of the spouse is described by the blue lines. The spouse has a shorter, lesser drop in income and returns to income levels that are similar to preillness levels.

including respite care and bereavement support. The patient and family caregiver journeys are described graphically in Figures 48-1 and 48-2.

GETTING PEOPLE OUT OF THE ILLNESS–POVERTY TRAP

Traditional Palliative Care

Palliative care programs in the United States provide bereavement support to families, usually for a year after the patient's death. Programs in many places provide charitable funds for the unemployed family caregiver to assist with training or retraining. Both these sources of support will assist the family caregiver in staying out of poverty or getting out of poverty through employment.

Supplementary Programs

Studies on poverty and workforce development note that households often need resilience in more than one or two domains. It may be insufficient to provide health care and employment to the family caregiver if employment outside the house means that children are under-attended. Quality public school, daycare, and other after-school programs may also be needed.

Capitalizing on Family Caregiver Experience

Home hospice in most settings relies on the family to provide a large proportion of the caregiving. Care for the terminally ill usually entails use of a skill set that comes from trained professionals in health care institutions. Those skill sets range from

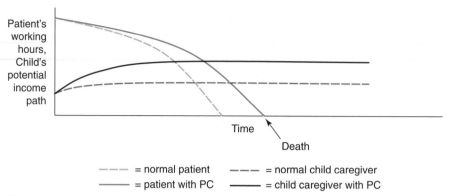

Figure 48-2. Describes the same case of a bread-winning parent getting sick. This time it is the child who stays away from school to provide care to the patient. The child's potential for earning stays minimal in the normal circumstance but is better with palliative care because the patient is less symptomatic and more independent. The potential income path of the child is shown in blue.

assisting with activities of daily living, as would be performed by a nurse's aide; to providing existential support, as would be done by a chaplain; to performing dressing changes, intravenous tubing or dialysis bag changes, and administration of medications, as would be done by a registered nurse. For the most part, these skills are acquired from the providers who visit from hospice.

In economic terms, these skills represent an infusion of human capital in the form of training. For those who are taken out of school or college to care for the patient, although they sustain an educational opportunity loss, they also gain an alternative type of training. For those who leave the workplace to care for the patient, although they sustain an income and career loss, they also gain a new type of skill. Those who were stay-at-home family members also gain a new type of skill.

The skill set gained by caring for a loved one is variable and not market employable without further training and certification. Programs that complete and certify the training and assist the family caregiver in securing employment as a paid home aide would leverage the infused capital. Similarly, programs for completing and credentialing the training for nursing, social work, or chaplaincy, or standard programs that accept hospice family care experience as an entry qualification have the potential to leverage the infused capital. Such programs are largely still not available.

Further, these programs are not a panacea; they become applicable only after the economic damage has been incurred—often after the patient has died—and they would not help those for whom such work is not a good aptitude match. Some who lose opportunities to care for their loved one have alternative better resources to leverage recovery. Others would find the emotional toll too high so soon after bereavement. But many find employment and turning their experience to assist others an important part of recovery.[13,14]

Overall, the potential for these programs is significant. They fall within the general health care system and so health care professionals can build such programs relatively independently. Providers of palliative care should offer such programs wherever relevant and possible as part of the core mission of the palliative care discipline.

Feasibility: Empirical Data from Three Different Areas

For such programs to be built, adequate evidence of their feasibility is necessary. Some critical conditions for program viability include the following:

- Households must have an interest in and need for such programs.
- Cultural acceptability of such programs must be adequate.
- An adequate economy must exist to provide employment opportunities for the new caregiver services.
- Capital must exist to finance the additional training and support the caregivers' securing employment.

Evidence exists that the first two conditions apply in relatively poor regions as far flung and distinct as Kampala in Uganda, Trivandrum in India, and Dupage County in Illinois, USA.[15–18] For governments such as the current United States government, which are interested in workforce development, safe loan programs should make a good fit for the population's needs and the government agenda. Similarly, safe loan programs would make a good fit for many foundations' missions.

Health Systems, Policy, Illness, and Poverty

Health insurance and social welfare policies have the capacity to greatly reduce the economic impact of illness on households and specifically to eliminate illness–poverty traps. The relevance for palliative care providers to attend to the economic impact of illness and its care varies with these policies. For example, in the United States one barrier to early palliative care is the choice individuals' families often make between skilled nursing facility placement and hospice benefits. If families can't provide 24-hour care, they often choose to send loved ones to nursing homes under Medicare A, which precludes hospice. Nursing facilities are not currently well equipped or reimbursed to provide palliative care, so those needs may go unmet until the person is no longer making progress in functional measures and is discharged from Medicare A. Responding to the financial/logistical incentive, families may push patients to work hard in rehabilitation so they can stay in the facility, which may take precious time away from the goals of palliation and the patient's dying process.

A second example is the reimbursement associated with placement of a new gastrostomy tube. This medical intervention is the only thing that will "skill" someone for the entire 100-day Medicare A benefit. That is, someone could, conceivably, place a feeding tube in a dying patient just to ensure them a nursing home bed for 100 days. In these situations, the economic incentives are working directly against the goals of hospice.

IMPACT OF HEALTH REFORM IN THE UNITED STATES

On March 23, 2010, President Obama signed the Patient Protection and Affordable Care Act. Although implementation carries unpredictable possibilities, the aim of this act is to ensure health insurance for an additional 25 to 30 million people, including those with a preexisting condition, and limiting household's exposure to unmanageable direct medical costs by limiting out-of-pocket expenditures.

The Affordable Care Act offers little relief for indirect costs and places more emphasis on home care. This will place potentially more economic burden on the household rather than less. To offset this, the Act provides a protection for recipients of home and community-based services against spousal impoverishment, and also requires that grants be allotted for training new and incumbent direct care workers in nursing homes and home-care settings. It also set up a National Health Care Workforce Commission to understand the supply and demand of future domestic health care workforce and State Health Care Workforce Development programs to assist in training the expected expansion in home care workforce. If implemented appropriately, the act will allocate money to rigorously develop a set of core rules, knowledge, and skills that caregivers must learn to be successful. Palliative care clinicians should remain alert to the emergence of such programs and take relevant opportunities to provide protection and training to family caregivers.[19] At the time of printing, political opposition to the Act has mounted.

CANADIAN INITIATIVES

In January 2004 the Canadian federal government launched an employment insurance benefit, the Compassionate Care Benefit, which provided 8 weeks of leave to employees to provide care or support to a family member with a significant risk of death within 26 weeks. The Canada Labour Code was also amended to provide federal employees with 8 weeks of job protection while on this leave. However, those not eligible for Employment Insurance benefits do not qualify. This ineligible group includes the unemployed (approximately 37% of Canadians who have no job or stay at home); self-employed (approximately 15%); and part-time, temporary, contract or seasonal employees with insufficient working hours to qualify. The majority of Compassionate Care Benefit claimants are women (71%).[20] This benefit has been underutilized even though eligibility criteria have been changed and the period of benefits increased. The reasons for this include the low level of compensation, the limited job protection, and the lack of public awareness.

EVALUATING DIFFERENT MODELS

Palliative care clinicians should insist on evaluation of programmatic and household outcomes as well as patient's medical outcomes. Programs should include efforts to minimize household economic impact and maximize resilience and should measure the success of these efforts.

Conclusions

Terminal illness causes severe financial impact on households not only because of illness-related inability to work but also because of the cost of medical care. This means that clinicians are obligated to treat economic devastation as an unwanted side effect of treatment that should be ameliorated as much as possible.

Palliative care is particularly obligated because the discipline professes to care for the social as well as other aspects of illness. It is also a type of service that is often provided in the home, when out-of-pocket and other indirect costs are high and when direct costs of care are also often high.

Palliative care has the capacity to ameliorate economic impact by optimizing symptom control so that the patient maintains function as long as possible and the family caregiver can stay in school or work longer as well.

It also has the built-in feature in home care services of infusing a tailored form of clinical education into the family caregiver. Some palliative care programs already offer retraining programs for the family caregiver to get back on her or his economic feet after bereavement. Programs that allow course credit to family members toward a training program in home-aide or nursing care might allow some people an additional boost as they try to regain their prior economic state.

Clinicians should be alert to these needs and to possible programs that family caregivers can be referred to.

References

1. Guerriere DN, Zagorski B, Fassbender K, et al: Cost variations in ambulatory and home-based palliative care, *Palliat Med* 24(5):523–532, 2010.
2. Cross ER, Emanuel L: Providing inbuilt economic resilience options: an obligation of comprehensive cancer care, *Cancer* 113(12 suppl):3548–3555. PMID: 19058152, 2008.
3. Miguel E: Health, education and economic development. In Lopez-Casasnovas G, Rivera B, Currais L, editors: *Health and economic growth: findings and policy implications*, Cambridge, 2005, MIT Press.
4. Kundu T, Reitschuler-Cross E, Emanuel L: Alleviating poverty: a proposal to mitigate the economic cost of disease. Poster presentation at the John & Gwen Smart Symposium, 2010. Available at www.northwestern.edu/aging.
5. Bell C, Devarajan S, Gerbach H: The long-run economic costs of AIDS: a model with an application to South Africa, *World Bank Econ Rev* 20(1):55–89, 2006.
6. Corrigan P, Glomm G, Mendez F: AIDS crisis and growth, *J Dev Econ* 77(1):107–124, 2005.
7. Russell S: The economic burden of illness for household in developing countries: a review of studies focusing on malaria, tuberculosis, and human immunodeficiency virus/acquired immunodeficiency syndrome, *Am J Trop Med Hyg* 71:147–155, 2004.
8. Lubitz J, Beebe J, Baker C: Longevity and Medicare expenditures, *N Engl J Med* 332(15):999–1003, 1995.
9. Langa KM, Fendrick AM, Chernew ME, et al: Out-of-pocket health-care expenditures among older Americans with cancer, *Value Health* (2):186–194, 2004.
10. Temel JS, Greer JA, Muzikansky A, et al: Early palliative care for patients with metastatic non-small-cell lung cancer, *N Engl J Med* 363:733–742, 2010.
11. Emanuel L, Scandrett KG: Decisions at the end of life: have we come of age? *BMC Med* 8:57, 2010.
12. Briguglio L, Cordina G, Bugeja S, Farrugia N: Conceptualizing and measuring economic resilience. Available at https://secure.um.edu.mt/__data/assets/pdf_file/0013/44122/resilience_index.pdf. Accessed August 18, 2010.
13. Li Y: Recovering from spousal bereavement in later life: does volunteer participation play a role? *J Gerontol B Psychol Sci Soc Sci* 62:S257–S266, 2007.
14. Hoppes S, Segal R: Reconstructing meaning through occupation after the death of a family member: accommodation, assimilation, and continuing bonds, *Am J Occup Ther* 64:133–141, 2010.
15. Emanuel RH, Emanuel GA, Reitschuler EB, et al: Challenges faced by informal caregivers of hospice patients in Uganda, *J Palliat Med* 11(5):746–753. PMID: 18588407, 2008.
16. Emanuel N, Simon MA, Burt M, et al: Economic impact of terminal illness and the willingness to change it, *J Palliat Med* 13(8):941–944, 2010.
17. Simon M, the Kellogg-Feinberg 2010 Economics and Illness Study Group,* Hajjar N, Emanuel L: Breaking the poverty trap: a feasibility study of training informal caregivers in DuPage County. Poster presentation at the John & Gwen Smart Symposium, 2010. Available at www.northwestern.edu/aging.
18. Simon M, the Kellogg-Feinberg 2010 Economics and Illness Study Group,* Hajjar N, Emanuel L: Breaking the poverty trap: a study of community stakeholder's opinions training informal caregivers in Chicagoland. Poster presentation at the John & Gwen Smart Symposium 2010. Available at www.northwestern.edu/aging.
19. This evaluation was provided by the Kellogg-Feinberg 2010 Economics and Illness Study Group.*
20. Osborne K, Margo N, Health Council of Canada: Analysis and evaluation: compassionate care benefit, Toronto, Canada, December 2005. Available at www.healthcouncilcanada.ca.

---

*Kellogg-Feinberg 2010 Economics and Illness Study Group Members:
Bautista J, Brown J, Clark B, Deane AL, Divan Y, Falson CC, Foley KE, Gopalan S, Harsch NL, Handel B, Holoyda B, Huang L, Hung S, Kang A, Morris A, Kannry SM, Litow MA, Lock J, Naik N, Nguyen K, O'Halloran M, Oustwani C, Paik K, Patel A, Polimeno A, Pomeranz C, Pordes E, Sanchez E, Sandberg J, Schulz J, Schweighofer E, Seth N, Sridharan L, Su A, Tang S, Tornheim R, Ueda Y, Walker K.

CHAPTER 49

Palliative Care in Developing Countries

LILIANA DE LIMA, ROBERTO DANIEL WENK, M.R. RAJAGOPAL, DANIELA MOSOIU, LIZ GWYTHER, and EDUARDO BRUERA

Except the United States, developed countries registered either a decline or no change in population during the last decade, whereas 99% of worldwide population growth took place in developing countries. As a result, by 2050, industrialized nations will record a population increase of only 4%, and the population in developing countries will expand by 55%.[1] Overall, the world population will reach approximately 9 billion by midcentury.

This population growth will burden developing countries with a greater demand for health care services. More individuals will require palliative care services, but funding is limited, infrastructures are inadequate, and there is limited access to preventive and curative measures.

The World Health Report, published by the World Health Organization (WHO), indicates that 57 million deaths occurred worldwide in 2004. Most of these deaths occurred in developing countries, where more than three fourths of the world's population lives. Infectious diseases such as human immunodeficiency virus (HIV), malaria, tuberculosis, and respiratory infections caused more than half the cumulative deaths in developing countries.

Cancer

Currently, 24.6 million people are living with cancer, and by 2020 it is projected that there will be 16 million new cancer cases and 10 million cancer deaths every year. Cancer is among the major noncommunicable causes of death worldwide, and it accounted for more than 12% of the total deaths in 2004, or more than 7 million cases.[2] The International Agency for Research on Cancer projects that global cancer rates will increase by 50%, from 10 million new cases worldwide in 2000 to 15 million new cases in 2020, primarily because of the aging of the population and increases in smoking. Fifty percent of the world's new cancer cases and deaths occur in developing countries, and approximately 80% of these patients already have incurable cancer at the time of diagnosis.[3]

HIV/AIDS

The number of people living with HIV has been rising in every region, with the steepest increases occurring in East Asia, Eastern Europe, and Central Asia. The increases in Asia are mostly the result of the growing epidemic in China. More than 60 million men, women, and children have been infected with HIV. More than 22 million people have died of acquired immunodeficiency syndrome (AIDS), and it is now the primary cause of death in Africa. Approximately 8% of the adult population is infected with HIV in sub-Saharan Africa, and global AIDS deaths totaled 3.1 million during 2003.[4] Initial efforts were aimed at prevention as the most realistic approach to reduce morbidity and mortality, but there is now an increased focus on care and treatment that stresses the importance of integrating prevention and treatment approaches into national health policies and priorities. Under this new approach, several government officials and activists have called for improving access to highly active antiretroviral therapy, prophylaxis, and treatment of opportunistic infections in people living with HIV/AIDS in developing countries. In addition, several authors have indicated that this should also include palliative care, pain relief, and support to families of patients who do not respond to the treatment or who do not have access to these expensive therapies.[5]

Palliative Care

WHO encompasses a broad definition of palliative care that includes the needs of patients, families, and caregivers, and also addresses the physical, emotional, and spiritual needs of those involved. The organization promotes a public health approach to palliative care and recommends that comprehensive palliative care programs be integrated into the existing health care systems and adapted to the cultural and social context of nations. Palliative care can be provided simply and inexpensively in tertiary care facilities, community health centers, and at home.

The key components of a national comprehensive palliative care program, as recommended by WHO, include policy development, education and training, the provision of good quality care, and drug availability.[5,6] To address the needs of patients with advanced disease, the World Health Assembly recently adopted a resolution that gives special emphasis to the development and reinforcement of comprehensive national cancer control programs that, for the first time, include palliative care as a main component of cancer control strategies.[7]

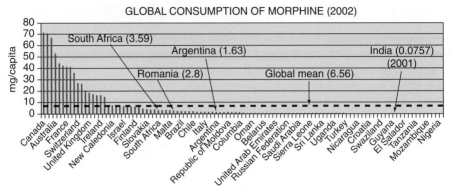

Figure 49-1. Global consumption of morphine. *(From the Pain and Policy Studies Group, 2005. International Narcotics Control Board and United National Demographic Group, 2002.)*

Opioid Consumption

For several years, morphine consumption has been used as an indicator of adequate access to pain relief. In 1986, the WHO developed the WHO analgesic ladder[6] for the relief of cancer pain. The method relies on the permanent availability of opioid analgesics, including morphine, codeine, and others. The WHO ladder has been widely disseminated throughout the world. Still, opioid analgesics are insufficiently available, especially in developing countries; prescription of morphine is limited to a small percentage of physicians; and the drug is unavailable in many countries of the world.

The International Narcotics Control Board (INCB) collects consumption data from government reports on a yearly basis. Although the supply of narcotic drugs for medical purposes remains inadequate, the consumption trends recorded by INCB indicate improvement. The global consumption of morphine has been doubling every 5 years since 1984. In 2002, global consumption amounted for 27.3 tons.[8] The trend is, however, mainly the result of increasing consumption in a few countries. For 2002, 82% of the total global consumption of morphine occurred in six countries: the United States, France, Canada, Germany, the United Kingdom, and Australia. The remaining 18% was consumed in the other 133 countries for which data are available. There are 51 developing countries with no registered morphine consumption at all. For that same year, the global mean of morphine consumption was 6.56 mg per capita. Figure 49-1 shows the consumption of morphine in selected countries of the world.[9] Highlighted are consumption rates for Argentina, India, Romania, and South Africa, countries discussed individually later in this chapter.

Palliative Care in the Developing World

Barriers to the adequate provision of palliative cancer care include the following: poverty; inadequate health care coverage; bureaucratic and inefficient processes related to the production or importation of opioids; restrictive laws and regulations related to the prescribing of opioids; centralized, ineffective opioid distribution methods that fail to reach rural regions adequately; insufficient drug availability; lack of knowledge and training related to palliative cancer care and pain management among health care workers; and insufficient support from national health authorities or low levels of political will to establish palliative cancer care programs.[10]

The cost of opioids has been identified as a significant barrier to adequate care in developing nations. A recent study of developing and developed nations demonstrated that the median cost of opioid medication was twice as high in developing countries. In U.S. dollars, a 30-day prescription was $112 in developing countries, compared with $53 in developed countries. Cost as percent of gross national product (GNP) per capita per month was 10-fold higher in developing countries, where patients have to spend more than one third of their salaries to cover pain therapy. Median cost was 31% of GNP per capita per month in the developing countries, compared with 3% of GNP per capita per month in the developed countries. Half of the opioid preparations cost more than 33% of monthly GNP per capita in developing countries, compared with only 4% in developed countries. There were also fewer programs to offset medication costs in developing countries. Only one of the five developing nations (20%) had a subsidization program or socialized medicine, compared with four of seven (57%) of the developed nations.[11]

A Latin American survey on advanced cancer care involved 667 physicians and demonstrated that, compared with other facilities or at home, most of the care given to persons with advanced cancer occurs in hospitals. However, the study also demonstrated that when the time of death approaches, most patients are discharged and die at home without receiving any type of medical care.[12] Several authors have called for the development of palliative care models fit to meet population needs and financial constraints. Home palliative care can be a cost-effective approach when relatives are able to provide care and there is sufficient capacity to train them to provide the required nursing care.

A large body of knowledge has emerged on the assessment and management of the physical and psychosocial problems that occur in patients who develop cancer and other progressive, incurable illnesses. Most of the available written material refers to the delivery of palliative care for diseases that occur mostly in the developed world and the use of resources available mostly in developed countries. However, patients in developing countries die younger and of conditions different from those in the developed world. In addition, certain socioeconomic and cultural issues pose particular challenges for the health care team.

Most of the research and advances published in the literature deal with medications or approaches that are not readily available in developing countries. Several treatment strategies and inexpensive technologies can be adopted and implemented in the developing world. Some of these include the following:

Proctoclysis: This simple and inexpensive alternative method of hydration may be helpful in situations where resources are limited. A small nasogastric nutrition catheter is inserted in the rectum for hydration daily or every other day. It utilizes the colon's intrinsic ability to absorb normal saline or tap water. Assessments of comfort showed that this technique is well tolerated, and family members can successfully administer proctoclysis at home.[13] This method may be especially helpful when technical difficulties make intravenous or subcutaneous infusion difficult or expensive. Such settings may include developing countries, rural areas, and situations where nursing care is limited.

Edmonton Injector: This simple, nondisposable, very low cost device allows patients to self-administer injections of opioids, metoclopramide, or other drugs intermittently into a subcutaneous needle. A bag contains 50 or 100 mL of medication, and pharmacists can prepare the medication from powder at a minimal cost. By a simple mechanical movement, patients are able to inject medication safely. The device does not require batteries, and little training is required for patients and families. The cost of this treatment is less than US$1 a day, and the device is not patented, thus allowing groups in developing countries to manufacture their own apparatus.[14] Unfortunately, in some countries this device is not available or has not been approved by health care authorities, mostly because of its extremely low cost, which makes it unattractive to manufacturers.

Methadone: A synthetic opioid and N-methyl-D-aspartate antagonist, methadone is a potent analgesic in treating cancer pain. Its characteristics include excellent absorption, high lipid solubility, high potency, long half-life, lack of known metabolites, decreased opioid cross-tolerance, and very low cost, thus making it suitable for developing countries. However, overly restrictive regulations do not permit access to methadone in many of these countries.[15]

Cultural Aspects

Recent publications address these issues and highlight the importance of a global approach sensitive to the different conditions, cultures, religious beliefs, ethnic backgrounds, and settings. Some of these include *Palliative Care in the Developing World: Principles and Practice*[16] and *Pain and Palliative Care in the Developing World and Marginalized Populations: A Global Challenge.*[17]

Communication, disclosure of the diagnosis, active participation in decision making and treatment, discussion of end-of-life issues, and other matters are all influenced by the context in which these occur. Research has shown major differences in attitudes and beliefs regarding issues such as the role of patients and families in the decision-making process, amount of information disclosed in the diagnosis and prognosis, spiritual aspects, discussion of end-of-life issues, and other related topics.[18] Professionals need to be aware of the need to recognize these differences, especially in multicultural environments or when traveling abroad to teach or work in another country.

The following are summaries of the status of palliative care in four different developing countries: Argentina, India, Romania, and South Africa. These sections were written by palliative care physicians who are actively working in their countries and are constantly facing many of the barriers discussed previously.

Argentina

Health care development in Argentina varies considerably. Some areas have excellent medical facilities, whereas others have insufficient basic primary care. A high percentage of the population, especially among the lower socioeconomic classes, has difficulty obtaining qualified and efficient medical attention. The economic resources allocated for public health are insufficient to solve the sanitary problems. In addition, poor administration and bureaucracy at the professional and administrative levels aggravate the problems.[19]

STATUS OF PALLIATIVE CARE

According to preliminary information from the National Directory of the Argentine Association for Medicine and Palliative Care (*Asociación Argentina de Medicina y Cuidado Paliativo*), there are approximately 90 palliative care teams in the private and public health systems in Argentina, and they are located mostly in urban areas.

Most programs provide partial care and consist of small teams from different disciplines with varying levels of participation. The care is provided either at home through home care services or by family members who receive training in patient care and follow up via phone calls; in outpatient facilities; or in institutions where patients can be hospitalized, although there are no beds dedicated to palliative care (mobile advisory teams).[20] Comprehensive palliative care programs with interdisciplinary teams that provide full-time care—in the consulting room, at home, in daycare, or at inpatient facilities—account for approximately 10% of the programs in the country.

SOCIOECONOMIC AND ADMINISTRATIVE CHALLENGES

In 2002, Argentinean mortality rates from cancer and AIDS were 126.6 and 4.4 per 100,000, respectively.[21] Despite the progress made in the last few years, the quality of assistance during the dying process is poor and has resulted in uncontrolled suffering and poor communication among professionals, patients, and families. Although there is limited information on the percentage of patients who receive palliative care, it can be estimated to be lower than 5% of the patients in need. Some of the reasons for this lack include insufficient support from health authorities, lack of rewards and incentives, and insufficient education. These are discussed in the following subsections.

Insufficient Support from the Health Authorities

Palliative care is not recognized as a specialty in Argentina, it is not incorporated within the health system, and no resources are assigned to the development of palliative care. In spite of the resolution adopted in 2000 by the Medical Obligatory Program, which established that all the country's health institutions must offer free palliative care (including opioid analgesics) for patients with cancer, the government has failed to implement this resolution.[22]

Lack of Rewards and Incentives

Palliative care workers, teams, and programs face financial constraints because the health system does not cover or underpays for the services. Many programs end up requesting donations from charity, hire workers on a pro bono basis, enroll volunteers, and request out-of-pocket pay from those patients who can afford it. A few private insurance programs in the country include palliative care in their coverage plans.

Palliative Care Education

Curricula for graduate health professionals are inconsistent, varied, and often inadequate. The results are predictable: Some professionals without training provide inadequate palliative care to patients; some clinicians are unable to recognize the final stages of illnesses or to provide effective interventions; the role of different specialties is performed by many, without regard to quality or standards of care; many palliative care workers still feel uncomfortable discussing end-of-life issues; and many clinicians are incapable of working in multidisciplinary teams.

A few programs offer teaching opportunities with clear objectives and methods targeted to practice and improve the teamwork approach. A sign of progress is the creation of concurrency posts (nonpaid training positions) and residency positions (paid training positions) in palliative care for recently graduated clinicians. In 2003, two concurrency positions per year for physicians were established in the Hospital Tornú in Buenos Aires. In 2005, five residency positions per year were established for clinicians at the Hospital Tornú and the Hospital Udaondo in Buenos Aires.

Opioid Availability and Accessibility

Although the use of opioids has increased in Argentina during the last 10 years, the registered consumption in 2002 was 1.63 mg per capita, much less than the global mean of 6.5 mg per capita (see Figure 49-1). Several opioids are available in urban areas, but high prices are a barrier to access.[11] The monthly cost of 180-mg equivalent doses of immediate-release oral morphine, methadone, and sustained-release oxycodone is US$136, US$57, and US$412, respectively,[23] whereas the minimum monthly salary in Argentina is currently equivalent to US$155.

India

SOCIOECONOMIC AND ADMINISTRATIVE CHALLENGES

In India, where 1 million people are diagnosed with cancer every year,[2] fewer than 1% of needy patients have access to palliative care. A few have access to curative treatment, but most either experience futile aggressive treatment modalities that are continued late into the course of the disease, or they are told, "There is nothing more we can do." There is no government-sponsored social security system. The overwhelming social problem of poverty is worsened by the cost of treatments. By the time the patient dies, families are often homeless and children may have dropped out of school.

In 1991, the government of India declared palliative care an essential component of cancer care, but health care delivery remained the onus of individual state governments. Policy did not become reality, and even now, very few cancer centers in India offer palliative care services. Even if they did, these services would still be grossly insufficient because most Indians live in rural villages with no access to cancer centers. Unless palliative care permeates primary health centers, coverage will continue to be inadequate.

Palliative Care Education

Only about 5 out of 200 medical colleges in India teach any palliative care to undergraduate students, and the situation is equally abysmal in nursing education. Preliminary educational efforts by many enthusiasts resulted in improved awareness of palliative care in at least in some pockets of the country. In addition to sensitization programs, short courses and distance education programs also have been started. In 2004, the only residential postgraduate course in palliative care started in the Amrita Institute of Medical Sciences, Kochi. It is a 2-year diploma course that offers a diploma in pain and palliative medicine, the first university-approved postgraduate course in the subject in the country. The International Association for Hospice and Palliative Care has supported this program with a faculty development grant. Pallium

India, a nongovernment organization that emphasizes education, was instrumental in persuading the National Board of Examinations (a government body that conducts national-level postgraduate examinations) to accept pain and palliative medicine as an independent postgraduate discipline.

Opioid Availability and Accessibility

Although India legally grows poppy and exports opium to many parts of the world, most suffering patients in India have no access to morphine. According to the INCB data, the consumption per capita in the country in 2001 was 0.07 mg (see Figure 49-1), lower than that of many countries with no palliative care programs. Fear of addiction among the public caused administrators to enact unrealistic narcotic regulations that effectively prevent medical use of the drug. The Narcotic Drugs and Psychotropic Substances Act of 1985 stipulated such strict penalties for even minor infringements that pharmacists all over the country stopped stocking potent opioids.[24] Because multiple licenses are required from different state agencies, it is not uncommon finally to obtain one license only to find that another has expired. To add to the confusion, individual states within the country have different narcotic regulations. Even where oral morphine is available, fear of addiction and respiratory depression prevent professionals from using it. The resulting downward trend in consumption of morphine in India means a progressive increase in unnecessary pain burden for millions.

Government efforts, unfortunately, have had limited success. Between 1991 and 1996, several workshops were conducted by the government of India in an attempt to improve access to opioids, but opioid consumption figures kept plummeting until the WHO Collaborating Center at Madison-Wisconsin joined forces with administrators and local organizations (including Indian Association of Palliative Care) to improve opioid availability.[25] Today, narcotic regulations have been simplified in 13 of India's 28 states, and morphine consumption has been rising steadily since 1999.

India has many systems of indigenous medicine, predominant among which is Ayurveda. Homoeopathy is also widely practiced. Theoretically, the availability of multiple systems of medicine should work to the patient's advantage, but there is seldom any scientific evaluation of the efficacy of these approaches, and they often add to patient's problems. Patients find it impossible to achieve a state of acceptance because there is always someone who offers a cure, no matter how hopeless the situation, and this contributes to the patient's emotional, physical, and financial burden.

THE LAST TWO DECADES

There has been a positive change in the last two decades. Inpatient hospices in some parts of the country have acted as beacons of care and have contributed to educational efforts. However, they did not have the potential for wide area coverage, and later efforts based on care at home reached more people. In the South Indian state of Kerala, a model of care generated by the Pain and Palliative Care Society in Calicut has now grown to a network of about 60 palliative care centers in the state, many of them in rural areas.[26] "The Calicut Model," as it came to be called, was a low-cost system designed to achieve coverage while maintaining quality. An extension of the model, called Neighborhood Network in Palliative Care, has taken it one step further by encouraging a greater role for volunteers and for getting closer to patients.[27] It seeks to ensure increased involvement of laypersons in ensuring the health of the community. Neighborhood Network in Palliative Care is currently being systematically evaluated.

THE WAY FORWARD

So far, development in India in palliative care has been mostly driven by Nongovernmental Organizations (NGOs); government participation has been minimal. This situation has resulted in programs and projects run by very committed groups and individuals, but they do not have the ability to reach many patients. As coverage improves, there is always a concern that the service is spread too thinly, thus compromising quality of care. To reach the length and breadth of India, it is necessary to integrate palliative care with both mainstream medical practice and the health care system. NGOs in India have repeatedly asked the government for a pragmatic palliative care policy; but change is often slow.

Pain relief and palliative care also need to be incorporated in the basic education of physicians and nurses. This requires the support and endorsement of the Medical and Nursing Councils of India.

Romania

SOCIOECONOMIC AND ADMINISTRATIVE CHALLENGES

Palliative care was introduced in Romania through an initiative of Graham Perrols, Chairman of the Ellenor Foundation in the United Kingdom. In 1992, a conference was organized with a group of supporters from the United Kingdom, and Romania's first service hospice, Casa Sperantei, was opened in Brasov.

Romania is an Eastern European country with 22.81 million inhabitants. Since the fall of the Communist dictatorial regime in 1989, it has struggled to overcome the consequences of 45 years under a totalitarian system and still faces problems such as a centralized economy, centralized distribution of funding, centralized decision making, a dictatorial political party, and extreme poverty.

The economy is going through a process of gradual reform, and since 2000 there has been a modest increase in the gross domestic product (GDP).[28] Romania has had 10 health ministers since 1992. This instability has seriously hindered coherent development in all areas, including palliative care services. The medical health care system is funded through a national state insurance body, and approximately 80% of the population is insured.[29] Despite the new legislative framework issued with the aim of decentralizing the health care system, most decisions are still largely under the responsibility of the Ministry of Health. In 2005, 4% of the GDP was allocated to health.

The leading causes of mortality are cardiovascular disease and cancer. These diseases are responsible for more than 50% of deaths in the persons up to the age of 64 years and for more than 85% of deaths among those older than 65 years. Two thirds of patients with cancer are diagnosed in the late, incurable stage of the disease.[2] AIDS is a problem, particularly in children, although there has been a steady fall in the number of new cases per year because of improvements in blood testing and safety measures.

Cultural aspects and traditions must also be considered for a complete picture of the founding of palliative care in Romania. According to the 2001 nationwide census, 87% of Romanians are predominantly Eastern Orthodox Christians. Traditional families with three generations living under the same roof are now rarely found in

Romania because of the migration and emigration of young couples. Community cohesion and rituals and traditions that surround major events in life (birth, marriage, death, grieving) are mainly preserved in the rural areas. Approximately 54% of the population lives in rural areas.

The main problems encountered in developing and providing palliative care services are lack of financial resources, lack of an appropriate legislative framework, low priority in the health care system for patients with incurable and terminal diseases, lack of trained staff, a hierarchical system that hinders team work, and lack of structures where these services could be provided.

Palliative Care Education

Since it opened in 1998, more than 2000 professionals, including health care professionals, managers, authorities, volunteers, and fundraisers from all over the country, have attended introductory or advanced courses at the Education Centre attached to the Hospice in Brasov. In 2000, palliative care was recognized as a medical subspecialty.[30] A 12-week program for doctors was nationally accredited by the Ministry of Health and is run by Hospice Casa Sperantei Education Centre. To facilitate access to courses involving a longer period of training, in 2004 Hospice Casa Sperantei opened branches of the training center in four other cities: Bucharest, Cluj, Oradea, and Târgu Mures. Most of the theoretical training is done at these regional centers, and the practical training takes place at the hospice in Brasov. To date, 128 doctors have received a diploma in palliative care.

Because nurses are vital members of the team, nursing education was another priority. On the national level, the Association of Nurses is in the process of reorganization. A continuing medical education system with credits was introduced in 2004 and has proved an ideal opportunity to offer introductory courses in palliative care. The nursing diploma is still in negotiation, and although the 6-week course for nurses was accredited nationally, it has not yet received the status of a diploma. Two universities offer optional palliative care courses at the undergraduate level for medical and nursing students in their final year: Brasov and Târgu Mures.

Opioid Availability and Accessibility

Romania has one of the lowest consumptions of morphine in Europe (2.8 mg per capita in 2002), less than the regional mean and global average (see Figure 49-1). This is the result of several existing barriers: the restrictive opioid law, inadequate training of physicians, patients' fears, and reluctance to use this medication. Legislation dates from 1969 and allows prescription of strong opioids only for patients with incurable cancer, peripheral vascular disease, and dyspnea resulting from terminal cardiac insufficiency. The procedure of obtaining the medication is lengthy and requires authorization, approval from the local health board, prescription with a dry stamp, and a triplicate prescription from the family doctor. Only one or two pharmacies per district dispense morphine and other strong opioids, and prescriptions must be renewed every 10 to 15 days. Because only one potent opioid is allowed at a time, patients receiving long-acting opioids cannot have breakthrough medication. A new authorization is required for any change in dosage or route of administration. General fear of morphine and lack of understanding by the general population are commonly encountered: morphine "equals death," "causes addiction," and is seen and used by doctors as a last resort.

Because of the interest the government showed toward pain control and palliative care, in 2002 Romania was selected to participate in a project by the Pain and Policy Studies Group at the University of Wisconsin. The old law was analyzed using WHO guidelines,[31] and a new law and regulations were drafted. The new law was passed by Parliament in the autumn of 2005. An implementation program was proposed, which includes dissemination (via booklets, news, and media) and an education program targeted to physicians, pharmacists, and the general public. The group of national and international experts will continue to work together to ensure smooth implementation of the new law. Most of the other drugs needed for palliative care are available.

ADOPTED AND PROPOSED MEASURES

Legislative changes have been proposed to foster the development of new services. The law regarding patients' rights was changed in 2003 and now includes articles about the rights of patients with advanced and terminal illnesses to receive appropriate care.

Since 2003, the health insurance law includes provisions that allow reimbursement through the insurance system for general home care services. Although palliative care services offered in inpatient units are included in the contract, no practical provisions were enacted to ensure that actual funding is made. As a result, funding for inpatient services is not possible from this source. The law also stipulates that hospitals can provide curative treatments, rehabilitation, and palliative care.

The Minister of Health appointed the National Palliative Care Commission in 2004 with the aim of developing palliative care services at the national level. The commission drafted the Regulations for Palliative Care Services after researching international documents, but it also took into account the national standards that were proposed in 2000 by the Romanian National Association for Palliative Care. The document includes several sections, including beneficiaries, type and level of palliative care services, requirements (staffing and equipment) for the authorization of palliative care services, authorization and accreditation process, national data collection, regional coordination of development, and funding for palliative care services. The document has not yet been adopted.

Despite all these obstacles, there has been considerable development of palliative care in Romania in the last 10 years, but a long, untraveled road is ahead. Hospice Casa Sperantei was and is the one institution leading the palliative care movement in Romania. The task now is to integrate palliative care into the main health care system to offer access and coverage for patients in need.

South Africa

Since 1980 in South Africa, the hospice movement has provided palliative care to patients and families faced with the diagnosis of life-threatening illness. Hospices started as volunteer organizations that filled the gap by providing palliative care, and especially end-of-life care, that was not available in formal health care services. The Hospice Palliative Care Association (HPCA) of South Africa was established in 1987 and has facilitated further development of hospices to provide professional palliative care services through an accreditation process and mentorship of member hospices to adopt recognized policies and procedures for clinical palliative care, management, and good governance.

SPECIFIC PROBLEMS IN THE PROVISION OF PALLIATIVE CARE

There are two significant challenges in the provision of palliative care. The first is the lack of financial resources. Hospices in South Africa are NGOs that rely on donations and grants to finance the service. Since 2003, the government has started providing grants to some hospices for the palliative care of patients with AIDS, but not for those with cancer and other terminal illnesses. On average, this contribution amounts to 10% of the hospices' budgets. Health insurance has generally been used for oncology treatment before patients come into the hospice service, where care is offered free of charge. With the emphasis on providing professional palliative care, HPCA has encouraged hospices to employ professional staff at market-related salaries. This has resulted in some tension in the local hospices because many hospice directors still feel strongly that hospice should be a volunteer service.

The second significant challenge is the lack of human resources. In South Africa, 31% of all health professional posts were vacant in 2003. Significant numbers of professional nurses and doctors have left the country to work in developed countries, where salaries are higher. Another concern is the impact of the HIV epidemic on health care workers, which is estimated to have 16% prevalence.[32,33] As antiretroviral programs are being implemented in South Africa, posts are being created in antiretroviral clinics for health care professionals, and staff shortages in palliative care are more pronounced as personnel move into these posts.

SOCIOECONOMIC AND ADMINISTRATIVE CHALLENGES

Until recently, palliative care in South Africa was provided only in hospices, and because these are NGOs, they depend on donations from the communities they serve, from corporate organizations, and from other funding sources. This means that hospices have been established in communities that are able to support the service financially and are capable of providing volunteer resources. Established hospices have expanded their services to include poor communities in their geographic areas, but many poorer areas have no palliative care services. Communities that identify a need for hospice services start the process by holding a public meeting to gauge public support for the project. Once financial support has been secured, a management committee is established with representation from health care professionals, management, and fundraisers. South African hospices provide home-based palliative care services, and a few hospices have also established inpatient facilities. It is an ongoing challenge to obtain sufficient funding to maintain hospice services, especially inpatient facilities.

International funds have recently become available for AIDS care, in particular funding from the U.S. government from the President's Emergency Plan for AIDS Relief. In South Africa, these funds have been granted to the HPCA to build capacity in member hospices. The Department of Health has identified the need to integrate palliative care into the formal health care system and has formed a collaborative partnership with the HPCA to develop further palliative care services. This collaboration with the Department of Health may promote sustainability of hospice services.

Hospices do not have their own pharmacies or medication supplies, but they have always worked closely with the local hospitals and clinics to provide medication for their patients through the local hospitals. Hospice services are nurse driven, and medical support is available only in the larger metropolitan hospices in South Africa. There are no full-time medical posts in palliative care. Physicians are employed seasonally, or they donate their time to support professional nurses and do not see many hospice patients. Nurses also work closely with the patient's general practitioner or oncologist.

Palliative Care Education

Medical schools and nursing colleges are integrating palliative care into the undergraduate curricula, and practical training takes place in local hospices. Before this recent initiative, many qualified professionals did not receive training in palliative care. In 1989, the HPCA developed a palliative nursing curriculum. The curriculum is accredited by the South African Nursing Council and is a 6-month day-release program that includes 132 practical training hours. Nurses qualify with a certificate in palliative nursing. Seven hospice training centers have been set up for professional nurses. The Cape Town Technical College initiated a degree program in palliative nursing in 2002.

The University of Cape Town offers postgraduate training in palliative medicine. These are distance-learning programs, an 18-month diploma course, and a 2- to 3-year master's program in palliative medicine. HPCA also has an introductory course in palliative care for the interdisciplinary team, a 6-month distance-learning program, and is developing training programs in psychosocial palliative care and pediatric palliative care.

Availability and Accessibility of Opioids

South Africa has a limited number of opioids available, but the South African Essential Drug List has medications available for each step of the WHO three-step ladder, and many adjuvant analgesics are also included on the list. Codeine is the most commonly used step 2 analgesic, and morphine (mist morphine, slow-release morphine tablets, and morphine sulfate injections) is the most commonly used step 3 analgesic. Tramadol and fentanyl are also available as alternate step 3 analgesics.

A recent study of the availability of essential palliative care medications in the state health system was very encouraging in that most recommended medications are available on the Essential Drug List. More medications are available in the private health system, although the only strong opioids available are morphine and fentanyl. Nonpharmacologic treatments are available but are not covered by medical insurance.

The Pain and Policy Studies Group at the University of Wisconsin reported that in 2002 the South African consumption of morphine was 3.6 mg per capita, and the global average was 6.56 mg per capita (see Figure 49-1), whereas pethidine consumption was 5.1 mg per capita.

PROPOSED OR ADOPTED SOLUTIONS

The following are the adopted or proposed solutions to the implementation of palliative care programs in South Africa:

- Increased public awareness in palliative care education, training, and research in palliative care
- Collaboration with medical and nursing schools
- Collaboration with the formal health care sector and emerging palliative care services
- Establishment of provincial palliative care development teams
- Access to funding
- Mentorship for developing palliative care services

Summary

The fact that a very large part of the world's population has either inadequate or no access to palliative care (including medications needed to alleviate pain and other symptoms) results in unnecessary suffering, especially among the poor and underprivileged. It has been estimated that one third of the world's population lacks access to the most essential medicines and curative treatments. Palliative care is and will continue to be the most cost-effective and, in many cases, the only possible care option for patients in developing countries. Governments, policy makers, health care professionals, and legislators should take the necessary steps to implement palliative care models suitable to fit the needs of the population. It is only through the designation of resources, allocation of space and beds, adoption of policies, education of health care workers, and increased awareness that patients will be able to have adequate care throughout the course of disease. The application of existing knowledge and resources is paramount to reach the majority of the population and patients around the world.

Resources

African Palliative Care Association
   www.apca.co.ug

Eastern and Central Europe Palliative Care Task Force
  www.oncology.am.poznan.pl/ecept/emenu.php
European Association for Palliative Care East
  www.eapceast.org
Hospice Palliative Care Association of South Africa
  www.hospicepalliativecaresa.co.za
Indian Association for Palliative Care
  Indian Association for Palliative Care Secretariat
  DNHP Memorial Palliative Care Clinic
  Bhuban Road, Uzan Bazar
  Guwahati-781001 Assam
  India
  Email: goswamidcg@sify.com and painassam@rediffmail.com
International Association for Hospice and Palliative Care:
  www.hospicecare.com
International Observatory in End of Life Care
  www.eolco-bservatory.net
Latin American Association for Palliative Care [Asociación Latinoamericana de Cuidados Paliativos]
  www.cuidadospaliativos.org

References

1. Population Reference Bureau: *World Population Data Sheet*, Washington, DC, 2004, Population Reference Bureau.
2. World Health Organization: *The World Health Report 2004*, Geneva, 2004, World Health Organization.
3. Stewart BW, Kleihues P, editors: *International Agency for Research on Cancer: The World Cancer Report*, Lyon, France, 2003, IARC Press.
4. United Nations: *AIDS epidemic update*, New York, 2004, United Nations.
5. Foley KM, Aulino F, Stjernsward S: Palliative care in resource-poor settings. In O'Neill J, Selwyn P, editors: *A guide to supportive and palliative care of people with HIV/AIDS*, Rockville, Md, 2002, Health Resources and Services Administration HIV/AIDS Bureau.
6. World Health Organization: *Cancer pain relief with a guide to opioid availability*, ed 2, Geneva, 2000, World Health Organization.
7. World Health Organization, Cancer Control Program: The 58th World Health Assembly Adopts Resolution on Cancer Prevention and Control. Available at www.who.int/mediacentre/news/releases/2005/pr_wha05/en/index.html.
8. International Narcotics Control Board: Consumption of the principal narcotic drugs. In *Narcotic drugs: estimated world requirements for 2003 and statistics for 2001*, Vienna, 2003, International Narcotics Control Board.
9. Pain and Policy Studies Group: *Consumption of morphine for 2002 in the world (from direct communication with staff)*, Unpublished document, Madison, Wis, 2005, Pain and Policy Studies Group.
10. Stjernsward J, Clark D: Palliative medicine: a global perspective. In Doyle D, Hanks G, Cherny N, Calman K, editors: *Oxford textbook of palliative medicine*, ed 3, Oxford, UK, 2003, Oxford University Press.
11. De Lima L, Sweeney C, Palmer JL, Bruera E: Potent analgesics are more expensive for patients in developing countries: a comparative study, *J Pain Palliat Care Pharmacother* 18:1, 2004.
12. Torres I, De Lima L, Wang X, et al: The availability of supportive care services and medications in Latin America: Preliminary findings from a survey of health-care professionals. In *Abstracts of the International Association for the Study of Pain (IASP) 10th World Congress on Pain*, Seattle, 2002, IASP.
13. Bruera A, Pruvost M, Schoeller T, et al: Proctoclysis for hydration of terminally ill cancer patients, *J Pain Symptom Manage* 15:4, 1998.
14. Pruvost M, De la Colina OE, Monasterolo NA: Edmonton injector: use in Cordoba, Argentina, *J Pain Symptom Manage* 12:6, 1996.
15. Davis MP, Walsh D: Methadone for relief of cancer pain: a review of pharmacokinetics, pharmacodynamics, drug interactions and protocols of administration, *Support Care Cancer* 9:2, 2001.
16. International Association for Hospice and Palliative Care (IAHPC), Bruera E, Wenk R, De Lima L, editors: *Palliative care in developing countries: principles and practice*, Houston, 2004, IAHPC Press.
17. Rajagopal MR, Mazza D, Lipman AG, editors: *Pain and palliative care in the developing world and marginalized populations: a Global Challenge*, Binghamton, NY, 2004, Haworth Press.

18. Bruera E, Neumann CM, Mazzocato C, et al: Attitudes and beliefs of palliative care physicians regarding communication with terminally ill cancer patients, *Palliat Med* 14:4, 2000.
19. Wenk R, Bertolino M: Argentina: palliative care status, *J Pain Symptom Manage* 24:2, 2002.
20. Wenk R, Monti C, Bertolino M: Asistencia a distancia: Mejor o peor que nada? *Med Paliat* 10:136–141, 2003.
21. Pan American Health Organization: Regional Core Health Data Initiative: Table Generator System. Available at www.paho.org/English/SHA/coredata/tabulator/newTabulator.htm.
22. Ministerio de Salud de la Nación, Superintendencia de Servicios de Salud: Programa Médico Obligatorio. Available at www.dasuten.utn.edu.ar/Documentos/PMO/Menu.PDF.
23. Kairos: Búsquedas y consultas de precios in Argentina: Available at www.kairosweb.com/medicamentos/buscaprecios.asp.
24. Rajagopal MR, Joranson DE, Gilson AM: Medical use, misuse and diversion of opioids in India, *Lancet* 358:139–143, 2001.
25. Joranson DE, Rajagopal MR, Gilson AM: Improving access to opioid analgesics for palliative care in India, *J Pain Symptom Manage* 24:2, 2002.
26. Rajagopal MR, Kumar S: A model for delivery of palliative care in India: the Calicut experience, *J Palliat Care* 15:1, 1999.
27. Kumar S: Learning from low income countries: what are the lessons? *BMJ* 329:1184, 2004.
28. Economist Intelligence Unit: Sceptic privind economia Romaniei Adevarul. Available at http://news.softpedia.com/news/1/2003/May/3277.shtml.
29. Casa Nationala de Asigurari de Sanatate: Raport 2003. Available at www.casan.ro.
30. Organizacion Mundial de la Salud [World Health Organization]: OMS Nr 254/9.06.2001 and OMS Nr 923/19.12.2001. In Monitorul Oficial 117 din 13.01.2002.
31. World Health Organization: *Achieving balance in national narcotics control policy*, Geneva, 2000, World Health Organization.
32. Padarath A, Ntuli A, Berthiaume L: Human resources. In Ijumba P, Day C, Ntuli A, editors: *South African Health Review 2003/2004*, Durban, 2004, Health Systems Trust. Available at www.hst.org.za/publications/423. Accessed March 27, 2007.
33. Shisana O, Hall EJ, Maluleke R, et al: HIV/AIDS prevalence among South African health workers, *S Afr Med J* 94:846–850, 2004.

CHAPTER 50

The Therapeutic Implications of Dignity in Palliative Care

BRIDGET MARGARET JOHNSTON and HARVEY MAX CHOCHINOV

Death is not the ultimate tragedy of life. The ultimate tragedy is depersonalization—dying in an alien and sterile area, separated from the spiritual nourishment that comes from being able to reach out to a loving hand, separated from the desire to experience the things that make life worth living, separated from hope.

**Norman Cousins,
Anatomy of an Illness**

DEFINING DIGNITY

The term dignity is widely used when discussing and debating various and sometimes contentious issues in end-of-life care. Dying with dignity has powerful and provocative connotations and yet, is rarely defined or fully explained.

The Oxford English Dictionary[1] defines dignity as "the state or quality of being worthy of respect." Thus the term is closely related to concepts like virtue, respect, self-respect, autonomy, human rights, and enlightened reason. The word dignity derives from the Latin word 'dignus' meaning worthy. The Universal Declaration on human rights[2] recognizes dignity as a condition closely associated with inherent human rights; "All human beings are born free and equal in dignity and rights ..." However, these definitions do not specify end-of-life circumstances and do not examine dignity from the perspective of seriously ill patients.

Dignity in health care is often presumed, yet rarely defined, in terms of its various components and targeted clinical outcomes. Without clarity on how to achieve or maintain dignity within the context of care, it is more at risk for being lost. When dignity is absent from care, people are more likely to feel devalued; they are more likely to sense that they lack control and comfort. The absence of dignity can undermine confidence, and patients may find themselves feeling less able to make decisions. At its worst, loss of dignity equates with feeling humiliated, embarrassed, and ashamed.

696

Table 50-1. Model of Dignity

MAJOR DIGNITY CATEGORIES, THEMES, AND SUB-THEMES		
Illness Related Concerns	**Dignity Conserving Repertoire**	**Social Dignity Inventory**

Level of Independence
Cognitive Acuity
Functional Capacity
 	
Symptom Distress
Physical Distress
Psychological Distress
  ○ medical uncertainty
  ○ death anxiety
	Dignity Conserving Perspectives
	  ○ continuity of self
	  ○ role preservation
	  ○ generativity/legacy
	  ○ maintenance of pride
	  ○ hopefulness
	  ○ acceptance
	  ○ resilience/fighting spirit
	
	Dignity Conserving Practices
	  ○ living "in the moment"
	  ○ maintaining normalcy
	  ○ seeking spiritual comfort
		Privacy Boundaries
		Social Support
		Care Tenor
		Burden to Others
		Aftermath Concerns

From Chochinov HM: Dignity-conserving care—a new model for palliative care: helping the patient feel valued, *JAMA* 287(17):2253, 2002.

A MODEL OF DIGNITY IN THE TERMINALLY ILL

Dignity has also been identified as one of the five most basic requirements that must be satisfied in caring for dying patients.[3] Empirical work by Chochinov et al studying dying patients and their families[4-6] has informed a model of dignity (Table 50-1). The model suggests that patient perceptions of dignity are related to and influenced by three major thematic areas termed: illness related concerns; the patient dignity conserving repertoire; and the social dignity inventory. For instance, illness related concerns relate to issues arising directly from the illness itself and has sub-themes that include level of independence and symptom distress. Level of independence is further subdivided into cognitive acuity, or ability to maintain mental capacity and functional capacity. The major category 'dignity conserving repertoire' includes those aspects of patients' psychological and spiritual landscape, often based on personality and internal resources, which influence the patient's sense of dignity, whether they are perspectives or practices. The social dignity inventory refers to social concerns or relationship dynamics that enhance or detract from a person's sense of dignity. The themes in this category are privacy boundaries, social support, care tenor, burden to others, and aftermath concerns.

In recent decades, the term dignity has become associated with the physician-assisted suicide (PAS) and euthanasia agenda (these topics are addressed elsewhere in this textbook). It is important that dignity be reclaimed within the lexicon of routine clinical and bedside care. Within this context, dignity should be considered an essential aim of quality, comprehensive palliative care. There is ample evidence, both from the perspective of patients and carers, that they crave dignity and fear its absence.[7-8] A recent qualitative study[9] (Table 50-1 and Table 50-2) addressing advanced cancer collected serial, triangulated data from patients within the last year of life, along with their families or friends and their health care providers. Six main

Table 50-2. Thematic Framework from Findings

Theme	Subtheme	Research Question
Maintaining Normality	Goal setting How others treat you Maintain normality Taking a break/holiday	1. From the perspectives of patients and carers, what is their experience of end of life care? 2. What self care strategies enable patient and carers to cope with their end of life care?
Preparing for Death	Euthanasia Getting worse Leaving family behind Planning funeral Process of dying	1. From the perspectives of patients and carers, what is their experience of end of life care? 2. What self care strategies enable patient and carers to cope with their end of life care?
Support from Family/ Friends	Carer support/information Talking about difficult issues Respite	1. From the perspectives of patients and carers, what is their experience of end of life care? 2. What support people with advanced cancer perceive that they require in order to self care?

From Johnston B, McGill M, Milligan S, McElroy D, Foster C, and Kearney N: Self care and end of life care in advanced cancer: literature review, *Eur J Oncol Nurs* PMID 19501021, 2009.

themes were identified, including: maintaining normality; preparing for death; support from family/friends; self care strategies/physical; self care strategies/ emotional; and support from health care professionals. Maintaining normality and preparing for death were the two most important areas identified by patients. Patients also valued support that enabled them to maintain their independence and remain at home. The overarching issue that came from the findings was that preserving and maintaining dignity and being treated with dignity was paramount to patients and permeated their experience of living with advanced cancer.

ADDRESSING DIGNITY IN CLINICAL CARE

The Model of Dignity in the Terminally Ill provides a clinically relevant, empirically based framework, which can inform and guide dignity-conserving care for patients nearing end-of-life. Every element of the model offers therapeutic possibilities to mitigate distress; in their entirety, these combined approaches could be described as a *Dignity Care Pathway (DCP)*. While the details of such a care pathway need to be elaborated and empirically tested (work is currently in progress by the authors), the following represent a sampling of what will eventually constitute elements of this novel approach (Table 50-3).

Table 50-3. Examples of Therapeutic Interventions to Conserve Dignity

Major Dignity Categories, Themes and Subthemes	Intervention/Action
Illness Related Concerns	
Symptom Distress	
Physical distress	• Assess identified symptoms using usual assessment tools • Address symptoms using usual guidelines • Seek help from relevant colleagues • Use communication skills of active listening
Psychological distress	• Refer to Palliative Care Network guidelines • Assess using HADs scale or similar. Discuss findings with the team and develop management plan • Refer to CPN colleagues if required • Use communication skills of active listening, open questions, appropriate body language • Check local symptom guidelines • Rectify highlighted problems as far as possible • Spend time discussing issues
Medical uncertainly Death anxiety	• Check with consultant/GP/Macmillan CNS what the patient has been told • Explore realistic goals and discuss day-to-day living • Emphasize what can be done • Show compassion and reassure patients that there will be plenty of support and that they will be cared for • Be prepared to talk about patients' death and fear about dying • Listen and acknowledge patients perceptions
Level of Independence	• Respect patient's decisions with regard to personal and medical care • Acknowledge the balance between providing care and patients' independency
Cognitive acuity	• Treat delirium; when possible, avoid sedating medication
Functional capacity	• Use of orthotics; physiotherapy, occupational therapy

Continued on following page

Table 50-3. Examples of Therapeutic Interventions to Conserve Dignity (Continued)

Major Dignity Categories, Themes and Subthemes	Intervention/Action
Dignity-Conserving Repertoire	
Dignity-Conserving Perspectives	
Continuity of self	• Treat patients with regard to the nature of the person, their feelings, their individuality, and their wishes
	• Support patients in maintaining even simple routines
	• If requested, help patients maintaining their grooming; make hair styling, shaving, and make-up available
Maintaining of pride	• Being with the person and show personal interest
Role preservation	• Listening to the patient's life history
	• Accommodate activities that are meaningful to the patient, such as hobbies, sports, or other interests
Hopefulness	• Support patients to refocus their hope onto things that can be realistically achieved
	• Do not give false hope but emphasize positive aspects
	• Accept denial as a way of coping
	• Emphasize the person's worth as a person
Generativity/legacy	• Encourage patients to talk about things they are proud that they have achieved
	• Listen to and acknowledge patient's perceptions on what they mean need to be done
	• Support patients in achieving these things
Autonomy/control	• Keep patients involved in treatment and care decisions
	• Advocate for patient's wishes with health care team and family if patient's is assert of own needs or wishes
	• Listen to patients and take them seriously
Acceptance	• Listen to patient's stories about the present and the past

Table 50-3. Examples of Therapeutic Interventions to Conserve Dignity (Continued)

Major Dignity Categories, Themes and Subthemes	Intervention/Action
Dignity-Conserving Practices	
Living in the moment	• Support patients in following what is going on in society by radio, TV, or discussions with others
Maintaining normalcy	• Emphasize patients to take advantage of moment when having the strength or not being in pain
	• Help patients to adjust usual routines to their health situation
Finding/seeking spiritual comfort	• See to it that patient has a personal connection to be comfortable in expressing spiritual needs
	• Enable the patient to participate in spiritual practices
Social Dignity Inventory	
Privacy boundaries	• Protect patients from unnecessary gaze from others
	• Protect patients from involuntarily viewing other patients in undignified situations
	• Listen to the patient's perception about being touched and uncovered (by unfamiliar or familiar persons)
Social support	• Encourage family members' presence and support family members
	• Maintain an active presence
	• Reassure that appropriate care will be available
Care tenor	• Be a good listener, take time and listen to the patient's story
	• Show respect for the patient by trying to comply with patients wishes, maintain confidentiality, be honest, and respect cultural, religious, and personal traditions
Burden to others	• Encourage discussion with those they fear are burdened
Aftermath concerns	• Attend to wills, advanced directives, naming a health care proxy; share information that might provide guidance or comfort for surviving family members/friends

Illness Related Concerns Symptom Distress

Of all areas pertaining to palliative end-of-life care, symptom management has the largest evidence base and is dealt with elsewhere in this textbook.

Level of Independence

There is evidence that many patients, more so than anything, fear loss of independence at the end-of-life.[10–12] Therapeutic interventions must therefore strive to preserve various elements of patient independence for as long as possible. These can be quite practical and operational, such as encouraging self care, using physical aids, and environmental modifications that facilitate access and maneuverability.[9] Psychological approaches must balance between helping patients accommodate to loss, while highlighting non-illness encumbered domains of independence and preserved function, which can be invoked well into advanced illness. These include partaking in clinical decision making; to the extent possible, directing daily care; and utilizing communications technologies to facilitate regular contact with, and extend roles within, various social or vocational networks. In addition, patients have indicated that living with dependency was made easier by caregivers (both carers and health professionals) who were knowledgeable, helped in a willing and pleasant manner, and established a comfortable climate with small talk, thereby establishing a trusting relationship.[13] Patients have also indicated that being in control is crucial for maintaining independence.[10]

Dignity Conserving Repertoire

DIGNITY CONSERVING PERSPECTIVES

Issues related to sense of self, hopefulness, acceptance, and generativity form part of a complex landscape defining individual personhood. Recognizing these issues, and the ability to elicit and broach them in a sensitive fashion, is a critical starting point. Exquisite communication and listening skills, along with an approach imbued with empathy and compassion, are core attributes for palliative care practitioners.[10] The research on dignity underscores the importance of a therapeutic stance, which provides patients a sense of affirmation. How patients perceive themselves to be seen is the strongest predictor of sense of dignity. This insight means that care providers have a responsibility, as well as an opportunity, to offer affirming reflections within every clinical contact.[14]

Life projects and activities are ways of being able to address issues of generativity, that is, a sense that one is leaving behind something of oneself. Generativity is a term that was coined by Eric Erikson. Erikson suggested that there are a series of development tasks we face during the course of our lifetime. Towards the end of life, we face a task he called generativity versus despair. He posed the question: "do we recognize that at some point, our contributions in life are in the service of those who will outlive us, or do we enter into a state of despair?"[15] This can take many forms, including videos, photographic projects, and various forms of narratives. The end of life is a natural time for reflection and for people to reflect on how they want to be remembered by those they will soon leave behind. Dignity therapy is a generativity oriented intervention, in the tradition of existential psychotherapies that are designed to

> **Box 50-1. *Dignity Therapy Question Framework***
>
> Tell me a little about your life history; particularly the parts that you either remember most or think are the most important? When did you feel most alive?
>
> Are there specific things that you would want your family to know about you, and are there particular things you would want them to remember?
>
> What are the most important roles you have played in life (family roles, vocational roles, community-service roles, etc.)? Why were they so important to you, and what do you think you accomplished in those roles?
>
> What are your most important accomplishments, and what do you feel most proud of?
>
> Are there particular things that you feel still need to be said to your loved ones or things that you would want to take the time to say once again?
>
> What are your hopes and dreams for your loved ones?
>
> What have you learned about life that you would want to pass along to others?
>
> What advice or words of guidance would you wish to pass along to your (son, daughter, husband, wife, parents, other[s])?
>
> Are there words or perhaps even instructions that you would like to offer your family to help prepare them for the future?
>
> In creating this permanent record, are there other things that you would like included?

address psychosocial and existential distress among terminally ill patients.[16] Dignity therapy allows patients to discuss issues that matter most to them or detail things they would want to be remembered. The outline for the dignity therapy interview guide (Box 50-1) is based on the themes and sub themes identified in the Model of Dignity in the Terminally Ill. These therapist-guided conversations are audio-recorded, transcribed, and edited. The resulting "generativity document" is returned to the patient for him or her to bequeath to a family member, friend, or anyone of their choosing. Dignity therapy has been shown to have positive subjective outcomes for patients, with the majority of patients indicating that it heightened their sense of dignity, meaning, and purpose and with 81% of patients completing the protocol reported that this novel intervention would help their family.[16]

DIGNITY CONSERVING PRACTICES

Dignity conserving practices include being able to maintain normalcy, live in the moment, and find spiritual comfort. Maintaining usual routines and living day to day—as long, and to the extent, possible—are ways of clinging to the familiar, and retaining ways of being that identify the person as part of the essence of who he or she is.[17] In considering dignity conserving practices, interventional options are as varied as the individual investment within each of its constituent domains. For some, music or poetry, for example, might provide a welcome and familiar ways of engaging life; for others, it might help them gain access into the realm of the transcendent; while for others yet, it may hold no resonance whatsoever. Therapeutic creativity and effectiveness depends on being able to identify specific practices that still resonate with individual patients, and finding ways to promote, preserve, or transform those practices in a fashion that remains viable and meaningful. For example, while attending congregational services may become less possible, personal prayer, or carrying out meaningful cultural and spiritual practices within one's home or hospital setting, may promote dignity up until the very end of life. Things such as hobbies, crosswords, and crafts have also been identified as key activities, which may suit patients nearing the end of life.[9]

Coming to know who people are, and not simply the ailments they have, is a way of affirming patients' sense of importance and enhancing their feelings of being whole persons. Sometimes a gentle and reassuring touch, specifically holding the patient's hand,[18] can reinforce that message. The focus of hope changes over time as illness progresses, with the challenge being able to help patients refocus their goals onto things that can be realistically achieved. It is important not to offer, or collude with, unrealistic expectations. Showing interest in the patient as a person and encouraging him or her to talk about their life are ways of providing hope. Patients indicate that when nurses and other health professionals make them feel valuable and important, this provides them with hope.[19]

SOCIAL DIGNITY INVENTORY

Interventions based on the social dignity inventory include maintaining and respecting patient privacy. This can be especially important in how care providers conduct intimate procedures or examinations. No one wants to be defined on the basis of what ails him or her; people, after all, are more than just their bodies. While bodies need attention, people need acknowledgement. Dignity conserving care provides acknowledgement, thereby minimizing patient vulnerability and a sense of being defined based on what they have rather than who they are. Warmth, compassion, and empathy are certainly key characteristics of palliative health care professionals.[10] These characteristics are however reliant on care provider attitudes and perceptions towards patients.[20] Within the social dignity inventory, this is referred to as the care tenor or simply, the tone of care; that is, providing a tone that is affirming of personhood.

Care tenor is impermanent; the patient may move settings, personnel may move, and eventually the patient will die. Continuation of dignity can be assisted by partaking in generativity measures, along with attending to unfinished business and personal affairs. Specifically, these are good ways of responding to aftermath concerns, i.e., those concerns patients anticipate might arise when they die, for those people that will soon be left behind.

Conclusion

It is important for health care providers to reclaim the language of dignity, which so aptly describes the ethos of state-of-the-art, creative, palliative care. The Model of Dignity provides empirical guidance and specificity on how to invoke dignity conserving interventions. Identifying and testing these various approaches will eventually yield a Dignity Care Pathway, used to achieve comfort and mitigate suffering for dying patients and their families. Eventually, helping patients to die with dignity will be associated with achieving comfort, finding peace, and receiving comprehensive, exemplary, dignity conserving palliative care.

> *The most important human endeavor is the striving for morality in our actions. Our inner balance and even our very existence depend on it. Only morality in our actions can give beauty and dignity to life.*
> —Albert Einstein

Summary

This chapter explores the concept of dignity, making reference to a body of empirical work on a model of dignity, dignity conserving care, and dignity therapy. It explores the recent use of the term dignity in the assisted suicide and euthanasia debate. Finally, this chapter examines why it is important to reclaim dignity as a term that is clinically relevant in the provision of palliative care.

References

1. *Compact Oxford English Dictionary of Current English*, rev ed 3, Oxford, 2008, Oxford University Press.
2. United Nations: *The universal declaration of human rights* (website). http://www.un.org/en/documents/udhr/. Accessed December 14, 2009.
3. Geyman JP: Dying and death of a family member, *J Fam Pract* 17(1):125, 1983.
4. Chochinov HM, Hack T, Hassard T, Kristjanson LJ, McClement S, Harlos M: Dignity in the terminally ill: a cross-sectional, cohort study, *Lancet* 360(9350):2026–2030, 2002a.
5. Chochinov HM, Hack T, McClement S, Kristjanson L, Harlos M: Dignity in the terminally ill: a developing empirical model, *Soc Sci Med* 54(3):433–443, 2002b.
6. Chochinov HM: Dignity-conserving care—a new model for palliative care: helping the patient feel valued, *JAMA* 287(17):2253, 2002.
7. Byock I: *The four things that matter most: a book about living*, New York, 2004, Free Press.
8. Seymour J, Gott M, Bellamy G, Ahmedzai SH, Clark D: Planning for the end of life: the views of older people about advance care statements, *Soc Sci Med* 59(1):57–68, 2004.
9. Johnston B, McGill M, Milligan S, McElroy D, Foster C, Kearney N: Self care and end of life care in advanced cancer: literature review, *Eur J Oncol Nurs* 13(5):386–398, 2009.
10. Johnston B, Smith LN: Nurses' and patients' perceptions of expert palliative nursing care, *J Adv Nurs* 54(6):700–709, 2006.
11. Seale C, Addington-Hall J: Euthanasia: the role of good care, *Soc Sci Med* 40(5):581–587, 1995.
12. Flanagan J, Holmes, S: Facing the issue of dependence: some implications from the literature for the hospice and hospice nurses, *J Adv Nurs* 29(3):592–599, 1999.
13. Eriksson M, Andershed B: Care dependence: a struggle toward moments of respite, *Clin Nurs Res* 17(3):220, 2008.
14. Chochinov HM: Dignity and the eye of the beholder, *J Clin Oncol* 22(7):1336, 2004.
15. Erikson EH, Erikson JM: On generativity and identity: from a conversation with Erik and Joan Erikson, *Harvard Educational Review* 51(2):249–269, 1981.
16. Chochinov HM, Hack T, Hassard T, Kristjanson LJ, McClement S, Harlos M: Dignity therapy: a novel psychotherapeutic intervention for patients near the end of life, *J Clin Oncol* 23(24):5520, 2005.
17. Johnston B, McGill M, Milligan S, McElroy D, Foster C, Kearney N: Self care and end of life care-patients' and carers' experience, *Palliat Med* [in press], 2010.
18. Doorenbos AZ, Wilson SA, Coenen A, Borse NN: Dignified dying: phenomenon and actions among nurses in India, *Int Nurs Rev* 53(1):28–33, 2006.
19. Clayton JM, Butow PN, Arnold RM, Tattersall MHN: Fostering coping and nurturing hope when discussing the future with terminally ill cancer patients and their caregivers, *Cancer* 103(9):1965–1975, 2005.
20. Chochinov HM: Dignity and the essence of medicine: the A, B, C, and D of dignity conserving care, *BMJ* 335(7612):184, 2007.

INDEX

Note: Page numbers followed by b indicate boxes; f, figures; and t, tables.